D1576448

k is to be return...
'3 s ...

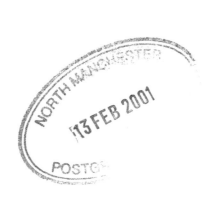
NORTH MANCHESTER
13 FEB 2001
POSTO...

MM02400

Bone Diseases

Macroscopic, Histological, and Radiological Diagnosis
of Structural Changes in the Skeleton

01-4553

Springer

Berlin
Heidelberg
New York
Barcelona
Hong Kong
London
Milan
Paris
Singapore
Tokyo

Claus-Peter Adler

Bone Diseases

Macroscopic, Histological, and Radiological
Diagnosis of Structural Changes in the Skeleton

With Forewords by F. Feldman and D.C. Dahlin

With 980 Figures and 6 Tables

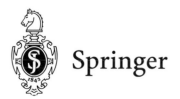

Springer

Univ. Prof. Dr. med. Claus-Peter Adler

Universität Freiburg, Pathologisches Institut
Ludwig-Aschoff-Haus
Referenzzentrum für Knochenkrankheiten
Albertstrasse 19
79104 Freiburg
Germany

Translated by:

Francis and Joyce Steel

Steinhalde 108
79117 Freiburg¯
Germany

ISBN 3-540-65061-X Springer-Verlag Berlin Heidelberg New York

CIP Data applied for
Die Deutsche Bibliothek – CIP-Einheitsaufnahme
Adler, Claus-Peter:
Bone diseases : macroscopic, histological, and radiological diagnosis
of structural changes in the skeleton ; with 6 tables / Claus-Peter
Adler. – Berlin ; Heidelberg ; New York ; Barcelona ; Hong Kong ;
London ; Milan ; Paris ; Singapore ; Tokyo : Springer, 2000
    Einheitssacht.: Knochenkrankheiten <dt.>
    ISBN 3-540-65061-X

This work is subject to copyright. All rights are reserved, whether the whole or part of the material is concerned, specifically the rights of translation, reprinting, reuse of illustrations, recitation, broadcasting, reproduction on microfilm or in any other way, and storage in data banks. Duplication of this publication or parts thereof is permitted only under the provisions of the German Copyright Law of September 9, 1965, in its current version, and permission for use must always be obtained from Springer-Verlag. Violations are liable for prosecution under the German Copyright Law.

© Springer-Verlag Berlin · Heidelberg 2000
Printed in Germany

Product liability: The publishers cannot guarantee the accuracy of any information about the application of operative techniques and medications contained in this book. In every individual case the user must check such information by consulting the relevant literature.

The use of general descriptive names, registered names, trademarks, etc. in this publication does not imply, even in the absence of a specific statement, that such names are exempt from the relevant protective laws and regulations and therefore free for general use.

Cover Design: de'blik Graphische Gestaltung, Berlin
Typesetting: K+V Fotosatz GmbH, Beerfelden
SPIN 10683525   24/3136-5 4 3 2 1 0 – Printed on acid-free paper

To my wife, Dr. med. Maria Adler,
and my children,
Elisabeth and Nikola-Maria

Foreword to the English Edition

It is a pleasure and an honor to have the opportunity of commenting on the English translation of the second German edition of *Bone Diseases* by Professor Dr. CLAUS-PETER ADLER. Dr. ADLER, an internationally renowned pathologist and a longtime member of the International Skeletal Society, has long-standing expertise regarding the many pathologic conditions afflicting the musculoskeletal system. He was a student of the eminent Professor Dr. ERWIN UEHLINGER of Zurich, Switzerland, and has also enjoyed postgraduate training at the Mayo Clinic.

The second edition of *Bone Diseases*, besides including microscopic and gross histopathological and immunohistochemical techniques, also incorporates newer imaging modalities. All of these tools prove mutually complementary in terms of understanding the nature and uniqueness of each entity. The book is divided into fifteen comprehensive sections as well as a separate section dealing with medical interventional techniques. Informative graphs, drawings and diagrams greatly contribute to the understanding of benign and malignant neoplasms as well as the normal processes of bone modeling and metabolism.

The illustrations are notable for their quality as well as their quantity and are easily accessed, conveniently appearing as they do on the same or facing page as the condition described. This arrangement is of great advantage to the reader: saving time and enhancing understanding.

This book, in addition to its intrinsic interest to pathologists, will serve as a valuable reference for radiologists, orthopedists, rheumatologists and, in fact, for all physicians interested in musculoskeletal diseases.

Frieda Feldman, M.D., FACR
Professor of Radiology and Orthopedics
Columbia University College of Physicians & Surgeons

Preface to the English Edition

This book on "Bone Diseases" first appeared in the German language in 1983, when it immediately aroused considerable interest among German-speaking physicians and medical students. It was presented at the Annual Conference of the *International Skeletal Society* in Geneva, at which time my American colleagues were already expressing their regret that, although the diagrams and illustrations were sufficiently familiar, they were unable to read the text. The wish was repeatedly expressed that the book should be translated. This proposal, however, met with the difficulty that no suitable native English-speaking translator who was familiar with the German language could be found. It had also been felt that a certain basic knowledge of medicine would be desirable. For this reason no English translation was forthcoming.

When the first edition of the book was sold out and the demand for it still continued, I began to work on a necessarily extended second edition. This was published by Springer (Berlin and Heidelberg), and it has already been well received by German readers. Once more the question of an English translation arose. Emeritus Professor D.C. DAHLIN, formerly Head Pathologist at the Mayo Clinic in Rochester, Minnesota, and an internationally renowned osteologist, had already written in his Foreword to the Second Edition: "I really hope that this book will soon be translated into English."

It was therefore a fortunate occasion for me when I encountered FRANCIS and JOYCE STEEL, both natives of England, who have been living for many years in Germany. Dr. STEEL is also a medically qualified anatomist, who worked for a number of years at the Anatomy Department of Freiburg University, where he helped to teach his subject to students of the Medical School. His wife has an MA degree in German.

With their assistance, it was possible to produce an English version of my book in a reasonably short period of time, especially since an extremely close, happy and cooperative relationship continued to exist between the author and his translators. During this time it was not only the strictly linguistic aspects of the task, but also the expression and display of technical matters which we were able to discuss and bring to a satisfactory and mutually acceptable conclusion.

Without the cooperation and commitment of Springer-Verlag the translation of the book would not have been possible. For this reason I would particularly like to express my gratitude to my Editor,

Professor Dr. D. Götze, for his support. I would also like to thank the staff of the Publishers, especially Dr. Agnes Heinz, Ms. Monika Schrimpf and Mr. Neil Solomon, to whom I am indebted for their constant advice on the production of the book and of its English translation.

The appearance of "Bone Diseases" in the English language will not only have satisfied the demands of my American and international colleagues, but will have made its appearance throughout the English-speaking world a reality.

Freiburg, Germany   *Claus-Peter Adler*
October 1999

Foreword to the Second German Edition

It is with great pleasure that I accepted the offer to write this foreword to the second edition of *Bone Diseases* by Professor Dr. CLAUS-PETER ADLER. This author published the first edition of the book in 1983. Its 387 pages include many excellent photographs, and it documents a great number of different bone diseases. When looking through the pages, I had the feeling that this obviously is an excellent and unique book that includes numerous kinds of bone diseases. The intention of the author was to write a book on these diseases that gives the reader all necessary information in comprehensive form. Radiologic images as well as histologic and macroscopic illustrations are included, enhancing the value of the text. In addition, more complicated processes of metabolism or bone remodelling are explained by informative diagrams and drawings. It is an excellent idea to face text and illustrations as in this book. This allows easy access to quick information.

The second edition of this book, written in the same manner, is largely expanded and includes many additional bone diseases in the different chapters. Some of them were missing in the first edition, others are new entities. New techniques in radiology (MRT, DSA) and in histopathology (immunohistochemistry) are considered, and a separate chapter deals with numerous kinds of medical exploration techniques.

The author of the book is a pathologist who has specialized in skeletal diseases, and he is an active member of the International Skeletal Society. He was instructed by Professor Dr. ERWIN UEHLINGER in Zürich/Switzerland and has trained several times at the Mayo Clinic in Rochester/USA in order to gain profound knowledge and experience on bone diseases. Repeatedly, he came to Rochester and has worked together with myself and my staff in our department of surgical pathology.

I am much pleased that Professor Dr. ADLER has written this excellent book, which deals with practically all relevant bone diseases. It belongs in the library of every pathologist, radiologist and orthopedic surgeon, and I am glad that it is new appearing in the English language. I wish the book a great success and acceptance.

D.C. Dahlin
Emeritus Professor of Surgical Pathology
Rochester, Minnesota, Mayo Medical School

Preface to the Second German Edition

The first edition of this book appeared fourteen years ago. Supported throughout by radiological, macroscopic and histological illustrations, it was intended to be a comprehensive work including a detailed presentation of all the relevant bone diseases, which could be used as a handy on-the-spot reference book for physicians from different specialties (radiologists, orthopedists, traumatologists, surgeons, faciomaxillary surgeons, internists, pediatricians, pathologists and even general practitioners), and from which they could rapidly obtain information about the various diseases of bone. To ensure this, each of the relevant illustrations (radiographs, macroscopic photographs and histological sections) was placed opposite the corresponding text. Factual information from the field of general osteology, backed up where necessary by diagrams, was also included, in order to clarify the various structural changes which take place in bone and to relate them to the manifold factors and disorders by which they are influenced. This resulted in the production of a book dealing with all the diseases of bone in a form which had not hitherto been available. It aroused considerable interest among both students and practitioners of medicine, and was soon out of print.

It is not easy for a book written in the German language to achieve international recognition, since the majority of foreign physicians are unable to read it. My professional colleagues and friends in the *International Skeletal Society* have therefore more than once requested me to publish the book in English, and this suggestion has indeed been seriously considered. Unfortunately, however, the money was simply not available.

Medical students and physicians can obtain and increase their knowledge of osteology in many ways. One of these is from books and professional conferences. Moreover, there are regular specialist meetings arranged by the *International Skeletal Society*, the *Deutsche Gesellschaft für Osteologie* and the *Arbeitsgemeinschaft Knochentumoren*, to mention only a few such organizations, which offer excellent opportunities for the exchange of views. It is also desirable that, in clinical practice, regular interdisciplinary discussions should take place between orthopedists, radiologists and pathologists – providing occasions when the diagnostic and therapeutic strategy for individual patients can be discussed and decided. Weekly meetings of this kind, where actual cases are discussed, have taken place regularly for over 20 years between the physicians engaged in osteological practice at the University Hospital, Freiburg. During these discussions we have become familiar with the various bone diseases and with all the diagnostic and therapeutic problems involved. In this way we gain increased experience which can be used for the benefit of our patients.

Since the appearance of the first edition of this book in 1983, there have been substantial and even revolutionary developments in the diagnosis of bone disease. It is, of course, particularly in the field of *diagnostic radiology* that the introduction of new techniques and apparatus has made it possible to obtain fresh insights into the structure of bone. At the same time, such methods of examination as computer tomography (CT), magnetic resonance tomography (MRT) and digital subtraction angiography (DSA), which did not even exist 14 years ago, have become established routine procedures. In the field of pathology also, new types of investigatory techniques have also emerged, and it is here that immunohistochemistry in particular has made a revolutionary contribution, especially to the diagnosis of bone tumors.

In addition to all these material advances, new concepts of bone disease, including the definition of new entities, have also come into being during this time. For example, several new tumorous entities have been defined and added to the recent classification of bone tumors by the World Health Organization (under the guidance of F. SCHAJOWICS, 1993), a matter in which I have myself been privileged to participate. Apart from neoplasia, new aspects of the diagnosis and treatment of other bone diseases have also emerged, and these must also be taken into account. An important example here is the use of osteodensitometry for analyzing the osteoporoses, and clinical examination has greatly advanced following the introduction of ultrasound and other similar procedures, none of which existed in 1983.

Nevertheless, in spite of all the modern technical developments in diagnostic methods and all that has been learnt in the field of osteology, one is still faced with the fact that bone diseases present their own particular diagnostic and therapeutic problems, and that these require highly specialized knowledge and experience. Unfortunately, the rather limited training in this subject given to medical students and physicians is in no way adequate. General practitioners also need to have their attention drawn to the modern approach to osteology and to modern methods of investigation in order to provide their patients with the best care available. This naturally applies with even greater force to specialists in the field – to radiologists, orthopedists, traumatologists, pathologists and others – who must ensure that they are familiar with all new developments in the diagnostic and therapeutic aspects of osteology.

For all these reasons it now seems the right time to produce a new and modern edition of my book: *Bone Diseases: The Diagnosis of Macroscopic, Histological and Radiological Structural Changes in the Skeleton*, particularly since there has been a considerable demand for it. In this edition, I have attempted to take all the new investigatory methods for diagnosing bone diseases into account. It is unfortunately true, however, that, as a consequence of the very large range of illustrations relating to each bone disease, some of the radiologi-

cal examination procedures (e.g. skeletal scintigraphy, DSA and sono-
graphy among others) have had to be rather more briefly handled
than I would wish.

As in the first edition, an effort has been made to ensure that the
figures are always printed to face the corresponding text, thus allowing the reader immediate access to the relevant information. To
make this possible, allusions to the literature have had to be omitted
from the text itself. References to related topics can be found in the
List of Subjects at the end of the book. Where appropriate, specific
directions for the treatment of the various bone diseases have also
been included.

However, notwithstanding all the technical progress in the field of
radiology during recent years, the plain radiograph is still the starting point and basis of all radiological diagnosis. In almost every case
it is neither sensible nor economical to turn directly to modern and
often very costly diagnostic procedures (e.g. MRT) without first having taken plain radiographs: normally an a.p. and a lateral view. It is
for this reason that the various bone diseases depicted in this book
are illustrated mostly with plain radiographs.

For the pathologist involved in the diagnosis of bone disease, the
hematoxylin-eosin (HE) section is what the plain radiograph is for
the modern radiologist. Such sections are in preparation the whole
time and continue to form the basis of all histological investigations.
Sophisticated histochemical procedures and other specialized techniques are only employed if there is a definite indication for them.
That is why I have deliberately included figures in this book which
have for the most part been taken from plain radiographs and routinely stained sections.

During the preparation of this second edition, I have relied once
again on those of my professional colleagues who have put illustrations of particular bone diseases at my disposal. I was most fortunate
in having access to the material collected by my revered teacher, the
late Professor Dr. Dr. ERWIN UEHLINGER. (This included some illustrations which he had already published elsewhere, the details of which I
have not been able to check). It is also a pleasure to express my gratitude to those other colleagues who have given their active support to
my work on this edition. Among these, Professor Dr. H.E. SCHAEFER,
Executive Director of the Department of Pathology, Freiburg University, deserves a particular mention. Privatdozent Dr. M. UHL, Physician in the Department of Radiology, University Hospital, Freiburg, offered me his expert advice on the selection and interpretation of the
radiographs. Dr. G. KÖHLER, Lecturer in the Department of Pathology, University of Freiburg, did a great deal of work on the presentation of the immunohistochemistry, and my doctoral student, Mr.
CHRISTIAN WEHR, worked out the statistical data and also drew up
the diagrams and skeletal schemata. Dr. G.W. HEGET, Lecturer in the
Department of Pathology, Freiburg University, undertook the coordination of the many activities involved. My special thanks are also
due to Mrs. X. LUDWIGS-KRAYER who, as photographer in our Department, was responsible for many of the illustrations.

Professor Dr. F.W. HEUCK, former Medical Director of the Department of Radiology at the Katharina Hospital, Stuttgart, has always

given me unlimited encouragement during my work on the second edition of the book, and it is he who was finally responsible for bringing it to the attention of the present publishers. I was most fortunate to find in Professor Dr. D. GOETZE of Springer-Verlag, Heidelberg, a publisher who has actively supported me during the production of the book, and I would like to express my particular thanks to both him and to his colleagues.

Freiburg im Breisgau,   *Claus-Peter Adler*
November 1997

Foreword to the First German Edition

„Je mehr wir können,
um so weniger kann der Einzelne alles"
(The more we are able to do,
the less can the individual achieve alone)
K.H. Bauer, 1953

From time immemorial, pathological changes in the skeletal system have been the domain of the surgeon, this today signifying predominantly the traumatologist and orthopedist. In the case of systemic diseases, however, such changes extensively involve all aspects of internal medicine and pediatrics as well as numerous other disciplines.

For the purposes of clinical diagnosis the radiograph, together with similar modern specialist techniques such as computer tomography, takes first place in clinical practice as the most important and least distressing method of examining the patient. However, although the technical work is done with such ease, the interpretation of the findings and their incorporation into the clinical jigsaw puzzle often presents much more difficulty. Not infrequently, the key piece is missing, which the pathologist is able to put in place by looking down the microscope.

Thus many people contribute to the processes of visualizing, classifying and appropriately treating pathological bone changes.

"To deduce the whole picture from a comprehensible synthesis is not to be achieved by a theoretical conference of specialists sitting around a table. This requires far more the work of one individual." *(Eine einleuchtende Synthese zu einem Ganzen gelingt aber nicht dadurch, daß sich die Spezialisten am grünen Tisch zu einer Konferenz zusammensetzen. Hier bedarf es vielmehr der Arbeit eines einzelnen Mannes).* This statement by the Nobel Prize Winner, Alexis Carrel, has been taken to heart by the author of the present work who, by his application of strict classifying criteria to the morphology, and by his visual portrayal, ranging from the clinical event and the radiograph to the histological background, has attempted to avoid a scattered and piecemeal approach to the numerous bone diseases. This attempt has, to my mind, succeeded in the highest degree; the book reflects the many aspects of countless discussions between clinicians, radiologists and pathologists which have taken place at demonstrations and lectures in Freiburg, at our University Hospital.

Thus, just as the goalkeeper in a team radiates security, calm and self-confidence, so the immense experience of the author makes clinical and radiological diagnosis of the skeletal system more secure and more exact for us in our professional circle; the recognition of essential findings will be swifter; the initiation of treatment will take place earlier.

The present book is far more than a mere text for the practicing pathologist, which is all the author modestly asserts. Its numerous tables relating to age distribution, predilection and special disease indications means that the clinician – whatever his provenance – and, to a particularly high degree, the radiologist, will have at his or her fingertips a valuable synopsis of clinical practice, radiographic images and fundamental morphological changes, which takes into account both routine and unusual cases. The advantages of its being a one-man work, namely, the editorial continuity and the diversity of its selected illustrative material, are of particular benefit to the book and testify to the author's extensive experience and far-reaching expertise in the field.

In addition, the author shows a decidedly thoughtful approach to indications for the extraction of biopsy material – thus, to surgical intervention. Similarly however, he names numerous lesions, such as the non-ossifying bone fibroma, which should be left alone. Indeed, the presentation of these particular lesions is so outstanding that it will become an essential source of help to any hesitant diagnostician. In the words, somewhat modified, of my old surgical teacher, K.H. Bauer, the morphologist shows more scientific knowledge and a greater sense of responsibility if, in cases of certain bone lesions, he advises, on clinical and radiological grounds, against a biopsy excision rather than in favor of implicit reliance on a diagnosis secured by means of the surgical extraction of tissue.

In this book, practically every known bone disease and both its morbid anatomical and radiological appearances are described and clinically classified; only very rare skeletal disorders have been omitted. Thus, this book differs from other published monographs in the field of osteology, which have, up to now, dealt solely with partial aspects of these diseases (e.g. bone tumors).

To my knowledge there is no other book in existence in which every bone disease is presented in such a clearly organized and comprehensive fashion, and which allows one such rapid access to information on current clinical and morphological topics. We have here a work which is in no way composed only for osteologists but is much more an aid to diagnosis and further treatment for all those practicing physicians who have patients with skeletal disorders under their care. This volume is a valuable source of information not only for pathologists and radiologists but also for surgeons, orthopedists, traumatologists, rheumatologists, oncologists and general practitioners. I wish for it a widespread acceptance.

Freiburg im Breisgau,   *W. Wenz*
April 1983

Preface to the First German Edition

Bone diseases present special diagnostic and therapeutic problems and demand comprehensive knowledge and experience in this field. It is extraordinary how many medical specialists have to do with disorders of the skeleton (pediatricians, physicians, surgeons, orthopedists, traumatologists, radiologists, faciomaxillary surgeons, and pathologists, among others), and there are enormous numbers of patients suffering from diseases of this sort.

As against this, however, the teaching on the subject of skeletal disorders is accorded only a secondary place in student and postgraduate training courses. It is assumed that particular expertise in this field is confined to "specialists" to whom difficult cases will be referred. Diseases of bone are often unfamiliar to the general practitioner, and the lack of a more intensive training means that he does not have the necessary knowledge and experience. Nevertheless, in most cases it is precisely the general practitioner who is the first to be confronted with a bone disease and the first to have to recognize it as such.

The preliminary clinical examinations are usually followed by radiological investigations, which can immediately provide crucial diagnostic information. The decision as to whether a bone biopsy is to be taken is based upon both the clinical and the radiological findings.

The tissue material taken from a bone lesion is then sent to the pathologist in anticipation of a final diagnosis. The proper course of treatment can then be planned accordingly. In a multitude of cases the radiological image is indispensable, since this is a quasi macromorphological representation of the bone lesion in question. The clinician should therefore make a point of sending the relevant radiological pictures along with the biopsy material. Only from a synopsis of the radiological and histological findings can a secure diagnosis be achieved.

This book has chiefly been written for practicing pathologists, who have to discern the differences between the various bone disorders as part of their normal routine diagnostic duties. Its place should be beside the microscope, since it offers a timely guide to the pathologist who has to make a judgement about a bone section and has perhaps additional access to the radiological pictures. For this reason, I have tried to present the most important bone diseases in their characteristic structural forms and, in the text, to concentrate on the corresponding descriptions. The text has intentionally been placed opposite the relevant figures. The description of the radiological, macroscopic and histological illustrations is a central point of the text. These details are marked in the figures by indicators.

In the first chapter and among the more general portions of each succeeding chapter some important osteological facts have been singled out which are helpful to the understanding of bone lesions. They do not in any way claim to deal comprehensively with osteological problems and queries and are no substitute for current information found in scientific research articles and books. Reference works of this sort are indicated in the literature lists.

The comparative contrast of the radiological, macroscopic and histological illustrations is perhaps of interest even to physicians whose field of work lies outside that of the pathologist. Radiologists and orthopedists in particular can get to know what the microscopic structural formation of so many radiologically diagnosed bone lesions actually looks like. The radiographs and the related descriptions in the book are there only to supplement the morbid anatomical findings and to complete the morphological spectrum in each of the bone diseases described. In no way does it claim to provide an expert radiological interpretation. Any pathologist, of course, who deals intensively with skeletal disorders and who has been required, over many years, to give a professional opinion in numbers of cases and sees the relevant radiographs, is bound to gain a certain amount of experience in the radiomorphology of bone disease. The regular collaboration with professional radiologists is here also a contributing factor. The final opinion on radiological structures must, however, be left to the expert radiologist. In practice, the pathologist does indeed describe the radiological features, but his diagnosis must be founded upon the histological appearance.

This book came about at the instigation of my esteemed teacher Professor Dr. Dr. ERWIN UEHLINGER, former Director of the Institute of Pathology at Zürich University in Switzerland. In order to provide the numerous illustrations for the various bone diseases it was necessary to collect together specimens from bone cases over a period of many years. In spite, however, of my long-lasting and intensive occupation with skeletal disorders, there are some extremely rare bone lesions for which I had no relevant illustrative material. Once again, it was Professor UEHLINGER who came to my aid by readily giving me access to his own extensive collection. His unexpected death in the spring of 1980 led to problems in this regard and substantially delayed the completion of the book. Many colleagues and friends helped me, however, by putting at my disposal the missing representative illustrations. At this point I wish to thank first and foremost Professors WENZ (Radiology), KLÜMPER (Radiology), MATTHIAS (Radiology) and KUNER (Accident Surgery) at Freiburg University. I also wish to thank my American friends, Professor D.C. DAHLIN (Mayo Clinic, Rochester), Professor H.D. DORFMAN (Baltimore) and Professor H.A. SISSONS (New York), who helped me out with illustrative material and with advice.

During the work on this book I relied on the active support of many colleagues and coworkers. Professor Dr. W. SANDRITTER, former Director of the Institute of Pathology at Freiburg University, gave me and my plans great encouragement, for which I am extremely grateful. My particular thanks are due to Ms. U. WIEHLE, a photographer at the Freiburg Institute of Pathology, who showed untiring diligence and great skill in preparing the photographs, and also to Ms. M. MEINHARDT, who, among other things, carried out the technical work. Dr. T. GENZ, Assistant in the same Institute, worked out the statistical data for the bone diseases and carried out the cytophotometric DNA measurements on bone tumors. Finally, I must thank Ms. H. EHRET and Ms. A. MÖLLER for their flawless typing and for the revision of the literature index.

In Dr. h.c. G. HAUFF, Georg Thieme Verlag in Stuttgart, I found a publisher who not only gave me both generous support and encouragement during the writing of this book, but also showed great understanding when its completion was affected by unexpected delays. My concluding thanks are due to Dr. HAUFF and the Georg Thieme Verlag.

Freiburg im Breisgau,   *Claus-Peter Adler*
May 1983

Contents

1 Bones and Bone Tissue

From many different points of view the skeleton plays a central role in the life of every man and woman. It gives every living body its individual form, is responsible for its *architectonics*, and also determines its *size*. The form of the skeleton is both proportional and symmetrical, so that the size of each of its parts is directly related to that of the structure as a whole. The skeleton is bilaterally symmetrical, the mid-sagittal plane dividing the body into two mirror images. For this to be possible, the proper formation and development of each individual bone during embryonic life and its subsequent continuous physiological growth during childhood and adolescence must be assured. It is at these times that various disturbances may take place which hinder or abnormally accelerate the growth and development of the skeleton. Such disturbances may be endogenous in kind (congenital or inherited) or brought about by outside influences (dietary deficiencies, radiation or drugs). They lead to malformations *(skeletal dysplasias)* which affect either the entire skeleton or single parts of it (arms, legs, skull, vertebral column etc.) or individual bones. This can also result in an overproduction of bones – hexadactyly, for instance. In every case this results in a change in the architectonics of the body, and in some cases in an alteration of its overall size.

The skeleton occupies a central position in the *locomotor system* of the body. Movement, which is an essential function of all living creatures, depends upon the action of the soft tissues – including the muscles, tendons, ligaments, fasciae and nervous system – but it is primarily the bones and joints that ensure the stability of the various parts of the body, as well as the flexion, extension and rotation of the joints that make movement possible. A variety of factors can also impair the function of the joints, and these may again be endogenous in nature (e.g. *joint dysplasias*). A close functional relationship exists between the movements of the skeleton and the morphological structure of the bones and joints themselves. The entire skeleton is constantly subjected to changes in structure which result from the demands made upon it and upon its functional loading. In this connection it is of great importance whether these influences act upon the growing or upon the fully developed skeleton.

The essential *supporting function* of the skeleton is influenced by the action of various extraskeletal factors. Embedded deeply within the soft tissues, bone is dependent on its blood and nerve supply. The skeletal muscles are inserted into the bones and control their movement. Various types of disorder of these extraskeletal tissues can have a detrimental effect upon the skeletal system itself.

Bone also plays a central role by contributing to life-supporting metabolic exchange, and the skeleton is an important *storage organ*, particularly for calcium and phosphate. It is essential for life that the serum calcium is maintained at a constant level, and it is here that the contribution of bone tissue is decisive. Under the influence of various hormones, calcium is removed from or deposited into bone according to the needs of the moment. For instance, parathyroid hormone → bone resorption; calcitonin, estrogens, androgens → inhibition of bone resorption; D-hormone, somatotropin → demand for bone resorption; insulin → new bone deposition; glucocorticoids → inhibition of new bone deposition + demand for bone resorption, thyroxin → stimulation for remodeling; estrogens → preservation of bone tissue; androgens, prostaglandin E2 → bone remodeling; β-TGF → demand for new bone deposition + inhibition of bone resorption, interleukin 1 → increase in bone formation + inhibition of bone resorption; α-interferon → inhibition of bone remodeling. In these ways, extraskeletal regulatory mechanisms control the metabolic exchange. The availability of calcium and phosphate is also controlled outside the skeleton (in the gut, for instance). Disorders of these metabolic processes lead to characteristic changes in the structure of bone, the diagnostic analysis of which is understood by radiologists and pathologists. The morphological picture of every bony lesion allows conclusions to be drawn about a great variety of local and systemic diseases.

The Function of Bones and of the Skeleton

Bone is the most highly differentiated of the mesenchymal tissues. It has two quite different functions to fulfil: (1) support and (2) storage. Both of these have in turn a decisive influence on bone, and only under the influence of these physiological functions can the skeleton and its component elements play their normal roles. In this way there exists a close reciprocal relationship between the structure of bone and its functional requirements.

The *supporting function* of the skeleton is made possible by the structure of bone, which resembles a composite building system. This structure can be adapted to every static or dynamic requirement by the metabolism of the tissue, while the remodeling and renewing processes take place most especially in the cortical bone. Under physiological conditions, remodeling is more intensive in the more heavily loaded regions of the skeleton (vertebral column, pelvis, long bones) than in regions which are less heavily loaded, such as the skullcap. The **cortex** is the most heavily stressed region of a bone, and it is able to resist pressure and tensile forces, responding to their action by physiological changes in shape. In spite of the greater density of its calcified tissue, the cortex (**compacta**) is malleable, this being ensured by the interpenetration of its Haversian canals. The different actions of mechanical forces on single bones is reflected in differences in the thickness of the cortex. In the long bones the cortex at the middle of the shaft is thickest and is rejuvenated from the end of the bone. The Haversian canals are narrower at the middle of the shaft than toward the end. Following the unphysiological action of pressure, tension or shear forces, this architecture can nevertheless be altered in a short time by remodeling. This kind of functionally controlled bone remodeling is most easily recognized in radiographs.

Apart from its supporting function, the cortex has to lay down the external contour of the bone, and to support and enclose the marrow cavity with its contents of spongiosa and soft tissue (hematopoietic bone marrow, fatty tissue

and vessels). Diagnostic assessment of the cortical bone includes observation of its width, bone density, structural homogeneity, and its periosteal outer and endosteal inner layers. Diseases which call forth a reactive remodeling of the bone can also lead to changes in the outer contour of the cortex, and this can be a very important diagnostic sign. Osteomyelitis, for instance, can lead to reactive new bone formation in the endosteum and particularly in the periosteum, and this can be seen radiologically. A bone tumor can cause erosion of the cortex from within, even to complete penetration, while at the same time stimulating an ossifying periostosis.

The **periosteum** constitutes a connective tissue sheath that completely covers all bones except over the articular cartilage and the many muscle attachments. This connective tissue layer is of great significance for the function of the skeleton and its individual bones, since it carries a dense network of blood and lymph vessels and predominantly sensory nerves which are necessary for the maintenance of the bone structure. The periosteum is more or less firmly anchored to the cortex by the bundles of Sharpey's fibers which penetrate into the bone. From the point of view of clinical symptoms it is important to be aware that it is only the periosteum which carries sensory nerve fibers with the ability to respond with pain to pathological processes, since the bone itself contains no sensory nerves. This means that "bone pain" is in fact always "periosteal pain". The essential significance of the periosteum for the biology of the bone lies in the pluripotence of its mesenchymal tissue structure. Most important is the fact that the periosteal connective tissue has the capacity to differentiate within a short time into bone, which then appears in the radiograph. There are many types of reactive periosteal change and also primary diseases which are bound up with new bone formation and which are correlated with functional disorders of the skeleton and must be analyzed morphologically.

The principal function of the skeleton is to make locomotion possible. This takes place in the various **joints** where adjacent bones are enabled to take up different relative positions with regard to one another. In joints with a limited range of movement (e.g. the ankle joint) stronger elasticity of the skeleton is possible. For every movement of the individual joints, the anatomical structure of the articulating surfaces, the form and structure of the joint capsule and ligaments and the insertions of those muscles which bring about and control the movements are all decisive. Any disorder of this system affecting the coordination of the parts, including the soft tissues, can lead to a disturbance of function, the reasons for which must be fully explored diagnostically.

Storage is the second main function of bone and of the skeleton. As can be gathered from the diagram shown in **Fig. 1,** the skeleton is both a **structural support** and a **metabolic organ.** It serves especially for the **storage of calcium and phosphate,** ensuring the equilibrium of these ions in the blood serum. A constant level of the blood calcium is essential for life and bone plays a decisive role in maintaining this level, the bone metabolism being under the control of extraskeletal regulatory mechanisms. For this purpose there is a particularly finely adjusted interaction between the parathyroids, kidneys, alimentary canal and the skeleton itself. The intake of calcium from the diet is controlled by the hormone "vitamin D_3" (1,25-dihydroxycholecalciferol). The parathyroid hormone (parathyrin) regulates the liberation of calcium from the bone in response to the serum calcium level, and calcium excretion is essentially a function of the kidneys. Any disturbance of this complicated and mutually interactive regulatory system involving a change in the level of the blood calcium has a morphological effect on the bone structure. As shown in **Fig. 1,** this results in bone remodeling which is expressed either as resorption or deposition of bone matrix. Such a remodeling process can be recognized and analyzed histologically (and often also radiologically), and the structural changes may provide a clue to the nature of the underlying metabolic disorder. Furthermore, there may be **changes in the mineralization** of the bone tissue which can be precisely assessed by means of microradiography. Serious disturbances of mineralization can also be recognized in the ordinary HE section by the relative increase or decrease in the amount of osteoid. For this purpose the use of undecalcified bone sections – not always available in every institute – is to be recommended. The experienced pathologist can, however, usually recognize such changes with sufficient certainty in EDTA decalcified sections. The various types of remodeling processes and mineralization defects are pathognomonic of the metabolic osteopathies.

Disturbances of bone function can on the one hand produce changes in the physical loading on the skeleton, and on the other have an influence on calcium metabolism.

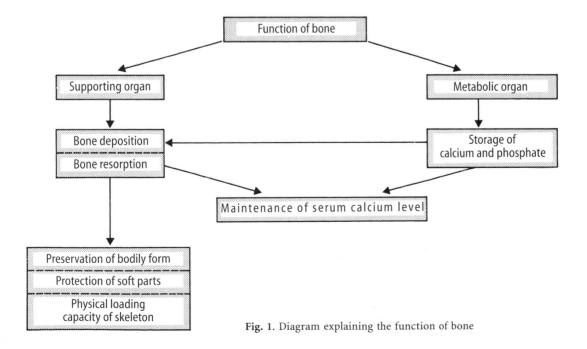

Fig. 1. Diagram explaining the function of bone

Bone as a Structural Support

An absolute prerequisite for the structural analysis of the skeleton and its bones as well as for the diagnosis of structural changes is the precise knowledge of the characteristics of normal bone. It is well known that the individual bones of the skeleton are very different in shape and size. There are short and long tubular bones, "irregular" bones (vertebrae, carpal and tarsal bones), flat bones (pelvis and skullcap) and bones of a highly specific form (skull base, facial skeleton), in all of which pathological processes produce very different structural effects. This is reflected in the supporting function of each type, but the **basic principle of bone construction** is well shown in the long bones. This is made clear in **Fig. 2,** which shows a diagram of the knee joint with the distal end of the femur *(1)* and the proximal end of the tibia *(2).* Topographically, one can distinguish the *epiphyses (3),* which are covered with articular cartilage *(4).* In the growing skeleton the adjacent *epiphyseal plate* (growth cartilage; *5),* which disappears from the adult skeleton, can be recognized. This is bordered by the *metaphysis (6).* The middle of the shaft, which constitutes the longest part of a tubular bone, is described as the *diaphysis (7).* Knowledge of these different regions of a bone ("first order structure") is important, since, corresponding to the various topographical and functional differences in the tissue, particular bone diseases are manifested predominantly in particular parts of the skeleton. The physiological growth in the length of a bone takes place at the epiphyses, and disorders of growth will therefore be associated with the signs of structural change in these regions. In particular, the form taken by certain bone tumors is dependent upon the predominating type of remodeling process normally found during ontogenetic development at the location of the swelling. In **Fig. 2** one can also see the dense structure of the *cortex (8),* which is covered on the outside with fiber-rich *periosteal connective tissue (9).* This is continuous with the *joint capsule (10).* The *marrow cavity* of the long bones *(11)* is occupied by a fine cancellous network which adapts itself structurally to the predominating bending stresses of long bones.

In **Fig. 3,** the mechanical structural principle is shown **diagrammatically** in the cortex (com-

pacta) of a long bone ("second order structure"). In the growing skeleton, periosteal osteoblasts lie upon the shafts of the long bones and lay down bone tissue from outside like the growth rings of a tree *(1).* During the second year of life, *Haversian osteons (2)* also begin to develop. The vascular canals running in an axial direction through the compact bone widen and become filled again with an orderly system of lamellar rings. The incorporation of Haversian osteons continues at a reduced rate even after the conclusion of skeletal growth. The resorption of old osteons *(3)* and the appearance of new ones *(4)* eventually produces a mosaic pattern of complete and incomplete or fragmented pieces of osteons with interspersed remnants of the periosteal lamellar ring system (the so-called intermediate lamellae; *5).* The more complete an osteon is in histological section, the younger it is; the more it is cut into complex shapes, the older. These remodeling processes produce a three-layered division of the compacta: the endosteal rings (internal general lamella; *6),* a middle layer of Haversian osteons *(7)* and a subperiosteal ring layer (the external general lamella; *8).* The necessary blood supply comes from the vessels of the periosteum, which pass through the perforating Volkmann's canals *(9)* to reach the bone.

The entire Haversian system of lamellar bone is elastically bound together by collagen fibers. As can be seen in the **diagram** of the *Haversian system* in **Fig. 4,** the fibrils of adjacent lamellae *(1* and *2)* run in opposite directions.

In **Fig. 5** *the border between cortex (1)* and *spongiosa (2)* is shown diagrammatically. Whereas the heavily loaded cortex is responsible for most of the supporting function, the spongiosa is the more frequent site of pathological changes; it provides a wide surface for calcium exchange and supports the cortex against mechanical loading.

The microscopic structure of bone is seen as a **"third order structure",** whereby the bone trabeculae with bone deposition (osteoblasts, osteoid seams) and resorption fronts (osteoclasts, Howship's lacunae) can be analyzed.

The **"fourth order structure"** is produced by the building materials of bone tissue, which consist of organic material (bone matrix) and inorganic material (hydroxyapatite).

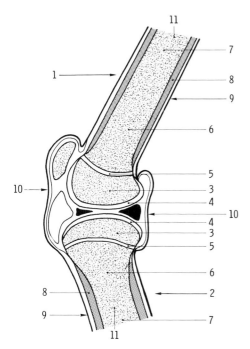

Fig. 2. Diagram of a normal knee joint (side view)

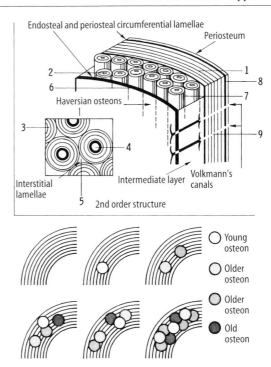

Fig. 3. The basic principles of bone construction

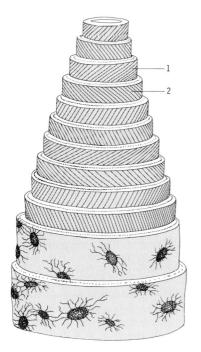

Fig. 4. Diagram of a Haversian system (after GEBHARDT)

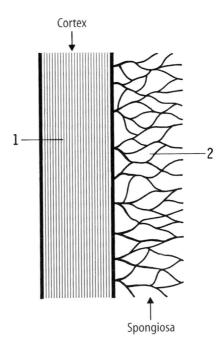

Fig. 5. Diagram of cortex and spongiosa (cancellous bone)

Bone as an Organ of Storage

The bone matrix consists of 77% inorganic and 23% organic material and is subject throughout life to constant renewal. The organic bone matrix – the *osteoid* – is 89% collagen and 5% protein, and is the site of bone mineral deposition. As illustrated in **Fig. 6a,** osteoid is produced by large polyhedral *osteoblasts (1),* which give rise to a layer 1 μm in width every day *(2).* This moves 1 μm daily away from the cell body. The total width of a normal osteoid seam amounts to 6 μm *(3).* Mineralization of the organic ground substance requires a maturation of the matrix of 10 days duration, so that the organic matrix is fully mineralized *(4)* only when it is 10 μm from the osteoblasts. Under the influence of the already mineralized bone tissue the osteoid becomes calcified up to 70% within the next 3–4 days, the rest of the mineralization following much more slowly over 6 weeks. The stepwise nature of the osteoid mineralization is marked by dark *cement lines* (or *reversal lines).* The appearance of wider osteoid seams indicates a functional disorder of the bone and is due either to excessive osteoid building (e.g. in an osteosarcoma, p. 274) or as a result of faulty mineralization (e.g. rickets, p. 50; osteomalacia, p. 86).

The ***inorganic component*** of the bone tissue consists of 90% calcium phosphate and 10% calcium carbonate. The most important mineral is calcium, which is deposited in the organic matrix as hydroxyapatite crystals. As can be seen in **Fig. 6b,** the crystals are hexagonal (5) and are embedded alongside the collagen fibrils at intervals of 68 nm. They stabilize the skeleton against pressure and shearing forces. In the entire skeleton, about 100 g ionic calcium is absorbed with carbonate or phosphate radicles. A rapid exchange of calcium ions with those absorbed onto the crystal surfaces is necessary to maintain a calcium level in the serum which is essential to life. The calcium ions embedded in the surface of the crystal lattice are responsible for the lesser and slower exchange. The greater number of the skeletal crystals are not available for ionic exchange, being deeply anchored in the bone tissue. The continuous physiological bone remodeling, which is 7 times faster in the spongiosa than in the compacta, serves to regulate the mineral "budget". About 5 g of skeletal calcium is always available for the steady exchange of ions.

Regulation of Bone Structure and Calcium Metabolism

Bone structure is subjected to a large number of regulatory mechanisms. Just as hormonal influences are of particular importance in connection with the storage of calcium and phosphate, so is their action able to alter the structure of bone. These factors maintain the constancy of the serum calcium level. In **Fig. 7** the interaction of organs and organ systems with bone is illustrated diagrammatically. Of first importance here are the **parathyroids** *(1),* which produce the *parathyroid hormone* (parathyrin). This increases the absorption of calcium from the **gastrointestinal tract** and the excretion of calcium and phosphate by the **kidneys** *(2).* In **bone** *(3),* the *osteoclasts,* which resorb the tissue and release calcium, and the *osteoblasts,* which build up osteoid and lead to bone deposition, as well as the *fibroblasts,* which produce collagen fibers, are activated. With this, parathyrin stimulates bone remodeling and finally leads to the histological picture of *dissecting fibro-osteoclasia* (see Fig. 148). *Calcitonin,* which is produced by the parafollicular cells (C cells; *4)* of the thyroid, acts antagonistically to parathyrin and inhibits the activity of the osteoclasts, bringing about simultaneous increase in the number of osteoblasts. A disturbance in its function leads to **hyperparathyroidism** (p. 80). There are also other systems which have an effect on bone deposition and calcium metabolism. The *somatotrophic hormone* (STH) from the anterior pituitary *(5)* controls skeletal growth, *the thyroid stimulating hormone* (TSH) stimulates the thyroid and *ACTH* activates the adrenals *(6).* Overproduction leads to developmental disorders of the skeleton or to atrophy of bone, and the *gonadal hormones (7)* can have similar effects. Finally, impairment of the blood supply to bone can have an important effect upon its structure *(8).* Arterial hyperemia leads to bone resorption (osteoporosis) and venous stasis may be responsible for increased deposition (osteosclerosis).

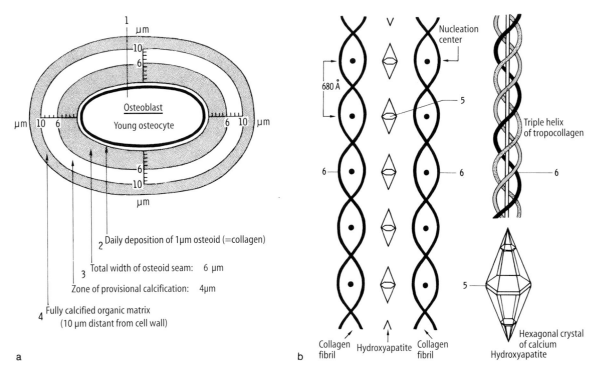

a   b

Osteoblast
Young osteocyte

2 Daily deposition of 1μm osteoid (=collagen)

3 Total width of osteoid seam: 6 μm

Zone of provisional calcification: 4μm

4 Fully calcified organic matrix
  (10 μm distant from cell wall)

Nucleation center

680 Å

Triple helix of tropocollagen

Collagen fibril   Hydroxyapatite   Collagen fibril

Hexagonal crystal of calcium Hydroxyapatite

Fig. 6 a, b. Formation of the organic and inorganic bone matrix

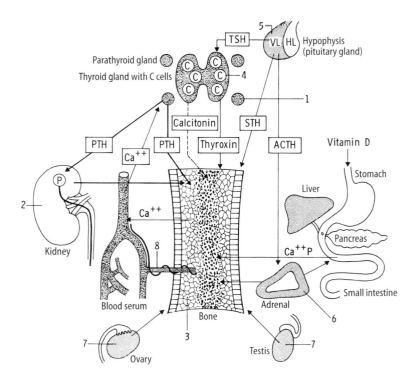

Fig. 7. Regulation of bone structure and calcium metabolism

Functional Bone Remodeling

The most pronounced physiological bone re-modeling takes place during particular periods of life. It is especially associated with skeletal development, when endochondral and intra-membranous ossification occurs and growth in the length, width and surface area of the bones takes place. During the first three decades of life the volume density of the spongiosa falls from 35% to 23%, with a further reduction to 10% in the eighth decade. In general the annual change amounts to 1%–2%. Within the space of 40 to 50 years the skeleton is completely re-newed. The loss of bone mass is associated with the reduction in the number of osteocytes and delayed mineralization, whereas resorption by osteoclasts remains unchanged throughout life. During normal maturation of the skeleton, slow bone remodeling leads, in spite of massive increase, to a harmonious growth of bone with the appropriate shape of the individual bones being strictly preserved throughout life.

The structures present during the remodel-ing of the shaft of a long bone are shown dia-grammatically in **Fig. 9.** Bone deposition at the periosteal surface *(1)* is due to the osteoblasts *(2)*, whereas in the Haversian canals *(3)* of the cortex the osteoblasts are responsible for an os-teosclerotic narrowing. At the endosteal surface *(4)* multinucleate and mononucleate osteoclasts *(5)* bring about resorption. Haversian canals can also be widened by osteoclastic bone re-sorption. In cases of *osteopetrosis* (p. 54) the osteoclastic activity is reduced and physiologi-cal remodeling inhibited; in *osteogenesis imper-fecta* (p. 54) the deposition process in the os-teons is severely inhibited by inadequate osteoblastic activity; in *Paget's osteitis defor-mans* (p. 102), on the other hand, the whole re-modeling process is greatly accelerated (activity of osteoblasts and osteoclasts).

As can be seen in the **histological photo-graph** of **Fig. 10,** such remodeling processes can also be easily recognized in histological sections. Here we see a lamellated cancellous trabecula *(1)* with well-marked osteocytes, which has, however, irregular outer borders *(2)*. Leading edges of deposition with rows of active osteoblasts *(3)* can be seen, and newly depos-ited, incompletely calcified osteoid bone tissue *(4)*. At the same time we can also recognize re-sorption fronts *(5)* with surface lacunae con-taining multinucleate osteoclasts *(6)*. The mar-row cavity contains loose connective tissue *(7)* in which trabeculae of fibrous bone *(8)* are dif-ferentiated, and where activated osteoblasts are also to be found.

The functional loading of a bone has a marked effect on its external form and internal structure. Through the remodeling process it adapts fairly quickly to the load. With long term abnormal mechanical loading or unphysi-ological joint function, deformation of the af-fected bone is more and more to be seen. In the vertebral column it is not uncommon to find a *kyphoscoliosis* (see Fig. 838) with marked osteosclerosis on the concave weight-bearing side and osteoporosis on the less loaded convex side. An example of the adaptation of bone structure is illustrated diagrammatically in a case of *tibia recurvata* in **Fig. 8.** As a result of the deviation of the axis and the long-term asymmetrical loading the cortex on the concave side *(1)* is greatly thickened, whereas on the convex side *(2)* it is equally severely narrowed. The spongiosa is also correspondingly remod-eled as a reaction to the pressure, tension and bending forces. Strong transverse trabeculae *(3)* which are orientated radially to the curvature have developed.

Such functionally conditioned bone remodel-ing as this can be recognized in the radiograph or on naked-eye examination of the specimen. **Figure 11** shows a macerated **tibia recurvata** that has been sawn through. As a result of the causative pressure stimulus the compacta at the vertex of the concave side *(1)* is greatly wid-

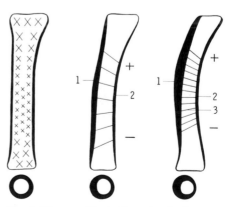

Fig. 8. Diagram illustrating adaptive bone remodeling (tibia recurvata) (after UEHLINGER)

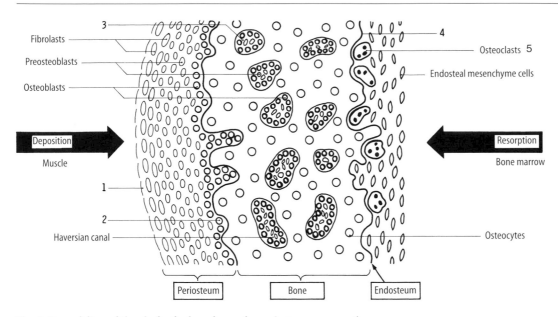

Fibrolasts

Preosteoblasts

Osteoblasts

Deposition

Muscle

1

2

Haversian canal

Osteoclasts 5

Endosteal mesenchyme cells

Resorption

Bone marrow

Osteocytes

Periosteum   Bone   Endosteum

Fig. 9. Remodeling of the shaft of a long bone shown in transverse section

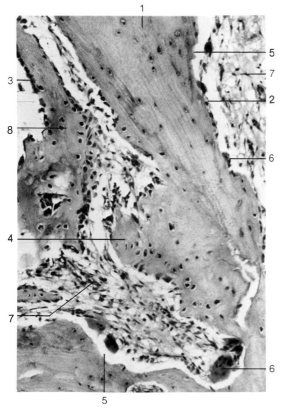

Fig. 10. Bone remodeling; HE, ×40

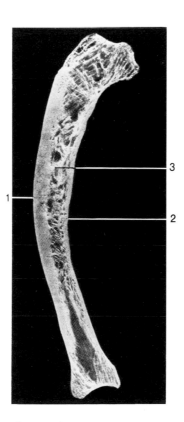

Fig. 11. Tibia recurvata (maceration specimen)

ened, whereas that on the convex side *(2)* is narrow. The spongiosa is undergoing remodeling as a *hypertrophic atrophy,* with thickened trabeculae *(3)* crossing the marrow cavity.

Physiologically, remodeling is taking place in bone weakened by osteoporosis. Because of the loss of cancellous structures which had contributed to the stability of the bone the remaining trabeculae have become more heavily loaded. This is a stimulus for osteoblastic remodeling by which the trabeculae have been thickened. The result is a spongiosa with fewer trabeculae which have at the same time become sclerotic. This remodeling can already be seen **radiographically.** In **Fig. 12** the cancellous framework is in general looser. The supporting trabeculae *(1)* are more pronounced and are separated by obvious gaps *(2).* Radiologically this is a so-called ***hypertrophic bone atrophy.***

Histologically this remodeling appears as bone trabeculae of varying width. In **Fig. 13** osteosclerotically widened trabeculae *(1)* lie next to narrow trabeculae *(2).* All trabeculae have smooth borders and show no leading edges of deposition or layers of osteoblasts, which is an indication of slow bone replacement.

According to FROST (1966) a threefold system of surface remodeling must be assumed, in which anatomically and functionally different types of bone cell take part: 1. periosteal deposition, 2. endosteal deposition and 3. deposition within the Haversian osteons. *Periosteal deposition* leads to growth and remodeling in length and thickness during skeletal development. This remodeling is greatly reduced in adults. *Endosteal bone deposition* on the other hand continues throughout life. It involves both the trabeculae of the spongiosa and the endosteal cortex, and on occasion gives rise to hypertrophic bone atrophy. *Bone deposition within the Haversian osteons* is, in practice, a continuation of endosteal deposition. FROST described the results of osseous modulation and the differentiation of particular bone cells as the "basic metabolic unit of skeletal remodelling" or the "bone remodelling unit". This "unit" is active in areas of bone in which either bone resorption or bone deposition at the surface is taking place. The "bone remodelling unit" includes the lifelong remodeling proce-

dures in terms of the bone volume, whereas the "bone metabolic unit" is a measure of the functional extent of the remodeling. This distinction is important, because the "bone remodelling units" refer to skeletal homeostasis and the "bone metabolic units" to mineral homeostasis. In general, the "bone remodelling unit" in man is completed within months, whereas the "bone metabolic unit" is usually, with wide variations, developed between a few months and over 10 years. Every "bone remodelling unit" has a characteristic life cycle. It begins in response to a stimulus – partly under the influence of the parathyroid hormone – which causes the mitotic division of the "precursor cells" and leads to the production of preosteoblasts. After a few hours or days, osteoclasts arise which initiate a resorptive phase of (on average) a month's duration. Within the next 3 months the newly formed osteoblasts replace the previously resorbed bone. The results of activating the bone cells – bone resorption and deposition – take place mainly in the endosteal region of the bone and less in the periosteal region. During life the external diameter of the long bones slightly increases, while the thickness and density of the cortex decreases.

Physiological bone remodeling is very much dependent on the functional loading of the total skeleton, as well as particular parts of it. It has important effects on the serum calcium level and is controlled in a very complicated fashion by hormonal factors. In addition to calcitonin and vitamin D (D hormone), the parathyroid hormone brings about bone resorption and hypercalcemia by stimulating the osteoclasts. The multiple interactions of the D hormone on the dynamics of metabolism of the skeleton, which regulates calcium homeostasis, is shown **diagrammatically** in **Fig. 14.**

Therefore vitamin D, which is taken in through the skin (cholecalciferol = vitamin D_1) and the intestine (7-dehydocholesterol = vitamin D_3), is converted in the liver and kidneys and finally acts to produce in the intestine an increase in calcium absorption, in the parathyroids inhibition of secretion of the parathyroid hormone and in the skeleton increased calcification. This dynamic bone remodeling is also histomorphologically demonstrable.

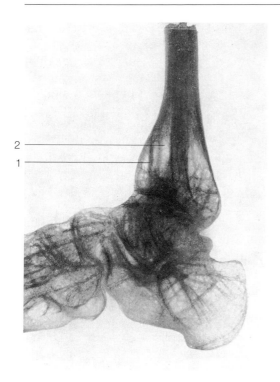

Fig. 12. Hypertrophic bone atrophy

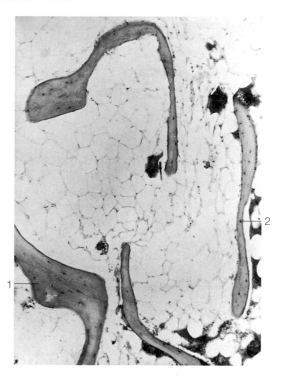

Fig. 13. Hypertrophic bone atrophy; HE, ×40

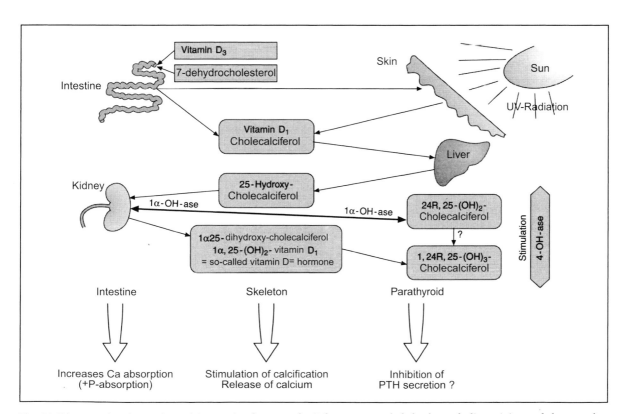

Fig. 14. Diagram showing reciprocal interaction between the D hormones and skeletal metabolic activity, and the part that this plays in the regulation of calcium homeostasis

2 Normal Anatomy and Histology

Macroscopic Structure

A variety of lesions can arise in any bone, or in different parts of the same bone, bringing about destruction or at least an alteration of the normal structure of the tissue. Depending upon their severity, these changes may be recognizable on a radiograph. The ability to assess a pathological lesion of bone naturally requires exact knowledge of the normal structure. At the macroscopic level, the distinction between the different types of bone change is first and foremost a matter of radiology, and it is by this means that the first examination is always carried out. The conventional radiograph, which is usually taken in two planes, provides the earliest and most conclusive information. The diagnostic value of such a radiograph is primarily dependent upon its quality. It must also be remembered that symptoms may be projected to a different part of the skeleton, remote from the actual lesion (a bone tumor, for example). In addition, other specific methods of examination are available to the radiologist – tomography, for instance, and scintigraphy, xerography, DSA, computer tomography, MR-tomography etc. – which are able to provide extra information and fundamentally influence the diagnosis. It is usually only after such an intensive radiological examination that a bone biopsy is taken to finally decide the diagnosis. The results of the radiological investigations should always be available to the pathologist, who should wherever possible obtain all the radiological reports (radiographs, tomograms, scintigrams, computer tomograms, and MRT findings) so that he can build up his own picture of the bone lesion. This information provides the pathologist who is assessing the lesion histologically with the macroscopic picture, and he uses it to supplement his histological evaluation. Indeed, it is only after combining the radiological, macroscopic and histological information with the clinical findings

that it is possible to achieve a reliable diagnosis.

The pathologist obtains the essential macroscopic picture from the accompanying radiographs. The macroscopic evaluation of specimens taken at operation or from autopsy material is in general only of secondary importance, since the primary diagnosis is most often made from a biopsy. Nevertheless, much can be learnt from comparing a macroscopic specimen with the corresponding radiological findings, since changes in the former can provide a better understanding of the latter.

In any case, whether one is dealing with the assessment of a radiograph, or analyzing bone removed at operation or at autopsy, complete understanding of normal bone development is absolutely essential. We must therefore know the density and structure of cancellous bone precisely in order to be able to recognize pathological changes. Whereas the spongy framework of a vertebral body, for example, is entirely regular, in the presence of *osteoporosis* (see Chapter 4) it shows a typical pattern of porosity. In cases of so-called *"eccentric atrophy"* we would expect to find the earliest and most pronounced rarefaction at the center of the spongy bone of the vertebra – something that can only be determined macroscopically (or in the radiograph). The same applies to osteoporosis of the neck of the femur with the development of the so-called *Ward's triangle* (see Fig. 117). It is possible to analyze osteolytic and osteosclerotic processes macroscopically and also radiologically in both the spongiosa and cortex, and to relate them to particular diseases.

When assessing lesions of bone we must begin with its normal architecture. Are the external contours of the bone regular? Is the external border of the cortex smooth? Is the periosteum visible? Is the shape of the bone preserved? Are the density and width of the cortex normal? Is it destroyed or fragmented? Is the endosteal surface of the cortex smooth?

Is the radiodensity of the spongiosa homogeneous? It is important whether a lesion develops in a compact bone (vertebra, long bone) or a flat bone (pelvis, scapula, skullcap).

The description of bone structure of the first order begins with that of the various topographical and structural elements, which are particularly discernible in the long bones. The external form and surface appearance of the **macerated femur** illustrated in **Fig. 16** are easily recognized. Proximally one can see the *femoral head* (caput femoris *1*), which makes up two thirds of a sphere, somewhat flattened at the top. It is covered by the smooth glistening cartilaginous articular surface. The central indentation or *fovea capitis femoris (2)* receives the insertion of the ligament of the head of the femur (ligamentum capitis femoris). The regular smooth spherical form of the head is normal; but it may become markedly deformed in diseases of the hip joint such as coxarthrosis deformans (see Fig. 807). Below this the **neck of the femur** (3) makes an angle with the shaft (4) of about 127° (Pauwels' angle). The sagittal diameter of the neck is less than the vertical, as can be seen from its height. The highly complex mechanical stresses acting here are reflected in the trajectorial pattern of the cancellous bone, which is illustrated diagrammatically in **Fig. 15**. The trabeculae in the cancellous bone are the most strongly developed and correspond to the maximal loading *(1)*, whereas the less heavily stressed regions of the neck contain only a supporting spongiosa which is much less dense *(2)*. It is this region which is first resorbed in the presence of osteoporosis, whereas the load-bearing trabeculae persist and become even more marked (so-called *hypertrophic bone atrophy*). Such changes can be seen in a radiograph. **Fig. 16** also illustrates the *greater (5)* and *lesser (6)* trochanters, which are united dorsally by the *intertrochanteric crest (7)*. The two trochanters often show the early and particularly well-marked signs of trochanteric atrophy, and isolated inflammatory or neoplastic processes can also develop here. By far the largest part of the femur is taken up by the *femoral shaft* (**diaphysis;** *8*). On the dorsal surface the *gluteal tuberosity (9)* can also be seen. This long bone becomes wider distally, leading into the *medial (10)* and *lateral (11)* condyles, which are separated by the *intercondylar fossa*

(12). The distal joint surfaces of the femur are normally covered with smooth articular cartilage. As can be seen in the **radiograph** in **Fig. 17**, all these structures can also be recognized radiologically. One can distinguish topographically between the *epiphysis (1), metaphysis (2)* and *diaphysis (3)*. The outer shape and internal structure of the *femoral head (4)*, the formation of the *femoral neck (5)*, both the *trochanters (6)*, the *shaft (7)* and the distal end of the bone with its two *condyles (8)* can be recognized. Special radiological methods can provide information about the internal structure (cortex and spongiosa). Insofar as the radiographs constitute very valuable records of the gross structure of bone for the pathologist too, they must always be available to assist in the diagnosis.

The proximal end of a **macerated femur** is illustrated in **Fig. 18**. The regular structures are easily recognized: the *head of the femur (1)* is clearly rounded and somewhat flattened above. The *femoral neck (2)* presents a smooth outline and a regular appearance. The *greater (3)* and *lesser (4)* trochanters are also regular in shape, and below these the smooth borders of the shaft are also seen. This region of the bone is normally covered with a more or less thickened periosteum, rich in fibers, which is absent from the maceration specimen, making the outer surface of the bone look somewhat rough. It is here that numerous muscles and ligaments are also attached.

As can be seen in **Fig. 19**, the contour *(1)* of the proximal end of the femur normally appears smooth and sharply outlined in **radiographs**. One can recognize the rounded form of the *head (2)*, the even joint space *(3)*, the slender *femoral neck (4)*, the *greater trochanter (5)*

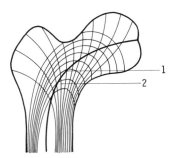

Fig. 15. Load-bearing spongiosa of the femoral neck (diagrammatic)

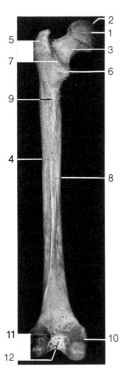

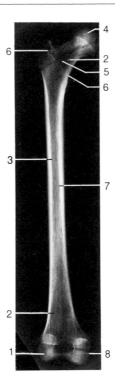

Fig. 16. Normal femur (maceration specimen)

Fig. 17. Normal femur (radiograph)

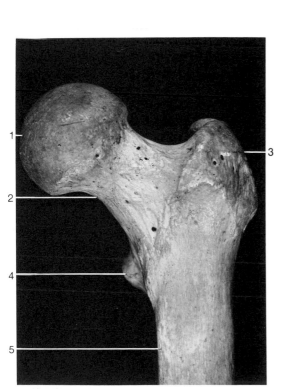

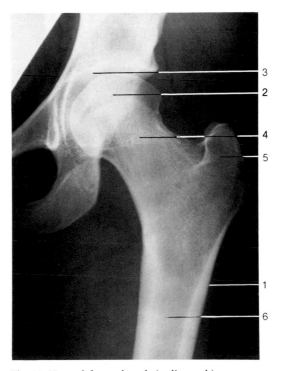

Fig. 18. Normal femoral neck (maceration specimen)

Fig. 19. Normal femoral neck (radiograph)

and, continuous therewith, the *shaft of the femur (6)*. The density of the cancellous scaffolding is remarkably homogeneous.

All bones are surrounded by a "frame" of cortical bone (compacta). Internally, the bone is filled with cancellous scaffolding, within which the narrow trabeculae intertwine with one another. In bone subjected to a particular stress the load-carrying spongiosa is more strongly developed than the rest of the "supporting spongiosa". In those bones where the load is equally distributed – the vertebral bodies, for instance – the components of the cancellous network are quite evenly developed. A **maceration specimen** of the cancellous scaffolding of a vertebral body is shown in **Fig. 20**. The bony trabeculae *(1)* are more or less equal in width and constitute a honeycomb formation that presents a wide surface for intensive metabolic exchange. It is here that the metabolic exchange of calcium continues to take place both in normal and even under pathological circumstances. Between the bony elements, spaces of very nearly equal size can be seen *(2)*, which contain the bone marrow. The bony trabeculae have completely smooth borders, and this produces the fairly uniform appearance in radiographs by which normal healthy bone can be recognized.

In **histological sections** the cancellous bone is also characterized by the homogeneous arrangement of the bony trabeculae. As can be seen in **Fig. 21**, these are of equal width *(1)*, and have smooth borders and internal lamellae. They contain small osteocytes *(2)*. The trabeculae are more or less evenly spaced and constitute a regular network. Between them lies the bone marrow *(3)*, which is filled with fatty tissue and through which very loose collagen fibers often run. Blood-forming cells are found in the fatty marrow *(4)*, representing the primitive stages of erythropoiesis and granulopoiesis, together with a few scattered megakaryocytes. The cell density of this blood-building bone marrow is variable, and depends upon the age of the subject. In the long bones of elderly people nearly all the marrow is fatty, with hardly any hematopoietic elements present.

The Blood Supply of Bone

It must always be remembered that bone is itself a living tissue, the life of which is dependent upon an adequate blood supply. Like any other tissue, bone undergoes necrosis if this supply is cut off. As is shown in **Fig. 22**, the most important supply of arterial blood to a long bone is through the nutrient artery *(1)*, which first passes through the cortical layer without branching, and which then on reaching its internal circumference divides into ascending and descending branches. At the ends of the bones the accessory arteries *(2)* supply the epiphyses and metaphyses with blood. They anastomose with the diaphyseal capillaries, and send terminal branches to the bone marrow, the cortical bone and the spongiosa, as well as to the articular cartilage *(3)*. The bone marrow is penetrated by a fine network of arteries of varying diameter. During the period of growth, the epiphyses are supplied separately. Clearly the outer layer of cortical bone is supplied by the numerous periosteal blood vessels *(4)*, which maintain connections with the cortical capillaries themselves. The arterial blood then empties into the sinusoids *(5)* of the marrow, and is subsequently drained through very thin-walled veins, either into the central vein in the diaphysis *(6)* or into the collecting veins *(7)* in the metaphysis. The blood is drained away from the bone either through the nutrient vein *(8)* or through a large tributary vein *(9)* or by the metaphyseal veins and small cortical perforating veins *(10)*.

This subdividing and complex vascular system within the bone can be well demonstrated by means of **intraosseous angiography**. In **Fig. 23** one can see how a contrast medium *(1)* introduced into the intraosseous vessels of the tibia spreads throughout the bone. It runs into a short proximally-directed stem vein *(2)* and then an abundance of subdividing vessels as far as the metaphysis *(3)*, which is connected to the nutrient vein by oblique venous anastomoses. The substantial central vein *(4)* is clearly seen. Venous drainage is largely through the metaphysis, where large caliber veins *(5)* arise. In this way it can be clearly shown that bones are provided with a complicated vascular system, and that they depend for survival upon having an adequate blood supply.

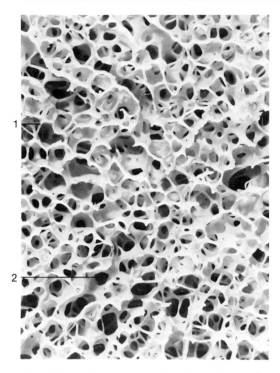

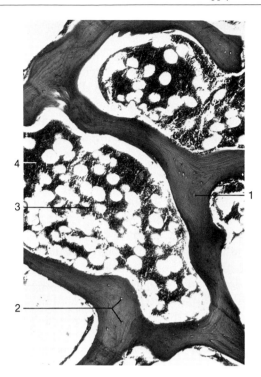

Fig. 20. Spongiosa of normal vertebra (maceration speci-men)

Fig. 21. Spongiosa of normal vertebra; HE, ×20

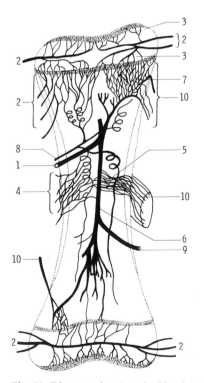

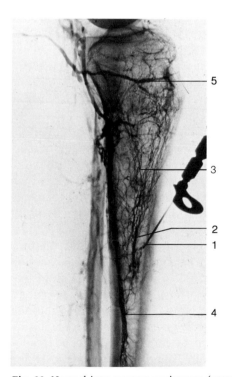

Fig. 22. Diagram showing the blood supply of a bone (after BROOKES 1971)

Fig. 23. Normal intraosseous angiogram (proximal tibia)

Histological Structure of Bone

Bone is a mesenchymal tissue the cells of which possess and retain the capacity for proliferation and differentiation. The **diagram** in **Fig. 24** illustrates the possible stages in development of bone cells. The *preosteoblasts*, which constitute those stem cells giving rise to all other bone cells, are derived from undifferentiated mesenchyme cells. They are small round or star-shaped cells with darkly staining nuclei, and they multiply by mitotic division. They mature to form *osteoblasts*, which are the true builders of bone. They produce collagen fibrils and especially osteoid, the initially uncalcified ground substance of bone, and each is capable of laying down approximately three times its own volume of bone matrix. The formation of collagen is a purely basal process, making the building up of an organized structure possible. The process of calcification of bony tissue requires a high concentration of alkaline phosphatase in the osteoblasts, and in the presence of osteoblastic activity this is also found in the serum. Resting osteoblasts are spindle-shaped, the active cells resemble epithelial cells. They have also lost the ability to proliferate by mitotic division. As a result of the production of osteoid in their neighborhood, which finally undergoes calcification, the osteoblasts are incorporated into the bone matrix and become *osteocytes*. These cells, which are responsible for the continued vitality of the bone, lie in the tissue in small lacunae bound together by cytoplasmic processes which pass through numerous canaliculi. They form within the calcified bone tissue a syncytial system of cells in which the vigorous processes of metabolic exchange can take place and which indicate the vitality of the tissue. The canaliculi do not, however, pass through the reversal line, which marks the outer border of the osteon. The canalicular system always begins close to a blood vessel and gives rise to a network of communicating tubes. Throughout the entire bony tissue of a human adult this network gives rise to a contact surface between the osteocytes and the intercellular fluid of about 250 m², which supports the rapid adjustment of the metabolic exchange of calcium. Young osteocytes continue to deposit new bone, whereas the activity of the older cells is predominantly osteolytic. The density of the osteocyte population in the tissue is age-dependent, the majority being found in infantile or newly deposited bone, whereas the older bony structures often contain only a few. As is indicated in **Fig. 24**, the origin of the *osteoclasts* has not been fully established. They are probably derived from the blood monocytes – the monocytic macrophage system. Mononucleated osteoclasts are spindle-shaped and lie in flat eroded spaces in the outer surface of the bone. The multinucleated osteoclasts are more striking in appearance, and are most often found in the deep *Howship's lacunae*. They are capable of amoeboid movements and contain the enzyme acid phosphatase. In spite of their rapid numerical increase during the osteolytic process (under the influence of parathyroid hormone, for instance) no mitotic proliferation can be definitely proved. Osteoclasts play an important part in bone resorption, although the exact mechanism is still unknown. What matters here is the fact that in unit time the osteoclasts can resorb 3 times as great a mass of bone as the osteoblasts are capable of depositing. This means that, when they are activated, osteoclastic resorption always predominates over osteoblastic deposition. On the other hand, osteoclasts have a much shorter lifetime than osteoblasts, and they can only resorb mineralized bony tissue, osteoid being invulnerable to their attack.

The laying down of bone constitutes a continuous process of maturation. In **Fig. 25** one can see a **histological specimen** of a newly developing trabecula of fibrous bone *(1)* that is still very loosely formed, and which contains many bone cells *(2)* and also narrow bands of osteoid *(3)*. This is (in fibrous bone dysplasia, see pp. 56 & 318) derived directly from myeloid tissue *(4)*.

Such a bone trabecula *(1)* is shown in **Fig. 26**. It is more densely formed and mineralized, but is still reticular in structure. This *fibrous bone trabecula* is embedded in a loose, highly cellular connective tissue stroma *(2)*. Fully mature and mineralized bone tissue is homogeneous in density and arranged in lamellae, an appearance which is especially clearly seen under polarized light or with increased dimming, and which shows up the basic structures with particular clarity.

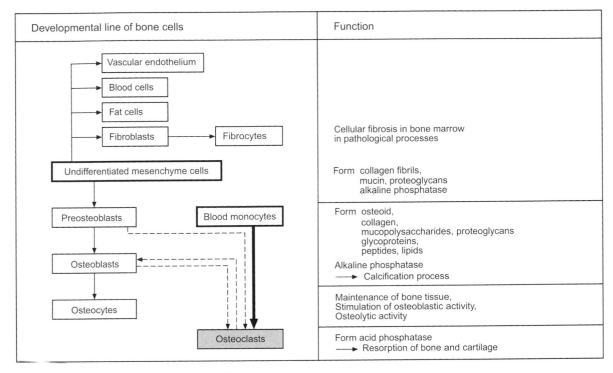

Developmental line of bone cells	Function

Vascular endothelium
Blood cells
Fat cells
Fibroblasts → Fibrocytes
 	
Undifferentiated mesenchyme cells
	Cellular fibrosis in bone marrow
	in pathological processes
	
	Form collagen fibrils,
	        mucin, proteoglycans
	        alkaline phosphatase

Preosteoblasts   Blood monocytes
 	
Osteoblasts
 	
Osteocytes
	Form osteoid,
	        collagen,
	        mucopolysaccharides, proteoglycans
	        glycoproteins,
	        peptides, lipids
	
	Alkaline phosphatase
	⟶ Calcification process

	Maintenance of bone tissue, Stimulation of osteoblastic activity, Osteolytic activity
Osteoclasts	Form acid phosphatase ⟶ Resorption of bone and cartilage

Fig. 24. Origin and function of the bone cells

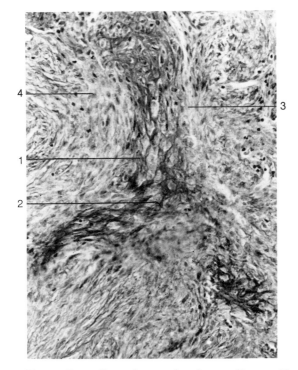

Fig. 25. Young fibrous bone trabecula; van Gieson, ×50

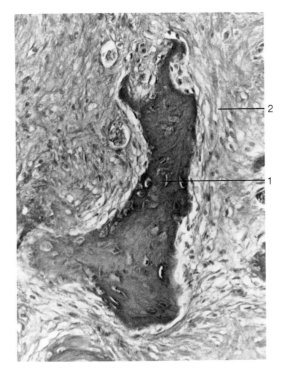

Fig. 26. Old fibrous bone trabecula; van Gieson, ×82

In the histological section of **Fig. 27** one can recognize cancellous bone trabeculae with very distinct lamellar layers *(1)* which appear double in polarized light. Osteocytes *(2)* with small dark nuclei can be seen between the lamellae, and these indicate that the bone tissue is vital. Toward the edges of the trabeculae *(3)*, where the bone is younger, the lamellae are more densely laid down than at the center. These normal cancellous trabeculae are outwardly quite smooth *(4)* and reveal no attached deposits of osteoblasts or osteoclasts, and there is usually no wide osteoid seam there. The deposition of osteoid *(5)* is to be regarded as physiological. In the marrow cavity there is loose connective tissue *(6)* with small isomorphic fibrocyte nuclei; in mature bone tissue, the marrow cavity is usually filled with fatty tissue (sometimes including hematopoietic foci).

According to whatever physiological or unphysiological stress may be acting on a bone, or in the course of a pathological bony lesion, a more or less vigorous reactive bone remodeling process will be taking place, sometimes with additional bone being added to the existing structure. This produces the picture of *osteosclerosis*, with the bone itself becoming more dense. **Figure 28** shows the classical **histological picture** of such an osteosclerotic bone remodeling. One can clearly recognize the original (autochthonous) bone trabeculae *(1)*, which show the regular layered appearance of lamellation. Nucleated osteocytes can be seen *(2)*, but quite a number of the osteocyte lacunae are empty because of decalcification (a possible artifact!). These trabeculae are covered on the outside by broad *tabular osteons (3)*, which have widened them enormously. They are separated from the autochthonous bony tissue by extended and very marked reversal lines *(4)*, which are already fully mineralized. Bone-depositing osteoblasts can no longer be observed. The leading edges of bone deposition can be recognized by their parallel orientated *reversal lines (5)*. The marrow cavity between the bony elements *(6)* is filled with fibrosed fatty tissue.

The lamellar deposition of the bone can be particularly clearly recognized under polarized light. In the **histological section** of **Fig. 29** the cortical bone can be seen. With phase contrast, one can observe transversely sectioned osteons

(1) with *Haversian canals* of varying width *(2)* and with smooth borders. The organic bone matrix contains parallel collagenous spirals in which the Haversian osteons develop. They gleam and emphasize the lamellation of the compact bone. Such well organized areas of deposition usually contain calcified mature bone. More or less numerous osteocytes with small dark nuclei are present, lying in small lacunae. These osteocyte lacunae *(3)* are also visible under phase contrast.

In **Fig. 30** one can see the **histological picture** of *woven bone* under polarized light. The bony elements *(1)* are completely unorganized, and the trabeculae vary in width. Collagen fibers *(2)* run irregularly through the marrow cavity and often form a reticulum. The varying translucency of the fibrous bone *(3)* indicates incomplete and irregular mineralization. A few indiscriminately directed reversal lines represent the leading edges of mineralization processes. A few osteoblasts *(4)* are deposited on the outside of the bony elements, and within the matrix several osteocytes can be seen *(5)*. The marrow cavity is filled with loose, moderately vascularized connective tissue. This is newly deposited immature bone, which may also be present during repair processes (e.g. fractures, p. 113) or during pathological deposition (e.g. fibrous bone dysplasia, p. 56).

It is possible to distinguish macroscopically and microscopically – particularly in the long bones – between the dense structure of cortical bone and the loose spongiosa. The majority of pathological processes take place in the spongiosa (cancellous bone). (Examples include osteomyelitis, p. 129; osteoporosis and osteopathies, p. 65; osteomyelosclerosis, p. 106; bone metastases, p. 396). They produce local or diffuse defects (areas of increased translucency in the radiograph indicate osteolytic foci) or irregular areas of increased density (osteosclerotic foci). Every change in the radiographic appearance must be precisely localized in order to make a histological diagnosis possible. A biopsy taken from the iliac crest which includes cortical bone and little or no spongiosa is not suitable for diagnosing a suspected disease of the bone or bone marrow.

Pathological processes in the cortical bone can also produce a defect in the structure of the bone that can be identified radiologically.

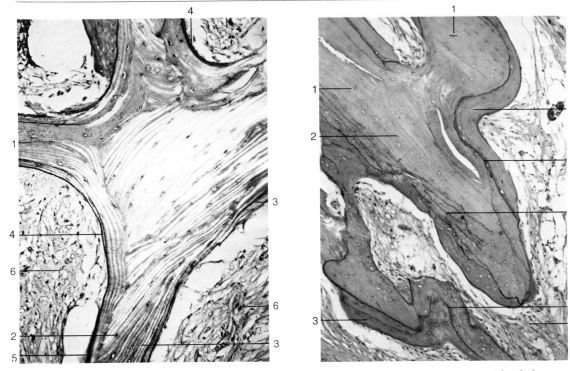

Fig. 27. Mature, fully mineralized lamellar bone tissue; HE, ×40 (under polarized light)

Fig. 28. Osteosclerotic bone tissue with tabular osteons; HE, ×40

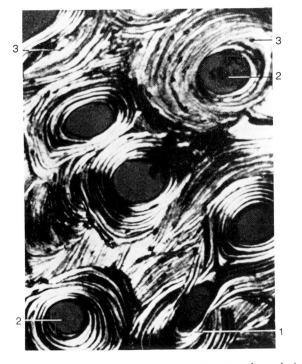

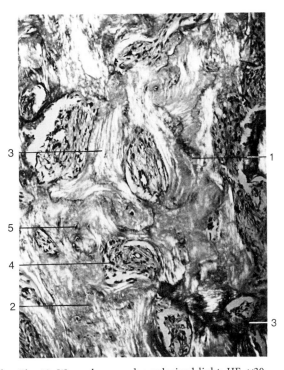

Fig. 29. Lamellar bone (Haversian osteons under polarized light); phase contrast exposure, ×40

Fig. 30. Woven bone under polarized light; HE, ×30

With lesions primarily affecting the marrow cavity (osteomyelitis, bone tumors) the endosteal layer, which is normally sharply delineated, should be particularly closely examined. An undulating or even jagged outline indicates intramedullary destruction. Furthermore, the cortical layer can be narrowed (in osteoporosis) or frankly interrupted (by a malignant bone tumor). The periosteal side of the cortical bone should also be examined, since periosteal irritation usually causes widening of the periosteum and reactive periosteal bone deposition (so-called periostitis ossificans: p. 160), which can show up on the radiograph as a shadow with or without bony elements (e.g. spicula). A biopsy taken from such altered periosteum is not informative, since only reactively changed tissue is obtained, and no structure pathognomonic of the actual bone disease is available for histological examination (a bone biopsy from Codman's triangle in a case of osteosarcoma, for example; see p. 276).

There are some bone lesions which attack the cortical bone preferentially (e.g. a cortical osteoid osteoma: p. 260; bone metastases from a renal cell carcinoma). Here the marrow cavity and the scaffolding of the involved bone may be unchanged, or similar foci may be seen within the bone. When foci of osteolytic destruction are present (e.g. osteolytic bone metastases), translucent areas may be seen radiologically in the cortical bone which may be accompanied by reactive local neoplastic periostitis ossificans. With osteosclerotic processes (e.g. a cortical osteoid osteoma) the cortical bone often shows increased density over a long distance and usually also a considerable widening, which can cause local narrowing of the marrow cavity or protrusion into the adjacent soft tissues, thus leading to distension of the bone. These changes can be easily recognized in the radiograph and diagnostically evaluated.

As can be seen in the **histological photograph** in **Fig. 31**, cortical bone is homogeneous and very densely structured. The typical lamellar structure of the bone is apparent in the onion-like arrangement of the osteons (1). The lamellae are emphasized by the so-called *reversal lines* (or cement lines 2), between which small nucleated osteocytes can be seen in their lacunae (3). These confirm the vitality of the tissue. Several empty lacunae (4) are the result of somewhat too severe decalcification. This can be largely avoided by using the much less violent decalcifying agent EDTA, although the time required for it to act is much longer. Nevertheless, when a large area of bone is free from osteocytes, this is a sign of bone necrosis. The Haversian canals (5) can be very narrow, smoothly outlined and containing loose stromal connective tissue and a blood-filled vessel.

In loaded regions of the skeleton (pelvis, long bones) continuous remodeling is taking place, involving 1% to 2% of the entire skeleton in the course of a year. This physiological (or also pathologically increased) remodeling can be precisely demonstrated by **intermittent tetracycline marking**. In **Fig. 32** an undecalcified bone section is viewed under fluorescent lighting, the leading edges of the deposition being clearly made visible by the tetracycline marking. This substance is laid down in the uncalcified osteoid and shows up as a bright yellow band (1). The Haversian canals (2), around which the deposited layers (3) are laid down like the bark of a tree, are easily recognized. The inner layer of the osteons consists of a wide, bright osteoid seam (4) without osteocytes. Here new bone is being laid down in the neighborhood of a Haversian canal.

Histological identification of cancellous bone depends upon the normally regular structural network of the bone trabeculae and the areas of marrow cavity, more or less of equal size, lying between them. As can be seen in **Fig. 33**, the cancellous trabeculae are almost equal in width (1) and the marrow cavity (2) is so wide that it and the bone tissue are virtually coextensive.

Under **higher magnification** (**Fig. 34**) it can be seen that the cancellous trabeculae mostly have smooth edges (1) and are not covered by osteoblasts or osteoclasts. The marrow cavity is filled with fatty tissue (2) and a few hematopoietic cells.

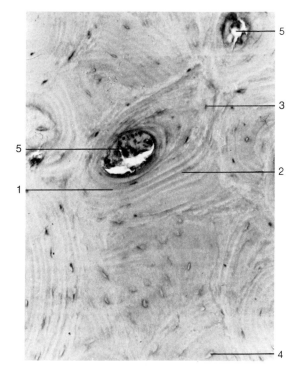

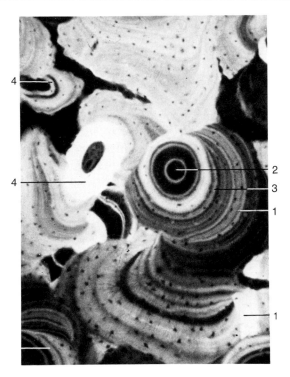

Fig. 31. Cortical bone tissue with Haversian osteons; HE, ×40

Fig. 32. Old and new osteons (tetracycline marking); fluorescent light, ×180

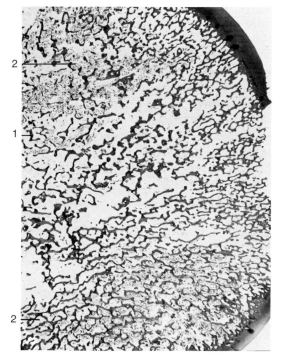

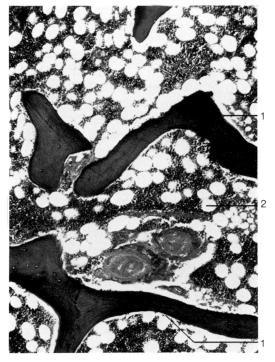

Fig. 33. Normal spongiosa, overall view; HE ×4

Fig. 34. Normal spongiosa; van Gieson, ×20

Bone Cells

The physiological and pathological deposition of bone is, like resorption, brought about by particular cells, and these can be identified in histological sections. Furthermore, the activity of these cells can be recognized morphologically, since the products of this activity (osteoid laid down by osteoblasts, for instance, and collagen fibers by fibroblasts) or its effects (e.g. the resorption lacunae of osteoclasts in the bone) can be seen in the histological section. By observing the cell population on the one hand and changes in the structure of the bone on the other, the extent of the remodeling can be evaluated.

The advanced **deposition** of bone is indicated in **Fig. 36** by the presence of rows of *osteoblasts*. **Histologically** the surface of the original bone structures *(1)* is seen to be densely lined with a row of osteoblasts *(2)*, which in places consists of many layers. These cells, which sometimes resemble epithelial cells, are very large and have large, uniformly dark, oval nuclei and a basophilic cytoplasm. Ultrastructurally they contain an extensive rough endoplasmic reticulum where protein synthesis takes place, a Golgi field and numerous intracytoplasmic vesicles. The mitochondria contain particles rich in calcium, and these represent an intracellular calcium reservoir. Basally, the osteoblasts lay down osteoid on the surface of the bone *(3)*, and, after subsequent calcification and widening, the various bone structures are then formed. These cells also control the primary mineralization of the newly formed osteoid partly by means of the alkaline phosphatase which they produce. They remain in contact with the osteocytes *(4)* through cell processes, thus constituting a transport path for calcium in and out of the bone. After the active phase is ended, small inactive osteoblasts with elongated spindle-shaped nuclei remain on the bone surface. The majority of osteoblasts, however, become embedded in the bone to form osteocytes *(4)*.

Bone resorption is brought about by the multinucleated *osteoclasts*, which have a brush border richly loaded with acid phosphatase. These cells produce proteolytic enzymes which make bone resorption possible. In the **histological section** shown in **Fig. 37** one can see a few

large osteoclasts *(1)* with several vesicular nuclei. One of these is lying in a deep Howship's lacuna *(2)* where calcified bone is being resorbed. This accounts for the undulating border of the trabecula. The rapid increase and high activity of these cells in response to particular stimuli is related to their short life. After resorption is complete, the empty lacuna shows that resorption is over. With advanced bone resorption large numbers of active multinucleated osteoclasts can be seen. As an alternative to this lacunar resorption, there is another and smoother process brought about in a much more concealed fashion by mononucleated osteoclasts, which can be identified enzyme-histochemically by their intracytoplasmic content of acid phosphatase. In this way the trabeculae are evenly narrowed without producing Howship's lacunae.

The presence of intact *osteocytes* in bone tissue confirms its vitality. Very often in sections of old bone **(Fig. 38)** only a few irregularly spaced osteocytes are visible *(1)*. Although these cells lie in small lacunae in the middle of fully mineralized bone tissue, they are interconnected by anastomoses and canaliculi which provide for the necessary metabolic exchange. They have both an osteoblastic and an osteoclastic function.

If empty osteocyte lacunae *(1)* are found in a **histological section** after decalcification with EDTA (see **Fig. 39**) we know we are dealing with necrotic bone tissue. In the presence of generally increased activity of the bone cells (with hyperparathyroidism, for instance: p. 80), the medullary mesenchyme cells are also activated. As can be seen in **Fig. 35**, activated fibroblasts *(1)* appear, which synthesize collagen fibers around themselves and produce **peripheral fibrosis** *(2)*.

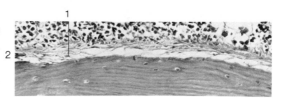

Fig. 35. Peripheral fibrosis with fibroblasts; HE, ×64

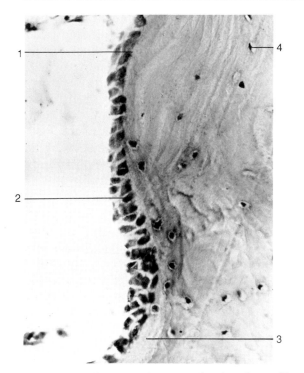

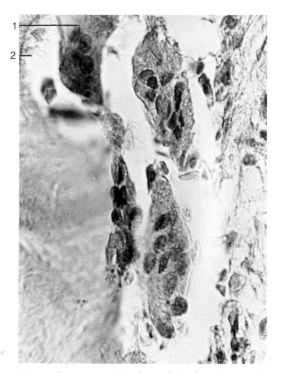

Fig. 36. Bone deposition by rows of activated osteoblasts; HE, ×100

Fig. 37. Bone resorption by multinucleated osteoclasts; HE, ×256

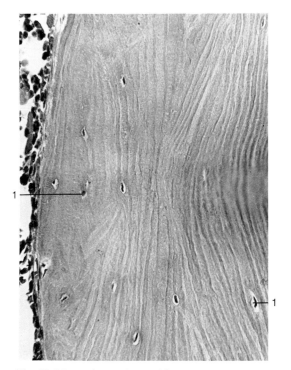

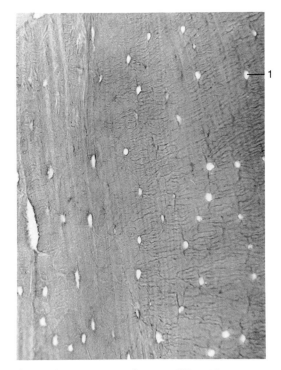

Fig. 38. Mature bone tissue with osteocytes; HE, ×100

Fig. 39. Empty osteocyte lacunae; HE, ×100

Endochondral Ossification

The essential physiological growth of bones is brought about by endochondral ossification, whereby cartilaginous growth of the epiphyses leads to growth in length. In addition to this, periosteal growth in thickness of the bones and maturation of the skeleton take place. Unphysiological variations in these complicated processes lead to disordered skeletal development (p. 31 ff.). During the early growth period endochondral centers of ossification (1) appear as illustrated in **Fig. 40**. These are later replaced by ossified epiphyseal centers, which contribute relatively little to the growth of the bone. Growth in length takes place mainly at the diaphyseal side of the epiphyseal cartilaginous growth center (2). Ossification always begins centrally and proceeds toward the periphery.

Endochondral ossification is illustrated **diagrammatically** in **Fig. 41**. The *reserve zone* (resting zone) (1) consists of the so-called stem cells: small mononucleated chondrocytes. In the zone of *proliferating cartilage (2)* the chondrocytes are larger, with small dark nuclei. Mitotic cell proliferation can be observed here, and this layer contributes to growth in length of the bone. The important region of growth is, however, the width of the layer of *hypertrophic zone* (maturation zone, columnar cartilage) *(3)*, in which the swollen chondrocytes lay down the cartilage matrix. In the adjacent *zone of provisional calcification (4)*, calcium is deposited in the cartilaginous ground substance, producing calcium spicules. In the contiguous zone, invading osteoblasts lay down osteoid around the spicules, and from this the *primary spongiosa (5)* develops. Later the osteoid becomes calcified, and the *secondary spongiosa* with its lamellar bone trabeculae appears.

Figure 42 shows the **histological** structure of the cartilaginous epiphyseal plate, which is responsible for the growth in length of the bone. One can recognize the various layers found during normal endochondral ossification (*1*, the reserve zone; *2*, the zone of proliferating cartilage; *3*, the hypertrophic [or vesicular] zone; *4*, the zone of provisional calcification; *5*, the primary spongiosa. The secondary spongiosa lies outside the picture). Disturbances in these regions of the growth zone lead to disorders of growth and skeletal malformations.

In the growing skeleton, the cartilaginous epiphyseal plates are easily recognizable radiologically, thus indicating the youth of the patient. The growth zones can also be recognized **macroscopically** when the bone is sawn through. **Figure 43** illustrates the sawn surface of the lower end of the femur of a 17-year-old man, showing the even spongiosa of the metaphysis (1), the more dense spongiosa of the epiphysis (2) and, in between, the sharply delineated epiphyseal cartilage (3) separating it from the spongiosa of the epiphysis (2). Close to this zone the bone structure is unevenly dense.

This can be observed in a **radiograph**. **Figure 44a** shows the lower end of the thigh with the femur (1) and tibia (2). The epiphyseal line (3) is clearly visible and shows the irregular density of the bone (4) in its immediate vicinity.

Bone remodeling can be impressively demonstrated by **skeletal scintigraphy**, since the activity is increased ($87^{m}Sr$). As can be seen in **Fig. 44b**, there is a considerable intensification of activity in the growth regions at the distal ends of the femora (5) and proximal ends of the tibiae (6) in a 14-year-old boy.

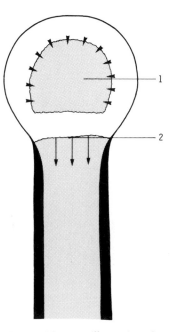

Fig. 40. Diagram illustrating the endochondral growth in length of a long bone

1 Reserve zone

2 Proliferating cartilage

3 Hypertrophic zone
(Maturation zone,
Columnar cartilage)

4 Zone of provisional
calcification

5 Osteoid production
(primary spongiosa)

Bone remodeling into
lamellar bone trabeculae
(secondary spongiosa)

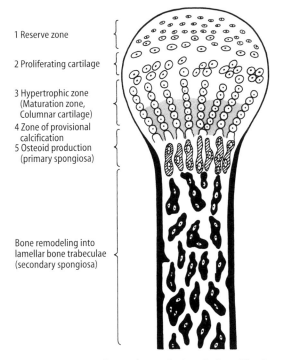

Fig. 41. Diagram illustrating endochondral ossification

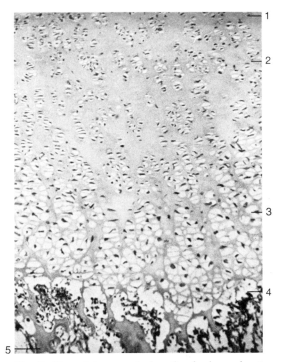

Fig. 42. Normal increase in length of a bone due to endochondral ossification in the epiphyseal cartilage; HE, ×63

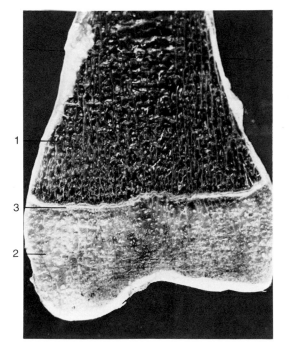

Fig. 43. Normal epiphyseal cartilage (distal epiphyseal line of femur)

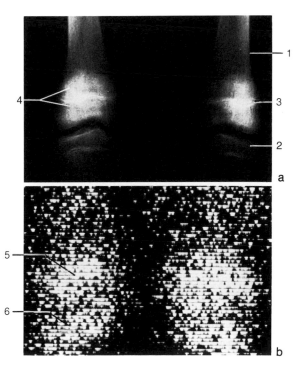

Fig. 44. a radiograph and **b** scintigram of a normal epiphyseal (growth) cartilage

Cartilaginous and Joint Structures

Both radiologically and macroscopically the evaluation of joint structures is of paramount importance to the pathologist, since it is here that numerous disease processes are found. Histologically it is often only possible to observe a small section of the joint component, which must nevertheless be macroscopically assessed in the context of the joint as a whole in each case. **Figure 45** illustrates a lateral **radiograph** of a normal knee joint. This specially soft film is also able to demonstrate the surrounding soft tissues. We can recognize the articulating bones (distal end of femur *(1)*; proximal end of tibia *(2)*; part of proximal end of fibula *(3)*) and also the patella *(4)*. All these bones are of normal appearance. In the region of the joint the radiolucent articular cartilage *(5)* is clearly differentiated from the denser bone, its layer being evenly bordered. The joint space *(6)* is fully present, and within it the menisci, synovial and fatty tissues [*(7)*, plica alaris] can be seen. The weak soft-tissue shadows include the patellar ligament *(8)*, the tendon of the quadriceps *(9)* and the muscles *(10)*.

As can be seen in the **macroscopic** and **histological photographs** in **Figs. 46a** and **b**, the cartilaginous joint surface *(1)* is completely smooth and shiny, with practically no irregularities or rough edges. It is evenly colored yellowish-white, and forms a homogeneous covering for the ends of the articulating bones *(2)*. In particular, irregularities of this part of the joint, sometimes accompanied by discoloration of the cartilage, indicate degenerative changes such as are found in arthrosis (p. 424).

Histologically, the articular cartilage *(1)* consists mostly of a hyaline layer of unequal width (**Fig. 46b**), with a superficial tangential section below in which a transitional zone, a radial zone and a calcified basal zone can be distinguished. In **Fig. 47** one can see fully homogeneous cartilaginous tissue *(1)*, within the weakly basophilic and virtually structureless tissue in which chondrocytes *(2)* are lying. These have spherical nuclei and a fine granular cytoplasm which may contain fat droplets and glycogen. After distortion due to fixation, the chondrocytes may shrink so that the cells appear to lie in a so-called "chondroblastic capsule". Occasionally multinucleated cartilage cells are seen. In aging cartilage, multinucleated chondrocytes are more numerous, and degenerative changes unmask and reveal the fine fibrils of the matrix, which may result in the appearance of so-called "asbestos-like degeneration". The ground substance has at this stage become eosinophilic.

A very important component of the joint is the *joint capsule,* which supports its function mechanically. As can be seen in the **histological photograph** of **Fig. 48**, it consists of tough fibrous connective tissue *(3)* with few fibrocyte nuclei. The collagen fiber bundles, which run parallel, are unequal in strength and leave weak places or gaps between them where a so-called hygroma or "ganglion" (p. 472) may develop. On either side of the joint the capsule blends with the periosteum of the articulating bones, the insertion of the capsule being at variable distances from the joint. This is significant for certain joint diseases (the spreading of osteomyelitis into the joint, for instance; see Chapter 7).

The connective tissue on the inside of the joint capsule is looser and passes gradually over into the *synovial membrane.* **Figure 48** shows a transverse section through the synovia. The stratum synoviale *(1)* consists of loose connective tissue with elastic fibers and contains capillaries and nerves. The synovial membrane is partly smooth and partly villous, and is covered by a single-cell layer of synovial epithelium *(2)*. Increase in width and vascularity of this membrane is a sign of irritation within the joint. On its outer surface the synovia is limited by the stratum fibrosum *(3)*.

Degenerative joint diseases (e.g. arthroses) develop primarily in the avascular articular cartilage and bring about secondary reactive changes in the subchondral bone. Inflammatory joint diseases, on the other hand, develop primarily in the vascular joint capsule and synovia, and only later cause damage to the articular cartilage. Degenerative changes of the capsule itself can, however, also occur. For the diagnosis of such diseases to be possible, accurate anatomical and histological knowledge of the individual joints is necessary.

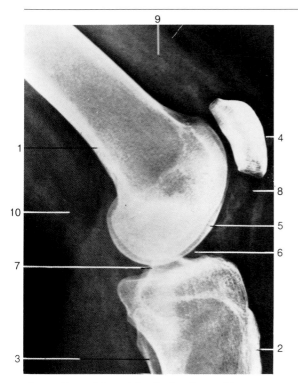

Fig. 45. Normal knee joint (soft radiograph)

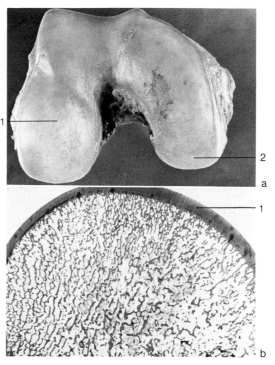

Fig. 46. a Normal cartilaginous joint surface; b normal articular cartilage, overall view; HE, ×8

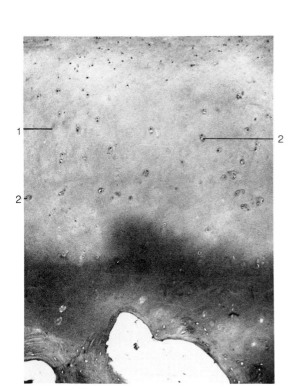

Fig. 47. Normal articular cartilage; HE, ×20

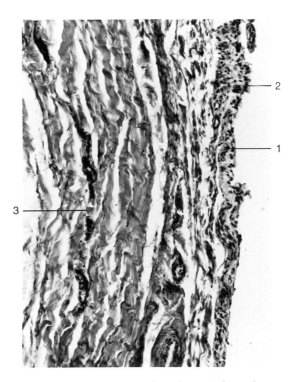

Fig. 48. Normal joint capsule and synovial membrane; PAS, ×40

3 Disorders of Skeletal Development

General

Developmental disorders of the skeleton appear in childhood and adolescence. They are sometimes hereditary, are often generalized and owe their immediate cause to an enzymatic defect or deficiency. Such disorders may also be acquired if important building materials (proteins, calcium, vitamin D) are absent, or not present in sufficient quantities, during the period of skeletal development. The bone tissue is incorrectly laid down either quantitatively (too much or too little) or qualitatively (e.g. fibrous bone instead of lamellar bone). Skeletal deformities are always due to disorders of growth. These diseases are known as the *osteochondrodysplasias*. The disorder can be located in the epiphyses, metaphyses, periosteum or endosteum. Many of the forms of this condition are only rarely seen, others appear more often and should therefore be recognized by the doctor.

Most of these developmental disorders can be diagnosed from the radiograph alone, and histological confirmation by a specific bone biopsy is not helpful and therefore contraindicated. We may, of course, encounter this type of bone or skeletal deformity at autopsy, and should then analyze it histomorphologically. There are, however, localized skeletal dysplasias which raise serious radiological problems for differential diagnosis, and which can only be recognized by histological examination. Of particular importance here are *fibrous bone dysplasia (Jaffe-Lichtenstein*, p. 56) and *osteopetrosis* (p. 54). Other bone dysplasias represent multiple primary bone tumors, including *enchondromatosis* (p. 60) and the so-called *exostosis disease* (osteochondromatosis, p. 62). These skeletal diseases can also be recognized with great certainty in the radiograph, although a histological assessment serves to confirm the diag-

nosis and, when proliferation is advanced, to predict the further progress of the condition. In a few instances these tumorous types of skeletal dysplasia can lead to the development of a bone sarcoma and follow a fatal course. With skeletal dysplasias the pathologist is sometimes also sent the radiographs for assessment, but he cannot be expected to identify each developmental disorder of the skeleton precisely. He should nevertheless at least be able to indicate that the case belongs to this group of diseases and that further radiological analysis is necessary.

So far at least 82 forms of skeletal dysplasia have been recognized and described, many of which are very rare. Up to now there is no uniform classification. SPRANGER and co-workers classify them according to their location and the nature of the original lesion. *Dysplasias which preferentially attack the epiphysis* are the chondrodysplasias (chondrodysplasia punctata, multiple epiphyseal dysplasia, hereditary arthro-ophthalmopathy, hypothyroidism). *Those which particularly affect the metaphyses* are the *metaphyseal chondroplasias* (e.g. achondrogenesis, hypophosphatasia, chondro-ectodermal dysplasia, achondroplasia, familial hypophosphatemic rickets). In the region of the vertebral column one finds congenital spondyloepiphyseal dysplasia, diastrophic or metatrophic dwarfism, or the Dyggve-Melchior-Clausen syndrome. A few skeletal dysplasias are based on a *mucopolysaccharidosis* or *mucolipidosis*. The true developmental disorders of bone include *fibrous bone dysplasia, enchondromatosis (Ollier)* and multiple *osteocartilaginous exostoses*. Finally, there are *idiopathic osteolyses* and *localized dysostoses* (dyschondrosteosis, ulno-fibular dysplasia, cleido-cranial dysplasia and osteo-onycho-dysostosis). Of particular significance for the pathologist are the disorders of bone development that depend upon *reduced bone deposition* (osteogenesis imperfecta, juvenile idiopathic osteoporosis) or involve an *increase in bone tissue* (osteopetrosis, melorheostosis).

As can be seen from the classification, there are very many developmental disorders of the skeleton and an enormous number of changes that may appear clinically or radiologically, the majority of which do not come to the pathologist for morphological analysis. However, the pathologist is asked to contribute to the diagnoses of some of them. In order to understand such skeletal changes, knowledge of the fundamentals of skeletal development and growth is essential.

Figure 49 represents a **schematic diagram of endochondral ossification and its disorders.** On the left the individual zones are shown which normally make up the region of endochondral ossification. The *reserve zone* (resting zone) consists of the so-called stem cells: small mononucleate chondrocytes. In the zone of *proliferating cartilage* the cells are larger and capable of dividing. This is followed by a wider *hypertrophic zone* (maturation zone), in which the cells are distended. Since they are arranged in columns, one also speaks of *columnar cartilage*. It is this bone which contributes particularly to growth in length, and it is here that these swollen cartilage cells give rise to the ground substance (matrix) of the cartilaginous tissue, the so-called chondroid. This is adjacent to the *zone of provisional calcification,* where calcium salts are laid down in the cartilaginous ground substance. Many capillaries sprout from the marrow cavity into the zone of endochondral ossification and break up the cartilage cells. The calcium spicules of the calcified ground substance remain in the *zone of initiation*. Osteoblasts wander into the region of the *primary spongiosa* and lay down osteoid around the calcium spicules. This is later calcified. It is here that the calcification centers appear, surrounded by a mantle of bone tissue. This is followed by resorption of the newly formed calcified bone by osteoclasts and the development of the definitive *secondary spongiosa,* while the primary spongiosa is resorbed and replaced by bone trabeculae aligned in the directions of the tension and pressure.

At every stage of this complicated endochondral ossification process some form of disturbance can arise which will lead to a developmental disorder of the skeleton. Some of these possible skeletal dysplasias are illustrated in the right half of **Fig. 49**. In the case of **achondrogenesis**, a rare autosomal recessive inherited condition, the resting cartilage is involved and no stem cells are differentiated. In most cases the child dies in the uterus or shortly after birth. In **achondroplasia** (chondrodystrophia fetalis, p. 248), an autosomal dominant inherited disease which is associated with dwarfism, there is underdevelopment of the proliferating cartilage. The action of ionized radiation on the proliferating zone can also inhibit cell division. If the development of the columnar cartilage is impaired or completely absent, this leads to a **chondrodystrophy** (p. 48). With *rickets* (p. 50) as with *osteochondritis luetica* (syphilis, p. 52), calcification is reduced or absent, and there is an abnormal accumulation of cartilaginous ground substance in the *zone of initiation*. If the osteoblasts lay down too little osteoid and bone in the primary spongiosa, the result is **osteogenesis imperfecta** (p. 54). Finally, there can also be a disturbance of remodeling of the lamellar bone if the resorption by osteoclasts is insufficient, and in this case it is exceeded by bone deposition, leading to the picture of **osteopetrosis** (p. 54).

Thus it can be seen that quite a number of developmental disorders of the skeleton are due to a disturbance of endochondral ossification. It is probable that the tumor-like skeletal dysplasias – such as **enchondromatosis** (p. 60) and **osteochondromatosis** (p. 62) – belong to this group. Other skeletal dysplasias can appear at a considerable distance from the region of bone growth (e.g. fibrous bone dysplasia, p. 56; arachnodactylia, p. 58). The mechanism of their development has not as yet been clarified.

Figure 50 is a schematic diagram showing the underlying disorders of ossification behind the most important skeletal dysplasias. All 5 diseases shown are the result of a disturbance of bone replacement, and therefore of endochondral ossification, which can be either epiphyseal or metaphyseal. In the case of rickets, osteogenesis imperfecta or osteopetrosis there is an additional disturbance of perichondral ossification. The deposition of the membrane bone is also disturbed in these latter diseases. This can be recognized both in the radiograph as well as in autopsy specimens.

Reserve zone
(stem cells)
Proliferating cartilage
(cell division)
Hypertrophic zone
(columnar cartilage,
matrix production)
Zone of provisional
calcification
Zone of initiation
Primary spongiosa
(osteoid production)
Osteoclastic
remodeling
Secondary spongiosa
Achondrogenesis
Achondroplasia
Radiation damage
Chondrodystrophy
Rickets
Syphilis
Rickets
Syphilis
Osteogenesis
imperfecta
Osteopetrosis

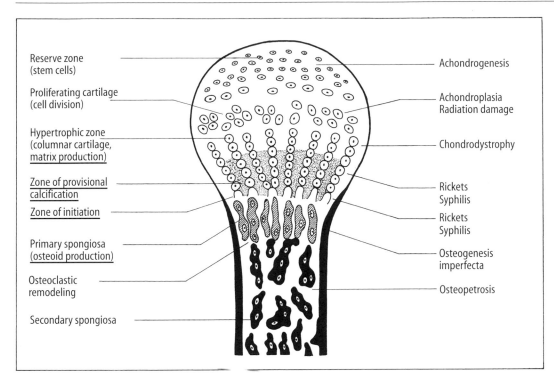

Fig. 49. Diagram illustrating disturbances of endochondral ossification

Chondro-
dystrophy
Rickets
Syphilitic
osteochondritis
Osteogenesis
imperfecta
Osteopetrosis
I. Replacement bone formation:
1. Disturbances of
endochondral ossification
a) Epiphyseal
b) Metaphyseal
2. Disturbances of
perichondral ossification
II. Membrane bone formation

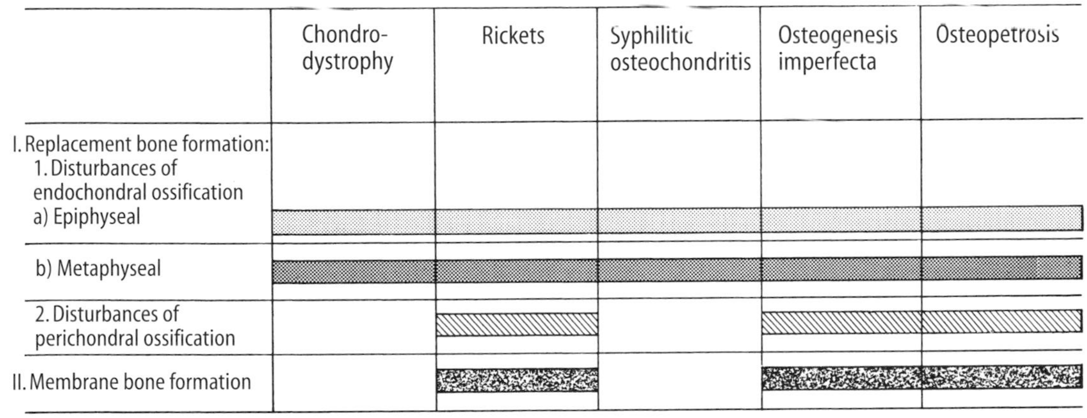

Fig. 50. Diagram illustrating the various types of ossification disturbances

The Classification of Skeletal Dysplasias

The most important dysplasias are listed in **Table 1** according to their intraosseous localization (epiphysis, metaphysis, vertebral column), their pattern of distribution throughout the entire skeleton, their developmental type (osteolysis, osteosclerosis), and the underlying etiology. What we are dealing with here is a heterogeneous collection of diseases which may be of genetic origin or acquired in utero, and which can in general lead to faulty development of the skeleton. A distinction can be made between dysplasias and dysostoses. By *skeletal dysplasias* one understands *generalized* defects of bone and cartilage development, which are principally manifested in the epiphyses and metaphyses of the long bones and vertebrae. *Skeletal dysostoses* are *localized* malformations of a single part of the skeleton (e.g. ulno-fibular dysplasia, cleido-cranial dysplasia). The classical radiological appearances are of decisive importance in their diagnosis, and here we refer particularly to pediatric radiologists with specialized experience in such matters. Account must also be taken of the whole clinical picture, the biochemical findings and the cytological and genetic criteria. This kind of comprehensive investigation of children with a skeletal dysplasia is essential in order to avoid foreseeable complications, to initiate appropriate therapeutic precautions and, finally, to be able to give genetic advice. When such cases come to autopsy, the pathologist also has his contribution to make to the morphological diagnosis by carrying out macroscopic and microscopic examination of the skeleton. Since, with many of the skeletal dysplasias (e.g. chondrodysplasia calcificans punctata, metaphyseal chondrodysplasia, the Ellis-van Crefeld syndrome, Jeune's disease etc.), other organs (heart, kidneys, gut, skin, eyes etc.) are also malformed or pathologically altered, one must also consider the possible complications involving these organs. Pathological changes in these diseased organs may, on the other hand, be the subject of pathological and anatomical analysis at autopsy.

At international conferences on nomenclature the skeletal dysplasias have been classified from various points of view. The criteria include 1. the localization of the developmental disturbance (osteochondrodysplasias), 2. its cause (chromosomal aberration, metabolic disturbances, idiopathic origin), 3. appearances at particular times of life (at birth, in later life), 4. nature of the osseous modeling disorder, (osteolysis, osteosclerosis). The clinical signs have also to be taken into account (e.g. hypercalcemia). In the meantime a large number of skeletal dysplasias have been described and precisely defined, and many of these are named eponymously for the discoverer. The great number and complexity of the individual symptoms of these diseases, the etiology of which is often unknown, has led to confusion and made it very difficult obtain an overall picture of the skeletal dysplasias. Various articles on the subject published by pediatricians (SPRANGER et al., 1974; WYNNE-DAVIES et al., 1985) have introduced different classifications. Moreover, they analyze the single lesions only by their radiological appearance. Articles and textbooks giving descriptions in terms of pathological anatomy (macroscopy, histology, AEGERTER and KIRKPATRICK, 1968; JAFFE, 1972; BÖHM, 1984) are incomplete, since only selected diseases were described.

In the present textbook no attempt is made to describe and illustrate more than a few skeletal dysplasias. These lesions are displayed in **Table 1** and listed in accordance with the *classification* of SPRANGER, LANGER and WIEDEMANN (1974). Eight groups are distinguished: dysplasias which mostly develop in the **epiphysis**, and others where the disturbance is predominantly in the **metaphysis**. Developmental disturbances mostly affecting the **vertebral column** make up a particular group of their own. Then come the **metabolic disturbances** affecting skeletal development, and constitutional bone disease with unchecked **abnormal tissue formation** and idiopathic **osteolyses**. A further group includes skeletal dysplasias which mostly affect **a single part** or only one side of the skeleton. A larger group comprises deviations from normal **bone density** or **bone remodeling**. In this table the most important skeletal dysplasias are arranged according to the recognized international nomenclature, and many eponymous names are therefore omitted. For descriptions of these diseases reference must be made to the specialized articles in the literature. These play a subordinate role in radiological and pathological diagnosis.

Table 1. Classification of the skeletal dysplasias (after J.W. SPRANGER, L.O. LANGER and H.-R. WIEDEMANN 1974)

I. **Skeletal Dysplasias with Predominantly Epiphyseal Involvement**
1. Chondrodysplasia punctata (=**Conradi's disease** [dominant, recessive])
2. Multiple epiphyseal dysplasia*
3. Hereditary arthro-ophthalmopathy
4. Hypothyroidism

II. **Skeletal Dysplasias with Predominantly Metaphyseal Involvement**
1. Achondrogenesis (types I and II)*
2. Hypophosphatasia (congenital lethal form, tarda)*
3. Thanatophoric dwarfism*
4. Asphyxiating thoracic dysplasia (= **Jeune's disease**)*
5. Chondroectodermal dysplasia (= **Ellis-van Creveld syndrome**)*
6. Short rib-polydactyly syndrome (**Majewski type, Saldino-Noonan type**)
7. Achondroplasia*
8. Hypochondroplasia
9. Metaphyseal chondrodysplasia (**Jansen type, Schmid type, McKusick type**)*
10. Metaphyseal chondrodysplasia with thymolymphopenia
11. Metaphyseal chondrodysplasia – malabsorption, neutropenia
12. Hypophosphatemic familial rickets

III. **Skeletal Dysplasias with Major Involvement of the Spine**
1. Spondyloepiphyseal dysplasia congenita (**Spranger-Wiedemann type**)*
2. Diastrophic dwarfism
3. Metatrophic dwarfism
4. **Kniest's disease**
5. Spondylometaphyseal dysplasia (**Kozlowski type**)
6. Pseudoachondroplasia
7. Parastremmatic dwarfism
8. Spondyloepiphyseal dysplasia tarda
9. **Dyggve-Melchior-Clausen disease**

IV. **Mucopolysaccharidoses and Mucolipidoses**
1. Mucopolysaccharidoses (I-H, I-S, II-IV, VI, VII)*
2. G_{MI} gangliosidosis type I
3. Mucolipidoses I, II, III

V. **Skeletal Dysplasias Due to Anarchic Development of Bone Constituents**
1. Dysplasia epiphysealis hemimelica
2. Multiple cartilaginous exostoses* (osteochondromatosis)
3. Enchondromatosis (= **Ollier's disease**)*
4. Fibrous dysplasia (= **Jaffe-Lichtenstein disease**)*

VI. **Osteolyses**
1. Idiopathic osteolyses

VII. **Skeletal Dysplasias with Predominant Involvement of Single Sites or Segments**
1. Dyschondrosteosis
2. Mesomelic dwarfism (**Nievergelt type, Langer type, Robinow type**)*
3. Ulno-fibular dysplasia (**Rheinhardt-Pfeiffer type**)
4. Tricho-rhino-phalangeal dysplasia (type I, type II)*
5. Pseudohypoparathyroidism
6. **Larsen's syndrome**
7. Oto-palato-digital syndrome
8. Cleidocranial dysplasia*
9. Osteo-onycho-dysostosis
10. Acrocephalosyndactyly, type I

Table 1 (continued)

VIII. **Skeletal Dysplasias with Abnormalities of Bone Density and/or Modeling Defects**

1. Osteogenesis imperfecta (congenital recessive form, dominant form)*
2. Juvenile idiopathic osteoporosis
3. Osteopetrosis (= **Albers-Schönberg disease**)*
4. Dysosteosclerosis
5. Pyknodysostosis
6. Sclerosteosis
7. Osteopoikilosis*
8. Osteopathia striata
9. Melorheostosis*
10. Craniometaphyseal dysplasia
11. Metaphyseal dysplasia (= **Pyle's disease**)
12. Craniodiaphyseal dysplasia
13. Frontometaphyseal dysplasia
14. Oculo-dento-osseous dysplasia
15. Osteoectasia with hyperphosphatasia
16. Endosteal hyperostosis (recessive type)
17. Pachydermoperiostosis
18. Diaphyseal dysplasia
19. Infantile cortical hyperostosis
20. Osteodysplasia
21. Tubular stenosis with periodic hypocalcemia
22. Idiopathic hypercalcemia

* Skeletal dysplasias documented in this chapter.

Those conditions which are described in detail are marked in **Table 1** with an asterisk (*). A few diseases which come under the skeletal dysplasias are found elsewhere in the book (e.g. osteopoikilosis, p. 108; melorheostosis, p. 108; fibrous bone dysplasia, p. 56).

Dysostoses are classified according to their location. Isolated malformations of the skull are all forms of *dyscephalia*. They are due to a primary closure of one or more cranial sutures (premature bony union, active synostosis) or developmental disorders of the brain affecting the shape of the skull (passive synostosis). These include the following malformations of the skull: 1. **Microcephalia** – an abnormal reduction in size, proportionate or disproportionate. 2. **Macrocephalia** – abnormal enlargement of the circumference or volume of the skull (megacephalus in premature infants, hydrocephalus, interstitial megalencephalus due to glial proliferation in the hemispheres). 3. **Turricephalia** – abnormal growth in height of the skull ("tower" or "steeple head", sometimes accompanied by hemolytic anemia). 4. **Scaphocephalia** – abnormal flattening of the parietal bones with premature synostosis of the sagittal suture ("boat skull"). 5. **Scoliocephalia** – asymmetrical skull due to premature synostosis of some of the sutures ("sloping skull"). 6. **Trigonocephalia** – wedge-shaped skull due to premature synostosis of the metopic suture ("triangular skull"). 7. **Hypertelorism** (Greig's syndrome) – inhibitory malformation of the skull base and frontal bone. 8. **Encephalocele** – bony defects of the skull due to incomplete ossification (often combined with brain malformations). Various types

of dyscephalia of the facial bones and neurocranium make up the *craniomandibulofacial dysmorphic syndromes*, which are autosomal dominant hereditary conditions. Several syndromes are recognized which are distinguished by the hypoplasia of particular bones of the face and skull.

Dysostoses of the limbs are known as *dysmelia*. Diplomelia (duplication of a limb) and **diplopodia** (duplication of a hand or foot) are very rare. On the other hand, **polydactylia** (an excess number of fingers or toes) appears more frequently (usually affecting thumb or great toe, little finger or toe). **Amelia** signifies the absence of a complete limb, and **hemimelia** the underdevelopment or absence of one proximal or distal limb segment (forearm, leg or upper arm, thigh). In **phocomelia** ("seal limb" or "flipper limb") the segmental bones (femur, tibia, fibula or humerus, radius, ulna) are absent, and the hands or feet articulate directly with the shoulder or pelvic girdle. These malformations are seen in *thalidomide embryopathy*, a condition due to the ingestion of thalidomide ("Contergan"). **Peromelia** refers to stump-like limbs following a disturbance of growth, and **micromelia** to short limbs due to shortening of the segmental bones. Absence of hands or feet is known as **apodia**, and absence of digital separation due to failure of the bone or soft tissue in hands or feet as **syndactylia**.

Dysostoses of the pelvic and shoulder girdles are very rare, and are usually only found where there are generalized dysplasias. Dysostoses of the ribs and sternum are also not very common. On the other hand, dysostoses of the vertebral column (vertebral hypoplasia, fused vertebrae = block vertebra, excess vertebrae, rhachischisis, spina bifida, spondylolisthesis) represent important lesions encountered in orthopedic practice. All these malformations can be either genetic in origin or have an exogenous etiology.

Arthrogryposis multiplex congenita

This malformation is characterized by numerous symmetrical contractures arising in the uterus. The pathological changes are primarily extraskeletal, involving the soft tissues, and working secondarily on the bones. It is due to a myopathy, with fibrotic contractures of the joint capsule and shortening of the flexor muscles. As can be seen in **Fig. 51**, the child's body is curved dorsally, the head turned to one side and the shoulders internally rotated. The thighs, however, are rotated externally and the arms and legs flexed. The musculature is underdeveloped and the skin is creased. The contraction of the soft tissues has caused deformity of the bones. **Figure 52** shows a femur which has a sharp bend proximally *(1)*, thus causing the limb to be shortened. The width of the shaft *(2)* and the contour of the joint *(3)* are normal. The soft tissue contractures often bring about multiple fractures within the uterus or during delivery.

These contractures have an effect on skeletal development. Within the uterus they prevent

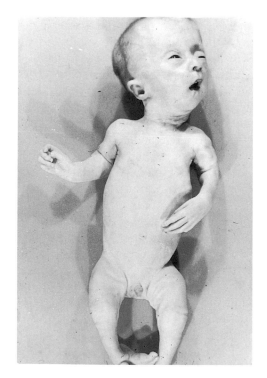

Fig. 51. Arthrogryposis multiplex congenita

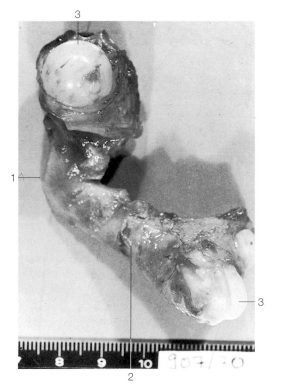

Fig. 52. Arthrogryposis multiplex congenita (femur)

the completion of endochondral ossification. **Figure 53** shows a **histological picture** of the growing regions of the femur. One can see that the height of the columnar cartilage *(1)* is significantly reduced. The zone of proliferating cartilage *(2)* is, however, normally laid down and hyperplastic. In the zone of provisional calcification *(3)*, which is considerably increased in breadth, the numerous wide blood vessels *(4)* are striking, and have invaded the cartilage extensively. Between these the chondroid *(5)* is quantitatively reduced and only minimally calcified. The structural changes in the growing regions indicate a growth disorder of bone which particularly affects the long bones.

In **Fig. 54** the widely dilated capillaries *(1)* shown under **higher magnification** in the zone of provisional calcification and zone of dilatation are striking. The vessels are pushing into the columnar cartilage *(2)* and reducing its volume. The chondroid *(3)* is moderately developed and poorly calcified. The pathogenesis of this growth disorder is still unclear, although possible neuropathic or myopathic etiologies have been discussed. The skeletal growth disturbances are secondary and must be regarded as a result of the soft tissue changes.

Multiple Epiphyseal Dysplasia (Ribbing-Müller Disease)

This is a hereditary autosomal-dominant condition, and is one of the most frequently occurring skeletal dysplasias. Growth is retarded, although the normal bodily proportions are maintained. The joints are stiff and painful, with contractures, and there is often a thoracic kyphosis with back pain. The symptoms usually appear after the second year of life, but sometimes not until early adulthood. There is a milder form **(Ribbing's disease)** in which hands and feet are not affected, and a more serious variety with severe mutilation **(Fairbank's disease)**.

Radiologically there is flattening, especially of the thoracic vertebrae, with irregular upper plates. **Figure 55** shows the leg of a 4-year-old child, in whom the epiphyses of the lower end of the femur *(1)* and upper end of the tibia *(2)* are too small and irregular in shape. The metaphyses *(3)* are also irregularly formed and raised up. The long bones *(4)* are too short, be-

cause of the disturbance of the growth zones, but normal in shape. The ossification centers usually appear late and are irregular and fragmented. The hip joints are also involved and the femoral heads flattened, and there may be dislocation with protrusion of the acetabulum. Similar changes are found in the short tubular bones of the hand. The joint changes lead eventually to premature progressive arthrosis, with severe limitations of movement in later life. This skeletal anomaly is not associated with any other malformations, and life expectation is normal.

Congenital Spondyloepiphyseal Dysplasia (Type: Spranger-Wiedemann)

This skeletal malformation is an inherited autosomal-dominant condition and is accompanied by more or less severe coxa vara, knock knees and/or progressive arthropathy. There is a disproportionate dwarfism with a shortened vertebral column, barrel chest, genu valgum and pigeon chest (pectu corinatum). The face is often flattened and there is a kyphoscoliosis. In 50% of cases there is also myopathy and retinal detachment. In the **radiograph** shown in **Fig. 56** one can see the pelvis and lumbar column of a 5-year-old child with this dysplasia. The vertebral bodies *(1)* are flattened and poorly ossified. There is a marked scoliosis. The pelvis *(2)* is also underdeveloped and poorly ossified. The acetabula *(3)* are unequal and horizontally aligned. Irregularities in the epiphyses and metaphyses of the long bones, particularly in the neighborhood of the hip joints *(4)*, are also apparent. The bony structures appear late (4th–5th year of life). They remain undeveloped and deformed with increasing age, and coxa vara develops. In general, bone development is reduced, particularly of the pelvic and hip bones. Osteoarthritis often appears, especially in the shoulder and hip joints. The locomotor activity in these patients is reduced, but their intelligence is normal. Hypoplasia of the spine of C2, loosening of the ligaments and muscular hypotonia can bring about atlanto-axial dislocation with compression of the cord at the C1-C2 level. The increased fragility of the bone may lead to cord compression appearing as the first clinical symptom.

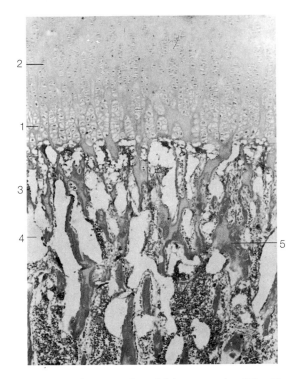

Fig. 53. Arthrogryposis multiplex congenita; HE, ×25

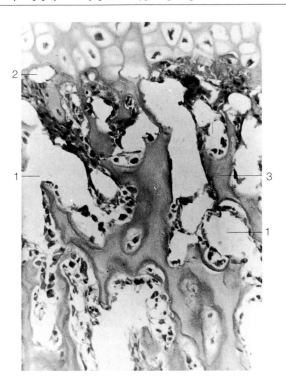

Fig. 54. Arthrogryposis multiplex congenita; HE, ×64

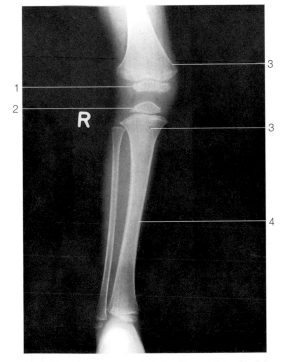

Fig. 55. Multiple epiphyseal dysplasia (tibia, fibula)

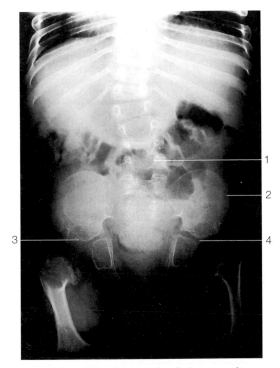

Fig. 56. Spondyloepiphyseal dysplasia congenita (pelvis, lumbar vertebral column)

Thanatophoric Dwarfism

There are a number of varieties of dwarfism which are present at birth and shortly afterwards, and lead to death by respiratory deficiency (short rib/polydactylia syndromes: type I **Saldino-Noonan**, type II **Majewsky**, type III **Neumoff**; achondrogenesis). These include thanatophoric dwarfism, which usually appears sporadically. In addition to the typical skeletal changes there are also cardiac and cerebral abnormalities.

As the **macroscopic photograph** in **Fig. 58** shows, there are, as a result of delayed skeletal maturation, disproportionate dwarfism with a somewhat shortened rump (1) and severe shortening of the limbs (2), which especially affects the proximal parts *(rhizomelic underdevelopment)*. The thorax (3) is severely narrowed and the abdomen is bloated. The head (4) is disproportionately enlarged. The root of the nose (5) is sunken with protrusion of the eyeballs (protrusio bulbi), and there is a so-called clover-leaf cranium with a deep sagittal furrow (6) in the middle of the forehead. This deficiency of growth is responsible for the circular creases in the skin and bulging soft tissues.

In the **radiograph** a large number of anomalies can be recognized. In **Fig. 57** the vertebrae (1) are flattened and have an H-shaped indentation; they show defective ossification. The ribs (2) are shortened and placed horizontally. The pelvic bones (3) are markedly underdeveloped, and the diameter is reduced. The long bones (4) are shortened, curved and relatively wide; they are shaped like telephone receivers and the metaphyses are distended. There is a relatively large skull (5) with small facial bones.

Figure 59 shows a **macroscopic specimen** of a femur from a case of *thanatophoric dwarfism*. This long bone is extremely crooked and of varying density (1). The proximal part (2) has the shape of a telephone receiver. The femoral head (3) is normally developed and covered with smooth articular cartilage.

The **histological picture** of the growing zone shows normal quiescent cartilage. In **Fig. 60**, however, it can be seen that in the layer of columnar cartilage the chondrocytes are not arranged in rows (1). This cartilage is at least reduced. These cells are diffusely dispersed and misshapenly distended. In the calcification zone of the specimen (2) only a few irregular blood

vessels can be seen. Here there are short, widened primary trabeculae (3) that contain a reduced number of osteocytes. In places the primary spongiosa immediately encloses the growth cartilage. The unlayered bone trabeculae are bordered by a few osteoblasts (4). In the marrow cavity there is loose connective tissue (5) infiltrated by round lymphoid cells.

In **Fig. 61** the growth zone is markedly underdeveloped. One can see the growth cartilage (1) with small cartilage cells grouped irregularly together. The cartilaginous layer is partially invaded by wide blood capillaries (2). Below the cartilage there are misshapen, irregularly placed, ungainly bone trabeculae (3) containing central islets of cartilage (4). The marrow cavity is filled with dense lymphoid cells (5).

Two forms of this congenital malformation can be distinguished. **Type I** is the classical form with a large skull cap and a small facial skeleton with a sunken nasal root. The limb bones are very bent and shortened. **Type II** has the so-called cloverleaf skull. The three-lobed skull configuration is due to premature union of the coronal and lambdoid sutures. The cranial fossae are greatly widened, and there is often a hydrocephalus. The limb bones are shortened, but not crooked. In both cases the malformation has a fatal prognosis.

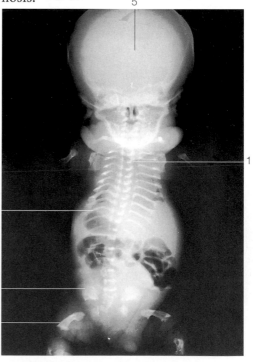

Fig. 57. Thanatophoric dwarfism

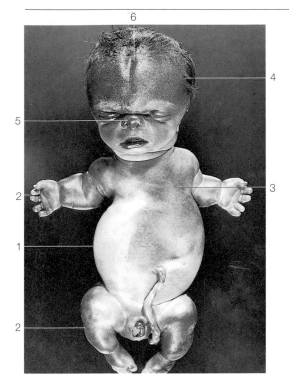

Fig. 58. Thanatophoric dwarfism
(rhizomelic underdevelopment)

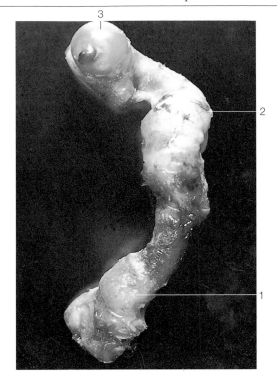

Fig. 59. Thanatophoric dwarfism (Femur)

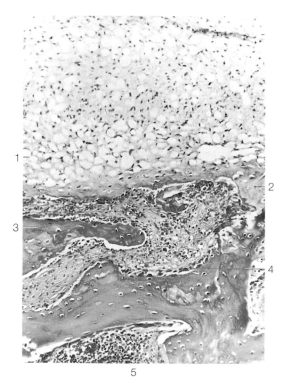

Fig. 60. Thanatophoric dwarfism; HE, ×40

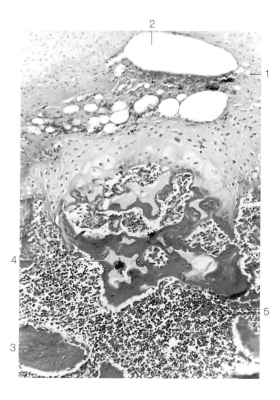

Fig. 61. Thanatophoric dwarfism; HE, ×64

Asphyxiating Thoracic Dysplasia (Jeune's Disease)

The principal finding with this autosomal-recessive skeletal malformation is the congenital narrowing of the chest to the point of respiratory insufficiency. The patients have a deformed thorax and die in early childhood. With the milder forms, however, they may reach adulthood. Then one sees impaired growth with disproportionately shortened limbs. Often there is an additional postaxial polydactylia. In later childhood chronic nephritis develops. These cases develop with dysplastic kidneys and liver changes.

A child with asphyxiating thoracic dysplasia is illustrated in **Fig. 63**. The skull (1) is normally proportioned, and the face (2) is unremarkable. The very narrow thorax (3) with its very short ribs is, however, striking. The internal organs are normally disposed and developed.

In the **radiograph** of **Fig. 62** it can be seen that the thorax is overall narrow. The ribs (1) are markedly shortened and aligned horizontally. The cartilage-bone borders are irregular. These changes regress somewhat in later childhood. The vertebral column develops normally and the vertebrae (2) themselves are normal. Radiologically one can also recognize underdeveloped pelvic bones (ilium, ischium, pubis), disproportionate shortening of the long bones with irregular metaphyses, shortened intermediate and terminal phalanges and frequently polydactylia of the hands and feet.

Macroscopically one can discern growth disturbances at the cartilage-bone borders. In **Fig. 64** these zones can be seen in a rib: the cartilage mass (1) is increased, so that these bones show lumpy swellings somewhat reminiscent of the "rickety rosary". The primary spongiosa of the zone of dilatation (2) is widely deposited and appears dark red. No changes are seen in the mature bone (3).

Histologically, a severe disturbance of endochondral ossification is evident. As can be seen in **Fig. 65**, the proliferation of cartilage is disordered and no longer under control. The maturation zone of columnar and vesicular cartilage is insufficiently developed. The cartilaginous columns (1) are narrowed and rarefied. In the vesicular cartilage one sees irregular foci of proliferation (2), indicating uneven hyperplasia.

This zone is deeply invaded by blood capillaries (3). The hyperplastic cartilage contains both grossly bloated and very small chondrocytes close together (4). The cartilaginous tissue shows degenerative changes and is incompletely calcified. This means reduced ossification of the osteoid. The osteoblasts are somewhat increased. There is also delay in the resorption of cartilage, the chondroclasts and osteoclasts being greatly reduced. At the costochondral junctions there is a very broad band of richly vascularized connective tissue between the hyaline cartilage and the zone of growing cartilage.

Figure 66 shows **histologically** the fully undeveloped zone of growing cartilage (1) with small chondrocytes irregularly distributed. The preparatory calcification zone and zone of dilatation are strongly reduced and are contiguous with an equally rarefied primary spongiosa (2). There are only slight changes in the epiphyseal cartilages of the long bones. Periosteal ossification, on the other hand, is not affected, and here relatively excessive bone deposition can occur. This leads to an incongruity of periosteal and endochondral ossification and to a spur-like structure in the radiograph.

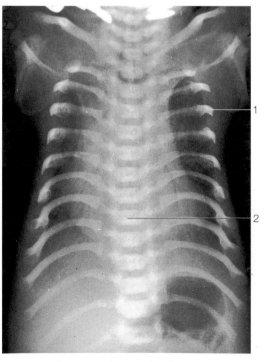

Fig. 62. Asphyxiating thoracic dysplasia (thorax)

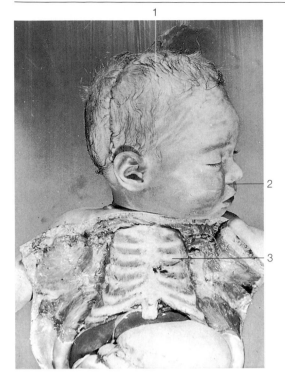

Fig. 63. Asphyxiating thoracic dysplasia

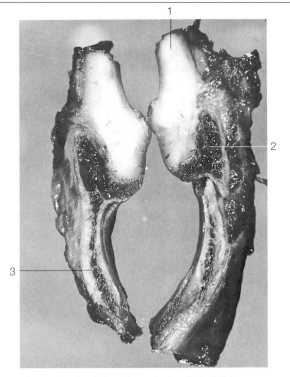

Fig. 64. Asphyxiating thoracic dysplasia (rib)

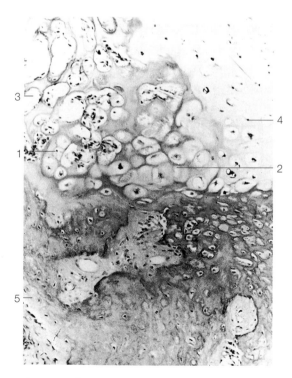

Fig. 65. Asphyxiating thoracic dysplasia; HE, ×64

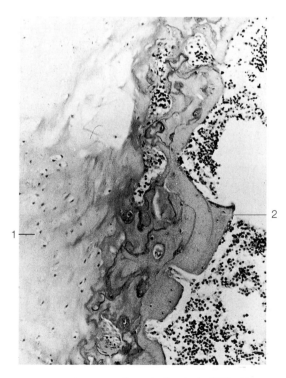

Fig. 66. Asphyxiating thoracic dysplasia; HE, ×82

Chondroectodermal Dysplasia
(Ellis-van Creveld Disease)

This very rare disorder of development, which is inherited as an autosomal-recessive condition, and is characterized by a skeletal dysplasia combined with an ectodermal dysplasia and a congenital cardiac defect. The *ectodermal dysplasia* manifests itself as complete alopecia, dental anomalies (dentitio tarda, absence of canines and lateral incisors, short teeth deficient in dentine) and hypoplasia of the finger and toenails. **Figure 67** shows the hand of such a child. The fingers, and in particular the terminal phalanges *(1)* are shortened and the fingernails *(2)* are underdeveloped. Postaxial polydactylia is also often present.

Radiologically there is a long narrow thorax with short ribs. The heart shadow is pathologically deformed. The vertebral column is unchanged. The long bones (**Fig. 69**) are markedly shortened and appear thickened *(1)*. The metaphyses of the femur *(2)* and tibia *(3)* are greatly widened. The proximal epiphyseal line of the tibia *(4)* runs an oblique course, which sometimes gives rise to a severe genu valgum. The neck of the femur *(5)* is much shortened. Furthermore, the pelvic bones are underdeveloped, with small iliac ala and a hook-shaped and downward protrusion of the acetabula. There are no skull abnormalities.

Macroscopically the most significant skeletal changes involve the meta-epiphyses. In **Fig. 70** one can see a specimen of the femur *(1)* and tibia *(2)* which has been sawn through to show massive cartilaginous development of the epiphyses *(3)* lying like a hooded border over the metaphyses *(4)*. The metaphyses are widened and club-shaped. The epiphyseal lines *(5)* are widened and indistinctly demarcated. They are blotched and fragmented, with an oblique course into the tibia *(6)*.

Under **higher magnification** one can see in **Fig. 68** the broad, fragmented epiphyseal line *(1)* with its fuzzy borders and the hyperplastic cartilaginous epiphysis *(2)*. The bony epiphyseal center *(3)* is underdeveloped and asymmetrical. Whereas ossification at the sides has lagged behind, in the middle it has pushed forward deep into the epiphyseal line *(4)*, thus producing here a three-pronged effect.

Histologically a marked disturbance of the proliferation and maturation of the epiphyseal cartilage can be seen. Whereas in **Fig. 71** the quiescent cartilage *(1)* appears to be normally developed, the large vesicular cells and columns of the maturation zone are underdeveloped and often seem barely viable. There are several nests of enlarged vesicular chondrocytes *(2)*, and here and there a few short cartilage columns *(3)*. The cartilaginous matrix is present in large amounts and is normally calcified. The zone of dilatation is reduced and contains only a few capillaries *(4)*. This leads to reduced resorption of the cartilage, with tongues of cartilaginous tissue *(5)* persisting and reaching far into the metaphysis. At the sides there is a covering of bone tissue *(6)* that has been produced by the rapidly proceeding periosteal ossification. As is shown in **Fig.**

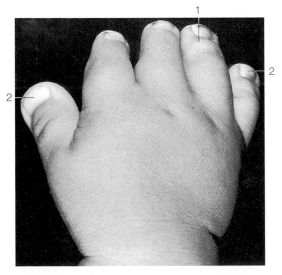

Fig. 67. Chondroectodermal dysplasia (hand)

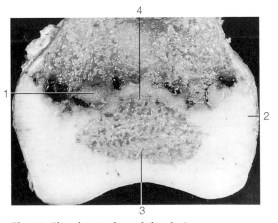

Fig. 68. Chondroectodermal dysplasia (distal femoral epiphysis and epiphyseal plate)

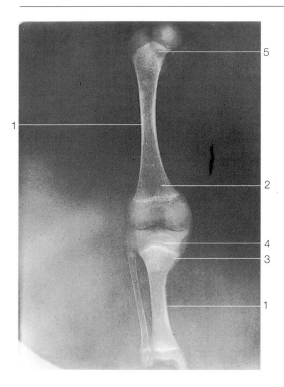

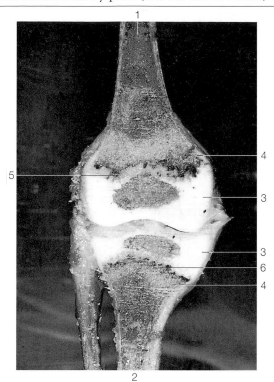

Fig. 69. Chondroectodermal dysplasia (femur, tibia)

Fig. 70. Chondroectodermal dysplasia (distal femur, proximal tibia)

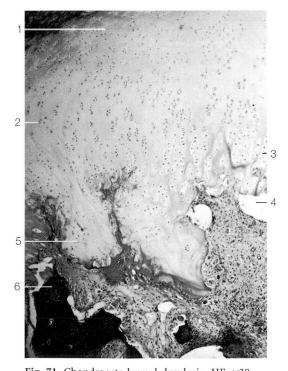

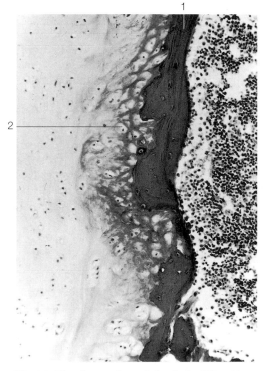

Fig. 71. Chondroectodermal dysplasia; HE, ×30

Fig. 72. Chondroectodermal dysplasia; HE, ×64

72, a wide plate of lamellar bone *(1)* has been pushed out from the periosteum under the carti-laginous growth zone *(2)*, so that no growth in length of the bone can take place. In the lateral region of the epiphyseal line there is in addition a disturbance of the nutrition of the cartilage, with cartilaginous necroses.

Mucopolysaccharidosis Type IV (Morquio's Disease)

Skeletal dysplasias may also be caused by congenital metabolic disorders. The various mucopolysaccharidoses are expressions of lysosomal storage diseases caused by enzymatic defects in the catabolism of the acid mucopolysaccharides (glucosamine glucocane, dermatan sulphate, heparan sulphate). The metabolic products which are not broken down are deposited in the mesenchymal tissues, nervous tissues and internal organs. In Morquio's disease, keratan sulphate is stored in bone tissue, which leads to typical developmental disorders of the skeleton. The disease is inherited as an autosomal-recessive condition. It manifests itself during the first four years of life with dwarfism, shortening and curvature of the vertebral column, pigeon chest, flail joints, dental anomalies and sometimes hepatomegaly.

Figure 73 shows a **radiograph** of the shortened vertebral column with marked platyspondylia of the vertebral bodies *(1)*, which are hookshaped owing to the ventral protrusion of bone. The intervertebral spaces *(2)* are widened. The odontoid process of the axis is frequently hypoplastic. The thorax is widely constructed *(3)* with paddle-shaped ribs. The iliac ala *(4)* are flattened. In the hip joint there are dysplastic changes in the epiphyses of the femoral head *(5)* and hypoplasia of the acetabula *(6)*. In adult life severe arthroses develop. *(Mucopolysaccharidosis I-H, Type Pfaundler-Hurler, p. 58).*

Mesomelic Dwarfism (Robinow's Fetal Face Syndrome)

Among the very rare mesomelic dysplasias that are inherited as autosomal-dominant conditions, **Robinow's Type** is characterized by a peculiar deformity of the face with a protruding forehead and hypertelorism resulting from a disproportionate enlargement of the neurocranium (the so-called "fetal face"). There is a short saddle nose. The extremities are shortened, the external genitals are hypoplastic. **Radiologically** there are incompletely developed thoracic vertebrae and

fusion of the vertebrae and the ribs with premature calcification of the costal cartilages. In **Fig. 74** one can see marked shortening of the radius *(1)* and ulna *(2)*. The bones appear enlarged at one end and narrowed at the other. The head of the radius *(3)* is dislocated. Similar changes are seen to a lesser extent in the leg. The skeletons of the hand and foot show no dysplastic changes. These patients have a normal life expectation.

Tricho-rhino-pharyngeal Dysplasia

This autosomal-dominant inherited condition makes itself apparent in the first year of life by the peculiar face with a wide mouth, pear-shaped nose, prominent philtrum and sparse hair. There is brachydactylia of one or more fingers. The interphalangeal joints are swollen and may show an axial deviation of the fingers distally. The stature is usually small. With *Type II* of this dysplasia (*Langer-Giedion syndrome*) there are also multiple osteocartilaginous exostoses. **Radiologically** the epiphyses of the long bones are underdeveloped and deformed, and there is premature epiphyseal closure. An aseptic bone necrosis (*Perthes's disease,* p. 176) often develops in the hip joint. In **Fig. 75** the epimetaphyses of the short bones of the hand *(1)* are conically enlarged. In this 8-year-old child one can see a few normal epiphyseal lines *(2)*, while others are closed *(3)* and no longer visible. In a few, some unusual dense strips *(4)* can be recognized. Life expectation is normal.

Cleido-cranial Dysplasia

This autosomal-dominant inherited condition consists of a developmental disorder of desmal ossification with inadequate formation of replacement bones. As a result there are skeletal changes in the clavicle and skull (cranium, facial skeleton). **Radiologically** one can see in **Fig. 76** the wide open fontanelles in a 2-year-old child (*1,* anterior fontanelle) and sutures *(2)* due to delayed ossification. Also in the skull base *(3)* disturbances of ossification have occurred. These produce an enlarged head with prominent frontal and parietal bones. Both clavicles *(4)* are only rudimentary formations. These aplasias can also be only parietal or confined to one

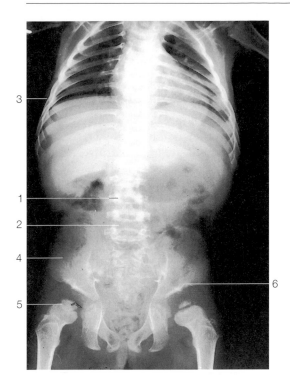

Fig. 73. Mucopolysaccharidosis Type IV
(thorax, lumbar vertebral column)

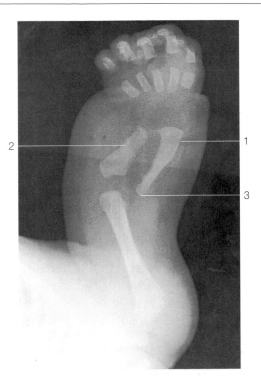

Fig. 74. Mesomelic dwarfism (radius, ulna)

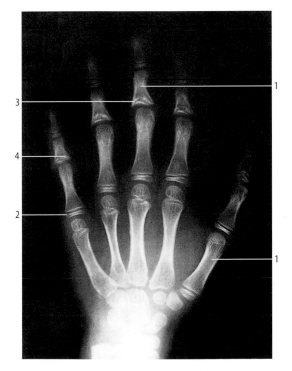

Fig. 75. Tricho-rhino-phalangeal dysplasia (hand)

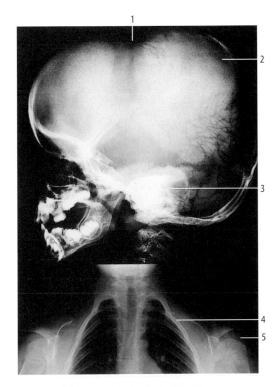

Fig. 76. Cleido-cranial dysplasia (skull)

side, and pseudarthroses can develop between these bones. This malformation also involves the attached muscles, which are inadequately developed. This leads to fallen shoulders. The scapulae *(5)* are small and deformed and loosely anchored. Life expectation is normal.

Achondroplasia (Chondrodystrophia fetalis)

This is a form of disproportionate dwarfism with short limbs (micromelia), the cause of which lies in an underdevelopment of the proliferating cartilage of genetic origin affecting the endochondral ossification. Diagnostically this type of dwarfism is classified in terms of the clinical and radiological findings, histomorphological examination being confined to autopsy material.

In **Fig. 77** a **radiograph** of such a newborn dwarf is shown in two planes. The vertebral bodies *(1)* are strongly flattened, and the intervertebral spaces *(2)* are seen to be much wider than normal. The vertebrae are curved outwards in the dorsal region *(3)*. In such patients there is also marked shortening of the long bones. In the **histological picture** of **Fig. 78** one can see in the zone of endochondral ossification the densely deposited and hypertrophic cartilage cells *(1)*, which are nevertheless not arranged in columns but lie together in groups. The normal long calcified spurs of the cartilaginous matrix which should be reaching out into the bone of the shaft are absent *(2)*. The proliferating cartilaginous tissue runs directly up against fully mineralized bone tissue with mature bone trabeculae *(3)*, thus making further growth in length impossible.

Chondrodystrophy

This skeletal malformation represents a fairly common autosomal-dominant inherited condition, but it also appears as a sporadic disease. *Since the chondroblasts no longer produce any columnar cartilage (Fig. 49), there is a premature cessation of endochondral ossification which results in a reduction in the growth in length of the bones.* Periosteal bone deposition and the laying down of covering bone (membrane bone) are, on the other hand, not affected (Fig. 50). The result is a *chondrodystrophic dwarf* with a completely disproportionate body (short thick limbs with a normally developed stem skeleton). The large head has, because of the growth disturbance of the skull base (replacement bones), the appearance of an "inverted pear".

As the **radiograph** of a chondrodystrophic individual in **Fig. 79** shows, there is a wide, weakly constructed pelvis *(1)*, with square iliac ala. The alignment of the lower border is horizontal. The long bones of the limbs *(2)* are severely shortened, and since the normal periosteal ossification produces a normal growth in width, they are remarkably stumpy. One often sees oval translucent areas at the proximal and distal ends of the long bones *(3)*, particularly the femurs.

The **histologically** demonstrable disorder lies in the region of the columnar cartilage, that is to say, in the epi-metaphyses of the long bones and the costochondral joints. As can be recognized in **Fig. 80**, the proliferation of the cartilage cells is only weakly discernible, and they are small and have small round nuclei *(1)*. The maturation zone is narrowed and the layer of columnar cartilage *(2)* has only 6 to 8 cells in a row instead of the normal 20 or so. The columns are therefore somewhat shortened, and in severe cases they can be completely absent. Calcification of the cartilaginous matrix and osteoid formation are also reduced and may be altogether lacking. At the bone-cartilage border one can see a few swollen chondrocytes *(3)* and hardly any contiguous layer of osteoid has developed *(4)*. The preparatory calcification layer and primary spongiosa are also affected by the disturbance of ossification. In the lower part of the picture one can see the structures of the secondary ossification layer with incompletely calcified bone trabeculae *(5)* and, between them, richly cellular hematopoietic bone marrow *(6)*.

Histological examination of chondrodystrophic bone is practically confined to autopsy material. The skeletal deformities restrict movement, but the intelligence is normal and the life expectation unaffected.

Chondrodysplasia punctata (**rhizomelic type**) is genetically am autosomal-recessive condition with a fatal outcome. In this rare disease, of which the definitive diagnosis is radiological, one sees symmetrical punctiform calcifications in the cartilaginous parts of the skeleton and bipartite vertebral bodies subdivided by a disc of cartilage. The long bones – and in particular the humeri – are short and stumpy, with metaphyseal distensions. The pathological-anatomical diagnosis is confined to autopsy material.

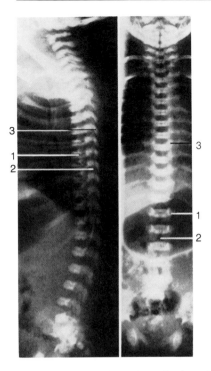

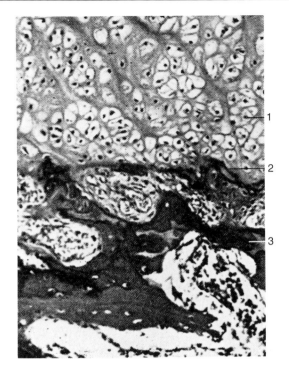

Fig. 77. Achondroplasia (spinal column).
(From SPRANGER et al. 1974)

Fig. 78. Achondroplasia; HE, ×64

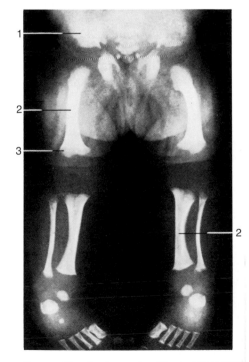

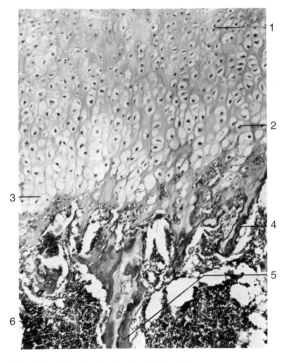

Fig. 79. Chondrodystrophy. (From SPRANGER et al. 1974)

Fig. 80. Chondrodystrophy; HE, ×25

Rickets

Rickets is characterized by defective calcification of the bony tissue in the growing skeleton which leads to a disturbance of endochondral ossification. In the preparatory calcification zone (Fig. 49) a great deal of uncalcified osteoid and cartilaginous tissue is laid down. This results in a disorganization of the whole endochondral ossification process. The cause of this is usually a *vitamin D deficiency* (hypovitaminosis) or a failure of the renal tubules to function properly (*vitamin D resistant rickets:* phosphate diabetes, Debré-de-Toni-Fanconi syndrome), disturbances of intestinal resorption or **hypophosphatasia**. Nowadays we seldom see rickets due to vitamin deficiency. On the other hand, cases of renal rickets are more frequent.

Figure 81 shows a **radiograph** of the right forearm of a 10-month-old child with active rickets. The ends of the ulna and radius show cup-like distensions *(1)*, particularly distally. The preparatory calcification zone is fuzzy, the pattern of the spongiosa is also unclear and shows reduced calcium density *(2)*. This so-called double growth in the wrist joint is known as *Marfan's sign* of rickets.

As can be seen in the **radiograph** of **Fig. 82**, the so-called *"bell-shaped thorax"* of rickets is found, together with Harrison's groove and the rickety rosary. Because of the reduced calcification the rib bones *(1)* are more translucent and their ossification centers *(2)* are distended. The **radiograph** in **Fig. 83** is a lateral view of the vertebral column of a 1-year-old child with active rickets. The parts of the vertebral bodies are indistinct and their outer contours fuzzy *(1)*. The vertebrae are somewhat flattened and the intervertebral spaces enlarged. There is an indistinct osteoporotic loosening of the vertebral spongiosa with the suggestion of three horizontal layers (the so-called *"rugger-jersey spine"*) *(2)*. The whole vertebral column is equally affected and noticeably stretched out. Since the bones are soft and flexible, curvatures of the column such as scoliosis and lumbar lordosis develop.

In **Fig. 84** the costochondral joint of a rib is shown in a **low-power histological section**. It is widened and distended (rickety rosary, *1*). Above this region *(2)* there is normal cartilage, and below it normal cancellous bone *(3)*. With-

in the widened ossification zone the layer of columnar cartilage has become lengthened *(4)* and poorly vascularized. The maturation of the proliferating cartilage (enlarged vesicular cartilage) is delayed, and it is inadequately resorbed by the myeloid capillaries. There is no typical preparatory calcification zone. Instead of this, it is immediately contiguous with a zone of chondro-osteoid *(5)*, which corresponds to the primary spongiosa. Here the penetrating myeloid vessels spread out in different directions and planes, instead of running in canaliculi parallel to the long axis of the shaft. In this way the chondrocytes are resorbed, and excessive osteoid irregularly deposited by the action of osteoblasts. This is not followed by calcification of the osteoid or cartilaginous matrix.

Under the **higher magnification** of **Fig. 85**, one can see between the penetrating myeloid vessels *(1)* in the primary spongiosa irregular tongues of cartilaginous tissue *(2)* and wide osteoid trabeculae *(3)*, which are not mineralized but are bordered by osteoblasts. Above that there is the zone of columnar cartilage *(4)*, the cartilaginous matrix of which is also not mineralized. In this "rachitic intermediate zone" a disorganized cartilage-bone tissue (chondro-osteoid) is laid down which is unstable and flexible and permits deformation of the bone. Not only endochondral but also perichondral and membranous ossification are disordered.

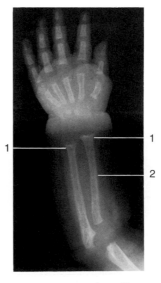

Fig. 81. Active rickets (forearm: Marfan's sign)

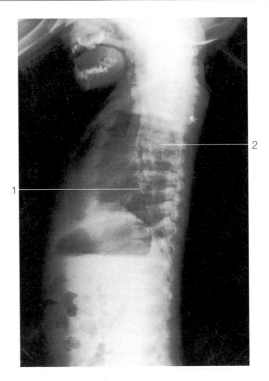

Fig. 82. Active rickets (thorax: rickety rosary)

Fig. 83. Active rickets
(vertebral column: rugger-jersey spine)

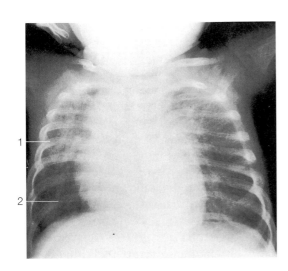

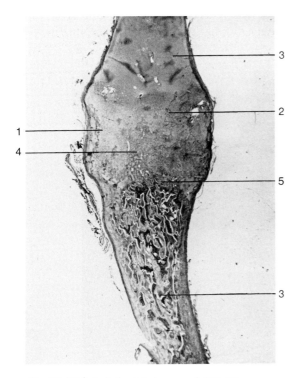

Fig. 84. Rickets (rib: rickety rosary) HE; ×5

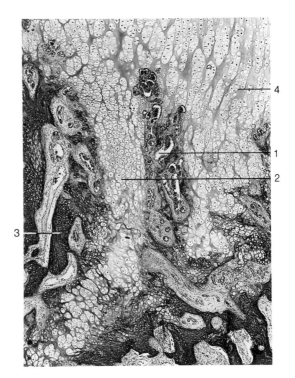

Fig. 85. Rickets; HE, ×50

Hypophosphatasia

This is a congenital disorder of bone formation and mineralization due to a reduced production and activation of alkaline phosphatase. The disease is genetically transmitted by an autosomal-recessive gene. In very rare cases it may lead to dominant inheritance and hypophosphatasia in the adult. The defect apparently lies in the osteoblasts, which produce alkaline phosphatase, and which may often be reduced in number or fail to form a functionally effective enzyme. Most neonatal cases of hypophosphatasia are already apparent by the 6th month of life and can sometimes be diagnosed in the uterus. Clinically the serum alkaline phosphatase is reduced and rachitic changes are present in the skeleton.

As is shown in the **radiograph** of a child who died 22 hours after birth (**Fig. 86**), the entire skeleton is incompletely developed. The long bones, such as the femur *(1)* and humerus *(2)* are shortened and only mineralized in the shaft. The mineralization is irregular, and one can see patchy translucent areas *(3)* in the bones. The femurs are curved *(4)*. The epiphyses *(5)* are lengthened and widened, and consist of increased but unmineralized osteoid. The cup-shaped widened and frayed metaphyseal endplates *(6)* are striking. The vertebral bodies *(7)* are only weakly developed. On the other hand the clavicles *(8)* are only poorly mineralized, but are fully developed (desmal ossification). **Figure 87** shows a **radiograph** of the forearm in a case of neonatal hypophosphatasia. One can see the widened growth zones *(1)* with cloudy shadowing of the increased and uncalcified osteoid. The metaphyseal plates of the radius *(2)* and ulna *(3)* are cup-shaped and widened and appear frayed. The absence of complete ossification of the epiphyseal lines is reflected in the tongue-shaped processes at the ends of the bones. Only a short proximal part of the ulna *(3)* is weakly mineralized. The short tubular bones of the hand *(4)* are very much underdeveloped, and some phalanges are not mineralized at all.

Figure 88 is a **macroscopic** illustration of the surface of a section through the growth region of the femur in a case of hypophosphatasia. In the epiphysis *(1)* one can clearly recognize a center of ossification *(2)*. The spongiosa of the metaphysis *(3)* is only poorly mineralized and most of the trabeculae consist of calcium-free

osteoid. The borders of the cartilaginous epiphyseal line *(4)* are undulating, with occasional tongue-like processes.

As can be recognized in **Fig. 89**, the **histological** appearance of the region of endochondral ossification is similar to that seen in rickets. The layer of columnar cartilage *(1)* has become lengthened and shows few blood vessels *(2)*, and the chondrocytes are distended. A zone of chondro-osteoid *(3)* lies up against the maturation zone.

In the **low-power histological picture** shown in **Fig. 90**, one can see the strongly developed and regularly formed layer of the growth cartilage *(1)*, where the layer of columnar cartilage *(2)* is widened. It is contiguous with a very broad layer of disorganized and uncalcified osteoid *(3)*, into which tongue-like processes *(4)* extend from the growth cartilage. Hardly any osteoblasts are present. In severe cases the child dies shortly after birth, in less serious cases it can reach later childhood or even adulthood. In this case delayed growth of the skeleton and cranial synostoses are to be expected. The urine of these patients contains phosphoethanolamine, and there is a hypercalcemia which can cause renal damage. Sometimes treatment with cortisone may alleviate the condition.

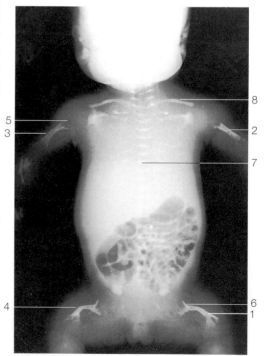

Fig. 86. Radiograph of a child with hypophosphatasia

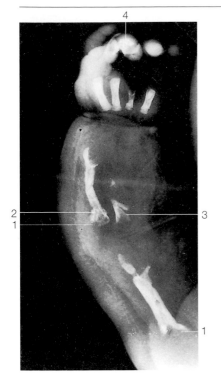

Fig. 87. Forearm in a case of hypophosphatasia

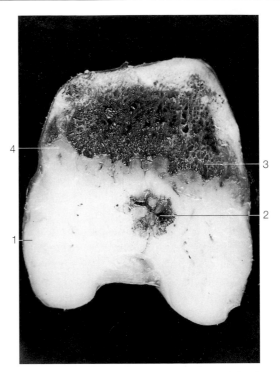

Fig. 88. Hypophosphatasia (growth region of the femur)

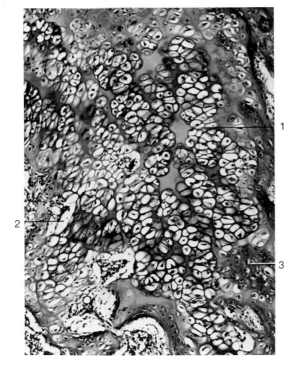

Fig. 89. Hypophosphatasia; HE, ×25

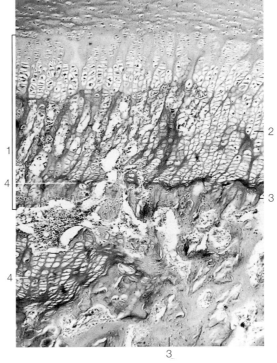

Fig. 90. Hypophosphatasia (overview); HE, ×5

Osteopetrosis (Albers-Schönberg Disease, Marble Bone Disease)

Osteopetrosis is an inherited disease of the skeleton which is accompanied by an increase in calcified bone tissue – namely osteosclerosis. Macroscopically the bones are heavy and inelastic, so that pathological fractures occur easily. The marrow cavity is almost completely filled with compact bone tissue and the cortex is thickened by periosteal bone deposition. Radiologically the bones are accordingly seen as complete shadows. These changes have led to the descriptive name *marble bone disease.* The pathogenesis is explained by an *insufficiency of osteoclasts,* whereby bone resorption, which plays an important role in endochondral ossification, is inadequate. Owing to the deficiency in osteoclasts, the primary spongiosa cannot be resorbed and a sufficient marrow cavity cannot develop. The primary spongiosa is not transformed into a secondary spongiosa. In newborn and young children the zone of proliferating cartilage in the regions of endochondral ossification is abnormally wide. The bars of calcified bone matrix cannot be resorbed, and these persist. Foci of calcified cartilaginous matrix are therefore found in the intramedullary bone tissue and even in the shafts of the long bones. Throughout the whole bone a lattice-work of calcified cartilaginous matrix remains behind, and in this metaplastic primitive bone tissue develops. Osteoclasts are only seldom found under the microscope, and the number of osteoblasts is also greatly reduced. However, the abnormal bone tissue does not arise because of increased osteoblast activity, but as a result of bone metaplasia in the cartilaginous matrix.

In **Fig. 91** one can see a **radiograph** of the lumbar column from a case of osteopetrosis. Typical findings include the dense sclerotic delimitation of the upper and lower plates of the vertebral bodies *(1)*, which frequently have a linear double outline *(2)*. In such cases one speaks of the so-called *"sandwich vertebra"*.

In the **histological picture** of **Fig. 92** one can recognize the close-meshed lattice-work of calcified cartilaginous bars *(1)* within the narrowed marrow cavity, in which irregular osteoid *(2)* has been deposited. Cartilage inclusions are to be found within the trabeculae. The absence of osteoclasts and osteoblasts is

striking. Because of this the levels of alkaline phosphatase, calcium and phosphorus in the serum lie within the region of normality.

Osteogenesis imperfecta

This is the result of a general defect of the mesenchyme which leads to a faulty synthesis of collagen and inhibits bone production. *Osteogenesis imperfecta is an inherited disease of the skeleton which is characterized by serious fragility of the bones.* Because of its underlying cause, this fragility is accompanied by excessive mobility of the joints, light blue sclerotics, otosclerosis, dental anomalies and a parchment-like thinning of the skin. Because of its genetic heterogeneity, the variable clinical picture and differing prognoses have been classified under the following types.

Type I: Blue sclerotics, dentinogenesis imperfecta, normal bone. Begins between 1st and 10th years of life. Autosomal-dominant inheritance. Mild course.

Type II: Multiple (intrauterine) fractures, deformed long bones, blue scleras. Begins at birth. Autosomal-recessive inheritance. Fatal outcome.

Type III: Reduced growth, thin bones, multiple (intrauterine) fractures. Begins at birth. Autosomal-recessive inheritance. Adverse course.

Type IV: Thin bones, moderate number of fractures, blue scleras. Commencement and course variable.

In the **radiograph** of the leg shown in **Fig. 93** one can see the extremely slender long bones of the tibia *(1)* and fibula *(2)*, in which the spongiosa *(3)* is highly osteoporotic and radiotranslucent, and the shadow of the cortex *(4)* almost reduced to a thread. As against this, the epiphyses *(5)* appear distended like a cudgel, but are of normal width.

In **Fig. 94** one can see **histologically** that, in the region of endochondral ossification, the layers of chondroblastic proliferation *(1)* are normal as far as the cartilage columns. In the preparatory ossification zone one observes fewer osteoblasts and osteoclasts than normal. Osteoid formation around the calcium spurs of the cartilage is greatly reduced. In the primary spongiosa we find only a dense network of bars

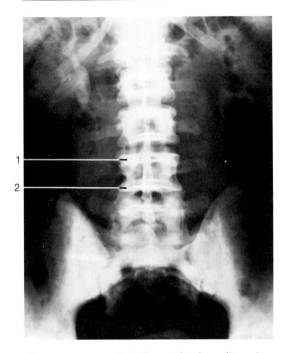

Fig. 91. Osteopetrosis (Albers-Schönberg disease); (lumbar vertebral column)

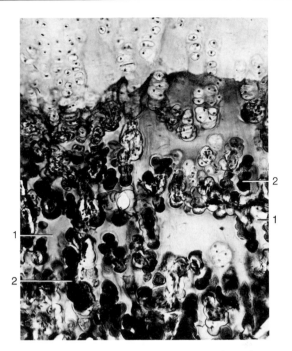

Fig. 92. Osteopetrosis (Albers-Schönberg disease); HE, ×113

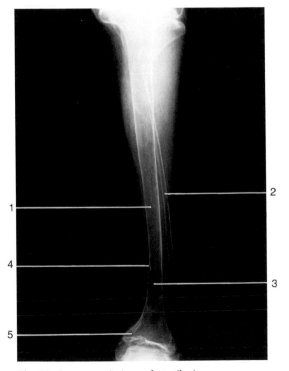

Fig. 93. Osteogenesis imperfecta (leg)

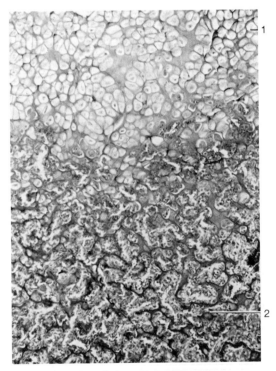

Fig. 94. Osteogenesis imperfecta; HE, ×25

of cartilaginous matrix *(2)*. For this reason the primary and secondary spongiosa cannot be fully developed, and this results in the picture of a high grade osteoporosis with a strong tendency to develop fractures.

Fibrous Bone Dysplasia (Jaffe-Lichtenstein)

One result of a local developmental disorder of the skeleton can simply be the differentiation of connective tissue instead of bone. *In cases of fibrous bone dysplasia the bone marrow is replaced by fibrous marrow with fibrous bone trabeculae, without any lamellar bone being laid down locally.* This common bone lesion is counted among the "tumor-like bone diseases" and is described in detail on p. 318.

In **Fig. 95** one sees a **radiograph** of a monostotic fibrous dysplasia with a focus in the 9th right rib. This change represents the most frequent tumorous lesion of the ribs. One can recognize a local distension of a limited region of the bone *(1)*, which is obviously cystic in appearance. The cortex bulges forward and is narrowed from within, but it is still intact.

Figure 96 shows a saw-cut through the resected rib. **Macroscopically** there is a central bony cyst with smooth walls. It is multiloculated and filled with a serous fluid. This portion of bone is greatly distended and covered outside with periosteum. Such lesions seldom show much increase in size after puberty.

In **Fig. 97** one can see a **radiograph** of polyostotic fibrous dysplasia which has involved almost the whole of the tibia. The bone is generally widened and distended *(1)*. Inside there is a "frosted glass" or "watch-glass" cloudy shadowing *(2)*. The cortex is narrowed from within *(3)* but still preserved. The lesion is not cystic and has no sharp border. It is often progressive after puberty.

The **histological picture** is characterized by connective tissue which is rich in fibers and relatively poor in cells, and in which numerous slender fibrous bone trabeculae have differentiated. In **Fig. 98** one can see that these trabeculae *(1)* are horseshoe-shaped and bound together in a kind of network. The collagen fiber-rich connective tissue *(2)* passes directly over into the bony structures, without any osteoblasts being present.

This is shown under **higher magnification** in **Fig. 99**. One can see that the fibrous bone has arisen directly from the fibrous stroma. In **Fig. 100** the indiscriminate irregularly disposed birefringent fibers within the immature trabeculae can be seen under polarized light *(1)*. The lamellar structures are absent. These immature bony structures with no osteoblast deposits are, together with the convoluted character of the connective tissue stroma, characteristic of fibrous bone dysplasia.

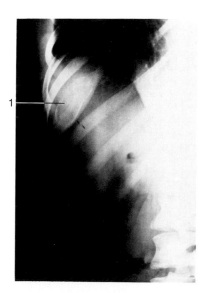

Fig. 95. Monostotic fibrous bone dysplasia (Jaffe-Lichtenstein) (9th right rib)

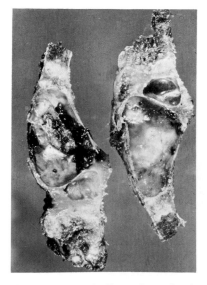

Fig. 96. Monostotic fibrous bone dysplasia (Jaffe-Lichtenstein) (saw-cut through resected rib)

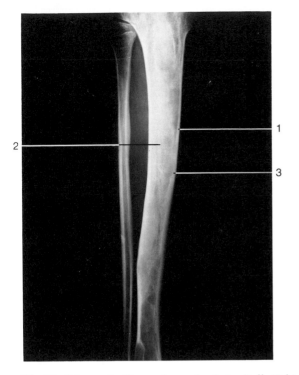

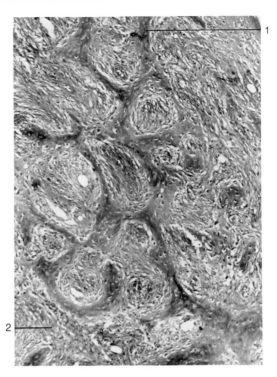

Fig. 97. Polyostotic fibrous bone dysplasia (Jaffe-Lichtenstein) (tibia)

Fig. 98. Fibrous bone dysplasia (Jaffe-Lichtenstein); HE, ×25

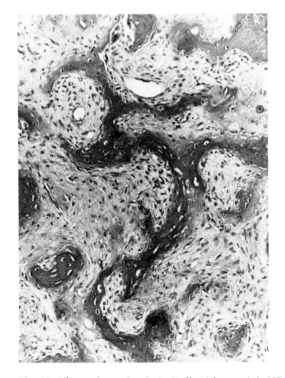

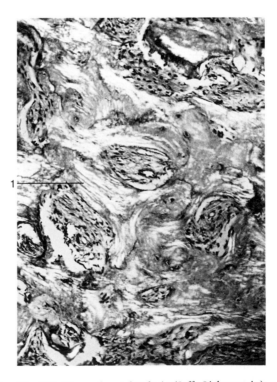

Fig. 99. Fibrous bone dysplasia (Jaffe-Lichtenstein); HE, ×40

Fig. 100. Fibrous bone dysplasia (Jaffe-Lichtenstein); polarized light, ×30

Arachnodactylia

This not particularly rare skeletal abnormality is often seen in cases of *Marfan's syndrome*, although it can be absent from this latter condition. *It is inherited as an autosomal-dominant condition, in which the long and short bones each grow to an excessive length.* This results in the so-called *"spider fingers"* and an asthenic bodily habitus with remarkably long limbs. Pigeon chest, a *"Gothic arch palate"* and a deformed vertebral column with scoliosis are included in Marfan's syndrome. Congenital subluxation of the lens can lead to *iridodonesis*. The scleras are blue and there are sometimes congenital cardiac abnormalities. The principal finding is the *Erdheim-Gsell idiopathic median necrosis,* with the appearance of vascular aneurysms, particularly in the aorta.

Experimental investigations have shown that β-aminoproprionitril can produce similar changes in the skeleton, which are known as *osteolathyrism.* In this case there is a disturbance of collagen matrix synthesis, leading to inhibition of bone deposition. Acid mucopolysaccharides are laid down in the collagen matrix, which can be histochemically identified by Alcian blue staining.

The diagnosis of arachnodactylia depends on the clinical and radiological findings. Histomorphological examination of a bone biopsy during life is not indicated and is exclusively confined to autopsy material.

As can be seen in the **radiograph** of the foot in **Fig. 101**, the extraordinarily long and slender short bones of the toes *(1)* and metatarsals *(2)* are striking. The spongiosa at the ends of the bones is somewhat loosened and straggly *(3)*. Otherwise there are no demonstrable skeletal alterations. **Histologically** too, normally developed bone is apparent *(1,* **Fig. 102**), and only a slight osteoporosis can be established. In the region of endochondral ossification the individual layers of cartilage are normally arranged *(2)*, although with Alcian blue staining the deposition of acid mucopolysaccharides *(3)* near the joint surface can be seen. The cartilage cells are normal in size and have small round nuclei. They are often shrunken.

Pfaundler-Hurler Dysostosis

This developmental disorder of the skeleton, which is also known as *gargoylism,* is due to a disturbance of metabolism. *There is a general disorder of endochondral ossification as the result of a genetically determined mucopolysaccharidosis, by which the enzymatic breakdown of acid mucopolysaccharides is impaired.* The disturbance of endochondral and periosteal ossification results in a shortened skull base, saddle nose, a widened face with a dull expression, a poorly formed body and lumbar kyphosis. There is also hepatosplenomegaly, corneal opacity and idiocy.

The diagnosis of this congenital condition depends on the outward appearance, the clinical signs and the radiological findings. Biopsy material from the liver, spleen and bone marrow contains large cells with mucopolysaccharide inclusions. Histomorphological examination of the skeleton is, however, mostly confined to autopsy material.

Figure 103 shows the **radiograph** of the hand of a child with Pfaundler-Hurler disease. The stumpy configuration of the tubular bones *(1)* and the sharply pointed proximal ends of the metacarpals *(2)* are typical. In places the density of spongiosa is increased *(3)* or shows irregular radiotranslucent areas *(4)*.

Histologically there is a narrowing of the bone trabeculae in the ossification centers of the epiphyses and metaphyses of the long bones, which is the result of reduced bone deposition. As can be seen in **Fig. 104**, within a cartilaginous layer including inconspicuous chondrocytes *(1)* there is a focus of swollen cartilage cells with pale cytoplasm and small nuclei *(2)*. These cells contain large quantities of mucopolysaccharides.

The signs of this so-called *"dysostosis multiplex"* progress greatly with increasing age and show themselves radiologically in various different bones. The skull is abnormally large, the frontal bone prominent and the back of the head flattened. The skull base and orbital roofs are sclerotically thickened. The vertebral bodies undergo a wedge-shaped deformation ("fish-hook vertebra"). In the region of the chest the clavicles and scapulae are shortened and stumpy, and we find so-called "paddle-ribs".

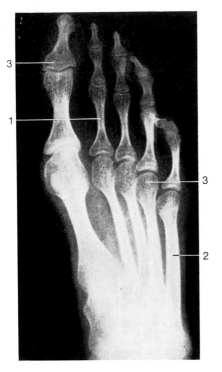

Fig. 101. Arachnodactylia (foot)

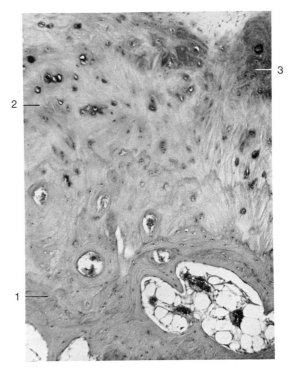

Fig. 102. Arachnodactylia; HE, ×25

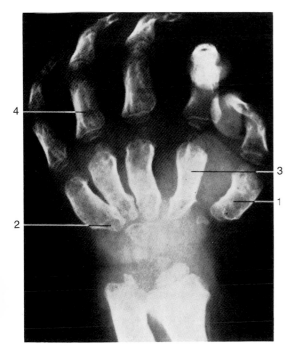

Fig. 103. Pfaunder-Hurler disease (hand)

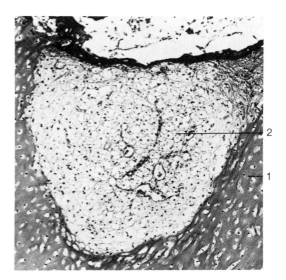

Fig. 104. Pfaunder-Hurler disease; HE, ×64

Enchondromatosis (Ollier's Disease)

Developmental disorders of the skeleton can also include tumor-like or even tumorous changes which are the result of a disturbance of normal endochondral ossification. *Enchondromatosis is an non-inheritable disorder of skeletal development in which multiple enchondromas can arise simultaneously in the metaphyses and diaphyses of several different bones.* This so-called *"Ollier's disease"* is usually confined to one side of the skeleton. As an expression of the disturbed ossification enchondromatosis is often combined with a fibrous bone dysplasia (p. 56). In the so-called *Maffucci syndrome* these dyschondroplasias appear together with hemangiomas of the soft tissues. Here also it has not been possible to establish an inheritable factor. Sometimes multiple enchondromas appear with generalized irregular lesions of the vertebrae, without the short tubular bones being affected. In about 50% of cases of enchondromatosis the development of a chondrosarcoma is to be expected.

Enchondromatosis leads to serious deformities of bones and of the whole skeleton (asymmetrical leg shortening, swellings of the hands and feet, pathological fractures) which require surgical corrective measures. The tumors arise in those bones which develop by the process of endochondral ossification, and therefore the bones of the face and skull are not affected. The tumors usually appear between the 2nd and 10th years of life and enlarge sporadically until puberty. No new enchondromas are to be expected after puberty.

Both radiologically and histologically, multiple enchondromas are seen which cannot be distinguished morphologically from the solitary form (p. 218). In the **radiograph** shown in **Fig. 105**, central regions of intraosseous osteolysis and tumorous swelling can be seen in the affected bones of the first three fingers of one hand [thumb *(1)*, index and middle fingers *(2)*], whereby the cortex is greatly narrowed and sometimes bulges forwards *(3)*, although it remains intact. No periosteal reaction can be seen. Also in the 2nd metacarpal bone one can see a large bulge *(4)*. Inside such a region of

bone there are irregular patchy and straggly dense areas *(5)*, and in between there are fine focal translucencies which are often cystic *(6)*. The adjacent joint contours *(7)* are faded or completely abolished. It is only when several such bone lesions can be demonstrated radiologically that a diagnosis of Ollier's disease is justified.

The **radiograph** of **Fig. 106** is the frontal view of two widened enchondromas in the distal part of the femur *(1)* and proximal part of the tibia *(2)*. The foci lie centrally in the long bones. They are relatively sharply limited, but without any recognizable marginal sclerosis. Within the foci there are numerous stain-like dense regions next to patchy translucent areas *(3)*. The cortex is completely intact and there is no periosteal reaction. **Fig. 107** shows enchondromatosis in a 2-year-old child. In the **radiograph** of the right leg one can see considerable curvature of the femur *(1)*, the proximal bony structures of which have become dense *(2)*. The distal part of the femur *(3)* shows a cup-like distension and a straggly appearance with longitudinal translucent areas *(4)*. Although in this case there are no dense circumscribed intraosseous foci that might suggest an intraosseous tumorous growth, such a bone deformation is characteristic of enchondromatosis.

The **histological** picture of an enchondroma is also typical in such cases. In **Fig. 108** one can recognize intraosseously deposited tumorous cartilaginous tissue, lobular in structure *(1)*, the lobes (or nodes) being separated by narrow connective-tissue septa. Within this region there are cartilage cells of different sizes *(2)*, most of which contain small isomorphic nuclei. Many focal calcium deposits may be present. Histologically it is very important to note the isomorphic character of the cartilage cells and their nuclei precisely, in order to be able to exclude a chondrosarcoma. As soon as such a focus increases in size, a bone biopsy is essential to decide whether or not a malignant transformation has taken place. From the point of view of treatment, all the tumorous cartilaginous tissue should in every case be carefully curetted surgically, since progressive growth is known to occur.

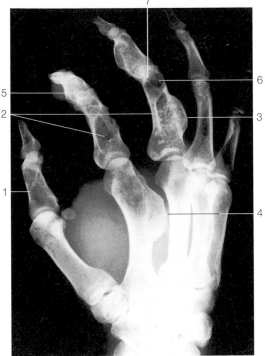

Fig. 105. Enchondromatosis (hand)

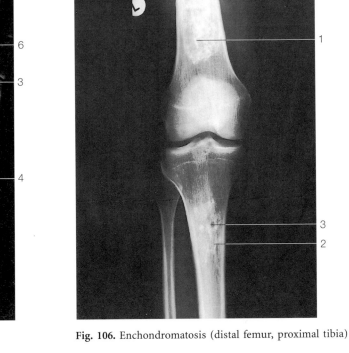

Fig. 106. Enchondromatosis (distal femur, proximal tibia)

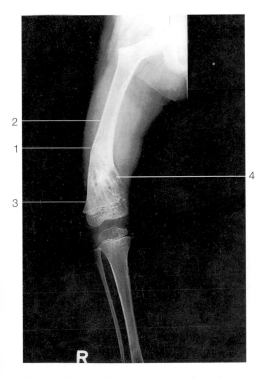

Fig. 107. Enchondromatosis (right femur)

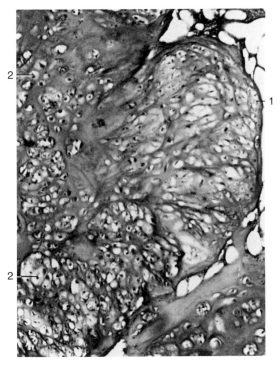

Fig. 108. Enchondromatosis; HE, ×25

Osteochondromatosis

Disordered skeletal development can also result in *multiple osteocartilaginous exostoses. This variety of exostosis is an inherited familial disease, in which multiple osteochromas arise, particularly in the region of the shoulder, knee and knuckles.* In about 10% of cases a chondrosarcoma develops in one of these tumorous bone lesions. It is this essential difference which distinguishes the disease clinically from the harmless solitary osteochondroma (p. 214).

Radiologically it is impossible to distinguish one of these exostoses appearing in a case of osteochromatosis from a solitary osteochondroma (see Fig. 292). In **Fig. 109** one can see several such exostoses in the distal part of the femur *(1)*. They are attached by broad bases to the bone, the spongiosa of the femoral bone being continuous with that of the exostosis, although sometimes there is a narrow sclerotic band between them *(3)*. At the end of the lesion the exostosis may be pushed up like a mushroom *(4)*; inside the bone the translucency and straggly increases in density give it a sponge-like appearance. One can easily see that this osteochondroma has been fractured *(5)*, although callus is not visible.

Figure 110 shows a **radiograph** of both legs of an 18-year-old patient with osteochromatosis. The long bones of the tibia and fibula appear shortened, and the fibulae especially are markedly thickened, otherwise the shaft seems normal *(1)*. In the region of the metaphysis one can see several osteochondromas. The largest exostosis is attached by a broad base to the proximal right tibial metaphysis *(2)*. It shows clear nodular formation and the border is lobulated. Within, there are flat wide areas of densification, and between them patchy translucent regions. This massive osteochondroma reaches deep into the soft tissues and showed a tendency to proliferate, so that it was chiseled away. A thorough histological examination is necessary here in order to exclude or confirm malignancy. A very much smaller osteochondroma has developed at the proximal left fibular metaphysis *(3)*. This is attached by a wide stem to the bone and is distended. One can see patchy calcification of the outer cartilaginous cap. At the lower two distal metaphyses large exostoses (*4* on the left, *5* on the right) can also

be seen. These are pictured in their long axes and are characterized by the band-like sclerosis of their stems.

Histologically it is the cartilaginous cap above all that must be very thoroughly examined in order to exclude a chondrosarcoma. As shown in **Fig. 111**, a highly cellular cartilaginous tissue may be present with the chondrocytes arranged in rows *(1)* or in groups *(2)*. They are distended and mostly have small pyknotic nuclei *(3)*. Binucleate cells may also be present *(4)*. No mitoses or polymorphic cells are visible. The cartilaginous cap is covered on the outside with periosteal connective tissue *(5)*, while below it, fingers of cartilage reach into the bone tissue *(6)*, which is here more highly vascularized. In osteochromatosis the osteochondromas often appear in the iliac ala, and there is a tendency towards a symmetrical occurrence. Because of the possible danger of one of the many exostoses undergoing malignant change, the patient should be put in the picture and kept under observation. Sudden increase in size, pain following any kind of trauma or a slow increase in size after puberty should awaken suspicion of malignant change and indicate the need for histological examination.

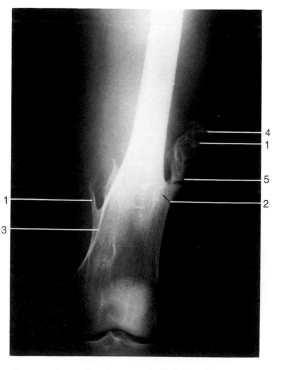

Fig. 109. Osteochondromatosis (left distal femur)

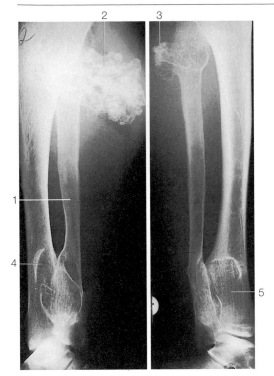

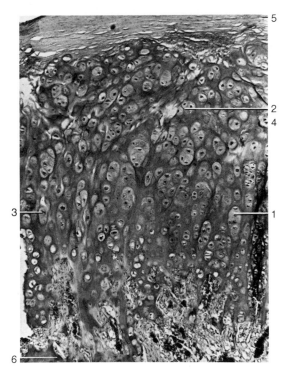

Fig. 110. Osteochondromatosis (both tibiae und fibulae)

Fig. 111. Osteochondromatosis; HE, ×16

With solitary or multiple osteochondromas, a biopsy to arrive at a histological diagnosis is of course not the correct procedure, it should rather be radiologically confirmed and any suspicious exostoses removed immediately if there are any local symptoms or evidence of a tendency to grow. At the same time all the cartilage (cartilaginous caps) must without fail be removed with them in order to prevent a recurrence. This material must then be histologically examined in order to exclude malignant change. In this connection serious diagnostic problems may arise, since the tumorous cartilage cells often show very few signs of malignancy.

4 Osteoporoses and Osteopathies

General

Osteoporosis is an atrophy of bone tissue in which the cortex is narrowed, the number and thickness of the trabeculae in the spongiosa are reduced, and the proportion of bone substance to marrow cavity is altered in favor of the latter. Because of the reduction of calcified bone substance, there is radiologically an increase in the translucency and porosity of the bone structure. Osteodensitometry, which measures the mineralization of the bone, shows that this parameter is also reduced. In radiological practice such findings very often lead to a diagnosis of "osteoporosis", meaning that the bone is less resistant to mechanical stress and that the risk of a fracture is correspondingly greater. One should, however, be aware that very different diseases of quite different etiology are covered by the term "osteoporosis", and that these require different forms of treatment. In other words, "osteoporosis" is a blanket term for various atrophic bone diseases. It is the task of the diagnosing physician – usually a radiologist or pathologist – to distinguish between these individual manifestations of bone atrophy on the basis of the particular morphological structure and other diagnostic findings.

The simple loss of mineralized bone tissue, in which no particular resorptive cellular activity is present, is a basic form of **osteoporosis** presenting in the guise of a straightforward bone atrophy. Here one can distinguish between **generalized osteoporoses**, which involve all or a large part of the skeleton (involutional osteoporosis. p. 72), and **localized osteoporoses**, which are confined to a particular part of the skeleton (immobilization osteoporosis, p. 74; Sudeck's atrophy, p. 96). Osteoporosis can have various causes. In most cases it is constitutional and appears late in life (senile osteoporosis). However, bone atrophy may be due to a substrate deficiency (starvation osteoporosis, vitamin C deficiency osteoporosis), hormonal insufficiency ("postmenopausal" osteoporosis, presenile osteoporo-

sis), inactivity (immobilization osteoporosis, p. 72), disease of the bone marrow (multiple myeloma, bone lymphoma) or reduced osteogenesis (juvenile osteoporosis, "fish vertebra disease", osteogenesis imperfecta, p. 54). In all these forms of osteoporosis a simple histological examination of the bone allows no conclusions to be drawn about the origin, since an identical microstructure is found in various types of osteoporoses, and a correct classification is only possible after taking the clinical and radiological data into account as well.

The precise classification of a case of osteoporosis in terms of its many possible causal and formal varieties of pathogenesis is difficult. On the one hand, reduced functional stimulation (reduced loading of the whole or a part of the skeleton) can lead to a consequent resorption of bone. On the other hand, alterations in the metabolism may have the same generalized or local effect. Finally, neurological disorders or an alteration in the blood supply can bring about bone resorption and thus lead to osteoporosis. Several factors working together may account for the appearance of the condition. When they are due to alterations in the bone metabolism, one can classify osteoporoses as *metabolic osteopathies*.

The term *osteopathy* includes all systemic diseases of bone, irrespective of their etiology and pathogenesis. We distinguish between *toxic osteopathies* (e.g. fluorosis, p. 100), *circulatory osteopathies* (e.g. bone necroses, p. 164; bone infarcts, p. 174), *infectious osteopathies* (e.g. osteomyelitis, p. 129), *neoplastic osteopathies* (e.g. medullary plasmocytoma, p. 348; bone metastases, p. 396) and metabolic osteopathies.

All these bone diseases are characterized by a general or local bone remodeling, which is reflected in the radiograph as a reduction ("osteoporosis") or increase ("osteosclerosis") in the bone material. Both bone-remodeling processes can occur simultaneously and side by side, thereby producing a patchy appearance on the radiograph.

To the *metabolic osteopathies* belong, in particular, generalized skeletal changes that have arisen because of a disturbance of the metabolism. It is known that the skeleton is a central organ for calcium metabolism, since it is a reservoir for the life-supporting serum calcium. The serum calcium level is one of the most strictly controlled and stabilized biological constants. If the serum calcium level (**normally 10 mg%**) falls below **9 mg%,** calcium is mobilized from the skeleton by a complicated regulatory mechanism and transferred to the blood. This naturally produces changes in the bone tissue which are radiologically recognized by the reduction in the density of the shadow. The cause of this radiological "translucency" of the bone structure is the characteristic bone remodeling. Calcium metabolism and bone remodeling are closely correlated with each other. This remodeling is controlled hormonally by the parathyroid hormone (parathormone), which both activates the osteoclasts in the bone and stimulates calcium and phosphate excretion by the kidneys. Parathyroid hormone increases the lifetime of the osteoclasts and their number, and also causes proliferation of fibroblasts. An increased secretion of the parathyroid glands activates a corresponding increase of remodeling in the skeleton, with a reduction in the amount of bone material. The picture of *"osteodystrophia fibrosa generalisata cystica" of von Recklinghausen* arises, with its characteristic structures, indicating the presence of *primary hyperparathyroidism*. The progressive bone resorption can cause local subliminal fractures to develop, in the region of which resorptive giant cell granulomas – the so-called *"brown tumors"* – can appear. Chronic renal insufficiency often leads to a **renal osteopathy.** This is a matter of bone changes resulting from *secondary hyperparathyroidism* and a disorder of vitamin D synthesis, which is structurally characterized by osteodystrophia fibrosa, osteomalacia (p. 86) and osteoporosis.

In addition to the parathyroid hormone (parathormone), other hormones can also have effects on the skeleton, most of which are expressed as an "osteoporosis". Of particular importance here is the influence of the steroids. With the increased release or long-term administration of corticoids there is a danger of the so-called *"Cushing's osteoporosis"* (p. 76) developing. Serious changes in the skeleton, together with fractures, can also arise in cases of diabetes mellitus. Furthermore, the thyroid hormones bring about a direct stimulation of bone resorption which can lead to "osteoporosis". Osteoporoses have been described in both *hyperthyroidism* and *hypothyroidism*. Increased activity of the growth hormone causes acromegaly, but can also bring about severe reduction of the bone mass and thus lead to "osteoporosis". All osteoporoses which arise as a result of an altered hormonal stimulation can be grouped under the description, **endocrine osteopathies.** To these belongs also the action of insufficient *sex hormones* (postmenopausal osteoporosis). Whereas the endocrine osteopathies have their structural origin in a disturbance of the bone modeling cells (osteoblasts, osteoclasts), disturbances in the production of the bone matrix can also lead to "osteoporosis". In particular, a general calcium deficiency, whether due to insufficient intake (dietary) or resorption, impairs the full mineralization of the organic bone matrix and leads to *rickets* (p. 50) in the growing skeleton and *osteomalacia* in the adult (p. 86).

A morphological diagnosis of the various forms of osteoporosis which allows conclusions to be drawn about the underlying condition is made possible by a *biopsy taken from the iliac crest*. In addition, clinico-chemical changes in the blood serum and urine are supportive. In the **schematic diagram** shown in **Fig. 112,** these changes are summarized. Radiological findings can also provide additional information.

Osteoporosis is not recognizable radiologically until at least 30% of the bone mass has been resorbed, but with osteodensitometry it can be diagnosed considerably earlier and also quantified. It is the most frequent bone change encountered in the skeletons of adults. The underlying cause is a negative balance of bone remodeling resulting from progressive resorption together with reduced deposition. The function of the osteoclasts is reduced. The reduction in the tissue is not associated with any change in the quality of the bone. The balance of bone remodeling is positive up to the 20th year, remains in equilibrium until the age of 50 and is thereafter negative. In advanced age one may expect the appearance of a so-called *involutional osteoporosis* (p. 72), which may be re-

	Blood serum		Alkaline phosphatase	Urine		Disease
	Ca^{++}	HPO_4^{--}		Ca^{++}	HPO_4^{--}	
Normal 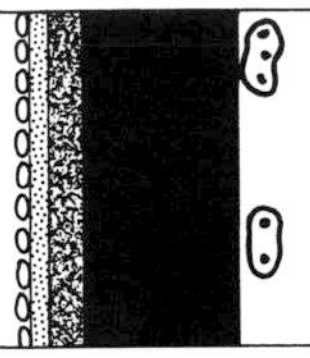	N	N	N	N	N	
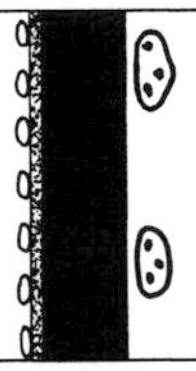 Osteoporosis	N	N	N	N	N	senile osteoporosis (Involutional osteoporosis)
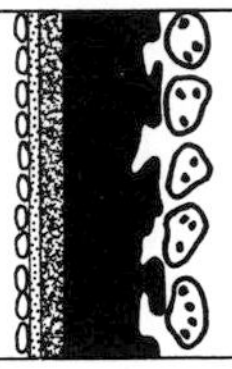 Osteodystrophy	↑	↓	↑	↑	↑	Primary hyperparathyroidism a) with skeletal involvement
	↑	↓	N	↑	↑	b) without skeletal involvement
	↑	↑	↑	↑↓	↑↓	c) with renal insufficiency
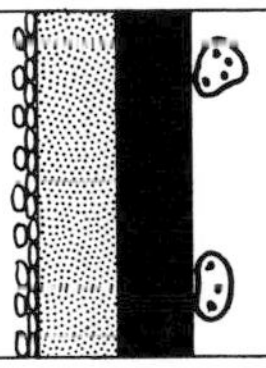 Osteomalacia	↓N	↑N↓	↑	↓N↑	↑	Osteomalacia
	↓(N)	↑	↑(N)	↓↑	↓↑	Renal osteopathy (secondary hyperparathyroidism)
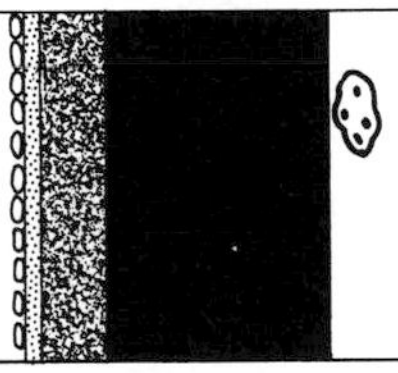 Osteosclerosis	↓	↑	N	↓	↓	Hypoparathyroidism
	N	N	↑	N	N	Paget´s osteitis deformans

■ = Older mineralized bone tissue
▓ = Newly formed bone tissue
░ = Uncalcified osteoid

= Osteoclasts
OO = Osteoblasts

N = Normal
↑ = Increased
↓ = Decreased

Fig. 112. Summary of the morphological and clinico-chemical changes found in various osteopathies

garded as physiological. Because of the frequency of these disorders of bone function and the possibility of a specific treatment, an understanding of osteoporosis is of tremendous importance for all physicians. Untreated osteoporosis leads to serious skeletal deformities, bone fractures and very severe pain with limitation of movement.

The reduction of bone tissue by osteoporosis begins on the side of the marrow cavity and extends outwards to the cortex, which is why we speak of *eccentric bone atrophy*. The breakdown of the bone structure begins in those bones which are normally subjected to much remodeling, namely, the vertebrae, ribs and also the pelvis. In the skull cap, where remodeling is slight, osteoporosis does not occur. Osteoporosis at first proceeds so that the ability of the skeleton to withstand loading is retained, and it is always the so-called "safety structures" which are sacrificed first, while the trabeculae along the tension and pressure lines are for a time still maintained. For this reason, the parts of the skeleton which make up its main framework are tremendously pronounced in the radiograph. The progressive course of osteoporosis can be very clearly followed in the vertebral bodies.

As an example, the **structural changes in the spongiosa** of a vertebral body are illustrated diagrammatically in **Figs. 113 a–d**. The corresponding **radiological changes** are placed alongside in **Figs. 114 a–d**. Whereas the structure of the framework of the spongiosa in a normal vertebral body is regular (**Fig. 113 a**) and radiologically shows a fine cancellous mesh (**Fig. 114 a**), with *grade 1 osteoporosis* the first translucencies in the bone structure appear in the center of the body (**Fig. 114 b**). First of all the transverse spongiosa (safety system) is sacrificed. The atrophy begins in the center of the bone and broadens out towards the periphery (**Fig. 113 a–d**). With *grade 2 osteoporosis* more transverse trabeculae have vanished, and even the vertical ones in the center are lost (**Fig. 113 c**). This is reflected radiologically as a further central translucency (**Fig. 114 c**). *Grade 3 osteoporosis* reveals itself by an extensive atrophy involving the tension and pressure structures (**Fig. 113 d**). Since the loss of the transverse spongiosa is much more marked than that of the supporting variety, which against a

background of so-called *hypertrophic bone atrophy* can even undergo compensatory thickening, the vertical structures of the spongiosa may show up in the **radiograph** very clearly (**Fig. 114 d**). With high grade osteoporosis even the cortex is also drawn into the atrophic process and becomes narrower. The Haversian canals in the cortex are widened, but still have smooth borders.

Figure 115 is a transverse section through a maceration specimen of a **normal vertebra**. It shows a fine cancellous network that is regularly distributed throughout the body. In such a normal vertebral body the supporting structures (vertical trabeculae) are more pronounced than the safety structures (horizontal trabeculae). As can be seen in the maceration specimen of a vertebral body shown in **Fig. 116**, the spongiosa has been greatly changed and irregularly remodeled by **advanced osteoporosis**. One recognizes the very irregular gaps in the spongiosa *(1)* where the trabeculae are absent. The supporting spongiosa *(2)* is considerably thickened by what is known as *hypertrophic bone atrophy*. Only remnants of the transverse spongiosa *(3)* remain, and the resistance of such a vertebra to pressure loading is considerably reduced.

Advanced osteoporosis of the vertebral column reduces its stability and gradually leads to a coalescence of the vertebral bodies or even to a compression fracture of single vertebrae. The skeleton becomes insufficient and breaks down. The form of vertebral compression, which can also be seen radiologically, is determined by the nature of the force applied. In the *thoracic column*, which shows a slight physiological kyphosis, the pressure forces from the upper parts of the body (head, pectoral girdle) are concentrated on the anterior part of the vertebral bodies. With advanced osteoporosis of the bodies of the thoracic vertebrae, this part is compressed and thus produces the so-called **wedge vertebra**. This change usually affects the 8th, 9th and 10th thoracic vertebrae. In most cases it involves a very slow coalescence of the ventral part of the vertebral body so that a wedge-shaped deformity slowly develops. Usually several neighboring vertebrae are affected. In rare cases a strong pressure loading can result in a sudden ventral compression fracture.

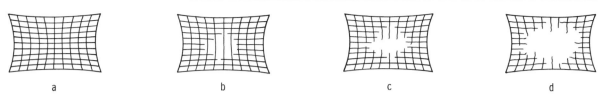

Fig. 113. **a** Diagram of normal vertebral spongiosa; **b** Diagram of grade I osteoporosis; **c** Diagram of grade II osteoporosis; **d** Diagram of grade III osteoporosis

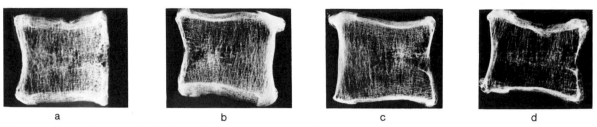

Fig. 114. **a** Normal vertebral body; **b** Grade I osteoporosis; **c** Grade II osteoporosis; **d** Grade III osteoporosis

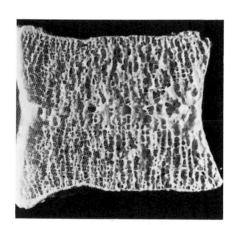

Fig. 115. Normal vertebral spongiosa
(maceration specimen)

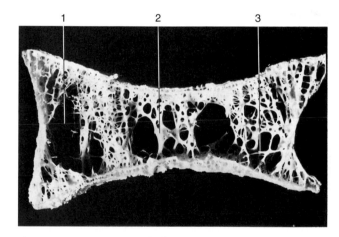

Fig. 116. Osteoporotic vertebral spongiosa
(maceration specimen)

Figure 118 is a lateral **radiograph** of an osteoporotic vertebral column in which the spongiosa of the vertebral bodies is highly porous *(1)*, so that the framework (cortex) is emphasized, as if drawn in with a pencil *(2)*. In the thoracic column there are three **wedge vertebrae** *(3)* which are strongly compressed, particularly in the ventral region. This has resulted in a more or less serious hump or kyphosis.

In the lumbar region the pressure due to the weight of the upper part of the body is fairly equalized over each entire vertebral body, the whole system having been compressed because of the advanced osteoporosis. This produces widening of the intervertebral discs (due to water uptake) and the upper plates of the vertebrae sink in. In **Fig. 119** one can observe these appearances very clearly in the **radiograph**. The lateral view shows a lumbar vertebra *(1)* which is deformed into a so-called **fish vertebra**. The upper plate *(2)* is sunken in and concave, producing a severe narrowing of the central part of the body. Here the spongiosa appears highly translucent because of bone atrophy *(3)*, although the outer framework *(4)* has been preserved and is sharply defined. The intervertebral bodies are greatly swollen and appear to be pressing into the vertebral bodies. Owing to the turgor of the nucleus pulposus the discs are widened and, if the upper vertebral plates break, they can herniate into the bone. These changes are known as *Schmorl's nodes* (p. 438).

With osteoporosis the systemic bone resorption is clearly seen in the *neck of the femur*. In **Fig. 120** one can see the cut surface of a **maceration specimen** of a normal neck of femur with a thick cancellous network in which both the supporting and safety trabeculae are fully developed. Radiologically the scaffolding is homogeneous.

In cases of osteoporosis, however, this scaffolding is irregularly porous, as can be clearly recognized in the **radiograph**. In **Fig. 117** one can see wide gaps in the femoral neck *(1)* and in the greater trochanter *(2)*. The supporting trabeculae *(3)* are strongly brought out. The macromorphological equivalent is also obvious in the **maceration specimen** of a femoral neck shown in **Fig. 121**. Here resorption of the safety structures has produced large gaps in the spongiosa of the greater trochanter *(1)* and in the

lateral triangle of the neck: *Ward's triangle (2)*. The supporting spongiosa is still preserved and clear *(3)*. When the resistance to loading is no longer sufficient a fracture of the neck will finally occur.

A fracture is the principal threat in cases of osteoporosis. It can either develop slowly (as in with coalescence of osteoporotic vertebral bodies) or take place suddenly (as with a medial fracture of the femoral neck). The physiologically more heavily loaded bones (vertebral column, femoral neck) are especially at risk, and these are bones in which osteoporosis is particularly common. Such an atrophy can, however, also arise in other stressed bones in which stability against the action of forces is more or less reduced. When marked osteoporosis arises in the humerus or tibia there is a risk that a *pathological fracture* may occur without any apparently adequate trauma. With serious reduction of the resistance of the bone tissue a so-called *creeping fracture* may develop which, particularly in the vertebral column, presents as pain.

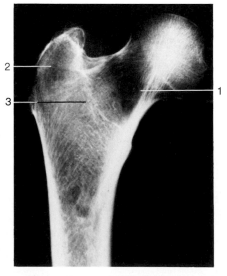

Fig. 117. Osteoporosis of the femoral neck

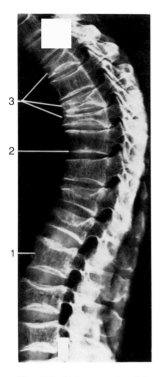

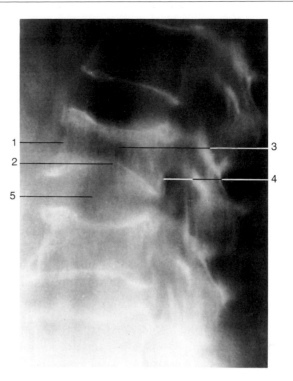

Fig. 118. Osteoporosis of the thoracic column (lateral radiograph)

Fig. 119. Osteoporosis of the lumbar column with "fish vertebra"

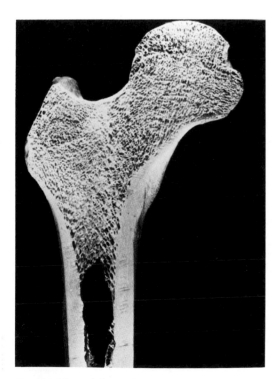

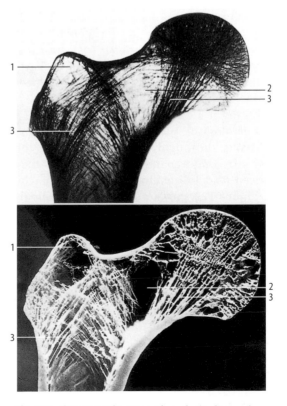

Fig. 120. Normal femoral neck (maceration specimen)

Fig. 121. Osteoporotic Femoral neck (radiograph, maceration specimen)

Involutional Osteoporosis

Involutional osteoporosis plays an important part in clinical practice, since it is very common, causes pain and limitation of movement and can greatly limit the ability to work. *Involutional osteoporosis is a very common generalized skeletal change which, because of the atrophy of the bone tissue, reduces the resistance of the skeleton to loading and carries the risk of pathological fractures.* We distinguish between **senile osteoporosis**, which slowly develops progressively in old age and is generally symptomless, from a postmenopausal or **presenile osteoporosis**, which appears particularly about 10 years after the menopause and usually involves the stem skeleton. It is accompanied by back pain, deformity of the vertebral column and fractured ribs. The cause of senile osteoporosis lies in a reduction in osteoblastic function, which in its advanced stage mostly attacks the ribs, femoral neck, ankle and wrist bones. Presenile osteoporosis results from estrogen deficiency and leads to rapidly progressive bone resorption in the vertebral column, thoracic cage and pelvis. The bones of the limbs and cranium usually remain unaffected. It must be emphasized that not every ageing person must necessarily develop involutional osteoporosis, and constitutional factors are here decisive. Only when this type of osteoporosis produces symptoms (pain, reduced mobility etc.) is it worth calling it a disease.

The **histological picture** of involutional osteoporosis is thoroughly "awkward", since the changes are only quantitative, although they can indeed lead to qualitative alterations in the tissue. **Figure 122** shows a **low-power histological section** through an osteoporotic vertebral body. Cranially and caudally one can see the contiguous discs *(1)*. The trabeculae *(2)* are greatly reduced in number, and those that remain are much narrowed. The cortex of the plates *(3)* and of the sides *(4)* is also narrowed, but remains intact. The proportion of calcified bone substance to bone-free marrow cavity is altered in favor of the latter. With regard to the total volume of bone the mineral content is reduced, as can be confirmed quantitatively by osteodensitometry. The reduction of the bone tissue begins in the middle of the vertebral body and extends outwards (so-called *eccentric bone atrophy*). It is always the "safety structures" (transverse spongiosa) which are first sacrificed, whereas the trabeculae along the tension and pressure lines (longitudinal spongiosa) remain for a time unaffected. The reduction of the bone tissue in involutional osteoporosis does not involve any change in its quality, that is to say, the remaining tissue is fully mineralized and functional. The risk of fracture depends entirely on the quantity of reduced stable bone material.

The histological diagnosis of involutional osteoporosis in a bone biopsy is made exclusively on the quantitative evaluation of the relationship between an enlarged marrow cavity and the bone material of the spongiosa, and on the narrowing of the trabeculae. The Haversian canals in the cortex are wider.

Under **higher magnification** one can see in **Fig. 123** the rarefied and greatly narrowed trabeculae *(1)*, which are nevertheless well mineralized. They are arranged in lamellae and the osteocytes *(2)* are intact. The outer contour is smooth and shows no signs of resorption lacunae. Osteoclasts cannot be seen, and the osteoblasts are sparse *(3)* and poorly developed. This loss of bone is to be attributed to a so-called *smooth bone resorption* (in contrast to the lacunar resorption by multinucleate osteoclasts in osteodystrophy. See Fig. 148). As a result of the decline in osteoblast activity in normal bone resorption there is a reduction in the amount of bone tissue. This negative remodeling is reflected by the relatively enlarged marrow cavity (with fatty marrow, *4*). As can be seen in **Fig. 124**, in osteoporosis one also encounters reparative and compensatory remodeling processes, in which the remaining bone trabeculae of the supporting spongiosa are thickened by deposition. Next to very narrow osteoporotic trabeculae *(1)* one can see the sclerotically thickened trabeculae of the supporting spongiosa *(2)*. This is the picture of so-called **hypertrophic bone atrophy**, which can also be seen in the radiograph.

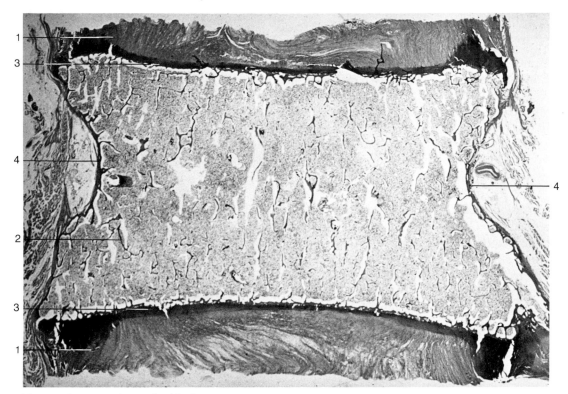

Fig. 122. Osteoporotic vertebral body; HE, ×10

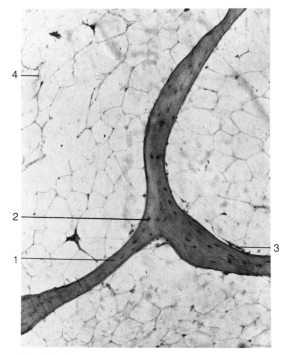

Fig. 123. Osteoporosis; HE, ×25

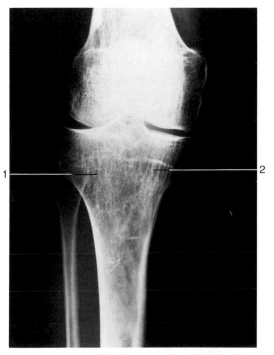

Fig. 124. Hypertrophic bone atrophy (tibial head)

Immobilization Osteoporosis

This variety of osteoporosis arises when a part of the skeleton is inadequately loaded for a prolonged period of time. *It is a localized osteoporosis that develops after resting a limb as the result of a fracture, inflammation or muscular paralysis.* In the early stages there is hyperemia of the osseous capillaries and sinusoids. The activity of the osteoblasts is doubled and that of the osteoclasts increased threefold. This results in a strongly progressive remodeling of bone (osteoclastic osteoporosis) that can produce a hypercalcinuria of up to 335 mg in 24 h. In the chronic stage the bone apposition and resorption processes become stabilized and the negative calcium balance is once again returned to equilibrium.

The *development of an immobilization osteoporosis* is represented diagrammatically in **Fig. 125**. With immobilization one finds morphologically that the spongiosa of the involved bone is reduced, beginning with a central atrophy which then proceeds outwards. It is always the safety structures (transverse spongiosa) which first disappear, whereas the supporting structures (longitudinal spongiosa) remain for a time unaffected. If normal mobilization of the limb is soon restored, a complete return of the original bony pattern is possible, and even though the trabeculae are narrowed their function as conducting structures is maintained. If, however, the immobilization persists and the osteoporosis progresses, there is a more or less serious loss of both transverse and longitudinal spongiosa, and after remobilization the bony scaffolding is only incompletely restored. Since the conducting structures have been lost, new bone tissue can only be laid down on those remaining trabeculae that are orientated along tension and pressure lines. This results in a bony scaffolding with fewer but thicker trabeculae. Such a type of remodeling is known as **hypertrophic bone atrophy.** This can be regarded as a form of defective healing, since the remodeled bone is less well able to withstand the forces which act upon it. In the case of immobilization osteoporosis there is no complete osteolysis. The bone resorption can neverthe-less progress so far that only the framework remains – a condition known as *bone cachexia.* Then even moderate loading can produce fractures. Mechanical overloading together with immobilization osteoporosis can lead to a completely disorganized type of bone remodeling in which the resorption reduces the bone to isolated fragments. The structure is such that it resembles Paget's osteitis deformans (p. 102) both histologically and radiologically, and is called Lièvre's *"remaniement pagétoide post-traumatique".*

Immobilization osteoporosis is normally diagnosed, and its severity analyzed, radiologically. No bone biopsy is required. The histological picture of this type of osteoporosis can nevertheless be studied by the pathological and histological examination of amputation material. A localized remaniement pagétoide can give the impression of a bone tumor, and this is an indication for histological examination.

Figure 126 shows the **histological picture** of an *immobilization osteoporosis* that cannot be distinguished from involutional osteoporosis (p. 72). One can recognize the greatly narrowed bone trabeculae *(1)* that show lamellation and contain small osteocytes. They have smooth borders, and no osteoblastic or osteoclastic activity can be seen. The enlarged marrow cavity *(2)* is filled with fatty tissue.

In **Fig. 127** the **histological appearance** of *remaniement pagétoide* is depicted. The bone trabeculae *(1)* are quite irregularly enlarged and show many drawn out undulating reversal lines *(2)*. There are layers of osteoblasts *(3)* and osteoclasts *(4)* and the bizarre bone tissue is unequally mineralized *(5)*. The marrow cavity is filled up with highly cellular loose granulation tissue *(6)*, which contains wide blood capillaries *(7)*. This shows a very considerable similarity to Paget's osteitis deformans (Fig. 188). Precise distinction between these two structurally similar bone diseases can be of importance when writing medical reports. In order to make a distinction, not only the history, but also the age of the patient, the histological structure and the radiological findings must be taken into account.

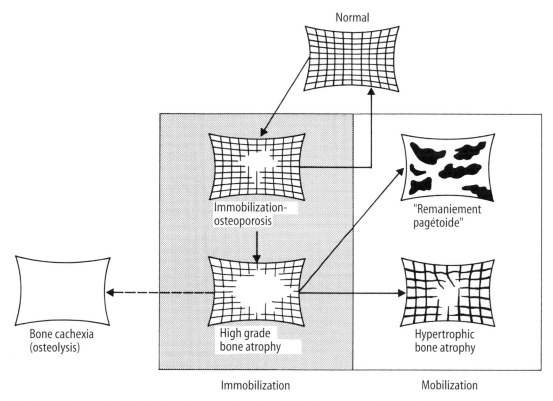

Fig. 125. Diagram showing the development of an immobilization osteoporosis. (After WILLERT)

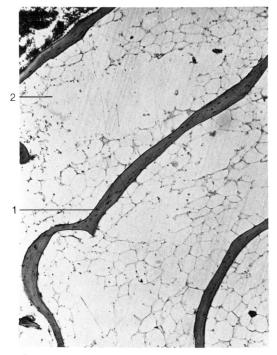

Fig. 126. Immobilization osteoporosis; HE, ×16

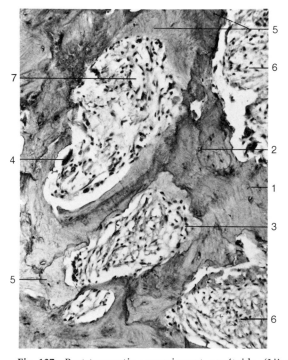

Fig. 127. Post-traumatic remaniement pagétoide (Lièvre); HE, ×40

Cushing's Osteoporosis

Cushing's osteoporosis belongs to the group of **endocrine osteopathies** *and arises endogenously following increased corticosteroid production (Cushing's syndrome with bilateral hyperplasia of the adrenal cortex or an adrenocortical tumor), or exogenously as a result of long term steroid therapy.* Under the influence of glucocorticoid there is an increased transformation of protein into carbohydrate and a decrease in protein anabolism. The protein available is therefore insufficient for osteoid production, and bone resorption predominates over bone deposition. At first there is a burst of osteoclastic activity with massive destruction of bone, which is then followed by reduced bone deposition. As we can recognize in **Fig. 128**, Cushing's osteoporosis *(steroid osteoporosis, adrenocortical osteoporosis)* is mostly concentrated in the stem skeleton, leading to spontaneous fractures of vertebrae and ribs that heal with hyperplastic building up of callus. After treatment of the endocrine disorder (e.g. Cushing's syndrome), complete restitution of the bone structure is possible in young people. In older people, however, hypertrophic atrophy of the cancellous scaffolding remains.

Figure 129 shows a **radiograph** of the vertebral column in a case of *Cushing's osteoporosis*. One can see the osteoporotic porosity of the vertebral spongiosa *(1)*, with the central layer *(2)* revealing itself as a translucent band. Near the vertebral plates *(3)*, as in the plates themselves *(4)*, the shadow is more dense. Such a radiographic structural appearance is known as *"marginal condensation"*, and is characteristic of this disease. Following vertebral compression the structure becomes more dense as a result of hyperplastic callus formation.

The **macroscopic picture** of Cushing's osteoporosis in the vertebral column is shown in **Fig. 130**. In this sawn specimen one can see that the vertebral bodies have been greatly narrowed by compression *(1)*. The framework and particularly the plates remain intact, but the latter have bulged into the body, giving rise to the so-called *fish vertebrae (3)*. The spongiosa cannot be evaluated macroscopically. The intervertebral discs *(4)* are swollen and widened.

In **Fig. 131** one can see the **histological picture** of osteoporosis with wide-mesh spongiosa.

The bone trabeculae are reduced *(1)* and those that remain are extremely narrow *(2)* and are arranged in a filigree pattern. There are deep resorption lacunae *(3)* which give the trabeculae a ragged, moth-eaten appearance. It is striking, however, that Howship's lacunae no longer contain multinucleate osteoclasts. The burst of osteoclastic activity is therefore already over, and what we can now see is the result of osteoclastic bone resorption. Bone deposition is also reduced and no active osteoblasts or osteoid seams are present. In active Cushing's osteoporosis the osteoblasts and osteoclasts are in equilibrium. In the center of the picture one can recognize an ***anemic bone infarct (4)***, in which the fatty marrow is necrotic and bordered by a seam of connective tissue *(5)*.

Under **higher magnification** one can again see, in **Fig. 132**, the reduced and narrowed bone trabeculae *(1)*. The marrow cavity is filled with richly cellular hematopoietic tissue in which fibrinoid necroses appear *(3)*. They probably represent early stages of the developing infarct.

With a long-standing Cushing's syndrome *fractures* or *bone infarcts* can also arise in the skeleton in addition to the typical *osteoporosis*.

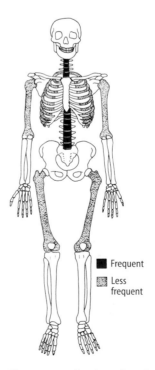

■ Frequent
▨ Less
   frequent

Fig. 128. Localization of Cushing's osteoporosis

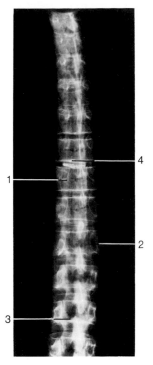

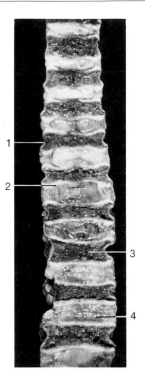

Fig. 129. Cushing's osteoporosis of the spinal column (radiograph)

Fig. 130. Cushing's osteoporosis of the spine (macroscopic specimen)

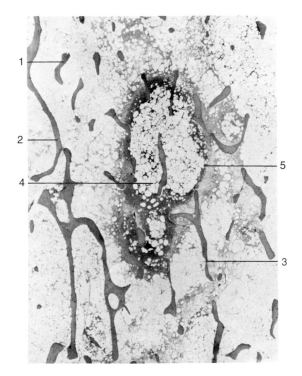

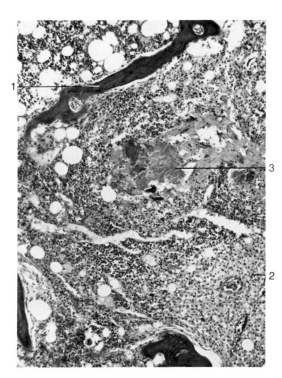

Fig. 131. Cushing's osteoporosis including anemic bone infarct; HE, ×20

Fig. 132. Cushing's osteoporosis; HE, ×45

These constitute a special complication of the condition. The *fractures occurring in Cushing's syndrome* result from the general instability of a skeletal osteoporosis, that is to say, from the loss of stabilizing bone tissue. Since it is especially the stem skeleton that is affected, the most frequent fractures involve the vertebrae. The fracture line is usually horizontal and parallel to the vertebral plates. Characteristically there is excessive callus formation. This dense fracture callus appears in the radiograph as a dark horizontal band with fuzzy edges and is recognized as the so-called *"marginal condensation"* of the vertebrae in this condition. Fractures due to Cushing's osteoporosis can, however, also appear in the proximal parts of the appendicular skeleton.

In **Fig. 134** one sees the **radiograph** of a fractured femoral neck in a case of Cushing's osteoporosis. The fracture line *(1)* is clearly recognizable, and the head *(2)* is displaced relative to the rest of the bone *(3)*. Although union has not yet taken place, the *hyperplastic callus formation* is already to be seen as a patchy and banded increase in density *(4)* between the trochanters and has also produced dark shadowing in the adjacent soft tissues *(5)*. Osteoporosis is clearly recognizable in the neighborhood *(6)*.

The hyperplastic fracture-callus of Cushing's osteoporosis has a very characteristic **histological** appearance. In **Fig. 135** one can see the fine-mesh, gnarled and ragged fibrous bone, consisting of both narrow *(1)* and broad *(2)* fibrous bone trabeculae with small osteocytes and drawn-out reversal lines *(3)*. Fragmented lamellae of the spongiosa may be embedded in the callus. Leading edges of bone deposition *(4)* are often encountered, and between these bizarre regions of new bone there is a loose fibrous marrow *(5)* in which only a few inflammatory cells are present.

The *bone infarcts of Cushing's syndrome* cannot be distinguished either morphologically on the radiograph or histologically from anemic infarcts with other etiological backgrounds (p. 174). In the vertebral bodies they are wedge-shaped, with the long side up against the disc. Because of calcium saponification they are bordered by a jagged linear pattern. However, symmetrical bone infarcts can also develop at the ends of long bones, and these are mostly paired by a similar lesion of the opposing bone.

Such infarcts can be seen in the distal part of the femur *(1)* and proximal part of the tibia *(2)* in the **radiograph** of **Fig. 133**.

Macroscopically these bone infarcts appear as in the saw cut through the femur and tibia shown in **Fig. 136**: a yellowish-gray map-like area of necrosis *(1)* which is surrounded by a hemorrhagic border *(2)*. The outer contour of the bone is unaltered.

Histologically one can see in **Fig. 137** that the trabeculae in the spongiosa *(1)* are still mostly preserved, even when many of the osteocyte lacunae are empty. There are no morphological signs of osteoclastic bone resorption. In the marrow cavity, however, the fatty tissue is necrotic *(2)*, which is clear from the eosinophilia of the fat cells and the absence of their nuclei. Old infarcts may be replaced by scar tissue, and dystrophic calcium deposition may be seen. Apart from a pathological fracture, a malignant bone tumor (usually a malignant fibrous histiocytoma – p. 324) may develop in a bone infarct. After the Cushing's syndrome has been successfully treated, local sclerosis of the spongiosa may remain.

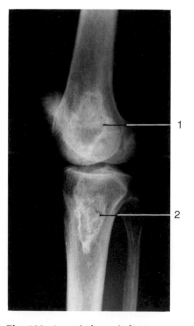

Fig. 133. Anemic bone infarcts (distal femur, proximal tibia)

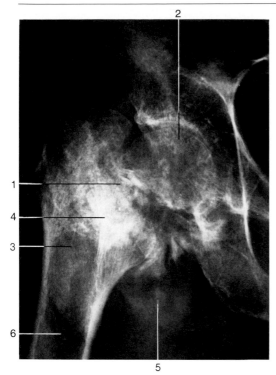

Fig. 134. Fracture of femoral neck with hyperplastic development of callus in Cushing's osteoporosis

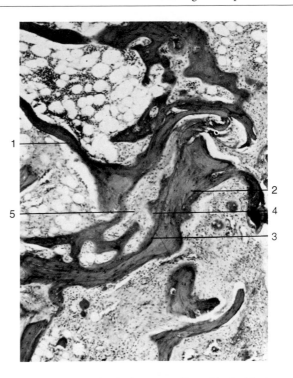

Fig. 135. Hyperplastic fracture callus with Cushing's osteoporosis; HE, ×30

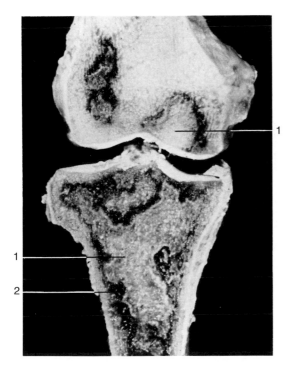

Fig. 136. Anemic bone infarcts (femur, tibia)

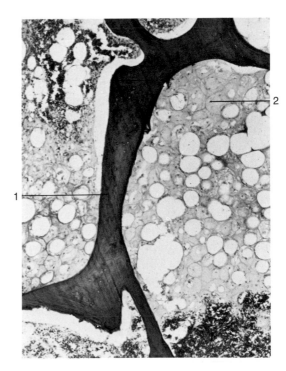

Fig. 137. Anemic bone infarct; HE, ×42

Osteodystrophy

Among the various organs and organic systems which have an active effect on bone the parathyroids have a particular significance. A disorder of their regulatory system (p. 6) can produce characteristic responses on the part of the skeleton. *Osteodystrophia fibrosa generalisata cystica (von Recklinghausen) is a condition in which localized focal, but also often generalized skeletal changes occur, and which is the result of increased parathormone secretion.* The fundamental cause is *primary hyperparathyroidism* due to a parathyroid adenoma (80%), a clear cell parathyroid hyperplasia (10%), a parathyroid oxyphil cell hyperplasia (8%) or a carcinoma of the parathyroid glands (2%). In about 25% of cases of primary hyperparathyroidism (HPT) osteodystrophy develops. As can be seen in **Fig. 138**, the disease manifests itself principally in the vertebral column and long bones, although the skull cap, maxilla and mandible are often affected. Early symptoms include erosions of the shafts of the intermediate phalanges of the fingers and atrophy of the lamina dura of the teeth (arrows). The diagnosis of HPT requires, apart from a clinical examination, the morphological examination of an iliac crest biopsy (see Fig. 112).

The increased activity of the parathyroid hormone (parathormone, parathyrin) brings about a generalized bone resorption and with it an "osteoporosis". There is typically an "exfoliation" of the cortex and the appearance of cortical cysts which are pathognomonic of this disease. In addition to the increased bone resorption there is also an increased deposition of fibrous and lamellar bone. This remodeling produces in the vertebral bodies the so-called *horizontal trilaminar layering* ("rugger-jersey pattern"), which can be clearly recognized in the **radiograph** of **Fig. 139**. One can see here a closely meshed, darkly shadowed spongiosa on both sides of the intervertebral disc *(1)* and a porosity (translucency) in the middle layer *(2)*. The rest of the vertebral column still shows signs of spondylarthrotic change *(3)*.

Figure 140 shows a lateral **radiograph** of a vertebral column with the generalized osseous appearance of primary HPT. This is a classical *"rugger-jersey spine"*. One can easily see the horizontal trilaminar layering with a wide, irregularly porous layer of spongiosa *(1)* in the center of the vertebral body. The upper *(2)* and lower *(3)* vertebral plates show a band-like sclerosity bordering the intervertebral space *(4)*. The lateral borders of the vertebral bodies *(5)* are osteoporotically narrowed and faded.

Radiological examination of a **maceration specimen** reveals the structural bone remodeling of osteodystrophy very clearly. **Figure 141** is again a lateral view of the thoracic column with the ribs attached. All the vertebral bodies show signs of a well-marked central osteoporosis *(1)* and band-like osteosclerosis of the upper *(2)* and lower *(3)* plates. The outer contours of the vertebral bodies are fuzzy, and the cortex very thin and exfoliated *(4)*. The ribs also show signs of advanced diffused osteoporosis. There are isolated creeping rib fractures *(6)*. The fracture line contains deposits of radiolucent fibrocartilage and appears in the radiograph as a gaping space. These creeping fractures appear in the so-called *Looser's transformation zones*.

Figure 142 is a **radiograph** of a **maceration specimen** of the proximal part of a femur with osteodystrophy. We can see the coarsened structure of the spongiosa *(1)* and the fine pat-

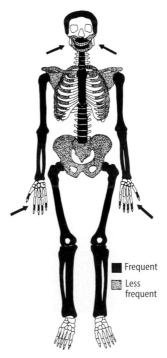

Fig. 138. Localization of osteodystrophy. → early manifestation

■ Frequent
▒ Less frequent

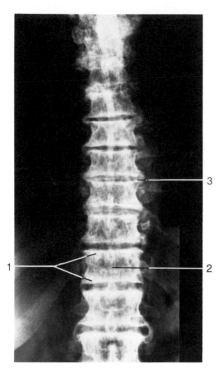

Fig. 139. Osteodystrophy (spine)

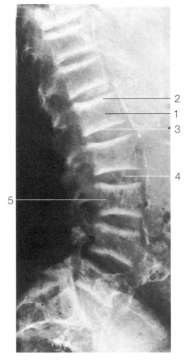

Fig. 140. Osteodystrophy: "rugger-jersey spine"
(lateral radiograph of lumbar column)

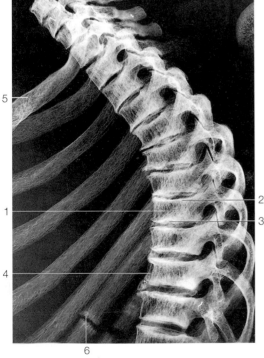

Fig. 141. Osteodystrophy: "rugger-jersey spine"
(lateral view of thoracic column, maceration specimen)

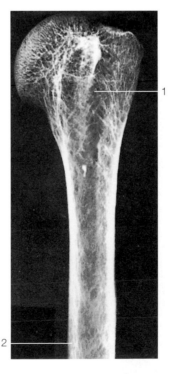

Fig. 142. Osteodystrophy
(proximal femur, maceration specimen)

chy porosity of the cortex in the region of the shaft *(2)*. All the structures are radiologically rarefied but sharply delineated.

In primary hyperparathyroidism all the bone cells are activated; but bone resorption brought about by the activated osteoclasts predominates over the merely partial deposition due to the osteoblasts. In the **tomogram** of an osteodystrophic vertebral column (**Fig. 143**) the adjacent bone deposition and resorption are only poorly seen. The outer contours of the lumbar vertebrae are retained. The central region *(1)* is osteoporotic, with zones of increased density above and below *(2)*. The border between the cortex and the spongiosa of the marrow cavity appears frayed. The irregular unphysiological bone remodeling of the affected vertebral spongiosa is well seen in the **maceration specimen.** In **Fig. 145** one sees the close-mesh scaffolding of the spongiosa, with trabeculae of varying width *(1)*, without smooth borders *(2)* and "pores" of various sizes *(3)*.

The **histological picture** of **Fig. 144** shows the irregular spongiosa with widened *(1)* and narrowed *(2)* trabeculae. These have undulating borders *(3)* on which numerous osteoblasts *(4)*

and osteoclasts *(5)* are lying. The fatty marrow *(6)* is loosely fibrosed.

In the early stages of osteodystrophy one sees only marginal fibrosis in the **histological picture** of an iliac crest biopsy. In **Fig. 146** there is a laminated bone trabecula *(1)* against which a narrow fibrous seam is lying *(2)*. **Figure 147** shows a wide-mesh network of spongiosa with irregularly bordered trabeculae *(1)* and deep resorption lacunae *(2)*. The bone *(3)* tissue is laminated and regularly mineralized, but only with the aid of tetracycline marking is the reduced mineralization recognizable. An important histological feature is the tunneling of the bone trabecula by a richly cellular and fibrous granulation tissue *(4)*.

As can be seen under **higher magnification** in **Fig. 148**, the intratrabecular spaces are filled with loose fibrous connective tissue rich in blood vessels and well-developed fibroblasts *(1)*. The undulating front of the bone tissue is covered with mono- and multinucleated osteoclasts *(2)* as well as rows of active osteoblasts *(3)*. Much endosteal fibrosis (marginal fibrosis; 4) can be seen in the transitional zone between bone trabeculae and marrow cavity.

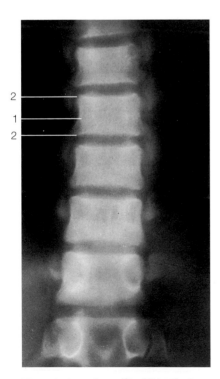

Fig. 143. Osteodystrophy (spinal column, tomogram)

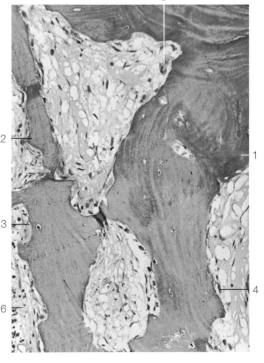

Fig. 144. Osteodystrophy; HE, ×100

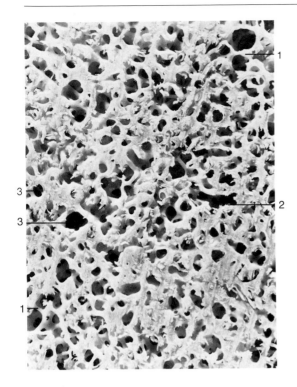

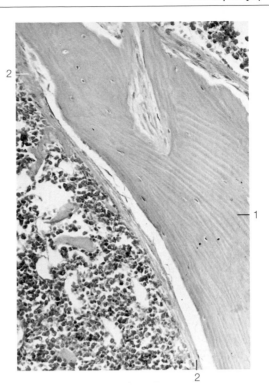

Fig. 145. Osteodystrophy (vertebral spongiosa, maceration specimen)

Fig. 146. Osteodystrophy; HE, ×100

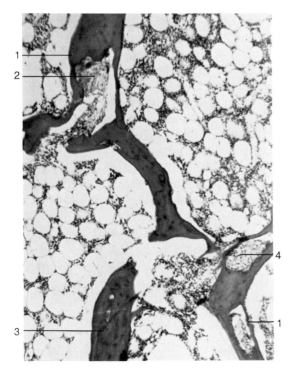

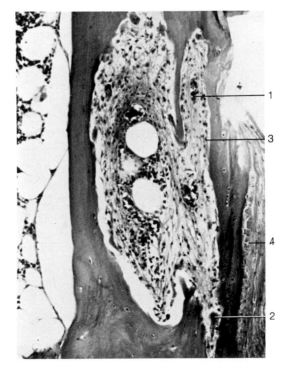

Fig. 147. Osteodystrophy; HE, ×25

Fig. 148. Osteodystrophy; HE, ×82

The osteoid is comparatively sparse. The histological picture of increased and activated osteoclasts with deep resorption lacunae under the influence of the parathyroid hormone is known as **dissecting fibro-osteoclasia**, because the trabeculae are actually cut into. This appearance, together with the marrow fibrosis, is pathognomonic of primary hyperparathyroidism.

When *primary hyperparathyroidism* is suspected, a radiograph of the hands and jaws should first be ordered, since it is here that the pathognomonic early symptoms appear. **Figure 149** depicts the **radiograph** of a hand in which the short tubular bones are greatly altered. Regions of *atrophy* due to periosteal bone resorption *(1)* are typically seen in the intermediate phalanges of the fingers. This is very characteristic of hyperparathyroidism. Indeed, the absence of such changes in the hand is usually sufficient to exclude the presence of the skeletal manifestations of hyperparathyroidism. The lamina dura of the teeth can be reduced, and the skull cap may present with a so-called *granular atrophy* ("pumice-stone skull"), owing to the loss of the lamina externa. Apart from the erosion of the intermediate phalanges of the fingers already mentioned, the hand in **Fig. 149** shows an irregular osteoporosis of the proximal phalanx of the index finger *(2)*, with straggly regions of increased density between the patchy translucencies. However, the most striking indication is the club-like tumorous distension of the 2nd metacarpal *(3)*, in which one can again see patchy translucencies (osteolyses) that are bordered by trabecular regions of increased density. The cortex of this bone is narrowed but preserved. These radiological findings, together with osteodystrophy due to hyperparathyroidism, suggest the presence of a so-called *"brown tumor"*.

Figure 150 shows the **radiological appearance** of such a *"brown tumor"* in the left iliac bone *(1)* and left femoral neck *(2)* of a patient with primary hyperparathyroidism. The defect appears as a circumscribed zone of osteolysis, surrounded by a narrow band of marginal sclerosis *(3)* and lying near the cortex. The cortex has not been penetrated and there is no periosteal reaction. Within the osteolytic area there is a discrete, dense cloudy region, and no true internal structure can be identified. Indicative of hyperparathyroidism and the presence

of "brown tumors", there are also single cortical cysts of a kind not seen in any other disease.

These so-called "brown tumors" are not true bony neoplasms, but rather a variety of **resorptive giant cell granuloma** *which can develop in an advanced case of primary hyperparathyroidism*. The osteolysis of hormonal origin in osteodystrophia generalisata cystica (von Recklinghausen) reduces the supporting capacity of the skeleton and leads to the random appearance of spontaneous fractures with indiscriminate bleeding. Under the influence of the parathyroid hormone the osteoclasts become particularly numerous and active in the neighborhood of the fractures. This produces a very marked local osteolysis which shows up on the radiograph as bone tumors or cysts. As a result of the earlier bleeding, macroscopic foci of iron deposits appear and are, because of their color, known as "brown tumors". As can be seen in **Fig. 151**, these lesions consist **histologically** of loose, highly vascular granulation tissue with bleeding and deposits of hemosiderin. The connective tissue stroma contains many similar slender fibrocytes and fibroblasts *(1)* with occasional mitoses. In the loose network of collagen fibers there are a striking number of multinucleate osteoclast-like giant cells *(2)*. They cluster together in unequal groups and are not regularly disposed throughout the tissue (thus differing from an osteoclastoma, Fig. 642). The spongiosa has largely disappeared, and only in the center can one recognize trabeculae *(3)* with poorly defined outlines.

One can see in **Fig. 152** under **higher magnification** that the loose stroma of a "brown tumor" contains numerous spindle cells with elongated isomorphic nuclei *(1)* and randomly distributed multinucleate osteoclastic giant cells *(3)*, as well as deposits of hemosiderin. "Brown tumors" develop in 12% of cases of primary HPT and appear mostly in the shafts of the long bones. Treatment must be aimed at the underlying hyperparathyroidism. This means that the hyperfunctional parathyroids must be surgically removed, after which the bone lesions will heal. Simple resection of the so-called "brown tumors" is pointless and is not indicated. In any case, the underlying disease should today be diagnosed early, before any question of "brown tumors" arises.

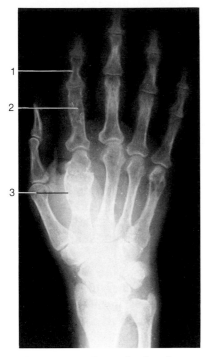

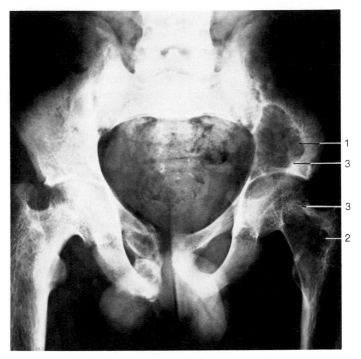

Fig. 149. Osteodystrophy (hand)

Fig. 150. Osteodystrophy, so-called "brown tumors" in a case of primary hyperparathyroidism (ala of left iliac bone, left femoral neck)

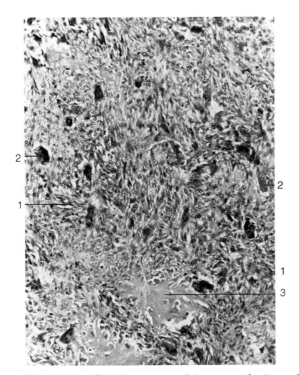

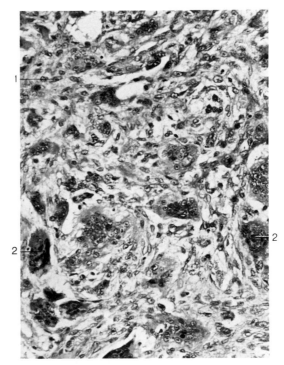

Fig. 151. So-called "brown tumor" in a case of primary hyperparathyroidism; HE, ×40

Fig. 152. So-called "brown tumor" in a case of primary hyperparathyroidism; HE, ×80

Osteomalacia

Every reduction in the calcium content of bone is reflected radiologically by a translucency of the structures. *Osteomalacia represents a disorder of calcification of the bone tissue in adults, and is therefore to be compared with the rickets of childhood (p. 50).* The cause may be due to a vitamin D deficiency, a *lack of calcium,* or *renal disease.* In the skeleton there is insufficient calcification of the bone tissue and an excessive increase in osteoid. As can be seen in **Fig. 153,** osteomalacia can appear in any bone, but is most pronounced in the stem skeleton (vertebral column, thorax, pelvis) and femur. The excessive osteoid building is particularly clear-cut in the skull cap, and leads here to the so-called *granular atrophy* ("pumice-stone skull").

Even under physiological loading the reduced mineralization can bring about skeletal deformation. The **radiograph** depicted in **Fig. 154** shows the curvature *(1)* of kyphosis leading to a hunchback. The spongiosa of the vertebral bodies is faded *(2),* with osteoporotic translucencies, although the framework is preserved. The ribs *(3)* also show an impaired and faded structure, and the weight of the upper part of the body itself is sufficient to cause a bell-like deformity of the thoracic cage. The so-called *Milkman's syndrome* frequently develops during the course of a hypophosphatemic osteomalacia. Here one finds symmetrical translucent areas in particular parts of the skeleton (**Fig. 153**), which may resemble fractures radiologically. They can be seen in several ribs in **Fig. 154** *(4).* These so-called *Looser's transformation zones,* which appear at highly stressed points in the skeleton, are regarded as permanent fractures, which begin with a cortical fissure and are held together by callus osteoid. The end result resembles a fracture that has simulated a pseudarthrosis.

Figure 155 shows the **radiograph** of advanced osteomalacia in the proximal part of the femur. The entire cancellous network is translucent and very faded *(1).* The typical trabeculae of the femoral neck are no longer recognizable. The cortex *(2)* is indeed preserved, but its outer contour is fuzzy, because osteoid is also being deposited in the periosteum. Below the trochanter one can recognize a Milkman's fracture in a Looser's transformation zone *(3).*

In the **histological section** the bone trabeculae are found to be rarefied (**Fig. 156**), mineralized centrally *(1)* and surrounded by extraordinarily wide osteoid seams (2; more than 10 μm wide). These seams are in general of varying width. Single osteoblasts *(3)* have been deposited, although the number of these cells can vary greatly. The decisive morphological features of osteomalacia are the wide osteoid seams, which can also be identified in decalcified sections stained with HE as wide, homogeneous pale red bands *(2),* clearly set apart from the laminar calcified bone tissue *(1).* The marrow cavity *(4)* is filled with fatty tissue and hematopoietic bone marrow. There is no medullary fibrosis.

Under **higher magnification** the morphological difference between the mineralized lamellar bone *(1)* and the wide, red, translucent band of osteoid *(2)* is clearly seen in **Fig. 157.** Occasional osteoblasts *(3)* are situated on the outside of the osteoid seam. The increased amount of osteoid gives the bone structure a faded appearance radiologically.

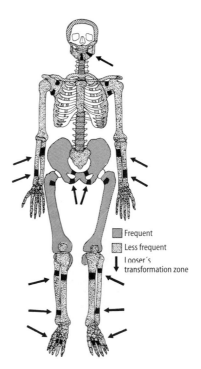

Frequent
Less frequent
Looser's transformation zone

Fig. 153. Localization of osteomalacia. → Looser's transformation zones

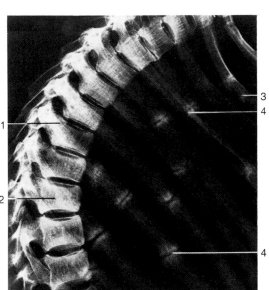

Fig. 154. Osteomalacia (thoracic column)

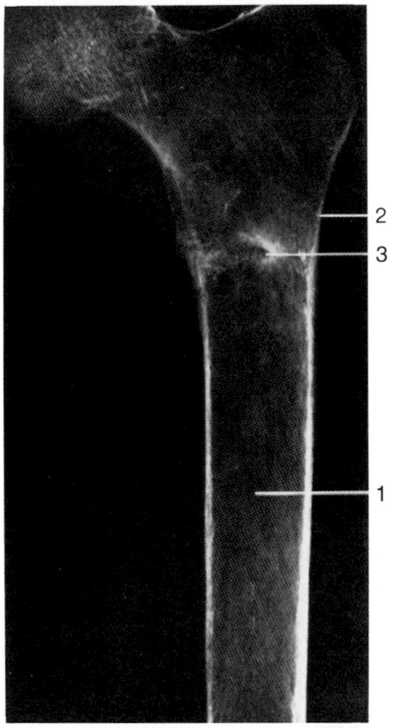

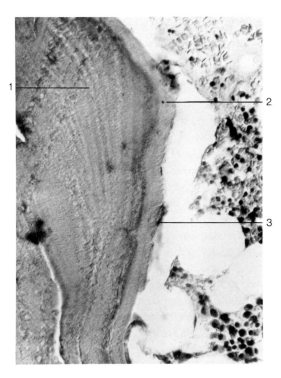

Fig. 155. Osteomalacia (femur)

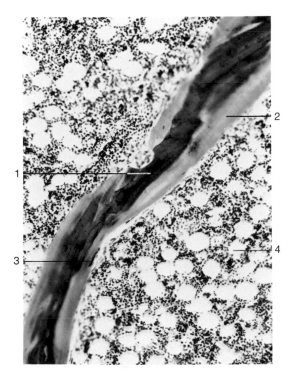

Fig. 156. Osteomalacia; HE, ×80

Fig. 157. Osteomalacia; HE, ×100

Renal Osteopathy

In the presence of chronic renal insufficiency a clinical condition of multiple etiology develops in the skeleton. This is known as renal osteopathy. *It is consists of bone changes resulting from endogenous factors* (secondary hyperparathyroidism, a disturbance of vitamin D metabolism, resistance to parathyroid hormone) *and exogenous factors* (restricted phosphate intake, an unphysiological uptake of cations and vitamin D or vitamin D metabolites), *so that the bone tissue reacts by producing the patterns of* **osteodystrophia fibrosa, osteomalacia** and **osteoporosis**. The diagnosis is based upon iliac crest biopsy. DELLING (1979), relying upon the histomorphometric analysis, put forward a classification of renal osteopathies in which he recognized three forms (Types I–III), corresponding to the degree of fibrous osteoclasia and osteoidosis present. He was able to correlate these osteopathies with the different types of renal disease. Such a specific analysis is, however, only possible with undecalcified material. Many pathologists have access only to decalcified histological specimens for routine diagnosis, but still have to be able to diagnose a renal osteopathy.

In chronic renal disease, however, there is **radiological** evidence of renal osteopathy. In **Fig. 158**, one can see a high degree of osteoporotic loosening of the cancellous scaffolding in the proximal part of the femur *(1)*, in which the contours – as in osteomalacia (Fig. 155) – are very faded *(2)*. One can see small cystic translucencies in the cortex *(3)*, and a *Milkman's fracture* is clearly recognizable near the proximal end of the femoral shaft *(4)*.

The **histological section** through an iliac crest biopsy seen in **Fig. 159** shows the appearance of adjacent regions of fibrous osteoclasia and osteomalacia. The trabeculae are unequally narrowed, with undulating contours *(1)* and central mineralization *(2)*. Outside one can recognize a broad layer of osteoid *(3)*, which varies in width, is internally homogeneous and shines with a bright red color. The rows of activated osteoblasts *(4)* deposited on this wide osteoid seam are plainly visible. They lay down the osteoid and raise the level of the serum alkaline phosphatase. These structures exemplify the picture of *osteomalacia (p. 86)*. The foci of myeloid fibrosis containing numerous fibroblasts are very clearly seen *(5)*. In a few places the bone trabeculae lack the osteoid coat *(6)*, while at others there are deep resorption lacunae filled up with highly cellular connective tissue and osteoclasts. The picture here is that of *osteodystrophy* with *dissecting fibro-osteoclasia (p. 83)*. Furthermore, the significantly narrowed bone trabeculae, indicating *osteoporosis*, are striking. In general, the spongiosa is widely meshed and the marrow cavity is enlarged and filled with fat and connective tissue, which leads to the appearance of osteoporotic translucencies in the radiograph. With the mixed type of renal osteopathy, the osteodystrophic, osteomalacial or osteoporotic component may predominate. Foci of osteosclerosis may also occasionally be found.

Under **higher magnification** one can see in **Fig. 160** a bone trabecula with central lamination *(1)* and small osteocytes *(2)*. A protracted reversal line *(3)* marks off the greatly widened osteoid seam *(4)* which is indicative of osteomalacia. Hardly any osteoblasts are present. One can also see deep resorption lacunae *(5)* which have burrowed into the trabeculae like tunnels, and which are filled with highly cellular connective tissue containing osteoclasts.

The **histological pattern** of *dissecting fibro-osteoclasia* is also seen in **Fig. 161**. In the deep resorption lacunae *(1)* activated osteoclasts *(2)* can be seen. In addition, the bone trabeculae include elongated reversal lines *(3)* and adjacent broad seams of osteoid *(4)* outside.

The changes in the histological structure show that renal osteopathy is essentially characterized by *secondary hyperparathyroidism* and a disturbance of vitamin D metabolism. The disease begins with a reduction in the glomerular filtrate, which leads to a reduction in phosphate excretion and consequent hypocalcinemia. The fall in the serum calcium level stimulates parathyroid secretion, thus calling a secondary hyperparathyroidism into existence. While the increased action of the parathyroid hormone produces a dissecting fibro-osteoclasia in the bone, the reduced synthesis of vitamin D is responsible for the disturbance of calcification.

Patients with impaired kidney function develop renal osteopathy to a varying extent. The reduced glomerular filtration found in ad-

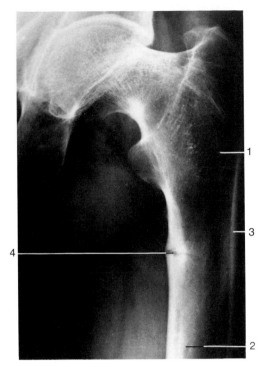

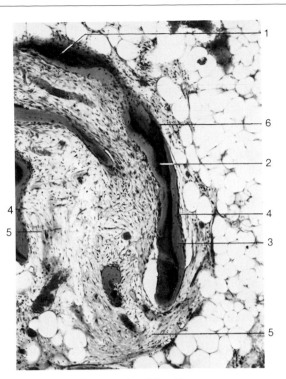

Fig. 158. Renal osteopathy (proximal femur with Milkman's syndrome)

Fig. 159. Renal osteopathy; HE, ×45

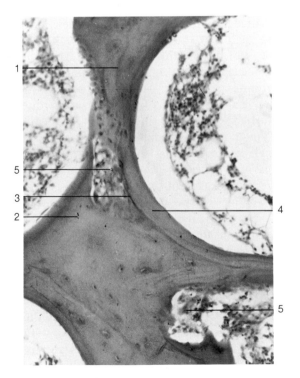

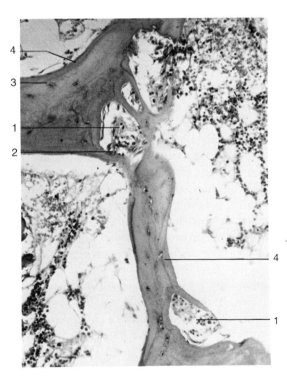

Fig. 160. Renal osteopathy; HE, ×80

Fig. 161. Renal osteopathy; HE, ×60

vanced renal disorders produces hyperphosphatemia and hypocalcinemia. This generates a secondary hyperparathyroidism with raised hormonal secretion and, finally, resistance to parathyroid hormone on the part of the skeleton. The synthesis of 1,25 dihydrocholecalciferol is reduced in the damaged kidney, and this again increases the secretion of the hormone. All the various factors influencing mineral metabolism in the presence of chronic renal insufficiency differ in their action on the bone structure, and this is displayed both in the radiograph and in the histology of the bone biopsy (iliac crest).

Figure 162 shows a **radiograph** of an advanced case of renal osteopathy. All the bones of the pelvis *(1)* and the femoral head *(2)* show an irregular osteoporosis with straggly regions of increased density and translucent patches in between. The structures are etiolated. In places, stronger resorptive remodeling processes have led to large areas of "osteolysis" *(3)*.

In **Table 2** the various **forms of renal osteopathy** are listed according to those histological criteria which, as affirmed by DELLING (1975, 1984), indicate the extent of the bone change. Three types are distinguished; they are histomorphologically described and allotted to each category of renal disease. *Classification of the renal osteopathies* is based partly on a quantitative histomorphometric analysis of iliac crest biopsies, and partly on clinico-pathological experience. The exact degree of mineralization disorder can only be evaluated in undecalcified specimens of bone. However, for most routine diagnosis, sections that have been carefully and completely decalcified with EDTA are adequate for the purpose; both the cellular components of the renal osteopathy (osteoclasts, osteoblasts, fibroblasts), the intramedullary connective tissue and also the widened osteoid seam being sufficient to categorize the various types of renal osteopathy. This classification of the renal osteopathies, based on the effect of renal insufficiency on the skeleton, has been applied in clinical practice for years and has guided physicians in their planning of the treatment. For this reason, it is important to specify the pathology in detail when diagnosing a renal osteopathy.

The histological criteria include; (1) fibro-osteoclasia (increased osteoclastic resorption), (2) disorders of mineralization, (3) surface and volume osteoidosis (extent of the osteoid seams), (4) reduction of the mass of calcified bone, (5) extent of the endosteal and myeloid fibrosis, (6) remodeling of the spongiosa and (7) deposition of new bone (fibrous bone trabeculae). In order to obtain exact and objective data on these indices it would be necessary to employ histomorphometry, which is mostly restricted to special laboratories. In clinical practice, however, it is usually sufficient to quantify the histological criteria subjectively and thus classify each case of renal osteopathy. It must be remarked here, however, that the exact degree of the renal osteopathy can be determined by histological examination.

Figure 163 shows the **histological picture** of a *Type 1* renal osteopathy. It can be identified by the increased osteoclastic resorption following a secondary hyperparathyroidism, with poor bone deposition and no mineralization. The structure of the spongiosa is preserved, although the bone trabeculae *(1)* nevertheless vary in width. They often show undulating borders containing flat resorption lacunae *(2)*. One can see single small osteoclasts *(3)*; osteoblasts are not present. Near the trabeculae there is a bandlike region of endosteal fibrosis *(4)* and focal fibrosis of the marrow *(5)* with dissecting fibro-osteoclasia, indicating increased parathyroid hormone secretion. Following a lengthy hemodialysis a disorder of mineralization due to disturbed vitamin D metabolism may appear. Type 1 renal osteopathy is seen in about 5% of all cases of renal insufficiency, and is particularly frequent in cases of rapidly progressive glomerulonephritis with acute renal failure. As far as the bone changes are concerned, no particular therapeutic precautions are necessary at this stage.

Type II renal osteopathy is characterized by an exclusively superficial osteoidosis without additional fibrous osteoclasia. One can distinguish two different reaction patterns created by the mineralization disorder. With *Type IIa* the osteoclastic resorption lacunae are filled with osteoid that is not mineralized. There is a complete cessation of mineralization. This **histological picture** is shown in **Fig. 165.** One can recognize the wide-mesh mineralized bone trabeculae *(1)*, against which lie osteoid seams of varying width *(2)*. Many resorption lacunae

Table 2. Classification of Renal Osteopathy. (After DELLING 1984)

Type of Renal Osteopathy	Histological Criterion	Frequency	Cause
Type I	Fibroosteoclasia Increased osteoclastic resorption No disturbance of mineralization	5%	Glomerulonephritis Acute renal failure (secondary HPT)
Type II	Isolated surface osteoidosis (without additional fibroosteoclasia) Volume and surface osteoidosis	20% 30%	Chronic renal insufficiency (without hemodialysis) Continuous hemodialysis
Type IIa	Reduced spongiosal remodeling Complete cessation of mineralization		
Type IIb	Narrow osteoid seams, with increase in their surface extension Reduction of bone mass		
Type III	Fibroosteoclasia and osteoidosis Endosteofibrosis	70%	Chronic renal insufficiency
Type IIIa	Reduced spongiosal remodeling		
Type IIIb	Normal spongiosal remodeling	60%	Continuous hemodialysis
Type IIIc	Complete spongiosal remodeling Massive development of fibrous bone Cuboidal osteoblasts		

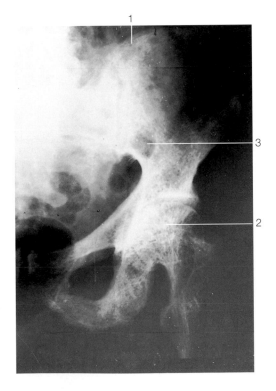

Fig. 162. Renal osteopathy
(left side of pelvis, femoral head)

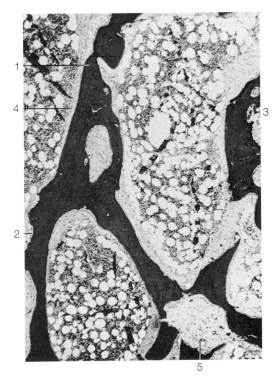

Fig. 163. Renal osteopathy, Type I, Azan, ×64

are completely filled with uncalcified osteoid
(3). No osteoblasts are seen. The enlarged marrow cavity is filled with fat and hematopoietic
tissue *(4)*. No endosteal fibrosis and no increase in the osteoclasts can be seen. The picture is characterized by wide areas of osteoidosis and reduced bone remodeling. Radiologically, there is an impression of "osteoporosis"
due to the reduction of mineralized bone tissue, so that spontaneous fractures may occur.
The serum concentration of parathyroid hormone is only slightly raised. This type of renal
osteopathy, accompanied only by a disorder of
mineralization (without secondary hyperparathyroidism), is found in 20% of patients with
chronic renal insufficiency who are not undergoing hemodialysis. Nevertheless, suppression
of the parathyroids can cause hypercalcinemia.

With *Type IIb* renal osteopathy the mass of
mineralized spongiosa is also reduced, which
can bring about radiological "osteoporosis". As
can be seen in **Fig. 166**, fully mineralized trabeculae *(1)* have been deposited, but there are
only very narrow osteoid seams *(2)* which present an increased superficial extension. No osteoblasts have been deposited. For the most
part there are no resorption lacunae present.
The mass of mineralized bone has been reduced, and in this case the final stage of mineralization has been greatly delayed. Bone
changes of this kind appear in 30% of patients
with kidney disease after long-term hemodialysis, in whom life expectation is reduced. Spontaneous fractures (vertebrae, ribs, extremities)
frequently appear, and fatal infections may
arise. The administration of vitamin D metabolites can bring about some mineralization of
the osteoid.

The **radiograph** in such cases shows osteoporosis with an etiolated cancellous structure.
In **Fig. 164** the spongiosa of the proximal end
of the femur is osteoporotic *(1)*. The femoral
neck shows some increase in density *(2)*, but
still appears faded. A so-called *Milkman's fracture (3)* is present. The renal osteopathy is radiologically identifiable by the fuzzy "osteoporosis".

With *Type III* renal osteopathy, both dissecting fibro-osteoclasia and endosteal and marrow
fibrosis are found as an expression of the increased parathyroid hormone activity, as well
as wide-spread osteoidosis resulting from a

mineralization disorder. The picture is that of
secondary hyperparathyroidism and a disorder
of vitamin D metabolism. **Histologically** one
can see in **Fig. 167** that the mineralized bone
trabeculae *(1)* are greatly reduced and have undulating borders. Wide osteoid seams *(2)* have
been deposited among the original trabeculae
of the spongiosa, together with deep resorption
lacunae *(3)*. *Type IIIa* renal osteopathy is also
histologically apparent in **Fig. 168**. The mineralized bone trabeculae *(1)* are reduced, and
wide osteoid seams *(2)* have been deposited
with discrete endosteal fibrosis *(3)*. Several
deep resorption lacunae *(4)* have tunneled into
the bone, indicating the increased influence of
the parathormone (secondary hyperparathyroidism). Nevertheless, the absence of osteoblasts
and osteoclasts is evidence of the reduced remodeling of the spongiosa. Changes of this
kind are seen in 70% of patients with chronic
renal insufficiency before hemodialysis.

In cases of *Type IIIb* renal osteopathy, *secondary hyperparathyroidism* with dissecting fibro-osteoclasia and marrow fibrosis is prominent among the changes in bone structure. In

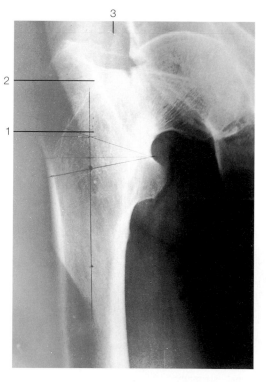

Fig. 164. Renal osteopathy, Type IIb (right proximal femur)

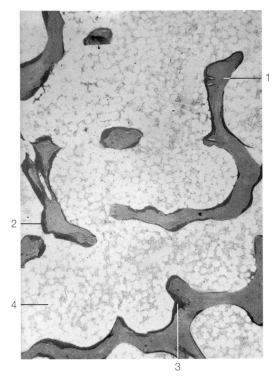

Fig. 165. Renal osteopathy, Type IIa; Azan, ×40

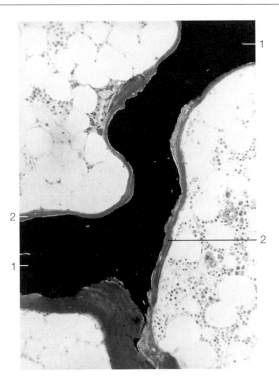

Fig. 166. Renal osteopathy, Type IIb; Kossa, ×80

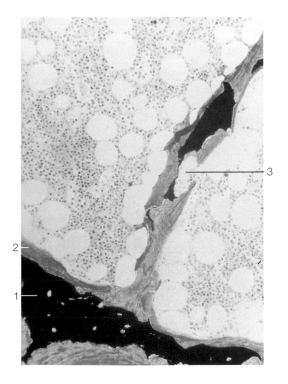

Fig. 167. Renal osteopathy, Type III; Kossa, ×60

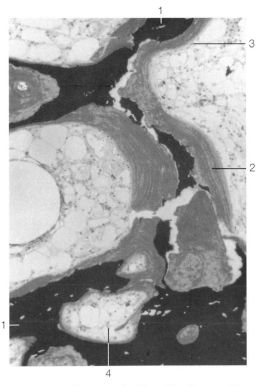

Fig. 168. Renal osteopathy, Type IIIa; Kossa, ×80

Fig. 170 one can see **histologically** an autochthonous, fully mineralized trabecula (1), into which an unusually large resorption lacuna (2) has sunk. It is filled with fibrous tissue containing strongly active fibroblasts and fibrocytes. The lacuna has an undulating border of bone, and one can see flat resorptive indentations containing osteoclasts (3). Furthermore, a row of activated osteoblasts (4) can also be seen here. The bone trabeculae are bordered by osteoid seams (5), some wide, some narrow. There is significant endosteal fibrosis (6). In this instance both dissecting fibro-osteoclasia ("osteodystrophy") and osteomalacia are found together. This is typical of renal osteopathy, particularly of Type IIIb.

In **Fig. 171**, *Type IIIb* renal osteopathy is again shown. Here the remodeling of the spongiosa is only slightly increased. In the immediate neighborhood of a mineralized trabecula (1) one can see broad seams of osteoid (2) and also a broad seam of collagenous connective tissue with many fibrocytes (3), indicating marked endosteal fibrosis. The mass of mineralized bone is greatly reduced, this being seen radiologically as "osteoporosis". This kind of structural change is very obvious in undecalcified iliac crest biopsies.

As seen in **Fig. 169**, careful preparation also makes it possible to demonstrate this type of structure in *decalcified biopsy material*. One can recognize a mineralized bone trabecula (1) that has been broken down centrally by a seam of connective tissue (2) (dissecting fibro-osteoclasia). Large single osteoclasts (3) are present in the resorption lacunae. The bone trabecula is bordered peripherally by a broad seam of osteoid (4) (osteoidosis). A few osteoblasts (5) have been deposited, and there is also peripheral fibrosis (6). Here in this decalcified specimen one can recognize all the criteria for a renal osteopathy of Type IIIb.

Type IIIc renal osteopathy is characterized by complete remodeling of the spongiosa with marked fibrous osteoclasia and moderate volume and surface osteoidosis. In **Fig. 172** one can see an irregular and incomplete cancellous scaffolding with trabeculae of varying width (1) which are adjacent to and intermingled with wider and narrower osteoid seams (2). There are also numerous wide and deep resorption lacunae (3) that are filled with connective tissue

and which contain a few multinucleate osteoclasts (4). The marrow cavity is filled with loose connective tissue and numerous fibrocytes and fibroblasts (5). One can see almost everywhere here strongly active deposition of fibrous bone. The trabeculae are covered by rows of numerous cubical osteoblasts. There is a marked dissecting fibro-osteoclasia with marrow fibrosis, indicating a severe secondary hyperparathyroidism. Such an osteological picture is an unmistakable indication for treating the parathyroids themselves.

Aluminum-induced Osteopathy

Patients with kidney disease who have been treated by long-term hemodialysis frequently develop a peculiar type of osteopathy which is caused by the deposition of aluminum in the bones. Aluminum hydroxide is either administered as a phosphate binder or is carried from the aluminum containing parts of the dialysing apparatus into the organism. This element is

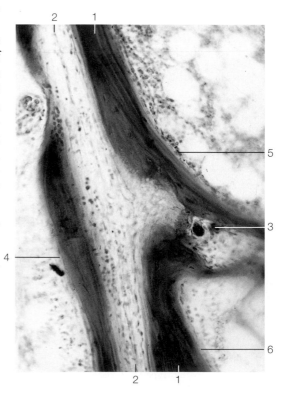

Fig. 169. Renal osteopathy, Type IIIb (decalcified biopsy material); HE, ×80

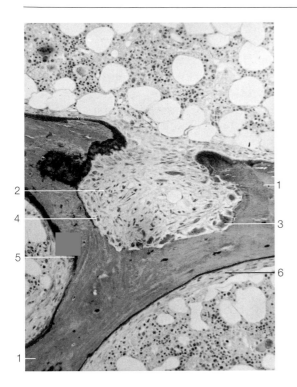

Fig. 170. Renal osteopathy, Type IIIb; Azan, ×80

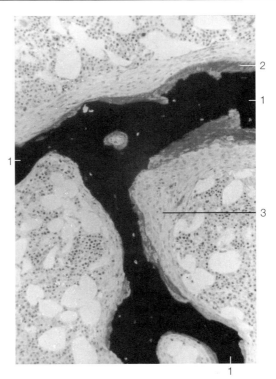

Fig. 171. Renal osteopathy, Type IIIb (undecalcified biopsy material); Kossa, ×80

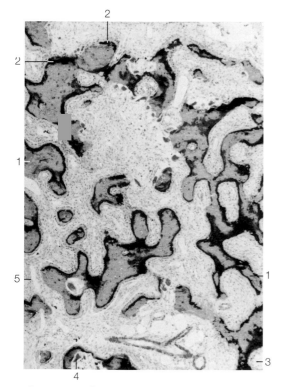

Fig. 172. Renal osteopathy, Type IIIc; Azan, ×40

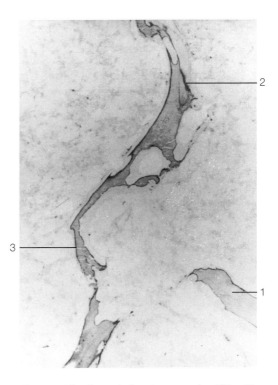

Fig. 173. Aluminum-induced osteopathy; HE, ×60

laid down at the leading edge of the mineralization in the bone, where it leads to impairment of the mineralization process and produces a severe osteoidosis. Multiple fractures may develop. In **Fig. 173** one can see **histologically** rarefied bone trabeculae *(1)* which are only partially calcified. Very wide osteoid seams *(2)* have been laid down which represent extended volume and surface osteoidosis. A narrow black band of deposited aluminum *(3)* lies at the leading edge of the mineralization process. By administering complex builders (Desferral) to the patient the aluminum can be bound and excreted.

Sudeck's Atrophy
(Sympathetic Reflex Dystrophy, SRD)

After injury to a limb and its subsequent resting period, venous stasis may develop because of the blood collecting in the sinusoidal spaces of the bone, and a painful osteoporosis may affect the region. *Sudeck's atrophy is an osteoporosis that is limited to a particular region of the skeleton. It can arise following a fracture, sprain or blunt injury, but it may also appear after an inflammatory process and produce very severe pain.* The etiology is not clear; probably the cause lies in injury to the nerves supplying the blood vessels in the bone. The affected extremity may be swollen and warm *(venous type of SRD)* or not swollen and cold *(arterial type)*.

The osteoporosis develops in the part of the bone lying distal to the fracture, and particularly affects the spongiosa. The compacta is preserved, since it is much more slowly broken down. Diagnosis depends on the clinical symptoms and the radiological changes, when a translucent area of the spongiosa can be recognized after about 4 weeks.

In **Fig. 174** one can see the **radiograph** of a hand with classical Sudeck's atrophy. All the small tubular bones reveal an irregular osteoporosis; the shaft appears to be more dense *(1)*, although it shows circular areas of translucency *(2)*. This is the picture of a so-called *patchy atrophy*. The extremely marked osteoporosis in the neighborhood of the joints is characteristic *(3)*, so that the joint spaces stand out with particular intensity *(4)*. The atrophy also appears early in the subchondral region. In the chronic stages of the disease (2–4 months after onset) the compacta also becomes involved. We can see the exfoliation and spongy appearance of the compacta in several places *(5)*. Patchy bone atrophy is also present in the carpal region *(6)*.

It is only infrequently that such a picture becomes apparent **histologically** in a bone biopsy. As can be seen in **Fig. 175**, the appearance is that of osteoporosis. The bone trabeculae are rarefied and irregularly narrowed *(1)*. They have smooth edges and show no resorption lacunae. No osteoclasts are present. The enlarged fatty marrow *(2)* is edematous. Capillary and venous stasis can be observed in the region of the myeloid vessels *(3)*. The bone atrophy can heal completely during the acute stage, but in chronic Sudeck's syndrome healing is defective, with the development of a "hypertrophic bone atrophy". In addition to *autonomic disturbances* (impairment of blood flow, soft tissue edema, hyperhidrosis or hypohidrosis), *motor disturbances* (reduced joint mobility, paralysis) and *sensory disturbances* (bone pain), the psychological condition of the patient (depression) is a significant feature of Sudeck's disease.

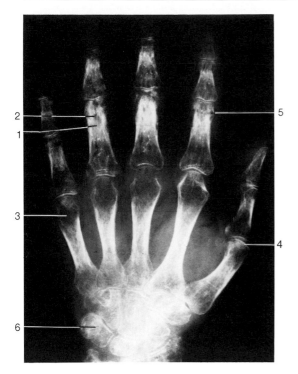

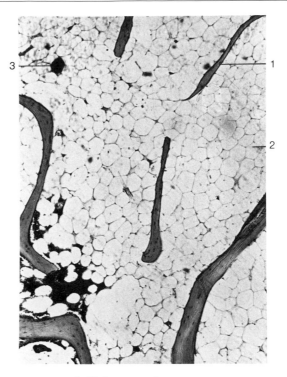

Fig. 174. Sudeck's bone atrophy (hand)

Fig. 175. Sudeck's bone atrophy; HE, ×16

5 Osteoscleroses

General

Whereas the osteoporoses (p. 65) are accompanied by a loss of bone tissue and produce translucency of the bone structure on the radiograph, with the osteoscleroses the exact opposite is the case. *By osteosclerosis, we understand an increase in density of the structures within a bone brought about by an increased mineralization of the tissue, leading to the appearance of darker shadowing on the film.* There are many types of osteosclerosis arising from different causes. In most cases there is a reactive increase of tissue in the neighborhood of a bone lesion. For instance, one frequently sees *marginal sclerosis* surrounding a benign tumor of bone (e.g. a *non-ossifying osteofibroma*, Fig. 581). Patchy foci of osteosclerosis can also appear inside a bone tumor (e.g. an *osteosarcoma*, Fig. 510). Osteosclerotic changes are often found near an old *fracture* (Fig. 211) or *chronic osteomyelitis* (Fig. 262). Single or multiple foci of osteosclerosis may appear in the skeleton or in single bones. Precise radiological analysis of such foci can permit far-reaching conclusions of diagnostic or differential diagnostic significance about the underlying disease to be drawn, and it is here that modern imaging procedures [tomography, scintigraphy, digital subtraction angiography (DSA), computer tomography (CT), MR tomography (MRT) etc.] may be helpful. In many cases, however, a diagnosis is only possible after the histological examination of a bone biopsy. When making a histological diagnosis, the pathologist must always include the radiological findings, for which representative radiographs are necessary. Nevertheless, local osteosclerosis may be so far advanced that the actual underlying bone lesion is hardly recognizable and is not apparent in the biopsy (in the case of an *osteoid osteoma*, for instance, Fig. 481). Diagnosis can then be very difficult, and only possible by taking all the clinical aspects into account.

Sometimes a systemic disease may lie behind solitary or multicentric osteosclerosis, a striking example being Paget's *osteitis deformans.*

Diseases of the bone marrow such as *osteomyelosclerosis* or *skeletal carcinomatosis* (multiple bone metastases) can bring about extensive osteosclerotic changes in the skeleton. There are also tumor-like congenital malformations of bone which are characteristically accompanied by osteosclerosis (e.g. *melorrheostosis, osteopoikilosis*). In these cases the radiograph is often pathognomonic, while the bone biopsy (which is by no means always indicated) only shows osteosclerotic tissue that does not provide a precise diagnosis. In many cases osteosclerotic and osteolytic foci appear in equal quantity and together in the same lesion (e.g. osteomyelitis, osteosarcoma).

Furthermore, osteosclerotic changes in the skeleton can also be caused by chronic intoxication with various substances. Lead, fluorine or phosphorus can either stimulate the osteocytes or, on the other hand, bring about bone

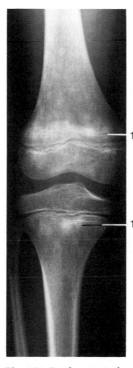

Fig. 176. Patchy osteosclerosis in lead poisoning (femur, tibia)

necrosis and stimulate the osteoclasts. In **Fig. 176** one can see a **radiograph** of the knee joint of a child with *chronic lead poisoning.* The patchy osteosclerosis in the metaphyses *(1)* is characteristic, and so are the broad dense bands (the so-called *"lead lines"* or *"lead bands"*). These are caused by the deposition of lead in the growing regions which can later bring about a bottle-shaped deformation of that part of the bone. If the poisoning is stopped, however, these structural changes may completely disappear.

Fluorosis

In bone, fluorine is a component of the hydroxyapatite crystals, and 94% of the fluorine taken in from the alimentary canal is laid down in bone. This leads both to a blockade of the alkaline phosphatase, with subsequent changes in the osteoid structures (protein, collagens, mucopolysaccharides), and to the development of a larger hydroxyapatite crystal than calcium, producing greater stability of the bone and its density. *Fluorosis is one of the most important exogenous toxic osteopathies resulting from excessive fluorine intake, leading to endostosis with spongiosclerosis (osteosclerosis) in all parts of the skeleton.*

This poison is mostly taken in with the drinking water. In children a dental disorder ("spotted teeth") develops, adults experience rheumatic pains reminiscent of ankylosing spondylitis. The earliest radiological signs appear in the vertebral column. In **Fig. 177** one can see a lateral **radiograph** of the spine in which the irregular density of the spongiosa *(1)* is striking. In some of the vertebral bodies *(2)* the framework of the spongiosa is almost completely sclerosed, in others there are still translucent regions. The outer contours of the vertebral bodies are undulating and poorly defined *(3)*, and here and there the edges are jagged *(4)*. The ligaments can also become less translucent, and a bony periostosis often develops.

Histologically there is marked irregular osteosclerosis. In **Fig. 178** one can see very wide, shapeless trabeculae *(1)* which are laminated, and the osteocytes are small *(2)*, although many of their lacunae are empty. In some places osteoblasts have been deposited on the

bony structures *(3)*. In some parts of the world, endemic fluorosis has been described, and this can be an occupational hazard for workers in aluminum or ceramic factories. Endemic fluorosis is seen in regions where the fluorine content of the drinking water is over 4 parts per thousand (the normal value is less than 1 mg per liter). In addition to the hyperostosis, simultaneous bone resorption may be seen alongside the osteosclerosis, leading to increased porosity. Radiologically, however, these osteopenic structures are masked by the hyperostosis.

Hypoparathyroidism

This is the opposite of hyperparathyroidism (p. 80). It results from reduced activity of the parathyroids, producing calcification of the soft tissues and sometimes osteosclerotic changes in the skeleton. *With idiopathic or postoperative hypoparathyroidism there is a diffuse osteosclerosis, which in children (idiopathic form) can lead to reduced growth, delayed tooth development and periarticular osteophyte formation. Postoperatively, after complete removal of all parathyroid tissue, osteosclerosis may arise in adults.* The cause may be primary anaplasia of the parathyroids or may follow the surgical removal of an adenoma which leaves insufficient tissue behind. Clinically there is hypocalcemia, hyperphosphatemia and hypocalcinuria.

In the **radiograph** of the skull shown in **Fig. 179** one can see an irregular, partly cloudy shadowing on the bone structure, which is very clear both in the skull cap *(1)* and in the bones of the jaws *(2)*. The outlines of these bones are irregular and indistinct, and the neighboring soft tissues may show signs of calcification. Typical of the condition is the appearance on the radiograph of calcium deposits in the stem ganglia. The reduction in bony tissue exchange (simultaneous falling off of deposition and resorption) can in the rarer cases lead to osteoporosis. In other words, the radiological findings with hypoparathyroidism are variable, non-specific and for diagnostic purposes not pathognomonic. In **Fig. 180** the biopsy from an osteosclerotic focus in a case of hypoparathyroidism shows **histologically** very dense sclerotic bone tissue, and sometimes widened *(1)*, some-

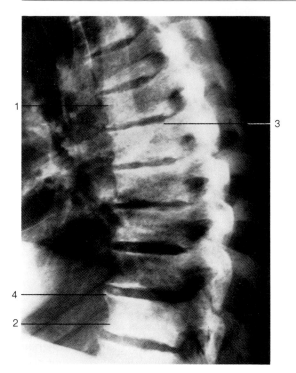

Fig. 177. Fluorosis (thoracic column)

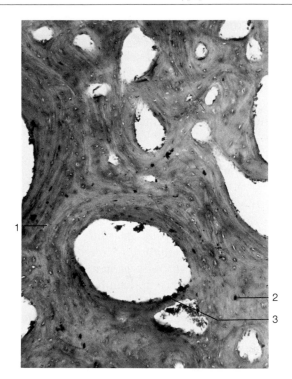

Fig. 178. Fluorosis; HE, ×25

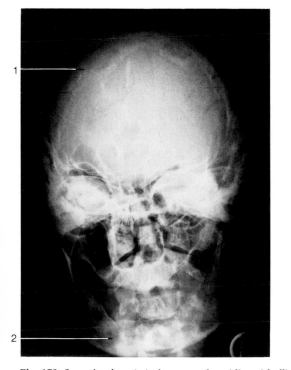

Fig. 179. Spongiosclerosis in hypoparathyroidism (skull)

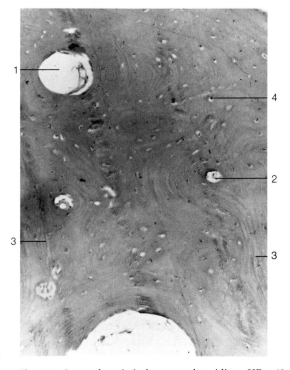

Fig. 180. Osteosclerosis in hypoparathyroidism; HE, ×40

times narrowed *(2)* Haversian canals with smooth walls. No deposited osteoblasts or osteoclasts can be identified. The bone tissue is strongly mineralized and irregularly laminated *(3)*, and contains relatively few and rather small osteocytes *(4)*. The osteosclerosis involves both the cortex and the cancellous scaffolding.

Osteitis deformans (Paget)

Paget's osteitis deformans ("Paget bone") is a bone dysplasia of unknown etiology that only affects older people on the far side of 40. It manifests itself as a monostotic, oligoostotic or polyostotic – but never as a generalized condition. In this age group it has been possible among 3% to 4% of hospital patients to identify a "Paget bone" which in more than half the cases has remained clinically silent. The monostotic form most often attacks the tibia and vertebral column, and 81% of all cases involve the stem skeleton (skull, spine, pelvis, femur or tibia). The *polyostotic form* (3% of cases) (**Fig. 181**) has a chequered distribution throughout the skeleton. Morphologically the condition is characterized by excessive bone remodeling.

One of the principal regions attacked by Paget's disease is the vertebral column. In the **radiograph** three changes are found: 1. a frame vertebra, 2. a trilaminate vertebra and 3. an ivory vertebra. In **Fig. 182** the development of a frame vertebra is much the most frequent. The outer contour of the lumbar vertebral bodies *(1)* is preserved. The spongiosa, however, is very irregular, having been remodeled by hypertrophic atrophy. One can observe the loss of the spongiosa from the large translucent foci *(2)* but also their replacement by very strong axially directed trabeculae *(3)*. There is also irregular sclerotic widening of the upper plate *(4)*.

This remodeling is particularly clear in the **maceration specimen** of the frame vertebra shown in **Fig. 183**. The central marrow cavity is framed by the marked thickening of the subcortical spongiosa *(1)*. The removal of the spongiosa from the middle layer is revealed both by the coarse gaps *(2)* and also by the single very strong vertical bone trabeculae *(3)*. In **Fig. 184** one can see the close-up of the **"Paget spongiosa"** of a vertebral body in which the

trabeculae are irregularly thickened *(1)* and to a large extent welded together into plate-like areas of bone *(2)*. It is striking that the outer bone structure *(3)* has an undulating and jagged border, which suggests the osteoblastic-osteoclastic bone remodeling that is in fact found. The marrow cavity is extensively narrowed by the excessive bone deposition *(4)*.

A diffuse cranial hyperostosis is extremely characteristic of Paget's osteitis deformans, and is particularly associated with the polyostotic form. In the **radiograph** of **Fig. 185** one can see that the bulge of the skull cap is greatly enlarged, and that its thickness has enormously increased (up to 5 cm, *1*). The lamina interna *(2)* is widened and its density sclerotically increased, due to a patchy osteosclerosis in which dense shadows with translucent edges can appear. The lamina externa is osteolytically loosened, thinned out and eccentrically displaced *(3)*. Such a radiological appearance is pathognomonic of Paget's osteitis deformans.

In the **maceration specimen** of **Fig. 186** one can clearly see the massive increase of the whole skull cap, which is overall greatly enlarged and thickened *(1)*. The normal spongio-

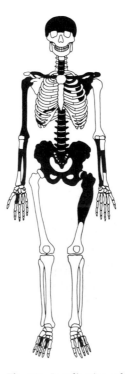

Fig. 181. Localization of osteitis deformans (Paget). (Modified from UEHLINGER)

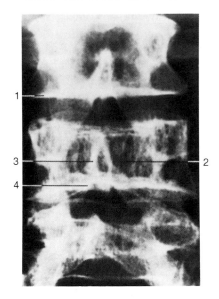

Fig. 182. Osteitis deformans (Paget)
(frame vertebra)

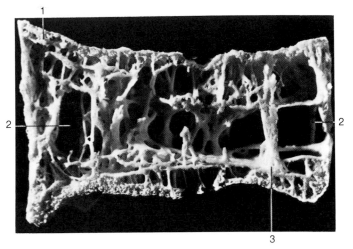

Fig. 183. Osteitis deformans (Paget)
(vertebra, maceration specimen)

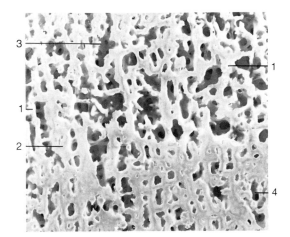

Fig. 184. Osteitis deformans (Paget)
(vertebral spongiosa, maceration specimen)

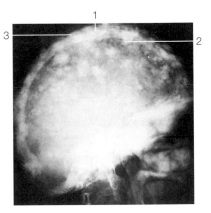

Fig. 185. Osteitis deformans (Paget) (skull)

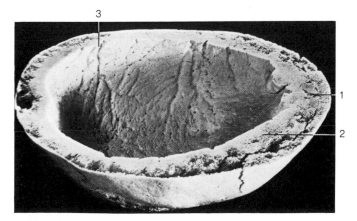

Fig. 186. Osteitis deformans (Paget) (skull cap, maceration specimen)

sa has been replaced by a light, finely porous pumice-like bone *(2)*. One therefore speaks of a "pumice-stone skull". Internally one can recognize the deeply embedded canals of the middle meningeal arteries *(3)*.

In the spongiosa, bone remodeling has led to *hypertrophic bone atrophy*. In the **radiograph** of **Fig. 187** one can see remodeling of the right femoral head *(1)* and neck *(2)*, that is reaching distally into the shaft. The angle of the neck is reduced; it can also bend to produce the so-called *"bishop's crook"* of the proximal part of the femur, leading to coxa vara.

The **histological picture** is characterized by excessive bone remodeling. This remodeling is accompanied by a raised vascularization of the cavity following the development of arteriovenous shunts, so that the blood supply of the bone can be increased up to twenty-fold. In this way the volume of the cardiac output of such patients is also increased. Histologically we can distinguish between 1. an initial osteolytic phase with numerous osteoclasts present, 2. an intermediate phase with reactive bone deposition by mononucleate polar osteoblasts and 3. a reconstructive end phase with the cementing together of bone fragments into a mosaic.

In **Fig. 188** one can see the **histological picture** of the intermediate phase of Paget's disease with its typical increased reactive bone deposition. There are irregularly widened bone trabeculae *(1)* in which the laminate structure is only partly preserved *(2)* and the numerous scattered cement lines are striking *(3)*. Rows of osteoblasts have been deposited on the bony structures *(4)*, next to which one can see resorption lacunae *(5)* laid down by osteoclasts. The marrow cavity is filled with loose fibrous tissue penetrated through by numerous dilated blood vessels *(6)*. **Figure 189** shows the **histological picture** of active Paget's disease. The bone trabeculae have only a partially regular lamination *(1)* among structures which have lost it altogether *(2)*. Rows of osteoblasts have been deposited on these bony structures *(3)*. In the deep lacunae there are many multinucleate osteoclasts *(4)*. The marrow cavity is filled with loose connective tissue *(5)* in which there are many isomorphic fibrocytes. Fibro-osseous trabeculae *(6)* can differentiate here.

In **Fig. 190** one can see a coarsely deformed bone trabecula with undulating borders *(1)* that

has been penetrated by irregular reversal lines *(2)* (so-called *mosaic structure)*. On one side it is being eroded by multinucleate osteoclasts (resorption) *(3)*, and on the other side new bone is being deposited by osteoblasts *(4)*. The highly vascularized marrow cavity is taken up by loose connective issue.

During the third stabilizing phase there is an osteosclerotic increase in the bone tissue. The trabeculae in **Fig. 191** are awkwardly enlarged and reveal a *mosaic pattern of reversal lines (1)* that have been produced by continuous bone deposition accompanied by simultaneous disorderly resorption. This confusion of short broken reversal lines is pathognomonic of Paget's disease, the bony tissue preserving its characteristic *"breccia" pattern* throughout. More osteoblasts *(2)* are arranged along the bony structures. The marrow shows signs of serous inflammation *(3)*. The bone tissue is incompletely calcified, and this leads to splinter-free fractures which heal with massive callus development. In 2% to 5% of cases an osteosarcoma (the so-called "Paget sarcoma") develops against the background of osteitis deformans. This is usually fatal within one year.

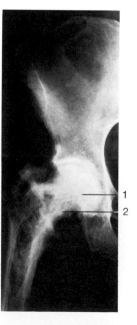

Fig. 187. Osteitis deformans (Paget) (right proximal femur, "bishop's crook")

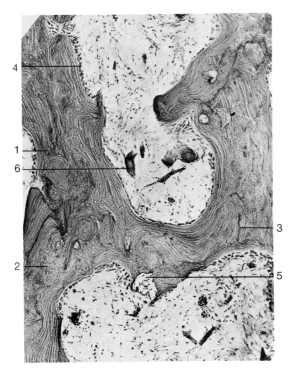

Fig. 188. Osteitis deformans (Paget); HE, ×40

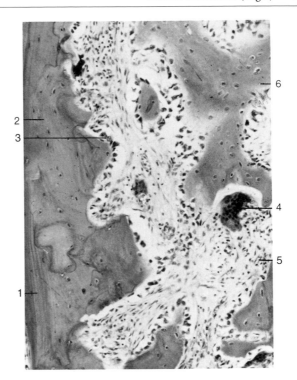

Fig. 189. Osteitis deformans (Paget); HE, ×64

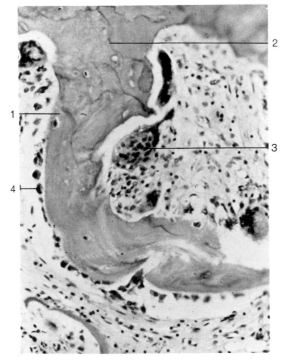

Fig. 190. Osteitis deformans (Paget); HE, ×82

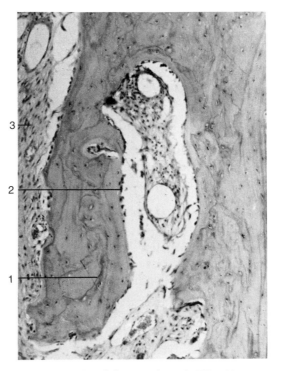

Fig. 191. Osteitis deformans (Paget); HE, ×64

Osteomyelosclerosis

An osteosclerotic increase in the density of the bony structures can result from a proliferation of the marrow in association with the development or deposition of new bone. *In cases of osteomyelosclerosis the marrow is generally replaced by connective and fibrous bone tissue, which leads to its continuing suppression and to insufficiency of the hematopoietic tissue itself.* Extramedullary hematopoietic foci develop in the spleen, liver and lymph nodes, and in other organs by which immature blood cells (normoblasts, myeloblasts, myelocytes) can be poured into the bloodstream. The liver and spleen are greatly enlarged (hepatosplenomegaly). These extramedullary hematopoietic foci are not able to make up for the suppression of the marrow, so that 10 to 20 years after the onset of the illness death follows from aplastic anemia. The terminal state of a third of the cases is a polycytemia or leukemia. No tissue substance is aspirated at sternal puncture. The diagnosis is confirmed by an iliac crest biopsy.

The bone remodeling in osteomyelosclerosis produces a patchy increase in the density of the spongiosa seen on the **radiograph**, with a scattering of cyst-like regions of translucency. In **Fig. 192** one can see a diffuse shadowing of the spongiosa in the whole of the proximal part of the tibia *(1)* which encroaches extensively upon the cortex *(2)*. The epiphysis *(3)* is significantly less involved in the sclerosing process. Fine patchy areas of translucency *(4)* are also found in the osteosclerotic bone.

Histologically one sees at first in the *fibro-osteoclastic initial phase* a focal transformation of the bone marrow into reticular connective tissue *(osteomyeloreticulosis)*. Later, an irregular network of collagen fibers develops which contains numerous capillaries. This stage of *osteomyelofibrosis* can be seen **histologically** in **Fig. 193**. Between the laminated cancellous trabeculae *(1)* the narrow cavity is filled with loose connective tissue consisting of collagen fibers of varying length and thickness *(2)*. Under polarized light the reticular connective tissue shows different degrees of birefringence. In the marrow cavity one can recognize a highly cellular marrow of lymphoid and reticular cells *(3)*, in which the megakaryocytes *(4)* are strikingly

increased. During the active medullary fibrosis the trabeculae are resorbed by osteoclasts and therefore display undulating borders *(5)*. In the *intermediate phase* a network of osteoid is laid down in the fibrous tissue of the bone marrow, and this will be transformed into fibrous bone in the final *phase of stabilization*. Rows of osteoblasts line the autochthonous sclerotic bone trabeculae *(6)*. **Figure 194** shows the complete picture of *osteomyelosclerosis.* The marrow cavity is filled with (sometimes dense, sometimes loosened) connective tissue *(1)* in which foci of immature erythro- and granulopoietic cells can be seen *(2)*. The giant cells with bizarre dark nuclei *(3)*, which are abnormal megakaryocytes, are striking. Whereas the osteoclasts are responsible for bone resorption during the stage of osteomyelofibrosis, with osteomyelosclerosis there are dense rows of active osteoblasts *(4)* lying along the trabeculae which bring about bone deposition. One can see bony structures which show no lamination and which contain strongly active osteocytes *(5)*.

In **Fig. 195** one can see an **osteomyelosclerosis** with autochthonous laminated bone trabeculae *(1)*, in which there are nevertheless fibro-osseous trabeculae *(2)* reaching into the marrow cavity. This intramedullary laying down of new bone projects a diffuse shadow of the marrow cavity onto the radiograph. This cavity is filled with erythro- and granulopoietic cells *(3)* among which numerous megakaryocytes are to be seen *(4)*, and near which myelofibrosis *(5)* can be recognized. The etiology of osteomyelosclerosis is unknown, possibly it is due to toxic damage to the bone marrow. It frequently follows a leucosis that has been treated with cytostatic drugs. On the other hand, acute leucosis can also often begin with osteomyelofibrosis, when it then becomes the initial form of a myeloproliferative bone marrow disease. After the normal hematopoietic bone marrow has been suppressed by a fibro-osseous proliferation process, a panmyelopathy with reduced production of erythro- and granulocytes (pancytopenia) ensues. The clinical course is that of progressive anemia and leucopenia with increasing displacement to the left in the peripheral blood. Sternal puncture produces an "empty bone marrow" *(punctio sicca)*.

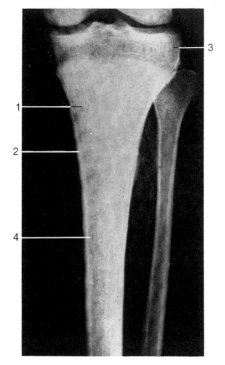

Fig. 192. Osteomyelosclerosis (proximal tibia)

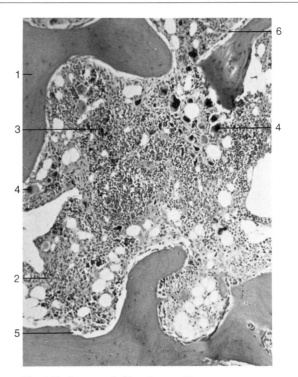

Fig. 193. Osteomyelofibrosis; van Gieson, ×25

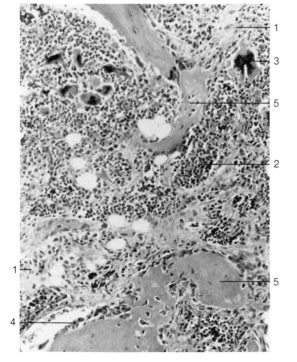

Fig. 194. Osteomyelosclerosis; HE, ×40

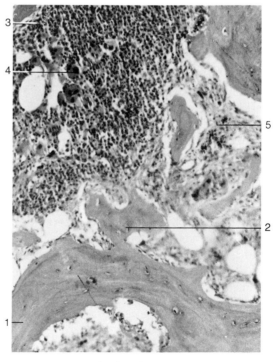

Fig. 195. Osteomyelosclerosis; HE, ×64

Melorheostosis

This rare osteosclerotic bone dysplasia was described in 1928 by Léri. He observed radiologically that an irregular mass of sclerotic bone was "flowing" in a limb, rather like congealing wax that had dripped from a candle. *Melorheostosis is a painful, non-inheritable progressive hyperostosis of unknown etiology, which usually appears in childhood in either the monostotic or polyostotic form, but usually affects only one limb* (**Fig. 196**). In a few cases it is without symptoms. The disease can follow a rapid course in childhood and then fade away in adult life, leaving behind painful joint contractures. Irregular bands of sclerotic bone tissue both line the endosteum and reach into the marrow cavity; or they can develop in the periosteum. Radiologically one finds long, wide, densely calcified bands running longitudinally in the limb bones. These changes most often affect the lower limb (**Fig. 196**).

In **Fig. 197** one can see the **macroscopic picture** of a classical melorheostosis of the distal part of the femur. A large tumor-like osseous mass *(1)* is attached to the outside of a long bone, where it appears as if it had flowed downwards like wax from a candle. The deposits vary in width and have transversely running notches *(2)*. The continuity is apparently interrupted *(3)*, and distally there is a more rugged mushroom-like hyperostosis *(4)* which gives the impression of a periosteal tumor. The periosteum opposite is also widened and ossified *(5)*.

Histologically such a lesion presents only osteosclerotic bone tissue without any kind of specific structure. In **Fig. 198** one sees this mature laminated bone tissue *(1)*. The Haversian canals *(2)* are narrowed, with smooth walls. There are no osteoblasts. In the adjacent marrow cavity one sees lightly fibrosed fatty tissue *(3)*, and sometimes metaplastic cartilaginous foci are also present. This is a congenital disorder of mesodermal development with a good prognosis, the progress of which mostly leads to a resolution. Only if the masses deposited on the bone cause symptoms is an operation necessary.

Osteopoikilosis

A peculiar form of osteosclerosis of the spongiosa in several bones was described in 1915 by Albers-Schönberg. *Osteopoikilosis is a harmless familial patchy spongiosclerosis, which is symptomless and most often discovered by accident radiologically.* It is not so much an actual bone disease, as an osteosclerotic bone dysplasia which is also known as *"osteopathia condensans disseminata"* or *"spotted bones"*. It can affect all the bones, most often in regions near the joints (**Fig. 199**). The skull is only exceptionally involved.

Figure 200 shows the classical **radiograph** of a case of osteopoikilosis. In this film of the knee joint one can see several round or oval foci of sclerosis *(1)* in the spongiosa of the proximal part of the tibia near the epiphysis and metaphysis, and similar foci are also present in the same region at the distal end of the femur *(2)*. The outer form of the other bony structures is unchanged.

Such numerous round densifications in the spongiosa, about the size of a lentil, can be met with at any age and in any bone, although they

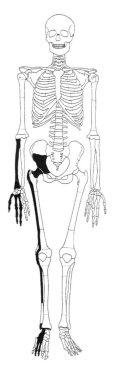

Fig. 196. Localization of melorheostosis

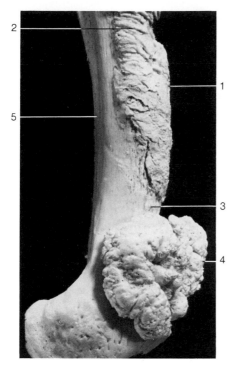

Fig. 197. Melorheostosis
(distal femur, maceration specimen)

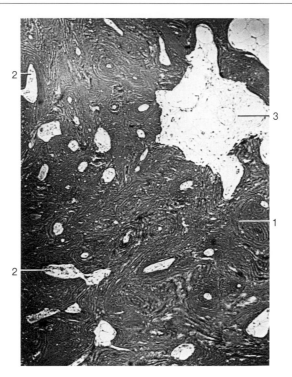

Fig. 198. Melorheostosis; HE, ×25

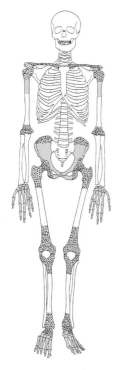

Fig. 199. Most frequent sites of osteopoikilosis foci

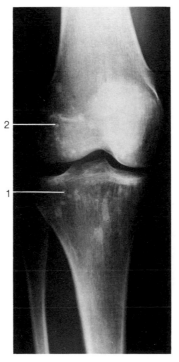

Fig. 200. Osteopoikilosis (distal femur, proximal tibia)

most frequently occur in the metaphyses of the long and short tubular bones and in the pelvis (near the acetabulum, **Fig. 199**). In the ribs and spinal column such changes are, however, only rarely encountered. Recognition of these patchy changes in the spongiosa is important; for one reason so that an unnecessary biopsy of such foci can be avoided, but also so that they may be distinguished from the osteosclerotic foci of metastases from a carcinoma of the prostate, from tuberous sclerosis and from sarcoidosis.

Figure 201 shows the **radiograph** of osteopoikilosis with multiple patchy focal scleroses in the bodies of the lumbar vertebrae *(1)* and the parasacral region of the pelvis *(2)*. The entire spongiosa of the imaged bones is spotty, because these foci frequently run together. They reach out into the cortex, which also appears pallid. The particularly marked increase in structural density near the sacrum is striking *(3)*. The lower ribs, on the other hand, show no such foci *(4)*.

The **radiograph** of osteopoikilosis in **Fig. 202** is particularly clear. One can see numerous coarse patchy densifications in the femoral head *(1)* and neck *(2)* and in the adjacent part of the pelvis *(3)*. Because of this the joint cavity of the right hip joint *(4)* is only incompletely identifiable. The femoral head of this 20-year-old man is obviously deformed. The intraosseous sclerotic foci are very close together and have partly united into large areas of sclerosis. This is an unusually well-marked case of osteopoikilosis. Since, however, all the signs of this condition are present, one should first undertake a scintigraphic examination before considering a biopsy. In this disease no increase in activity is to be expected, and therefore a diagnostic bone biopsy is only indicated when activity in one of the foci has been found on the scintigram, most particularly to exclude a possible bone metastasis.

The **radiograph** of **Fig. 203** shows the classical findings in osteopoikilosis, where all the wrist bones are involved *(1)*. There is a coarse patchy sclerosis of the spongiosa, which is often extensively confluent. The outer contours of these bones have been preserved. Coarse sclerotic patches can be seen from regions near the joints in the adjacent bones: radius *(2)*, ulna *(3)* and metacarpals *(4)*. In some places *(5)* the joint cavity is obscured by the osteosclerosis.

Histological examination of such bone changes (**Fig. 204**), which is not indicated during life, shows irregularly bordered foci of sclerotically densified laminated trabeculae in the cancellous framework. Peripherally the bone tissue is more dense, inside the foci it is markedly porous. Between these bony structures there is fatty marrow.

If it is necessary in such a case to exclude the differential diagnosis of osteoblastic bone metastases, a scintigram can be helpful. Unlike the metastatic foci, no increase in activity is found in the scintigram of osteopoikilosis. A biopsy is not necessary.

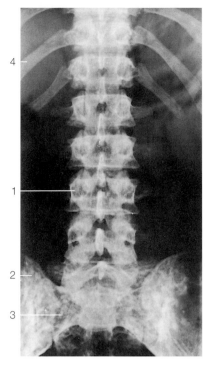

Fig. 201. Osteopoikilosis (lumbar column, lateral mass)

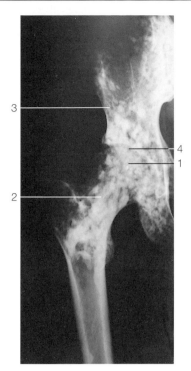

Fig. 202. Osteopoikilosis (right hip joint)

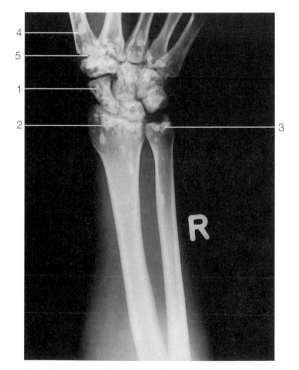

Fig. 203. Osteopoikilosis (right wrist joint)

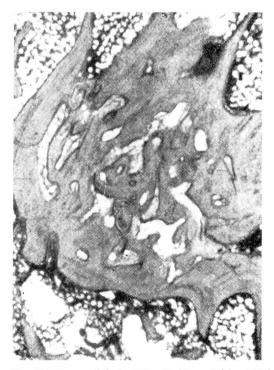

Fig. 204. Osteopoikilosis; HE, ×64. (From Schinz 1952)

6 Bone Fractures

General

Fractures, in all their variety, are very frequent events. Diagnosis normally depends upon clinical examination and the radiological findings. In many cases, because of the treatment or because of some particular indication (a so-called "pathological" fracture, for instance), tissue is removed from the region of the injury for histological examination in order to obtain information about a possible underlying bone disease. *A fracture is a complete or incomplete solution of continuity of a bone that has been brought about by direct or indirect violence.* As is well known, a fracture is immediately followed by severe pain (periosteal pain) and the affected area is incapable of active movement.

We distinguish between a *traumatic fracture* (immediate fracture) and a *long-term fracture* (fatigue fracture, stress fracture or spontaneous fracture type I; **Fig. 211**) and a *pathological fracture* (spontaneous fracture type II; **Fig. 212**). A traumatic fracture involves a supraliminal trauma with a degree of local violence that exceeds the natural elasticity of the bone. This is usually accompanied by simultaneous injury to the soft tissues and very often the skin. With *closed fractures* the adjacent soft tissues (periosteum, fascia, muscles, vessels, nerves) may also be injured, but the covering soft parts are largely preserved. In this case the damaged bone is given a certain amount of protection against bacteria entering through a wound, and the risk of infection is less. With an *open fracture* (earlier known as a "compound fracture") the broken ends of the bone are freed by extensive soft tissue injury, so that pathogenic bacteria from outside can enter the wound directly. Basically every open fracture should be regarded as infected, since it carries with it the risk of a secondary purulent osteomyelitis. For this reason antibiotic treatment is begun immediately.

From the surgical point of view fractures are classified according to the mechanical nature of the break. This is responsible for the different radiological appearances (p. 115), the diagnostic evaluation of which is very important for specialist reports and also for matters of practical treatment. The dislocation (or displacement) of the bone ends must be taken into account. With *incomplete fractures* only fissures or cracks without displacement are seen in the radiograph. These include the so-called *"greenstick"* fractures of children, in whom the extremely elastic periosteal tube keeps the bone ends together, allowing at most bending (axial deviation) to occur. Such bone injuries are revealed by the radiograph, the removal of tissue is unnecessary.

A fracture initiates natural reactions in the local tissue which lead to a reconstitution of the bone continuity. Essential for fracture healing are: (1) internal contact of the bone ends, (2) uninterrupted immobility of the part, and (3) an adequate blood supply. If these three conditions are present, *primary healing* will take place. The break will be invaded by longitudinally directed osteons without any intermediate intervention of connective tissue or cartilage, and no distorting changes in shape due to resorption will occur (contact healing). The minimal space is filled primarily with bone tissue, but without supporting tissue – which is later remodeled by lamellar bone – differentiating. With all conservative fracture treatment, constant rest and internal contact of the bone ends is absent, and ossification takes place indirectly, with the temporary formation of connective and cartilaginous supporting tissue *(callus)* which later differentiates secondarily into bone. During *secondary bone healing* a characteristic cartilaginous callus develops. The presence of metaplastic cartilaginous tissue in a callus is always a sign that the bone ends have been inadequately immobilized.

Types of Bone Fracture

Depending on the structural characteristics of the fracture seen in the **radiograph**, various types and forms of fracture can be distinguished, both by the course of the fracture line and the position of the ends or fragments of bone. These radiological differences are of technical and surgical significance. The different forms of fracture are determined by the way the violence was applied and by the simultaneous action of the local muscles.

In the **radiograph** of **Fig. 205** one can see an *oblique torsion fracture* of the distal part of the tibia. The fracture line *(1)* is clearly seen to be slightly gaping and rather smooth. The two bone ends *(2)* have been displaced sideways from each other and also pressed together in the long axis. In addition to the oblique fracture, the bone ends have moved so that the point of the lower fragment *(3)* lies behind that of the upper fragment *(4)* and to one side of it. One can also see that the proximal end of the fibula *(5)* is fractured. This is a recent fracture, so that no shadow of callus appears on the radiograph.

In **Fig. 206** a simple *transverse fracture* through the tibia *(1)* of a child is displayed. The epiphyseal lines *(2)* are still present. The fracture crosses the tibial shaft, and the fracture line is gaping slightly. Both ends of the bone lie in the long axis, and have not been driven into each other. They are held together within the elastic sleeve of the periosteum. The bone tissue near the injury is somewhat sclerotic. In children such a *closed fracture* heals under conservative treatment with callus formation.

Figure 207 shows a *comminuted fracture* of the distal ends of the radius and ulna. Just below the wrist joint *(1)* all that remains of the long bones is a group of coarse fragments *(2)* that have escaped from the bone as a whole. A large piece of bone *(3)* appears to have undergone sclerotic change. Such a destructive bone injury suggests severe trauma, as a result of which the adjacent soft tissues would also have been damaged *("open fracture")*. The single pieces of bone may become necrotic and would then have later to be removed surgically as so-called sequestra (p. 164).

Figure 208 shows the **radiograph** of a typical *fractured femoral neck,* of the kind frequently encountered in old people. One can see the wide fracture line *(1)*, with the bone ends – the femoral head *(2)* and the intertrochanteric region *(3)* – driven together distally and impacted on one side *(4)*. The head shows signs of arthrotic deformity and an irregular sclerotic increase in density. The periosteum is widened near the fracture *(5)*, but with no signs of callus formation. The bone outside the region of the break shows signs of osteoporosis *(6)* (p. 72), which is often the cause of a spontaneous fracture of the femoral neck.

As can be seen in **Fig. 209**, a *compression fracture* is very obvious in the vertebral column. The undamaged bodies of the lumbar vertebrae *(1)* show signs of advanced porosity of the spongiosa; the supporting bone appearing fairly strong, whereas the transverse component is rarefied (p. 68). Because of this osteoporosis, one of the lumbar vertebrae has collapsed under the weight of the body. The vertebral body *(2)* is greatly narrowed, and the density of the spongiosa increased by compression. Here and there wide gaps in the spongiosa *(3)* are still to be seen. The intervertebral spaces adjacent to the compressed vertebra *(4)* are much wider. *A series of rib fractures* following an accident is mostly observed in patients who are already shocked. This means that the radiological examination has to take place with the patient in bed, and the radiographs are consequently less satisfactory. Several fractured ribs can be seen in **Fig. 210**. The fracture lines gape somewhat and the bone ends are displaced *(2)*.

To bring about uncomplicated healing as quickly as possible, it is absolutely essential to keep the ends of the broken bones immobile. Continued mobility can cause a *pseudarthrosis* to develop in such a fracture; it remains unhealed, and the function of the part involved is severely impaired or even destroyed. Immobility is ensured either by plaster bandages or osteosynthetic treatment, and this leads to bony union and stability. In the case of fractured ribs, complete immobility is impossible because of respiration, and it is here that a characteristic cartilaginous callus develops.

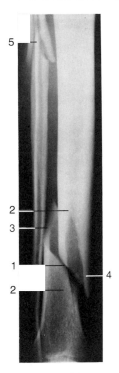
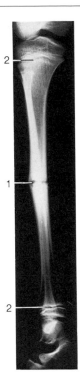
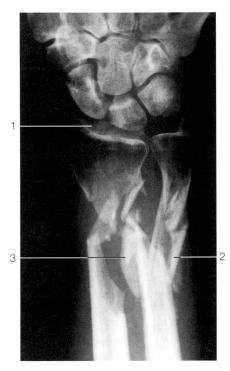

Fig. 205. Oblique torsion fracture (distal tibia)

Fig. 206. Transverse fracture (mid-shaft tibia)

Fig. 207. Comminuted fracture (distal radius and ulna)

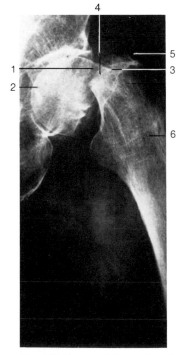
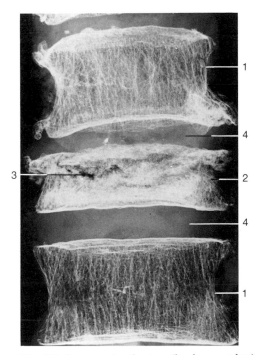
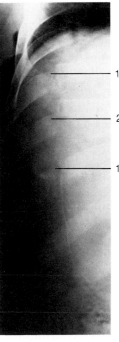

Fig. 208. Fractured femoral neck

Fig. 209. Compression fracture (lumbar vertebra)

Fig. 210. A vertical series of fractures involving several ribs

Figure 211 shows a *creeping fracture* (fatigue fracture) *(1)* of the proximal part of the tibia of a child. The affected region of the bone is sclerotic and very dense, with a particularly dark shadowy band of osteosclerosis *(1)* running transversely across the long bone. This is the fracture itself, the line of which is invisible or only indicated by a fissure. The reactive osteosclerotic apposition of bone occupies most of the radiograph, and reactive thickening of the periosteum is developing, mostly with periostitis ossificans. The creeping fracture is developing very slowly in a region of bone which has been subjected to continuous overloading (*"stress fracture"*). A similar lesion in a metatarsal is known as a *"march fracture"*. Fractures which appear in connection with the so-called *Milkman's syndrome* in "Looser's transformation zones" (osteodystrophy, p. 80) also represent creeping fractures in shattered regions of the skeleton. Following removal of the load and intermittent rest for the affected limb, spontaneous healing of the fracture may occur.

A **pathological fracture** arises spontaneously, without there being adequate trauma to account for it. From this it may be inferred that the bone has been previously damaged, either by systemic disease (e.g. osteoporosis, osteodystrophy, Paget's osteitis deformans) or by a local bone lesion (e.g. metastasis, radio-osteonecrosis or a bone tumor). Bone metastases are a common cause of spontaneous pathological fractures. **Figure 212** shows such a fracture in the proximal part of the femur *(1)*. The rather smooth ends of the bones are very characteristic. The fracture itself is gaping, and the bone ends are only slightly displaced relative to one another. No developing callus can be seen. The other parts of the femur show the typical loose structure of an involutional osteoporosis (p. 72), without any signs of intraosseous lesions. There is also severe arthritis of the hip-joint. In cases of pathological fractures, it is essential to remove tissue for histological examination from the neighborhood of the fracture during operation (and if necessary from the iliac crest) in order to diagnosis the underlying disease.

Normal Uncomplicated Fracture Healing

The healing of a fracture starts with proliferation of the local mesenchyme and the development of a *fracture callus*. The regular chain of events within the tissue is diagrammatically illustrated in **Fig. 213**. The fracture tears the vessels of the bone, producing bleeding into the space and the development of a *fracture hematoma* between the ends of the bones (**Fig. 213a**). On the second day, fibroblasts, osteoclasts and capillaries invade and begin to organize the blood clot, in which young connective tissue is being laid down. Within a week (between the 2nd and 8th days) a *temporary connective tissue callus* (**Fig. 213b**) is built up between the bone ends, which is, however, incapable of weight-bearing. Between the 7th and 9th days, together with the development of fibrillar connective tissue, hydroxyapatite is deposited on the collagen fibers. Undifferentiated mesenchyme cells are transformed into osteoblasts, and these produce osteoid, which then becomes mineralized. Fibrous bone trabeculae appear, without osteoblast deposition, and these form a mechanical connection between the bone ends. This *temporary bone callus*, which is also still incapable of weight-bearing, remains until the 4th week (**Fig. 213c**). If, during this stage of fracture healing, pressure or shear forces act on the bones, cartilaginous tissue may form in the callus by endochondral ossification (*"cartilaginous callus"*). During this phase of healing the debris at the fracture site is removed by osteoclasts. After 4 to 5 weeks the *definitive callus* develops, in which the fibrous bone is gradually broken down by *"creeping substitution"* and replaced by lamellar bone (**Fig. 213d**). During fracture healing, which accompanies development of the fracture callus (secondary bone healing), the fracture hematoma will first be replaced by granulation tissue. The fibrous connective tissue differentiates into fibrocartilage and finally into fibrous bone, which brings about fixed contact between the bone ends. In this way the two bones become temporarily united, which is a good precondition for secondary fracture healing. At this stage, however, the bone still remains unstable.

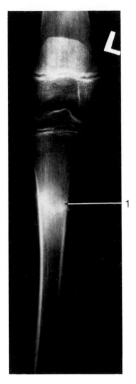

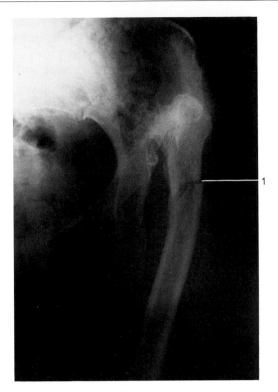

Fig. 211. Creeping or fatigue fracture (proximal tibia)

Fig. 212. Pathological fracture (proximal femur)

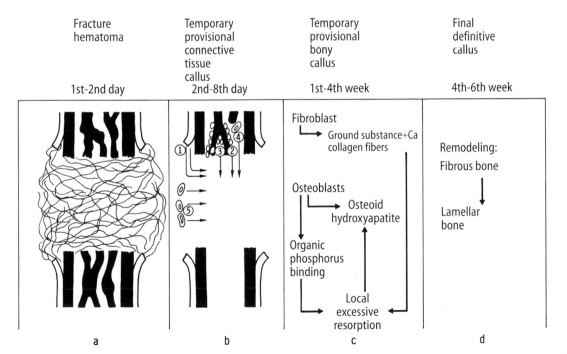

Fig. 213 a–d. Fracture healing (diagrammatic): *1* periosteum, *2* endosteum (osteoblasts), *3* Haversian canals, *4* blood vessels in marrow cavity, *5* blood vessels in soft parts

Figure 214 shows a low-power section through a fibular fracture in which a *temporary connective tissue callus* has developed. One can recognize the two sideways displaced bone ends *(1)*, with cortex *(2)* and a marrow cavity *(3)* that is filled with fatty tissue, and which contains only a few cancellous trabeculae. Signs of osteoporosis are also present. The fracture line has been bridged over by loose connective tissue *(4)*. This consists partly of granulation tissue with complete and sprouting capillaries, together with some infiltration of lymphocytes, plasma cells and histiocytes. Inside the connective tissue – and particularly around the edges – slender fibrous trabeculae *(5)* which are irregularly connected with one another have developed. They form a "bony shell" around the connective tissue callus and also appear outside the actual fracture in the region of the periosteum *(6)*, where they constitute a radiologically identifiable sign of reactive *periostitis ossificans*.

In the **diagrammatic illustration** of **Fig. 215** the bony structures of the fibular fracture are emphasized with Indian ink. One can recognize the two bone ends *(1)*, which are displaced sideways. The spongiosa *(2)* contains only a few trabeculae, and the cortex *(3)* is relatively porous with Haversian canals. Therefore osteoporosis is present. The pure connective tissue fracture callus *(4)* is hatched in the diagram. It is bridging over the fracture and binding the two bone ends together. It is only in the peripheral region of this connective tissue callus *(5)* that one can see incompletely mineralized bony structures (fibrous bone), which have not yet, however, bridged over the fracture. It is obvious that such a "filling tissue" offers no support against pressure or bending forces, and even the strong periosteal new bone *(6)* has only a limited stabilizing effect.

A biopsy of the active fracture callus can sometimes present the most enormous diagnostic difficulties histologically if a radiograph is not to hand, and if one can only observe a single section through the proliferative process. **Figure 216** shows such a **histological picture** of a temporary connective tissue fracture callus. One can recognize the loose connective and granulation tissue, which has been invaded by numerous blood capillaries *(1)* and which is often considerably spread out and filled with blood *(2)*. One can see collections of lymphocytes, plasma cells, histiocytes and a few granulocytes, especially around the blood vessels *(3)*. Within this connective tissue, fibro-osseous trabeculae have differentiated *(4)*, forming a network which contains well-developed osteocytes. Rows of active osteoblasts *(5)* have been deposited on these trabeculae, and a few osteoclasts, most of which are lying in flattened resorption lacunae. Vigorous bone remodeling (simultaneous deposition and resorption) is taking place. In unstable fractures (e.g. fractured ribs) additional newly developed areas of cartilage can also be seen within the fracture callus.

The maturation of fibro-osseous trabeculae and their mineralization is most advanced in the periphery of the connective tissue callus. In the **histological photograph** of **Fig. 217** one can see on one side lamellar bone *(1)* which is probably autochthonous bone tissue. The broken ends of the bone are increasingly resorbed by osteoclasts *(2)*. Next to this, fibro-osseous trabeculae *(3)* have developed along which rows of osteoblasts *(4)* have been deposited. Between these bony structures there is loose and moderately cellular connective and granulation tissue *(5)*, with capillaries and a few inflammatory cells. This inflammatory granulation tissue, of a kind that one can recognize histologically in biopsy material from a healing fracture, is reactive in nature and part of the secondary healing process. It has nothing to do with the true osteomyelitis that can – especially after an open fracture or operation – certainly appear as a complication of fracture healing when bacteria from outside produce a local wound infection. In cases of severe local inflammation the expression "osteitis" is frequently employed.

During *primary fracture healing* a direct union of the two bone ends takes place, with the narrow gap being bridged over by osteons from both sides and without any inflammatory reaction. *Secondary fracture healing*, however, involves local inflammation and the development of a callus. Osteoid seams are laid down near the sprouting vessels of the granulation tissue, and bone-building cells (osteoblasts) must first differentiate from the pluripotent mesenchyme cells before the callus is finally replaced by mature bone tissue.

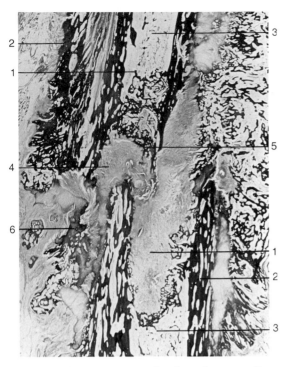

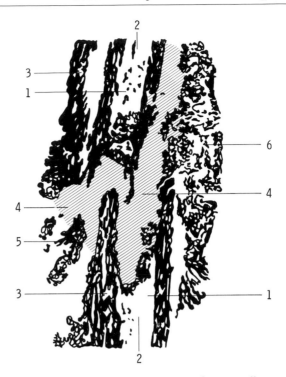

Fig. 214. Temporary connective tissue fracture callus; HE, ×20

Fig. 215. Temporary connective tissue fracture callus (diagrammatic)

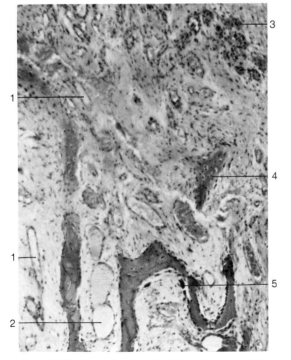

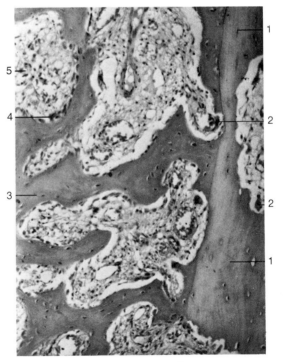

Fig. 216. Temporary connective tissue fracture callus; HE, ×25

Fig. 217. Fibro-osseous fracture callus; HE, ×25

Figure 218 shows the **histological picture** of a *temporary bony callus*. In the upper part of the picture one can see newly differentiated fibro-osseous trabeculae *(1)* with numerous osteocytes and a layer of deposited osteoblasts. In between, there is loose connective and granulation tissue *(2)* which has been invaded by blood capillaries. These structures represent immature bone tissue from the transitional zone between the temporary connective tissue callus and the true bone callus. New bone formation then progresses, and one can see wide, clumsy structures *(3)* which are largely mineralized. The osteocytes are prominent and irregularly deposited. It is still not possible to discern lamination of the bone tissue. Rows of osteoblasts *(4)* have been deposited, and here and there wide seams of osteoid *(5)* can be observed. This formation of new bone, together with bone apposition, is taking place simultaneously with osteoclastic resorption within a pattern of creeping substitution. In particular, the autochthonous bridging elements of the fracture are being resorbed.

Sometimes a proliferating hyperplastic fracture callus may have a polymorphic appearance which recalls that of a malignant tumor, and a biopsy from such a callus may easily be mistaken for an osteosarcoma. In **Fig. 219** one can see the **histological picture** of a proliferating hyperplastic fracture callus. There is a confusing network of fibro-osseous trabeculae *(1)* along which osteoblasts have been deposited. In places this new bone tissue is heavily mineralized and seems to have a laminated appearance *(2)*. Between the bony structures there is a highly cellular stroma of connective tissue *(3)* in which one sees darkly nucleated fibroblasts and mitoses. The atypical cellular cartilaginous tissue *(4)* that has differentiated among the bony structures is striking. It contains polymorphous and multinucleated cartilage cells (so-called *cartilaginous callus*). The whole picture reminds one of the checkered distribution of the variously differentiated tissues in an osteosarcoma (p. 274). Only by taking into account the clinical findings, the radiographic appearance and the histological picture can a reliable diagnosis be ensured.

In **Fig. 220** one can see a **maceration specimen** of a very large hyperplastic fracture callus

(callus luxurians). This is an old fractured femoral neck which healed while the bone ends remained apart. The femoral head *(1)* has been included in the mass of the callus *(2)*, the spongiosa of which has undergone hypertrophic atrophy (p. 72). Parts of the callus have reached out well into the surrounding soft parts, and they reveal a completely disorganized construction, characterized by a dense cortex-like bony shell *(3)* and an assemblage of ungainly trabeculae *(4)*, together with large cystic spaces *(5)*. Distally, the cortex of the adjacent part of the shaft *(6)* has been drawn into this thoroughly disorganized bone remodeling process. Both radiologically and macroscopically such a hyperplastic fracture callus can give the observer the impression of a bone tumor.

Figure 221 presents the **histological picture** of an old bone callus in a fracture that is already consolidated. The bony structures are widely distributed and contain large numbers of osteocytes *(1)*. The bone tissue is fully mineralized and organized into lamellae. The original fibrous bone has already been replaced by lamellar bone. Rows of osteoblasts *(2)* and a few osteoclasts in flattened resorption lacunae *(3)* nevertheless provide evidence of continuing bone remodeling. The marrow cavity is filled with a loose connective tissue *(4)* that has been invaded by wide blood capillaries *(5)*. During the subsequent course of fracture healing, this residual callus becomes included in the Haversian system of osteons, and the original cancellous structure with fatty marrow is again restored. Under satisfactory conditions (an uncomplicated fracture with adequate immobilization) the fracture is healed by callus formation as described above in about six weeks. It is laid down upon the extensive inner surface of the spongiosa, which favors the regular deposition of callus. The degree of dislocation also plays an important part here. A pertrochanteric fracture with marked dislocation is only ready for weight bearing after 10 to 14 weeks. Lengthy oblique fractures of the long bones of the limbs are ready to take up the load earlier than short oblique or transverse fractures. A compression fracture of a vertebral body, in which the whole of the spongiosa is jammed together, needs to be kept free of pressure for many weeks.

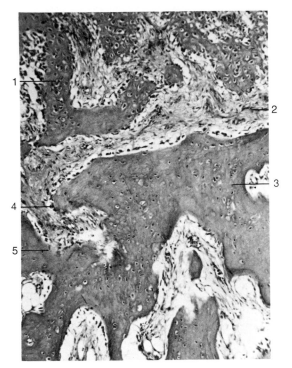

Fig. 218. Temporary bony fracture callus; HE, ×25

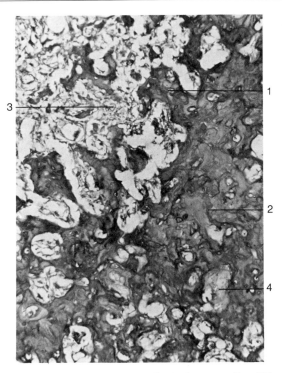

Fig. 219. Proliferating hyperplastic fracture callus; HE, ×25

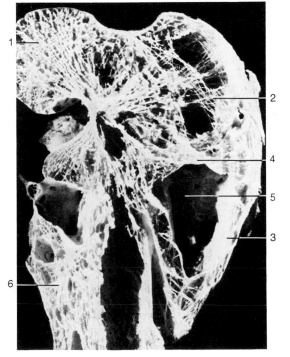

Fig. 220. Hyperplastic fracture callus
(proximal femur, maceration specimen)

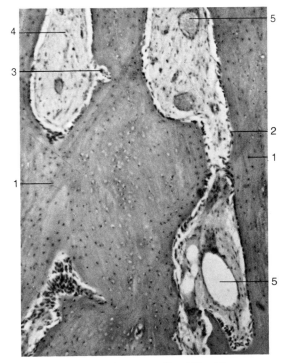

Fig. 221. Old bony fracture callus; HE, ×25

Complications of Bone Fractures

Spongiosal Plastic Treatment. Modern accident surgery includes many procedures designed to accelerate fracture healing and allow the patient to become mobile again with minimal delay. At the same time, these make it possible to avoid many of the dreaded complications associated with a broken bone. The most important of these are the various osteosynthetic procedures by which the bone fragments are brought into their original relationship and anchored there with nails, plates or screws. In cases of delayed fracture healing or pseudarthrosis, *transplants of spongiosa* are also often introduced around the fracture site. In this way bony union across the fracture line can often be accelerated. After the curetting of a pathological area of bone (e. g. tumor, osteomyelitis) the remaining cavity is filled up with autogenous spongiosa. This encourages the formation of organized tissue or temporary connective tissue callus. The cancellous implant is finally resorbed by creeping substitution and replaced by stable bone tissue.

Figure 222 shows the **radiograph** of a fracture of the distal part of the femur, which has been stabilized by applying a plate *(1)* which is then fixed to the bone with screws *(2)*. A cancellous transplant was also inserted into the fracture *(3)*, which can be recognized radiologically by its rather fainter shadow.

In **Fig. 223** one can recognize **histologically** within the cancellous scaffolding *(1)* the remains of an earlier implant of foreign spongiosa *(2)*. This is blue because of the uptake of calcium salts; no more lamellar layering is to be seen and there are no osteocytes. This devitalized bone tissue is being surrounded by newly deposited young bone tissue *(3)* in the course of the healing process. Within this formation one can recognize drawn out reversal lines *(4)* which mark the various leading edges of the bone deposition. The exogenous spongiosa is built into the appositional bone production, and this is followed by the gradual integration of the foreign tissue into the deposition process. No osteoclastic resorption of the exogenous bone is to be seen.

Metallosis. *By metallosis one understands the production of local soft tissue and bone damage in the neighborhood of a metallic bone implant, where the metal acts as a foreign body and releases a non-specific inflammatory process.* It represents a frequent complication of osteosynthetic treatment and has a negative influence on the process of healing. Today nearly 5% of osteosyntheses lead to metallosis. These reactive inflammatory processes in the neighborhood of a metallic prosthesis can lead to its becoming loose. In the **radiograph** shown in **Fig. 224** the condition of the right hip joint is shown after the implantation of a total endoprosthesis (TEP). The implanted prosthesis is easily recognized in the radiograph *(1)*. The surrounding bone tissue in the upper part of the femur shows an osteosclerotic increase in density around the prosthesis *(2)*, which almost reaches up to the prosthesis itself. One can, however, observe a narrow translucent region *(3)* between the prosthesis and the bone. Furthermore, there are several osteolytic foci *(4)* within the femur near the prosthesis. The radiological changes are evidence of vigorously reactive bone remodeling near the prosthesis and also indicate that it is becoming loose.

In **Fig. 225** one can see the **histological substrate** of this tissue in the neighborhood of the implanted prosthesis. It consists of very fibrous scar tissue *(1)* in which large and small particles of iron have been deposited *(2)*. In their neighborhood the scar tissue has become organized and replaced by highly cellular connective tissue *(3)*. The coarse iron fragments appear as brownish foreign bodies *(2)*; the fine iron deposits are stained by the Berlin blue and appear blue. These iron particles produce local tissue damage (tissue necrosis) with subsequent loosening of nails implanted into the marrow, or of an endoprosthesis. The metallic foreign bodies have a mechanical action (damage to the vitality of the tissue), and a physico-chemical action by which electrophoretic effects that corrode the metal are induced in the tissue fluids. In about 80% of cases there are signs of metallosis in the surrounding tissue after the metal has been removed.

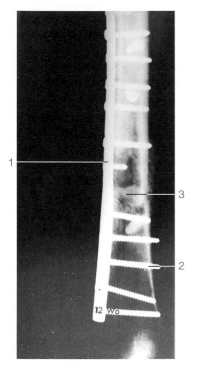

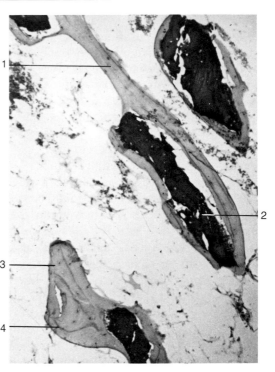

Fig. 222. Fracture treated by osteosynthesis and a cancellous implant (distal femur)

Fig. 223. Old cancellous implant which has become embedded; HE, ×25

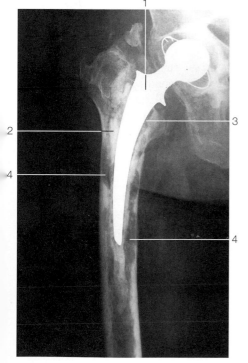

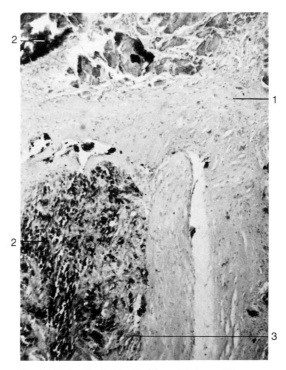

Fig. 224. Hip prosthesis which has become loosened due to metallosis (right hip joint)

Fig. 225. Metallosis; Berlin blue staining, ×25

Pseudarthrosis. If, following a fracture, insufficient callus is formed and after a long time no bony union is established, the two bone ends form a kind of joint and are able to move relative to one another. *One uses the term pseudarthrosis if for a long time after a bone is fractured the two ends fail to form a bony union, and a joint-like mobility persists in the region of the original fracture.* This development of a "false joint" is always a complication to be feared after a bone has been broken. It is a defective healing with serious functional consequences, since such a bone is naturally not able to bear weight.

The classical **radiological appearance** of a pseudarthrosis can be seen in **Fig. 226.** It deals with the condition of a fracture of the lower part of the leg. One can still clearly recognize a wide and gaping fracture line *(1)* in the tibia and in the adjacent fibula *(2)*. The bone ends are slightly angled to one another. On both sides of the fracture the density of the bone is sclerotically increased *(3)*, and the fracture line is undulating and poorly defined. One can clearly recognize the excessive callus formation *(4)* which has been built up beside the fracture. Obviously the fracture was insufficiently stabilized by an osteosynthetic plate, since one can now see the screw holes which held the plate in position *(5)*. Distal to the pseudarthrosis there is an immobility osteoporosis *(6)* of the bone.

In **Fig. 227** one can see the **radiograph** of an old comminuted fracture of the distal part of the tibia *(1)* on which osteosynthesis had been carried out. In spite of this treatment no adequate callus developed. A wide, gaping fracture line *(2)* passes through the bone, the fragments *(3)* of which are easily recognized. Both bone ends show signs of an inactivity osteoporosis (p. 74). Since the smaller bone fragments of the comminuted fracture show a faded irregular density, it must be assumed from the radiograph that we are here probably dealing with necrotic bone tissue that may well have contributed to the development of the pseudarthrosis.

Figure 228 shows an *overall* **histological section** which offers an overall view of such a pseudarthrosis. The cancellous trabeculae of the bone ends *(1)* are irregularly distributed and, because of the reactive bone remodeling, of unequal thickness. There is no building up of bone callus. The fracture line is bridged over only by highly fibrous connective tissue *(2)* in which degenerative gaps *(3)* have appeared. It is necessary to remove this connective tissue surgically in order to stimulate bone deposition within the fracture. To this end one attempts to induce more vigorous deposition of the host bone by implanting autogenous or heterogenous spongiosa. Then, while a fibro-osseous callus is developing, new bone tissue is laid down and at the same time the cancellous implant is resorbed. The original fracture or pseudarthrotic line is then bridged over by bone, and this leads to a stable union of the fracture (secondary bone healing).

Post-fracture Osteomyelitis. A greatly feared complication of fractures is infection of the region accompanied by the development of osteomyelitis. This applies particularly to *open fractures*, which are potentially infected and must therefore be treated from the start with antibiotics. In **Fig. 229** one can see the **histological picture** of post-fracture osteomyelitis. The autochthonous trabeculae *(1)* in the region of the fracture are fragmented and often present only as small pieces *(2)*. In between, one can see a highly cellular inflammatory granulation tissue *(3)* which has been infiltrated by plasma cells, lymphocytes and granulocytes, together with many blood-filled capillaries *(4)*. The tissue in a fresh fracture also contains blood and fibrin. Sometimes bacterial invasion can also be demonstrated histologically.

There is a whole collection of complications which may appear after a bone has been fractured. *Increased bone remodeling* may produce a coarse straggly spongiosa or *Sudeck's bone atrophy* (p. 96). Partial *osteonecrosis* may be found in the region of a fracture, leading to the development of sequestra. This impairs bone healing and can lead to a pseudarthrosis. In some cases *excessive callus development* (**callus luxurians**) may take place, and fractures through joints may be followed by *post-traumatic arthrosis*.

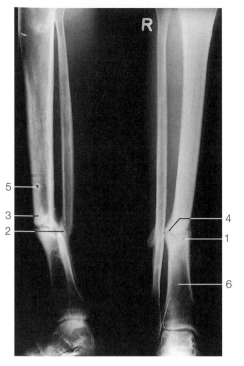

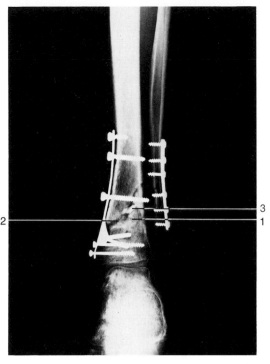

Fig. 226. Pseudarthrosis (distal tibia and fibula)

Fig. 227. Pseudarthrosis following a comminuted fracture treated by osteosynthesis (distal tibia)

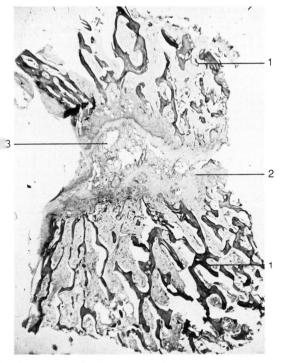

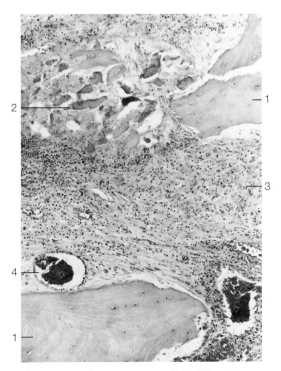

Fig. 228. Pseudarthrosis (overall view); HE, ×2

Fig. 229. Post-fracture osteomyelitis; HE, ×40

Pathological Bone Fractures

A normally developed and properly formed bone is able to resist the physiological action of pressure, shear and bending forces and can, for a short time, withstand an excessive degree of these forces without being in any way damaged. It is only when a traumatic force exceeds the resistance threshold of the bone tissue that the bone breaks. *A pathological fracture is a fracture that has been brought about by inadequate trauma, the underlying cause being a pathological alteration of the bone tissue.* When absolutely no traumatic violence has led to a fracture, we call this a ***spontaneous fracture.*** The underlying bone disease is diagnosed by radiological and histological examination. There are many local and generalized skeletal diseases that involve breakdown of the tela ossea or changes in the bone quality, and can thus be the cause of a fracture. A general reduction of the bone tissue is present in all forms of osteoporosis, and this is more local in the presence of osteomyelitis, a bone tumor or bone metastases. The quality of the bone tissue can also be damaged by insufficient mineralization in osteomalacia or by Paget's osteitis deformans.

In **Fig. 230** the **radiological appearance** of a pathological fracture in the distal part of the leg can be seen, and one can recognize a large bone defect *(1)* that has arisen in the distal third of the tibia. Although the fracture has been treated osteosynthetically with a plate and screws *(2)*, a pseudarthrosis has developed. The cancellous structure of the bone is very indistinct, particularly in the distal part of the fracture *(3)*. Here there are osteolytic defects which also involve the cortex. These bone changes and the following fracture are due to a *purulent osteomyelitis* that is persisting. In addition to this, we can also see a fracture of the distal part of the fibula *(4)*, which has itself been treated by osteosynthesis.

A primary bone tumor may lie behind a pathological fracture. It is not always visible radiologically, and tumorous tissue in the middle of fractured bone tissue, together with the tissue of the callus itself, can also be difficult to recognize in a bone biopsy. In **Fig. 231** one can see the **histological appearance** of tissue from a pathological fracture, with loose connective and granulation tissue *(1)* that has been invaded by blood capillaries *(2)*. Fibrous bone trabeculae have also developed *(3)*, against which rows of osteoblasts *(4)* and some osteoclasts *(5)* have been deposited. Near to this fibro-osseous fracture line we can see tumorous cartilaginous tissue *(6)* with some limp deposition and isomorphic chondrocytes. Here it is an enchondroma that has brought about the pathological fracture.

In **Fig. 232** we can see the **radiograph** of a pathological fracture of the humerus. The long bone is broken at the middle of the shaft *(1)*, and the bone ends are somewhat angulated and slightly displaced. The rather smooth and splinter-free edges of the bones are striking, and this suggests a pathological fracture. Furthermore, throughout the whole spongiosa of the humerus *(2)*, but most particularly clearly shown near the fracture *(3)*, there are irregular patchy areas of translucency that suggest a destructive process.

In the **histological picture** of **Fig. 233** one can see in the region of the fracture a fibro-osseous fracture callus with a loose connective tissue stroma *(1)* and newly differentiated fibrous bone trabeculae *(2)*, against which rows of osteoblasts have been deposited. Furthermore, complex epithelioid tumor cells *(3)* with polymorphic nuclei are also lying in the stroma; they sometimes resemble an adenoid pattern. With the aid of *immunohistochemistry* these can be identified as epithelial cells, since they express cytoceratin, which is an epithelial marker (**Fig. 959**). This is a ***bone metastasis*** from a carcinoma of the breast which has brought about a pathological fracture of the humerus (**Fig. 232**).

The so-called pathological fracture represents a fracture in a diseased bone. Very often such a sudden event is what first draws attention to the primary bone lesion or the underlying disease (e.g. bone metastases from a carcinoma of the breast), and histological examination of tissue from the region of the fracture frequently leads to the correct diagnosis. In some cases (e.g. with juvenile cysts of bone, p. 408) the spontaneous fracture has a positive effect in that healing of the bone after sufficient immobility also leads to healing of the lesion.

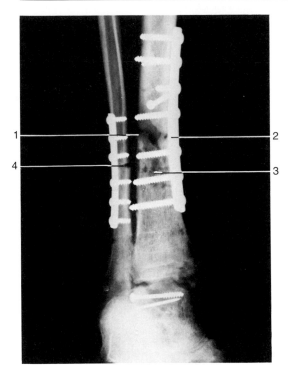

Fig. 230. Pathological fracture due to osteomyelitis (distal tibia)

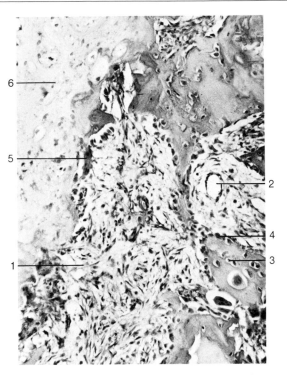

Fig. 231. Pathological fracture due to an enchondroma; HE, ×40

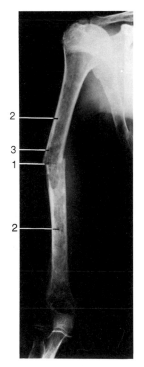

Fig. 232. Pathological fracture due to a bone metastasis (mid-shaft humerus)

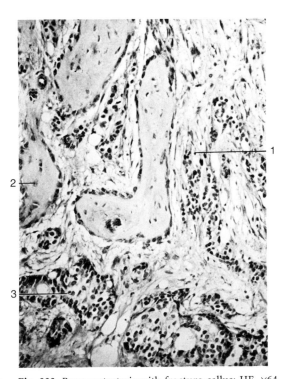

Fig. 233. Bone metastasis with fracture callus; HE, ×64

7 Inflammatory Conditions of Bone

General

Bone inflammation develops primarily in the marrow cavity, from which it can secondarily attack the bone tissue itself. When the responsible pathogens reach the marrow and damage the local tissue, *osteomyelitis* arises. Many different pathogenic organisms – they are mostly bacteria – can cause *osteomyelitis*. Some of them can, as with inflammatory conditions outside the skeleton, produce a characteristic histological pattern. In these cases there is a *specific osteomyelitis* (e.g. tuberculosis, typhoid, syphilis, fungal infections).

Most frequently the *osteomyelitis* is histologically *non-specific,* and in 90% of cases it is due to infection with Staphylococcus aureus. Hemolytic streptococci are only involved in 3% of cases, and these are mostly found in newborn infants and children. In none of these inflammatory reactions in the marrow cavity is it possible to draw conclusions about the causative organism histologically. The pathogens invade the bone by direct contact (per continuitatem), in the region of an open fracture, for instance *(post-traumatic osteomyelitis)*. In the majority of cases, however, the infection is blood borne *(hematogenous pyogenic osteomyelitis)*, and the portal of entry is often unidentifiable. Acute hematogenous osteomyelitis appears in 7% of cases in children of less than 1 year of age. Infection most frequently occurs between 2 and 16 years of age (80%), that is to say, during the period of most intensive skeletal growth. It most often attacks those parts of the skeleton where growth is fastest: the metaphyses of the femur, tibia and humerus (**Fig. 234**). 13% of cases of hematogenous osteomyelitis are found in adults, in whom the short bones, and most especially the vertebrae, are affected. 75% of all cases are found at the upper and lower ends of the femur and tibia.

Localized secondary osteomyelitis *(osteomyelitis circumscripta)* is often met with in the bones of the jaws – particularly the mandible – where the origin lies in an inflammatory dental condition.

Bacteria (mostly staphylococci) that reach the marrow cavity via the bloodstream call forth a leukocytic inflammation with the development of small abscesses (**Fig. 235 a**). As a result of damage to the vessels a hemorrhagic outer seam is formed, and perifocal edematous fluid is driven under the periosteum by way of the Haversian and Volkmannn canals. Elevation of the periosteum causes local pain. Osteomye-

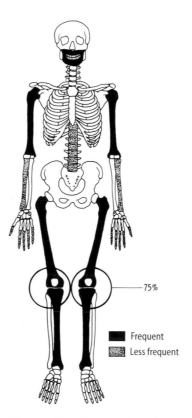

Frequent
Less frequent

Fig. 234. Most frequent sites of hematogenous osteomyelitis

Fig. 235 a, b. The development of hematogenous osteomyelitis (diagrammatic)

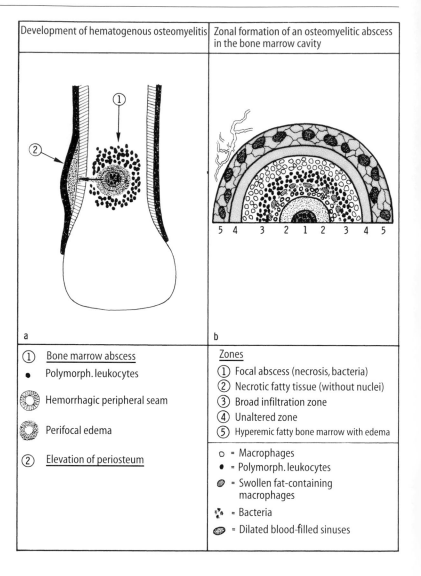

Development of hematogenous osteomyelitis	Zonal formation of an osteomyelitic abscess in the bone marrow cavity

a   b

①   <u>Bone marrow abscess</u>

•   Polymorph. leukocytes

    Hemorrhagic peripheral seam

    Perifocal edema

②   <u>Elevation of periosteum</u>

<u>Zones</u>
① Focal abscess (necrosis, bacteria)
② Necrotic fatty tissue (without nuclei)
③ Broad infiltration zone
④ Unaltered zone
⑤ Hyperemic fatty bone marrow with edema

○ = Macrophages
• = Polymorph. leukocytes
◉ = Swollen fat-containing macrophages
⁝ = Bacteria
⬭ = Dilated blood-filled sinuses

litic abscesses in the marrow cavity present a *zonal pattern* (**Fig. 235 b**). The center of the abscess *(1)* contains cell detritus with edema and collections of bacteria. Then comes a zone of necrotic fatty tissue without nuclei or inflammatory infiltrate *(2)*. This is followed by a wide infiltration zone *(3)* that consists internally of the remains of dead cells without nuclei, bacteria and granulocytes, and externally of a dense assemblage of macrophages. Further out lies a zone of unchanged fatty tissue without hyperemia or exudate *(4)* that is surrounded by hyperemic fatty marrow with dilated sinuses *(5)*. This zonal pattern of the osteomyelitic abscess reflects the virulence of the bacteria on one hand and the resistance of the organism on the other.

The likelihood of the inflammation spreading into a long bone depends on the *age of the patient* (**Fig. 235 c**). In infants, in whom the blood vessels run through the epiphyseal cartilage, the bacteria can enter the epiphysis and finally reach the joint space. A *pyarthrosis* then develops. An extensively ossifying periostitis is common in infants. In *childhood* the avascular epiphyseal cartilage prevents the inflammatory process reaching the joint. Only in joints where the insertion of the capsule reaches over the epiphyseal line (hip, knee) can direct invasion of the joint cavity occur.

Fig. 235 c, d. The development of hematogenous osteomyelitis (diagrammatic)

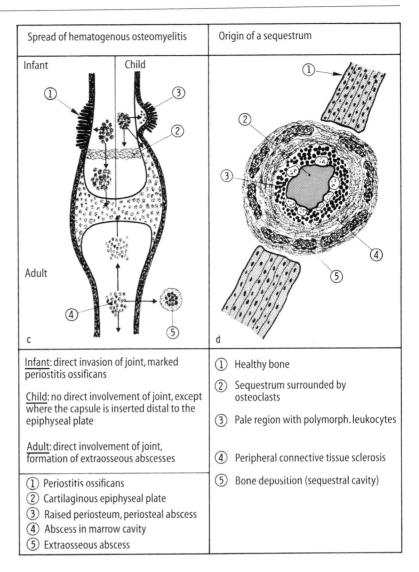

Spread of hematogenous osteomyelitis	Origin of a sequestrum
Infant: direct invasion of joint, marked periostitis ossificans	① Healthy bone
Child: no direct involvement of joint, except where the capsule is inserted distal to the epiphyseal plate	② Sequestrum surrounded by osteoclasts
	③ Pale region with polymorph. leukocytes
Adult: direct involvement of joint, formation of extraosseous abscesses	④ Peripheral connective tissue sclerosis
① Periostitis ossificans	⑤ Bone deposition (sequestral cavity)
② Cartilaginous epiphyseal plate	
③ Raised periosteum, periosteal abscess	
④ Abscess in marrow cavity	
⑤ Extraosseous abscess	

Furthermore, periosteal abscesses often arise, which in childhood characteristically lead to the production of cortical sequestra.

In *adults* again, the inflammation in the marrow cavity of the diaphysis can spread and, because of the absence of an epiphyseal cartilage, easily invade the joint directly. The firmly bound down periosteum is not usually raised, but is broken through by masses of pus to produce abscesses outside the bone and to form fistulas.

In the neighborhood of an osteomyelitic abscess the blood supply to the bone is cut off by the compression of the vessels. The staphylococci destroy the osteocytes, so that the bone dies (**Fig. 235 d**). The osteoclasts are activated and separate the living from the dead bone. In the center of the inflammatory lesion, with dense collections of polymorphonuclear leukocytes, the dead bone tissue remains behind as a *sequestrum.* The sequestrum, which is released from the spongiosal network, is enclosed by edema and with masses of polymorphonuclear leukocytes and, later, a connective tissue capsule inside which new bone deposition is taking place. After a few days or weeks one can recognize the dense radio-opaque sequestrum surrounded by a translucent region and, outside that, by dark marginal sclerosis: the so-called *sequestral cavity.*

Paronychia (Panaritium Ossale)

With purulent inflammation of the soft parts of the fingers and toes there is always the danger that pus formation will reach the periosteum of the phalanges, metacarpals or metatarsals and attack the bone. It is usually a staphylococcal infection. The periosteum is destroyed by the inflammation, and this is followed by rapid destruction of the cortex and a purulent coalescence with the cancellous bone marrow. At the forefront of this purulent osteomyelitis there is a pronounced osteolysis. **Figure 236** shows an advanced paronychia in the distal phalanx of a finger, which developed as the result of a stab injury. The soft parts *(1)* show an inflammatory swelling, and the bone is extensively damaged from outside *(2)*. We can see a wide zone of osteolysis in which the bony structures are necrotic and soaked through with pus. No reparatory processes can be recognized, but they may nevertheless be present and can even lead to restoration of the bone, although this is mostly necrotic and structureless.

If the articular cartilage is involved we speak of a *panaritium* (paronychia) *ossale et articulare.*

Osteomyelitis of the Jaws

Inflammation of the teeth and oral cavity generally is very common and often involves the bone of the jaws. Most frequently there is a *primary chronic osteomyelitis of the jaw* with a strong tendency to recur. This kind of osteomyelitis can be recognized by the appearance of bone abscesses together with simultaneous reparatory osteosclerosis. *Acute purulent osteomyelitis of the jaw* is usually staphylococcal in origin. In the lower jaw it has a tendency to spread, but remains more often localized in the upper jaw. The starting point is a dental root granuloma (dental root abscess) resulting from a purulent pulpitis. In **Fig. 237** one can recognize a dentogenous osteomyelitis that has involved the entire mandible. The vigorous remodeling processes show themselves in the association of irregular zones of sclerosis *(1)* with patchy foci of osteolysis *(2)* which are in fact abscesses. At one point an active dental granuloma *(3)* can be seen. Such abscesses are characteristically found in both alveolar processes.

Osteomyelitis in Infants

Hematogenous osteomyelitis particularly attacks growing bones, and even more so the most actively growing parts of such bones. If the inflammation spreads from the metaphysis to the epiphyseal cartilage and epiphysis there is a danger that growth may be impaired. An invasion of the joint with the development of a pyarthrosis is possible. In **Fig. 238** one can see an osteomyelitis that has developed in the distal metaphysis of the femur in an infant. There is a cloudy increase in density in the long bone with a tiny radiodense sequestrum *(1)*. The metaphysis has become club-shaped, and the epiphysis has also become involved in the destructive remodeling process *(2)*. The outer contours of the cartilaginous joint surface are indistinct and jagged. Characteristically an extraordinarily marked *periostitis ossificans* *(3)* has developed, and this makes the contour of the bone appear double. Later the ossifying changes in the periosteum disappear and the small sequestra are completely resorbed.

Osteomyelitis in Children

In later childhood the avascular epiphyseal plate presents a barrier to the spreading of inflammation into the epiphysis. As a result of the increased blood supply to the metaphysis, growth of the epiphyseal cartilage is stimulated and it is therefore wider than usual. **Figure 239** shows a pronounced purulent osteomyelitis in the tibia of a child. The entire long bone is involved and its structure altered, the destructive process extending exactly as far as the two epiphyseal plates *(1)*, which are somewhat widened. The epiphyses *(2)* are unaffected. As a result of the inflammatory osteolysis and reactive osteosclerosis the bone presents a chequered appearance. In the widened proximal metaphysis, which shows the most pronounced changes, one can recognize a large *coalescent focus of osteomyelitis (3)* which is incompletely demarcated by marginal sclerosis. Characteristically there is an extensive *periostitis ossificans (4)*, against which *cortical sequestra* can develop. There has been a *spontaneous fracture (5)* of the osteomyelitic bone, and a sequestral cavity can be seen. Osteomyelitis such as this most frequently appears in the 8th year of life and in the majority of cases involves the tibia or femur.

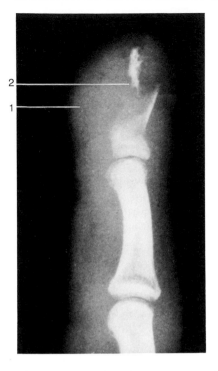

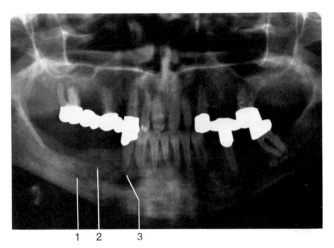

Fig. 236. Paronychia (panaritium ossale, whitlow) with bone involvement (terminal phalanx of finger)

Fig. 237. Dentogenous osteomyelitis (mandible)

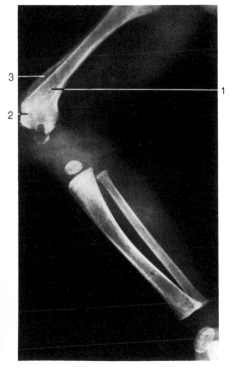

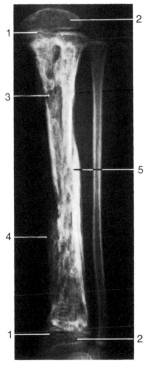

Fig. 238. Infantile osteomyelitis (distal femur)

Fig. 239. Osteomyelitis in a child (tibia)

Acute Purulent Osteomyelitis in Adults

The **radiograph** (**Fig. 240**) shows a large osteomyelitic lesion in the proximal part of the tibia *(1)* together with a cortical *sequestrum (2)*. The bone tissue in the center of the abscess has been completely broken down to form a purulent mass, and the adjacent cortex is severely damaged and penetrated. No periosteal reaction can be seen. The density of the spongiosa around the osteomyelitic focus has been increased by reactive sclerosis *(3)*, which has demarcated the abscess cavities. The inflammation has spread into the epiphysis *(4)*, and here the association of increasingly porous bone destruction and reparative osteosclerosis has produced the patchy appearance. No involvement of the knee joint is detectable. The reactive osteosclerosis is limited to the region around the osteomyelitic focus; the more distant bone shows signs of acute *bone atrophy (5)*. Radiologically, acute osteomyelitis will be first demonstrable in this case after three weeks, until then the bone findings remain negative.

Macroscopically (**Fig. 241**) one can see a highly active osteomyelitic focus of destruction in the marrow cavity, and in a few places this has spread to the cortex. In the long bones these lesions are especially to be found in the metaphysis, from where they can extend into the diaphysis and epiphysis. It is a region with map-like edges in which the network of the spongiosa has been destroyed. It contains a dirty yellowish-gray mass of soft consistency. The focus is bounded on the outside by a reddish hemorrhagic seam. The cortex is irregularly narrowed, and has in places been broken down by fistulas through which the pus can get under the periosteum and reach the soft parts. In **Fig. 241** one can recognize osteomyelitic changes in a tibia, from which the soft parts can only be incompletely dissected free *(1)*. In the metaphyseal region of the diaphysis there is a large reddish-gray defect in the cortex *(2)* where an intramedullary focus of inflammation has broken through and produced a fistula.

In **Fig. 242** one can see the typical **histological picture** of an *acute purulent osteomyelitis*.

The whole of the marrow cavity is filled up with highly cellular granulation tissue and soaked through with inflammatory edematous fluid *(1)*. Densely packed collections of *polymorphonuclear leukocytes* which have destroyed the original fatty marrow can be recognized. Fibrin is present within this coalescent mass of tissue, and the cancellous trabeculae are necrotic *(2)*. The typical lamellar layering of the bone has been lost, and osteocytes are no longer found in their lacunae. Owing to the massive purulent inflammation of the bone marrow the trabeculae have been deprived of their nourishment and are dead. They have formed small *cancellous sequestra*. Here and there one can see typical *marrow abscesses*, and there are many collections of *bacteria* within the highly cellular granulation tissue which show up with HE staining as tiny bluish specks (cocci). These can be more clearly seen if stained with methylene blue. The retention of bone sequestra in the marrow cavity supports the inflammatory process and prevents healing, so that finally a chronic recurring osteomyelitis develops. For this reason it is essential that all sequestra are removed surgically.

Under **higher power** (**Fig. 243**) the excessively granular polymorphs with their deeply lobed nuclei are clearly seen *(1)*. They are distributed – sometimes very densely, sometimes more loosely – throughout the marrow cavity. Many of them are necrotic. The whole space is soaked with inflammatory edematous fluid. The trabeculae are necrotic, and the lacunae no longer contain osteocytes. The lamellar layering is extremely faded and often undetectable *(2)*. The trabeculae have irregular jagged edges, although in this acute stage of the inflammatory process no osteoclastic bone resorption is to be seen. One has the impression that these necrotic trabeculae have disintegrated into thin plaque-like sheets.

Although this type of purulent osteomyelitis is practically always due to bacterial infection, active bacteria are not often seen on histological examination. The surgeon who undertakes the bone biopsy should also remove a sample for bacteriological analysis.

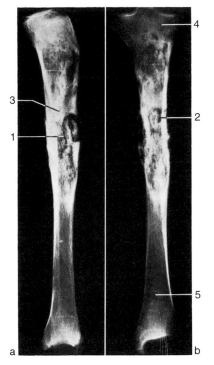

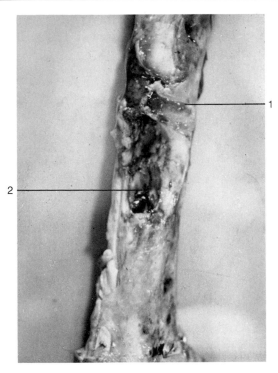

Fig. 240 a, b. Acute purulent osteomyelitis in an adult (tibia)

Fig. 241. Acute purulent osteomyelitis (tibia)

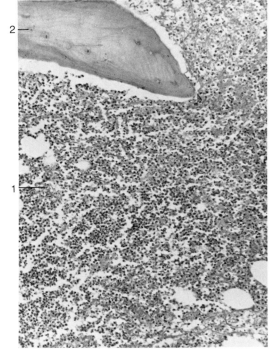

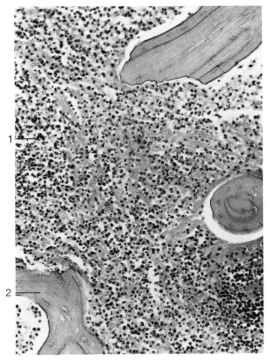

Fig. 242. Acute purulent osteomyelitis; HE, ×25

Fig. 243. Acute purulent osteomyelitis; HE, ×40

Fig. 245 shows active osteomyelitis of the femur with an *intramedullary bone sequestrum (1)*. The bone tissue has been irregularly destroyed by the osteomyelitic process, which shows up **radiologically** in the long bone as a patchy area of translucency with an indistinct border *(2)*. In the middle of this pale area of granulation tissue and demineralized bone, the sequestrum is sharply delineated by its undulating border. It is also strongly mineralized and therefore dark.

In **Fig. 244** one can recognize **macroscopically** a similar osteomyelitic focus in the distal part of the tibia. The marrow cavity has been taken over by a large map-like area of necrosis *(1)*, with a dirty grayish surface in section which is surrounded by a region of grayish-red hyperemia *(2)*. Clearly demarcated dense white calcified sequestra are lying in the abscess cavity *(3)*. **Histologically (Fig. 246)** the richly cellular infiltration of the marrow cavity is again striking *(1)* and leukocytes with heavily lobulated nuclei are present. Between them lie necrotic trabeculae without osteocytes *(2)*.

If an acute purulent osteomyelitis overcomes the tissue of the cortex and reaches through to the periosteum, the periosteal connective tissue reacts by widening and laying down new trabeculae. After this new bone has been mineralized it can also be seen in the **radiograph. Figure 247** is the picture of a tibia with patchy porous osteomyelitic changes in the marrow cavity *(1)*. The outer surface of the long bone shows a double contour *(2)*, and at one point *(3)* the cortex has been penetrated. A bony shell – known as a *sequestral cavity* – has been reactively laid down around the inflamed bone. With a long smouldering osteomyelitis, several such bony shells can lie one upon the other, and these are also visible in the radiograph. In contrast to the radial "spicula" (p. 162 and **Fig. 304**) which may arise, for instance, with a tumor, the bony shells in osteomyelitis are arranged parallel to the surface of the bone.

If the granulation tissue and the purulent exudate are driven through the Haversian and Volkmann canals as far as the periosteum, this is at first raised up from the cortex, causing a characteristic local periosteal pain. The inflammatory irritation originating from the marrow cavity causes the connective tissue of the periosteum to thicken (**Fig. 248**). Osteoblasts are differentiated and begin to form fibro-osseous trabeculae *(1)* which contain many osteocytes and osteoblasts. This is a typical **reactive periostitis ossificans**. After a while the newly formed bony structures mature and become calcified. They lie radial to the bone surface and are bound together in the form of arcades. The mineralization front is rendered visible by dark undulating lines *(2)*. Between these newly formed subperiosteal bone trabeculae there is loose or dense connective tissue *(3)*, and sometimes an inflammatory infiltrate.

These morphological observations show that the inflammatory processes of bone attack and damage not only the bone marrow (osteomyelitis) but also the bone itself (osteitis) and the periosteum (periostitis). The ways in which the tissues react to the inflammatory stimulus are limited, the resistance of the body playing a deciding role here. The radiological appearance of osteomyelitis depends on the association of bone resorption (osteolysis) and deposition (reactive osteosclerosis), as well as on reactive periostitis (the so-called *involucrum*).

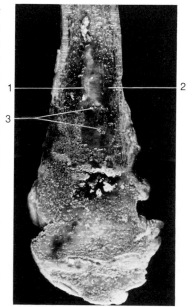

Fig. 244. Acute purulent osteomyelitis with sequestra (distal tibia)

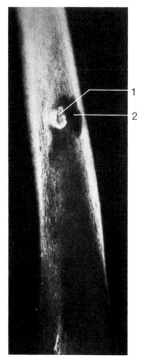

Fig. 245. Acute purulent osteomyelitis with sequestra (femur)

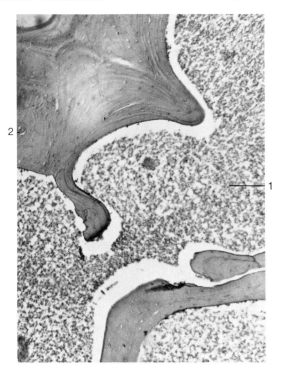

Fig. 246. Acute purulent osteomyelitis; HE, ×25

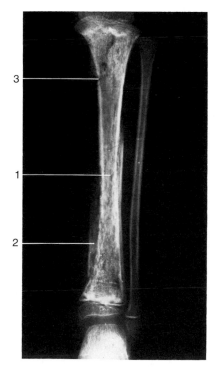

Fig. 247. Reactive periostitis ossificans in a case of osteomyelitis (periosteal involucrum, tibia)

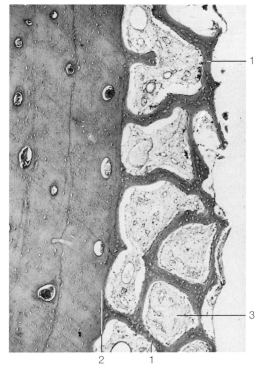

Fig. 248. Reactive periostitis ossificans (periosteal involucrum); HE, ×25

Chronic Osteomyelitis

An acute purulent granulating osteomyelitis can remain active for a long time (weeks or months), especially when a sequestrum is left in position. During this time advancing reactive processes are proceeding in the bone which are associated with pronounced remodeling. Near the destructive osteomyelitic lesion there are irregular regions of osteosclerosis which can be seen in the **radiograph**. Chronic osteomyelitis involving the neck of the right femur can be seen in **Fig. 249**, reaching distally into the long bone. The innermost parts of the bone have mostly undergone an osteosclerotic increase in density *(1)*, with patchy foci of translucency in between *(2)*. The cortex is in places lighter *(3)*, in places thickened and casting a dense shadow *(4)*. The outward contours of the bone are smooth, and the periosteum appears in some places to be widened *(5)*. Radiologically osteomyelitis can sometimes simulate a bone tumor. The association of osteolytic and osteosclerotic bone remodeling processes gives the impression of a proliferating tumor, especially when there is subliminal inflammation of the bone without any of the clinical signs of inflammation (fever, leukocytosis, raised ESR etc.), and when the presence of bacteria cannot be proved. Equally well, a bone tumor (a bone lymphoma, for instance, or a Ewing's sarcoma) may lurk behind the supposed radiological appearance of an acute osteomyelitis.

In cases of chronic osteomyelitis the extensive bone remodeling is also **macroscopically** very striking. In **Fig. 250** one can see a saw cut through the proximal end of a femur that is very much distended and deformed. The greater trochanter appears to have been greatly enlarged by bone deposition *(1)*. The cortex is considerably widened *(2)*, and contains small patchy holes and wide zones of irregular osteosclerosis which also reach into the femoral neck and head *(3)*. The marrow cavity is filled with a coarse dense network of bone *(4)*. In several places one can recognize dark grayish-red map-like regions of coalescing masses of blood and pus *(5)*.

As with every case of bacterial infection, increasing scar tissue also develops with chronic osteomyelitis and leads to an advancing fibrosis of the marrow cavity. The osteomyelitic process intensifies and bursts into flame again and again. This has now become a *chronic recurrent osteomyelitis* that even with modern antibiotic treatment is difficult to deal with. In **Fig. 251** it can be seen that the marrow cavity is completely filled with scar tissue *(1)*. The original cancellous framework is no longer present, and instead the progressive bone remodeling has led to the development of clumsy, thoroughly irregular bone trabeculae which are in no way arranged to correspond to the pressure and tension lines of the bone *(2)*. These bony elements lie indiscriminately here and there within the scar tissue. In some places the connective tissue in the marrow cavity has become porous and is invaded by capillaries *(3)*. Here one finds collections of plasma cells, lymphocytes and histiocytes, as well as a few polymorphonuclear leukocytes, which confirm the presence of a raging inflammatory process. The sporadic outbreaks of inflammation can lead to severe bone defects and bring about a pathological fracture. Fistulas may break through the cortex and reach the soft parts, until finally amyloidosis develops.

Under **higher magnification (Fig. 252)** an osteosclerotically widened bone trabecula can be seen *(1)* in which the deposition front is marked by extended reversal lines. The marrow cavity is filled with fibrous tissue *(2)*, which in the neighborhood of the trabeculae is dense and rich in fibers. The layers of osteoblasts also confirm the advancing osteosclerosis *(3)*. One can also see loose, highly cellular granulation tissue in the marrow cavity, with developed and sprouting capillaries *(4)*, together with infiltrates of plasma cells, lymphocytes, histiocytes and a few polymorphonuclear leukocytes, which indicate the continuation of the inflammatory process.

The recurrence of a chronic osteomyelitis can sometimes take place after ten or more years, either at the original site or in some other region. To this extent the condition may produce late effects. If the recurrence of an earlier osteomyelitis is found at the site of the original inflammation, one speaks of *late osteomyelitis*, which is mostly accompanied by a pronounced osteoporosis and sometimes involves joint changes as well. In a tomogram it often is possible to demonstrate many small sequestra.

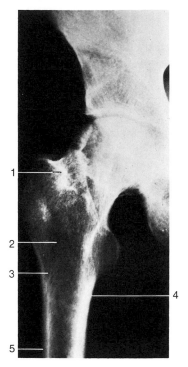

Fig. 249. Chronic osteomyelitis (femoral neck)

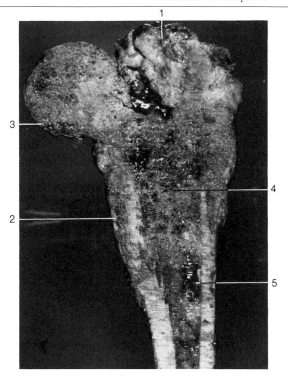

Fig. 250. Chronic osteomyelitis (proximal femur)

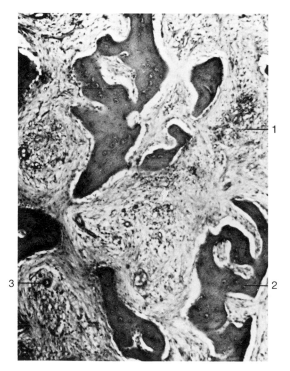

Fig. 251. Chronic osteomyelitis; van Gieson, ×40

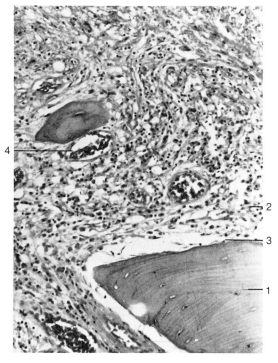

Fig. 252. Chronic osteomyelitis; HE, ×64

A chronic osteomyelitis that develops over several years may lead to pronounced bone remodeling which extends into the bones involved and destroys their structure, so that even a malignant tumor may have to be considered during the differential diagnosis. In children, and therefore in the growing skeleton, such bone remodeling can also appear in a relatively short space of time.

In **Fig. 254** one can see the **radiograph** of a severe osteomyelitis in the right humeral shaft of a 5-year-old child. The entire long bone seems to have increased in size. Inside there is an area of translucency *(1)* which looks like a cavity and which probably contains pus and bacteria. The surrounding spongiosa is dense and sclerotic *(2)*. The pronounced increase in width and density of the periosteum is particularly striking *(3)* and extends over almost the whole of the bone. In places it is raised up from the cortex. The thickened periosteum is layered like the skin of an onion. In the **radiograph** of **Fig. 255** the chronic osteomyelitis of the same humerus is shown in another plane. The entire shaft of the bone shows an extensive increase in osteosclerosis *(1)* which involves both the spongiosa and the cortex. Inside this zone of sclerosis there are fine moth-eaten foci of osteolysis *(2)*. The shaft of the humerus is slightly enlarged. Externally one can see the widened and densely shaded periosteum *(3)*. Such a radiological appearance in a child must be distinguished from a Ewing's sarcoma (p. 352), and for this a bone biopsy is required.

The **histological picture** of the biopsy makes it easy to confirm the chronic osteomyelitis. In **Fig. 253** one can see the loose granulation tissue, with only a few fibers *(1)*, which completely fills the marrow cavity. It is loosely infiltrated by lymphocytes and plasma cells *(2)* and has been invaded by numerous dilated capillaries *(3)*. Many trabeculae of fibrous bone *(4)* have developed within the granulation tissue. The possibility of this being a malignant tumor can be excluded.

If chronic osteomyelitis develops in the body of a vertebra, we speak of a *chronic spondylitis*. It usually affects one or more adjacent vertebral bodies, and only rarely involves the transverse or spinous process. If the inflammation invades the adjacent intervertebral discs and destroys them, this gives rise to a *spondylodiscitis*. The

corresponding radiological changes in structure are due to the destructive and reparative activity of the inflammatory process.

Fig. 256 is a lateral **radiograph** of the thoracic column. The 7th *(1)* and 8th *(2)* thoracic vertebrae are extensively destroyed and fused together. The intervertebral space *(3)* is no longer recognizable. Next to the large areas of osteolysis there are regions showing a diffuse increase in density. The lateral cortex *(4)* is completely destroyed.

The **histological** appearance of the material obtained by a needle biopsy is that of chronic osteomyelitis. In **Fig. 257** one can see a sclerotically thickened trabecula *(1)* with active osteocytes *(2)* which are lining the deposition front *(3)*, and here a few osteoblasts *(4)* have also been deposited. The marrow cavity contains loose inflammatory granulation tissue *(5)* with a sparse infiltrate of lymphocytes and plasma cells *(6)* and dilated capillaries *(7)*. This is a chronic, histologically non-specific spondylitis, and the search for bacteria is often negative.

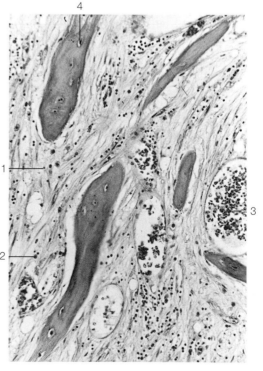

Fig. 253. Chronic spondylitis; HE, ×64

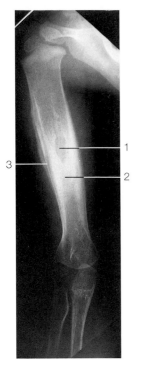

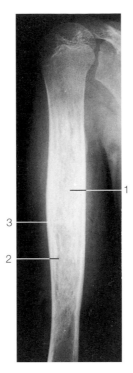

Fig. 254. Chronic osteomyelitis (shaft of humerus)

Fig. 255. Chronic osteomyelitis (shaft of humerus)

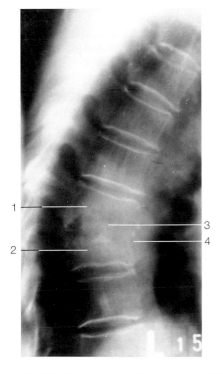

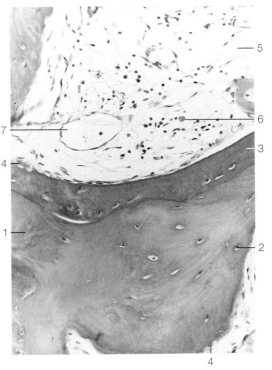

Fig. 256. Chronic spondylitis and spondylodiscitis (7th and 8th thoracic vertebrae)

Fig. 257. Chronic spondylitis; HE, ×64

Brodie's Abscess

If the virulence of the pathogens is low and the patient's resistance good, an osteomyelitic bone abscess may develop – usually in the metaphysis or epi-metaphysis, and most often in the proximal or distal part of the tibia – which produces only a slight degree of pain. It most commonly appears in connection with an attack of chronic osteomyelitis in young people (14th–24th year of life) which has been overcome. Such a Brodie's abscess can be seen at the distal femoral metaphysis in **Fig. 258**. In the **radiograph** one sees a well-defined elongated oval "bone cyst" *(1)* lying centrally in the bone and extending in its long axis. Within, the bone tissue has been destroyed and the cavity filled with pus. Unlike other "bone cysts" (e.g. juvenile bone cyst, aneurysmal bone cyst or osteoclastoma), a Brodie's abscess is surrounded and sharply demarcated by a narrow marginal osteosclerotic shell *(2)*. It differs from bone tuberculosis in that the surrounding osteosclerotic zone is clearly marked. Periostitis ossificans may also develop. Large bone abscesses my lead to a pathological fracture *(3)*. There are no sequestra.

Plasma Cell Osteomyelitis

If resistance is good and the virulence of the organisms restricted, a type of localized chronic osteomyelitis can develop in which there is no pus. Macroscopically there is a cavity in the bone from which it is possible to evacuate a mucoid, whitish mass *(osteomyelitis albuminosa)* consisting almost entirely of plasma cells *(osteomyelitis plasmacellulare)*. Very often it is impossible to detect the presence of bacteria. It usually attacks children and young people, the most frequent site being the metaphysis of a long bone.

In the **radiograph** a plasma cell osteomyelitis very often appears as a bone cyst. Such a focus can be seen in **Fig. 259** at the distal tibial metaphysis of a 15-year-old boy. There is a cyst-like central translucent region of bone tissue *(1)* that is surrounded by an osteosclerotic border *(2)*. The boundary zone can sometimes appear more faded, or the osteosclerosis may include a large part of the neighboring bone. A reactive periostitis ossificans may develop, although this is not present in the case depicted. The osteolytic zone is orientated in the long axis of the bone and reaches as far as the epiphyseal line *(3)*.

In the overview of **Fig. 260** one can recognize **histologically** a mass of highly cellular granulation tissue that has taken up the whole of the marrow cavity *(1)*. Next to the dense cellular areas there are porous regions that have been soaked through by edematous fluid. Numerous capillaries are running or sprouting throughout the underlying granulomatous framework *(2)*. The trabeculae near the walls of the bony cavity *(3)* are osteosclerotically widened and in many places have a jagged outline. The osteocytes are preserved, and in this case no sequestra have developed. Peripherally one often sees newly formed bony structures consisting of fibro-osseous trabeculae which are patchy in appearance and contain many osteocytes and osteoblasts.

Under **higher magnification** (**Fig. 261**) the cellular structure of the inflammatory granulation tissue stands out clearly. The marrow cavity is soaked through with edematous fluid, and only a few thin collagen fibers can be seen *(1)*. In between, large numbers of plasma cells are loosely distributed *(2)*, their eccentric nuclei and the distribution of the chromatin, resembling the spokes of a wheel, are clearly seen. In most cases their cytoplasm is strongly eosinophilic, and they can be distinguished by their monomorphic appearance from the cells of a plasmocytoma. Active bacteria cannot be seen. The adjacent bone tissue *(3)* is vital and contains intact osteocytes. One can recognize a wide region of bone deposition *(4)* and a few deposited osteoblasts.

It is often impossible to diagnose a plasma cell osteomyelitis with any certainty from a plain radiograph, and one is sometimes unable to distinguish it from a Ewing's sarcoma. Various different bone diseases may lie hidden behind such a "bone cyst" – amongst others, an eosinophilic granuloma, non-ossifying osteofibroma or enchondroma. In such cases the final diagnosis must depend upon the histological examination of a bone biopsy. This type of bone inflammation is known to run a protracted course and to have a strong tendency to recur. When the spinal column is involved it is particularly important to exclude tuberculosis.

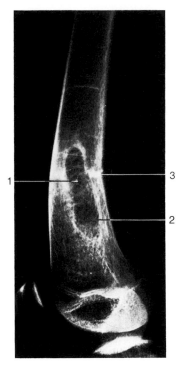

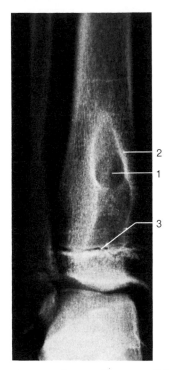

Fig. 258. Brodie's abscess (distal femur)

Fig. 259. Plasma cell osteomyelitis (distal tibia)

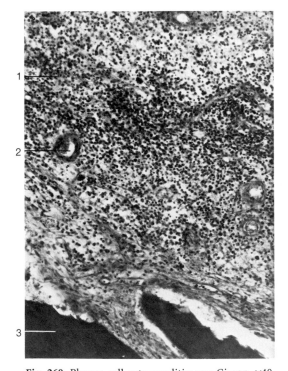

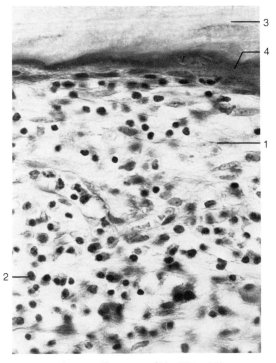

Fig. 260. Plasma cell osteomyelitis; van Gieson, ×40

Fig. 261. Plasma cell osteomyelitis; HE, ×160

Non-purulent Sclerosing Osteomyelitis (Garré)

This is an unusual form of chronic bone inflammation in which the virulence of the invading organisms is restricted from the beginning, and which often appears several years after an incidental sepsis. It does not occur as frequently as acute or chronic osteomyelitis and mostly attacks children or young adults. It mostly involves the shafts of long bones, and in particular the bones of the jaws. In the **radiograph** (**Fig. 262**) the extensive and very dense osteosclerosis – with occasional small translucent areas – is the most striking feature *(1)*. The proximal metaphysis of the tibia is involved and the marrow cavity has been filled with newly formed bone tissue. The cortex is thickened *(2)* and new bone tissue has differentiated even in the periosteum. No sequestra have been formed. In the jaw bones a similar kind of osteosclerotic distension can put one in mind of a bone tumor (a Ewing sarcoma, for instance), particularly if the surface of the cortex has become severely roughened.

As can be seen in **Fig. 263**, only a very few – if, indeed, any – polymorphonuclear leukocytes are found in cases of sclerosing osteomyelitis. The principal event is the formation of a highly fibrous, dense connective tissue that occupies the entire marrow cavity of the metaphyseal region involved *(1)*. Here new irregular bone trabeculae develop *(2)* and are haphazardly distributed. These trabeculae show many thick and thin drawn out reversal lines *(3)* and are often covered by rows of osteoblasts. These structures indicate the progressive bone formation and apposition which constitute the sclerosing process. It is noticeable that, alongside this extraordinarily vigorous new bone formation, the original bony structures are preserved. The osteocytes have not been destroyed. Regions of coalescence, sequestra and marrow cavity abscesses form no part of the picture of sclerosing osteomyelitis, and bacteria cannot usually be identified in the inflamed tissue. Inflammatory cells (plasma cells, lymphocytes, histiocytes) are only sparsely represented. Clinically, this condition is accompanied by a rheumatoid type of pain. The course and prognosis are benign.

Tuberculous Osteomyelitis

Even today this is still the most frequently occurring *specific inflammatory disease of bone*. It often attacks both bones and joints simultaneously *(osteoarthropathia tuberculosa)*. Since the introduction of antibiotic treatment, bone tuberculosis has declined in young people, but those of more advanced age are increasingly affected. There is no such thing as primary bone tuberculosis; it is always blood borne (from a pulmonary focus, for instance) during the hematogenous phase, or in the phase of organic tuberculosis. In 3% to 5% of cases of generalized tuberculosis the skeleton becomes involved. The appearance of bone tuberculosis and the involvement of particular bones depends on several factors. Failure of resistance to infection particularly favors the development of bone tuberculosis, and its spread is determined by the distribution of the active red bone marrow. It is known that in early childhood the entire marrow cavity is involved in blood building, whereas in later adult life it is concentrated in the axial skeleton. This is responsible for the different skeletal distribution of tuberculosis in childhood and in adult life. As is illustrated in **Fig. 264a–c**, the most frequent localization of bone tuberculosis (40%) is in the spinal column (particularly from Th 6 to L 3), followed by the hip joint (25%) and knee joint (20%). In children, over 20% of cases involve the short bones of the hand or foot, but in adults the pelvis is a more frequent site. The inherited constitution can also be decisive for the development of bone tuberculosis. This is confirmed by observing the incidence of cases of multiple bone tuberculosis in uniovular twins (**Fig. 264a–c**). Since the introduction of protective inoculation with BCG and the use of tuberculostatic drugs, the number of cases of bone and joint tuberculosis in children has markedly decreased. Adult tuberculosis has been displaced into a higher age group, and has increased in the elderly. A very important factor in tuberculosis is the time which elapses between the spread of the disease and the first symptomatic focus. This so-called latent period varies with the different skeletal manifestations: it is about 1–2 years for tuberculous spondylitis (minimal 2–8 months), 6–19 months for tuberculosis of the knee joint and 16–36 months for the hip joint. Synovial tuberculosis has a very short latent period (1–3 months).

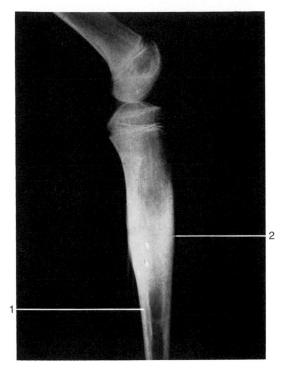

Fig. 262. Sclerosing osteomyelitis Garré (proximal tibia)

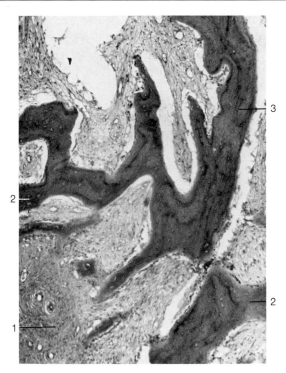

Fig. 263. Sclerosing osteomyelitis Garré, HE, ×25

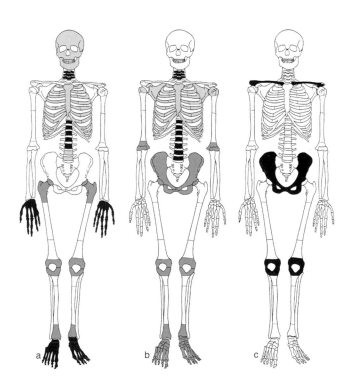

Fig. 264 a–c. Localization of skeletal and joint tuberculosis in children (a), adults (b) and in old age (c). (after UEHLINGER, 1979) [black – very common, >20%; dark gray – common, >10%; light gray – rare]

Bone tuberculosis is only clearly recognizable **radiologically** after at least three months. In **Fig. 265** there are large tuberculous lesions in the body of a thoracic vertebra (1) which have extensively destroyed the bone. One can observe large areas of translucency (tuberculous cavities) which in places have run together. In between one can recognize surrounding regions of sclerosis. The roof plate has been destroyed (2) and the intervertebral disc narrowed. The surrounding bone shows signs of an atrophy (perifocal osteoporosis) which is typical of tuberculosis. There are no signs of periostitis ossificans or sequestra, and these are rare in tuberculosis.

In **Fig. 266** tuberculous spondylitis of the 3rd and 4th lumbar vertebrae is illustrated **macroscopically**. In L4, near the intervertebral disc, one can see a large cavity (1) filled with a mass of "caseation". The disc itself (2) has been destroyed. Collapse of the upper plate has led to a prolapse of the nucleus pulposus into the cavity and to narrowing of the intervertebral space, which is an important early symptom of tuberculous spondylitis. The tuberculous process has also extended into the adjacent 3rd lumbar vertebra (3). The extension of the tuberculous granulation tissue from this so-called saddle cavity continues outwards parallel to the disc (4) as far as the short intervertebral lateral fibers of the anterior longitudinal ligament (5). This leads to the development of a so-called hypostatic abscess. Central vertebral cavities do not usually show up in the conventional radiograph, but can be seen in the tomogram (CT, MRT). Destruction of the vertebral bodies has severe consequences for the spine. In the thoracic region this may lead (as seen in **Fig. 267**) to collapse of the anterior part of the bone so as to produce a wedge vertebra (1), and this can result in a gibbus angularis (hump). In this **maceration specimen** one can also see coalescence of the spongiosa with complete bridging over of the intervertebral space by bone (2). Two small cavities can still be seen here (3). In **Fig. 268** one can see such a block vertebra where two lumbar vertebrae (1) have completely fused together and the disc has been replaced by bone tissue (2). These changes in the macroscopic structure of the spinal column, which can also be recognized radiologically, are very typical of tuberculous spondylitis.

Fig. 269 shows **histologically** typical tuberculous granulation tissue within a tuberculous bone lesion, where it has destroyed the local bone tissue. Large regions of "caseation" have developed (1) which nevertheless have a nodal appearance. In these it is often possible to demonstrate tubercle bacilli histochemically (Rhodamin-Auramin staining, fluorescence). Close by there is a small tubercle (2), which is surrounded by epithelioid cells, lymphocytes and Langhans' giant cells. The spongiosa is extensively destroyed and practically no osteosclerotic reaction is to be seen. Similar tubercles are seen in the synovia. The diagnosis of bone or joint tuberculosis cannot, however, be made from the histological picture alone, it is also necessary to establish the presence of tubercle bacilli.

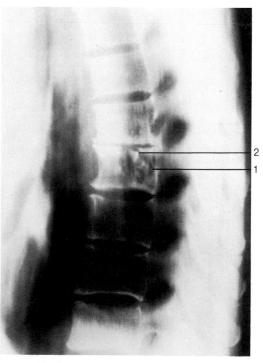

Fig. 265. Tuberculous spondylitis (thoracic vertebrae)

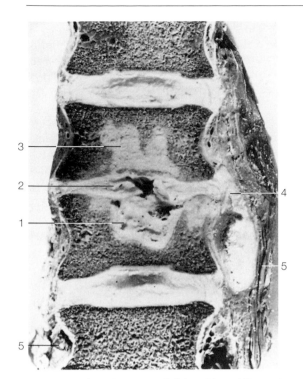

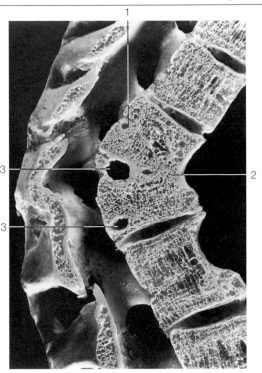

Fig. 266. Tuberculous spondylitis with saddle cavity and hypostatic abscess (3rd and 4th lumbar vertebrae)

Fig. 267. Tuberculous spondylitis with development of wedge vertebrae and gibbus angularis (thoracic vertebrae, maceration specimen)

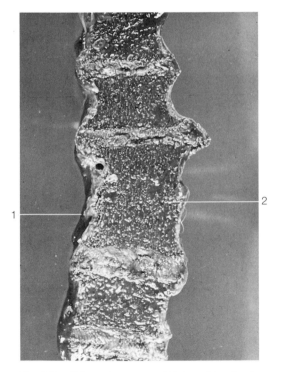

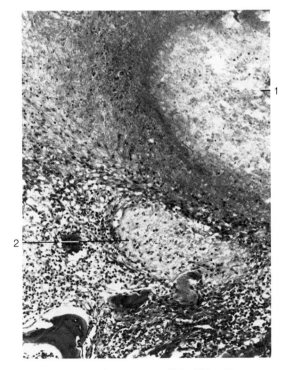

Fig. 268. Tuberculous spondylitis with development of block vertebrae (lumbar vertebrae)

Fig. 269. Tuberculous osteomyelitis; HE, ×40

Fig. 270 illustrates a **maceration specimen** of tuberculous spondylitis of the lumbar column. The 3rd (1) and 4th (2) lumbar vertebral bodies are partly fused to form a block vertebra. The intervertebral space (3) is narrowed and partly eliminated. In the center we can see a large cavity (4) that reaches into both bodies and contains the usual infective material. The preserved perifocal spongiosa (5) shows signs of irregular osteoporosis. These structural changes are clearly demonstrable radiologically. Such advanced destruction of bone invaded by the tuberculous cavity on one side and by the osteoporosis on the other can easily result in a compression fracture of the vertebral body with narrowing of the spinal canal, eventually complicated by pressure on the cord.

In **Fig. 271** one can see a **radiograph** of tuberculous osteomyelitis of the proximal part of the left femur. There is a large area of osteoporotic loosening of the spongiosa in the femoral neck and trochanteric region (1). There are no circumscribed osteolytic foci (cavities). The hip joint is not very clearly seen, and the joint cavity (2) is narrowed. A fracture (3) has appeared in the femoral neck. **Histological examination** of the biopsy material revealed the presence of tuberculous osteomyelitis. In **Fig. 272** one can see granulation tissue with several tubercles in the marrow cavity (1) which show central caseation (2) and are surrounded by a wall of epithelioid cells (3) and Langhans' giant cells (4). The spongiosa is extensively destroyed and only the remains of trabeculae are to be seen (5). This typical histological picture also leads one to consider tuberculosis very seriously, but proof must depend upon confirming the presence of tubercle bacilli.

Treatment requires that the bone cavity is curetted and the tuberculous granulation tissue removed. Sometimes stabilization by osteosynthesis is also necessary. In these cases tuberculostatic treatment is naturally indicated, and that is usually rather a lengthy process. Patients with bone tuberculosis must be kept constantly under observation in order to recognize a recurrence as soon as possible and to prevent the disease from spreading.

BCG Osteomyelitis

As a result of the introduction of BCG inoculation and the use of tuberculostatic drugs the incidence of tuberculosis has been greatly reduced. However, BCG inoculation, like every other aggressive therapy, does on rare occasions have its complications. A few patients show an extreme pathological reaction to such an inoculation, and the picture of bone tuberculosis develops. This applies particularly to children with a lowered resistance. In **Fig. 273** one can see a **radiograph** of the right humerus of a one-year-old child after BCG inoculation. The proximal part of the humerus (1) is extensively damaged, and there is a pathological fracture. In the shaft one can see a sclerotic increase in density (2) and a cavernous region of translucency (3). The periosteum is elevated over a wide region, and appears widened and cloudy (4). The **histological picture** of the bone biopsy seen in **Fig. 274** shows the structures which are virtually pathognomonic of active tuberculosis. There are tubercles with necrotic centers (1), and in the neighborhood a highly cellular granulation tissue (2) with epithelioid

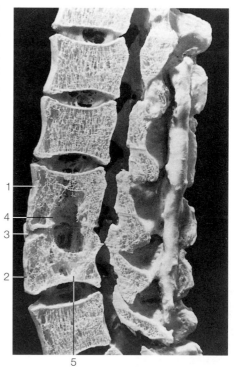

Fig. 270. Tuberculous spondylitis with cavitation and block vertebrae (maceration specimen)

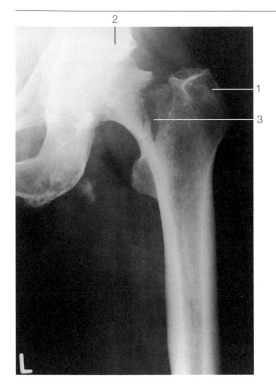

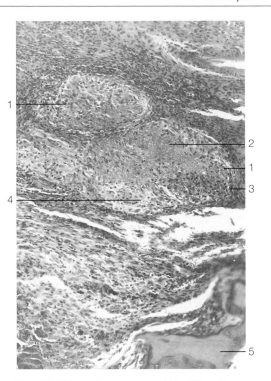

Fig. 271. Tuberculous osteomyelitis with pathological fracture of the femoral neck (left femur)

Fig. 272. Tuberculous osteomyelitis; HE, ×40

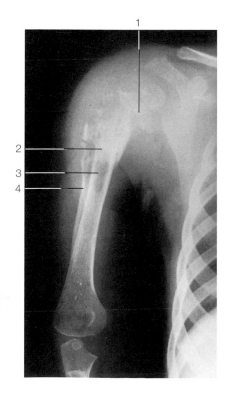

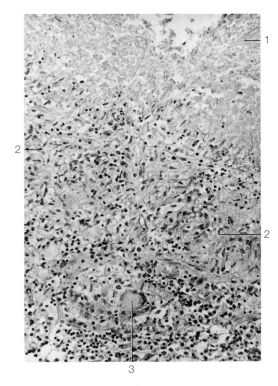

Fig. 273. BCG osteomyelitis (right proximal humerus)

Fig. 274. BCG osteomyelitis; HE, ×80

cells and multinucleate Langhans' giant cells (3). It is not, however, possible to confirm the presence here of tubercle bacilli either histologically or bacteriologically.

Boeck's Sarcoidosis of Bone (Jüngling's Ostitis Cystoides Multiplex)

Boeck's sarcoidosis is a granulomatous inflammatory condition of unknown etiology that particularly affects the reticulo-endothelial system (lymph nodes, spleen, liver, bone marrow). The disease can therefore appear in bone and lead to radiological changes, which are, however usually without subjective symptoms. It is only if the granulomas in the bone marrow produce reactive osteolysis or osteosclerosis that the condition can be detected radiologically. Bone involvement is to be expected in about 14% of cases of Boeck's sarcoidosis, and in 2.2% there is *hypercalcemia*. It is most often the intermediate and terminal phalanges of the fingers and toes that are affected *(Jüngling's ostitis cystoides multiplex)*. Less frequently lesions are found in the metacarpals and metatarsals, carpals and tarsals, the epiphyseal lines of the long bones or the axial skeleton. Very often they can appear simultaneously in several different bones.

In **Fig. 275** one can recognize a destructive lesion **radiologically** in the intermediate phalanx of the right little finger (1), which contains a sharply bordered, patchy translucent area. The surrounding bone tissue is porous (2). There is no perifocal osteosclerosis or reactive periostitis, and the neighboring joints are not affected. The lesion could regress spontaneously.

Skeletal sarcoidosis can give rise to multifocal osteosclerosis with corresponding radiological changes, of which sclerosis of the medial third of the iliac wing is particularly characteristic. The **radiograph** of **Fig. 276** shows such a finding. There is a massive band of osteosclerotic spongiosa (1) in the medial third of the wing of the left iliac bone, and one can also see round sclerotic foci in the iliac crest (2) and the pubic ramus (3) on the left side. It is not possible in this case to distinguish this from the sclerosing osteomyelitis of Garré (p. 144). Such osteoscleroses are, in cases of sarcoidosis, without any symptoms.

With progressive reactive bone remodeling due to sarcoidosis, one finds an increase of activity near the bony foci in the **skeletal scintigram**. In **Fig. 277** one can see a case of multifocal Boeck's sarcoidosis with the "hot points" particularly in the short tubular bones of the hands (1) and feet (2), in the bones of the carpus (3) and tarsus (4), in the proximal tibial epiphyses (5) and in the left elbow joint (6).

The **histological picture** contains multiple avascular nodes of highly cellular granulation tissue (1). As appears in **Fig. 278**, the nodes are often sharply bordered by the surrounding connective tissue (2) and consist almost exclusively of epithelioid cells. There is no central caseation. **Figure 279** shows that they fill up the marrow cavity and in places coalesce. The bony spongiosa (1) in this granulation tissue has been destroyed, dispersed and resorbed. These are tuberculoid granulomas which – unlike the lesions of bone tuberculosis – have no central areas of necrosis (caseation). The nodes consist essentially of a loose collection of epithelioid cells with oval shoe-shaped nuclei, between which lie a few lymphocytes and isolated Langhans' giant cells (2).

Unlike the tubercle of bone tuberculosis, the sarcoid granuloma consists of a loose arrangement of peripherally placed epithelioid cells without any central region of caseation. Usually

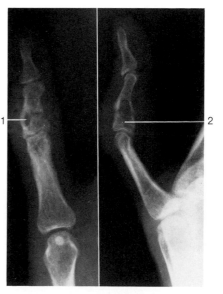

Fig. 275. Boeck's sarcoidosis (middle phalanx of right little finger)

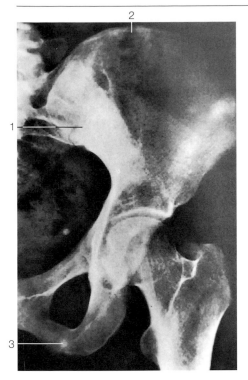

Fig. 276. Boeck's sarcoidosis (left iliac bone)

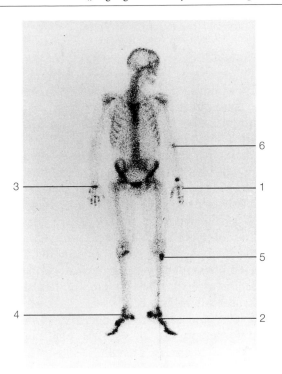

Fig. 277. Multifocal Boeck's sarcoidosis (scintigram)

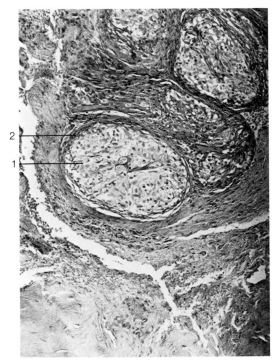

Fig. 278. Boeck's sarcoidosis; HE, ×40

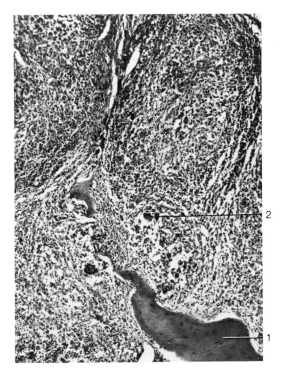

Fig. 279. Boeck's sarcoidosis; HE, ×80

there is no closed lymphocytic surrounding wall. In the active phase of sarcoidosis the Kveim reaction is positive and the tuberculin reaction negative. Associated joint inflammation, fistulas and sequestra do not belong to the picture of sarcoidosis.

Syphilitic Osteomyelitis (Syphilis of Bone)

This infectious disease, which is caused by the spirochete Treponema pallidum, can be transmitted to the fetus across the placental barrier or can be acquired in adult life. We can therefore distinguish between *congenital syphilis* and *acquired syphilis*. The skeletal manifestations of these two forms can be distinguished both radiologically and histologically. *Congenital syphilis* is principally characterized by trophic disturbances of cartilaginous growth: *syphilitic osteochondritis* or *osteochondritis luetica*. The **radiological appearance** of syphilis is not specific enough to provide a certain diagnosis. The epiphyseal cartilages are usually widened with fine irregularities on the epiphyseal and diaphyseal sides. The epiphyseal plates are faded and torn, and seem to be detached from the brighter metaphyses. In **Fig. 281** one can recognize the increase in breadth of the preparatory calcification zone *(1)* in a syphilitic child. The layer of spongiosa adjacent to the epiphyseal cartilage is weakly developed and therefore translucent *(2)*. It encloses a feebly sclerotic layer of the spongiosa *(3)*. The remaining spongiosa is mostly atrophic. A region of marked *periostitis ossificans (4)* is also striking.

Histologically in **Fig. 282** one first recognizes in the widened preparatory calcification zone the proliferating columnar cartilage *(1)*. Adjacent to this the irregular cartilaginous matrix is more strongly calcified than normal, so that a regular scaffold of calcium has developed *(2)*. This is characteristic of syphilitic osteochondritis. As a consequence of the reduced osteoblastic activity hardly any bone tissue has been deposited in the calcified matrix. The marrow cavity contains highly vascular granulation tissue without any foci of hematopoietic activity.

In *acquired syphilis* one most often observes defects in the nasopalatine region, with saddle nose and palatal defects. Syphilitic osteomyelitis is mostly found in the long bones, predominantly in the form of *syphilitic periostitis ossificans*. In the later stages, gummatous cavities develop within the bones. In **Fig. 280** one can see the **radiograph** of syphilitic osteomyelitis in the distal part of the radius. This region of the bone is elevated and shows signs of extended sclerosis *(1)*. Inside the lesion there are numerous small *(2)* and large *(3)* osteolytic defects, which are sharply delineated and have indented the cortex *(4)*. The preceding periostitis ossificans is structurally drawn into the cortex. Such a radiological appearance is reminiscent of a bone tumor. Typical syphilitic periostitis ossificans can be seen in the **radiograph** of the femur in **Fig. 283**, where one observes marked widening and cloudiness of the periosteum *(1)*, the outline of which is unclear and feathery. It is in some places fused with the cortex *(2)* and in others separated from it by a translucent region *(3)*. Within the bone, there is diffuse sclerosis of the spongiosa with fine patchy regions of translucency *(4)*. Distal to this a wide sclerotic demarcation can be seen *(5)*.

The **histological picture** of an intraosseous gumma is shown in **Fig. 284**. There is highly cellular granulation tissue with confused foci of a dense infiltrate of lymphocytes and plasma cells *(1)*, most of which surround a central vessel *(2)*. This is a specific syphilitic gumma, and it is decisive for the diagnosis if found in a biopsy. These days it is extremely rare to encounter acquired syphilis in an adult, and the diagnosis should only be made if the presence of syphilis has been confirmed serologically.

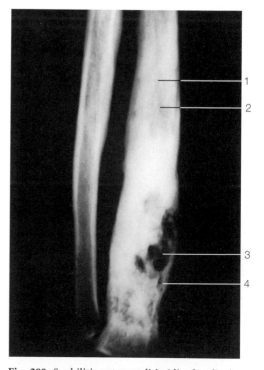

Fig. 280. Syphilitic osteomyelitis (distal radius)

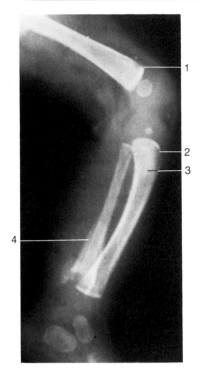

Fig. 281. Congenital syphilitic osteomyelitis (femur, tibia, fibula)

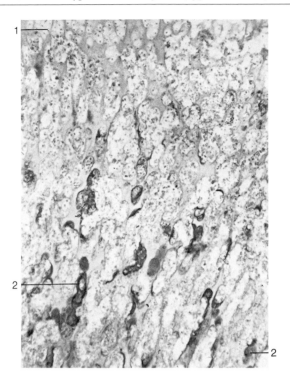

Fig. 282. Syphilitic osteochondritis; HE, ×25

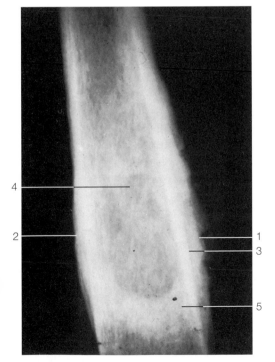

Fig. 283. Syphilitic osteomyelitis in an adult (femur)

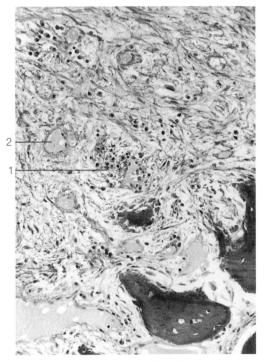

Fig. 284. Syphilitic osteomyelitis; HE, ×64

Typhoid Osteomyelitis

Involvement of bone in a Salmonella infection is very much less common than in a staphylococcal infection, but osteomyelitis accompanying typhoid fever is being increasingly observed as more and more people travel. Children are more frequently affected than adults. Typhoid osteomyelitis is particularly to be seen accompanying typhoid in patients with sickle cell anemia. The disease is more serious than staphylococcal osteomyelitis. The mortality rate is 19% among children and young people, and can even reach 58% in those over 25 years old. Multiple lesions appear simultaneously in several bones. In the **radiograph** of **Fig. 285** such a typhoid lesion is to be seen in the patella *(1)*. One can recognize a circumscribed zone of destruction that is fairly sharply delimited by marginal sclerosis. Internally there is a fine, patchy, cloudy appearance. The cortex is also completely destroyed on one side *(2)*, and here a discrete bony periosteal reaction can be recognized. The remaining bone tissue of the patella is given over to irregular sclerosis.

In the bone biopsy shown in **Fig. 286** one can recognize **histologically** loose fibrous tissue *(1)* in the marrow cavity with slender fibrocyte nuclei and a lymphocytic infiltrate. There are also small nodes with unclear borders *(2)* which consist of a loose collection of histiocytic cellular elements. These granulomas contain macrophages with irregular dark nuclei *(3)*, known as *Rindfleisch cells* (or "typhoid cells"), which have phagocytosed nuclear debris and erythrocytes. In the outer regions of such a typhoid node one finds mostly lymphocytes and a few plasma cells. Polymorphonuclear leukocytes are not demonstrable in this granulation tissue. In the periphery of such an osteomyelitic typhoid focus the bone trabeculae show regions of deposition and several drawn out reversal lines *(4)* as signs of a reactive osteosclerosis.

Bang's Osteomyelitis (Osteomyelitic Brucellosis)

This late manifestation of *Bang's undulant fever* particularly attacks the vertebral column *(Bang's spondylitis)*, but can also arise in the ribs and long bones. In the vertebral column it is especially the lumbosacral region (including the sacroiliac joint) that is affected. The causative organism is the Brucella bacterium (Brucella abortus, suius, melitensis), which gains entry into the organism through the skin, gastrointestinal tract or respiratory passages. It lodges in the liver, spleen, lymph nodes, bone marrow, joints or kidneys. In the bones and joints the inflammatory foci require a few weeks or months from the initial infection to cause pain. In **Fig. 287** a focus of Bang's osteomyelitis is shown **radiologically** at the proximal femoral metaphysis of a 20-month-old child *(1)*. The lesion lies in the center of the bone marrow and is sharply bordered by a thin layer of marginal sclerosis. The spongiosa inside the focus has been extensively destroyed to produce a "bone cyst". Apart from slight perifocal osteosclerosis *(2)* the remaining bone shows no other changes.

Histologically (**Fig. 288**) the marrow cavity is filled with highly cellular loose granulation tissue. Within it, there are poorly delineated nodular granulomas *(1)* consisting of collections of numerous mononucleated macrophages between which no – or only a very few – polymorphonuclear leukocytes are to be seen. One can also see lymphocytes, plasma cells and occasional multinucleate giant cells within the granulomas. These are mononucleated or multinucleated macrophages which have phagocytosed the bacteria and most of which will perish. In the small granulomas the spongiosa can remain unchanged. In the case shown here, the spongiosa in the neighborhood of the osteomyelitic lesions has, however, been extensively destroyed by the inflammatory process. Reactive osteosclerosis has developed peripherally, as indicated by the widened bone trabeculae *(2)*.

In the spinal column Bang's osteomyelitis develops in the vertebral bodies. The lesions lie mostly near the intervertebral discs and can attack the adjacent bodies. This may lead to deformation of the spinal column and sometimes to compression of the cord. Bang's spondylitis can imitate tuberculous spondylitis (p. 146, **Fig. 265**) radiologically in every detail. The osteoporosis in Bang's disease is, however, less marked. A biopsy can settle the diagnosis.

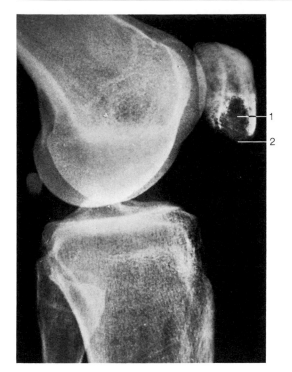

Fig. 285. Typhoid osteomyelitis (patella)

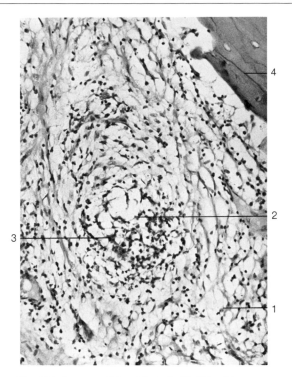

Fig. 286. Osteomyelitis with typhoid; HE, ×64

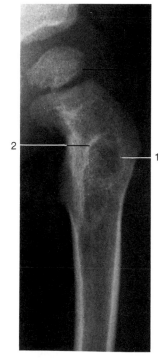

Fig. 287. Bang's osteomyelitis: *Brucella abortus* (proximal femur)

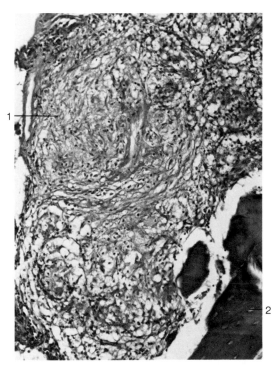

Fig. 288. Bang's osteomyelitis: *Brucella abortus*; HE, ×71

Fungal Osteomyelitis

Osteomyelitis can develop as a result of a fungal infection, with the fungus subsequently settling in the bone marrow. Even if bacterial osteomyelitis occurs much more frequently, fungal osteomyelitis always crops up from time to time and can cause serious diagnostic difficulties. Basically speaking, any fungus may be responsible, although the most usually encountered are Actinomyces bovis (*actinomycosis,* truly bacterial), Coccidioides immitis *(coccidioidomycosis),* Blastomyces dermatiditis (blastomycosis) and Sporotrichum schenckii *(sporotrichosis).* Fungal infections of this kind occur much more often and primarily in the soft parts, but they can sometimes secondarily attack the skeleton. Usually a fungal osteomyelitis is a late manifestation of a fungal infection, but it can also sometimes be the first sign of the disease.

Radiologically a fungal osteomyelitis produces no specific structural changes in the bone, so that this cannot be a basis for the diagnosis. **Figure 289** is a picture of a fungal osteomyelitis of the ulna, shown on histological examination to be coccidioidomycosis. In the proximal part of the diaphysis one can recognize a small translucent osteolytic area *(1)* which has an unclear and slightly jagged border. There is no marginal sclerosis. The adjacent bone tissue, including the cortex, has undergone an osteosclerotic increase in density *(2).* No periosteal reaction can be recognized.

Diagnosis depends upon **histological examination** of a bone biopsy (confirmed by bacteriological and immunological tests). The marrow cavity usually contains highly cellular granulation tissue which can be mistaken for a nonspecific or specific osteomyelitis or even a bone tumor – an osteoclastoma, for instance. The presence of a fungus can best be confirmed by Grocott staining, or PAS.

The histological structure of a fungal osteomyelitis is illustrated in **Fig. 290.** The marrow cavity is filled with loose granulation tissue in which collections of eosinophil leukocytes and a few neutrophils can here and there be seen *(1).* In addition, one can recognize with PAS staining small cordlike structures *(2)* which are pathognomonic of a fungus. They consist of septate hyphae which frequently subdivide di-

chotomously to form a network (the mycelium). In between there are numerous conidia ("pistils") *(3).* The organism here is the fungus *Aspergillus,* which has attacked the wall of the maxillary sinus. This fungus is found all over the world, and usually enters the body by inhalation of the spores. If resistance is lowered, the mycosis can spread through the bloodstream to reach the bone and initiate a fungal osteomyelitis.

In **Fig. 291** a highly cellular granulation tissue can be seen that originated in the marrow cavity. The numerous microabscesses *(1)* consisting of dense collections of polymorphonuclear leukocytes are striking. In between one sees a large number of multinucleated giant cells *(2),* the nuclei of which lie close together or are arranged in rows around the cell periphery. There are also many histiocytic cellular elements *(3).* Such giant cell granulation tissue can lead to serious diagnostic difficulties. In the presence of existing inflammatory changes with giant cells that closely resemble foreign body giant cells, the possibility of a fungal osteomyelitis must be borne in mind.

The higher magnification of **Fig. 292** shows inclusion bodies within the giant cells which stain red with PAS. These are the sporocysts of *coccidioidomycosis (1),* which are empty, or the endospores *(2)* of this fungal disease. The sporocysts are round and 30–60 μm in diameter. The endospores leave the fungal cells and lie in the cytoplasm of the giant cells. A fungal osteomyelitis such as this can resemble tuberculoid granulation tissue, and the macroscopic changes are also similar to those of tuberculosis. Coccidioidomycosis, which is found particularly in the southwest states of the USA and in Middle and South America, is especially liable to attack the lung. If the skeleton is involved, lesions are usually found in several bones, mostly near to the joints.

A whole host of organisms can settle in the bone marrow and give rise to skeletal inflammation. *Actinomycosis* of bone may produce cavities and scleroses with fistulas in the bones of the jaws, where the organisms can usually be clearly demonstrated histologically. In cases of *echinococcosis* of bone, the parasites (Ecchinococcus cysticus or alveolaris) can give rise to single or multivesicular hydatid cysts in bone (spinal column, pelvis, long bones).

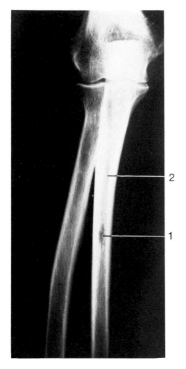

Fig. 289. Fungal osteomyelitis: aspergillosis (ulna)

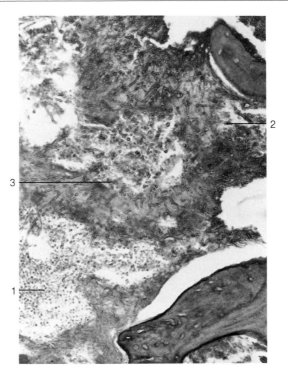

Fig. 290. Fungal osteomyelitis: (aspergillosis); PAS, ×64

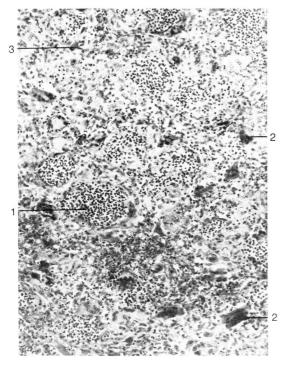

Fig. 291. Fungal osteomyelitis: (coccidiodomycosis);
HE, ×40

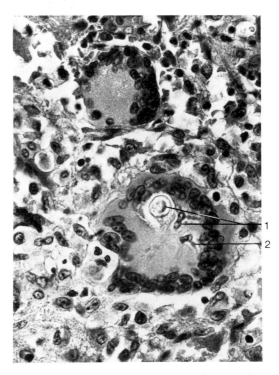

Fig. 292. Fungal osteomyelitis: (coccidiodomycosis);
PAS, ×160

Echinococcosis of Bone

Bone diseases due to parasites are rare. *Bone echinococcosis is due to a parasitic invasion of the tissue by the cysticercus of the canine tapeworm (Taenia echinococcus) following contamination with the feces of infected dogs, cats or rabbits.* Infection most often occurs by mouth and in childhood. The embryos reach the bloodstream from the gut and settle in 65% of cases in the liver, and in 10%–15% in the lung. Bone is involved in only 1%–3% of cases, usually by Echinococcus granulosus. As illustrated in **Fig. 293**, the most frequent sites are in the axial skeleton (vertebral column, pelvis). The long bones (humerus, tibia, fibula) are also often attacked, the femur and skull only rarely.

The **radiological structure** of echinococcosis is distinguished by multicystic bone remodeling which involves large regions of the bone attacked and may recall the picture of a malignant bone tumor. In **Fig. 294** one sees a case of echinococcal involvement of the proximal part of the left humerus. More than a third of this long bone is showing signs of multicystic remodeling. Near the large intraosseous bony cysts *(1)* there are several smaller cysts *(2)*, none of which have any internal structure. The cysts are only incompletely separated by narrow septa *(3)*. The affected region is slightly elevated. The cortex appears to be narrowed from within, but is completely intact. One can recognize an obliquely-running pathological fracture *(4)* within these lesions. This has already united after immobilization, which is why the bone here has expanded *(5)*. The lesion is clearly bordered distally by a region of marginal sclerosis *(6)*.

The **radiograph** of **Fig. 295** also shows a case of bone echinococcosis which involves the proximal part and neck of the left femur. In the neck one can see large cysts *(1)* which are bordered by narrow septa *(2)*. These cysts have no internal structure. The affected region is slightly elevated. The cortex appears to be narrowed from within, but is completely intact, and no periosteal reaction can be observed. Similar intraosseous cysts are present in the left side of the pelvis *(3)* above the hip joint.

The **histological picture** of the material from a curettage or biopsy of such a bone cyst includes membranous cystic structures which are easily recognized as belonging to an echinococcal cyst. In **Fig. 296** one can see loose scar tissue *(1)* with foci of inflammatory cells *(2:* lymphocytes, plasma cells) and numerous cystic hollow spaces *(3)*, which are empty and which resemble the gaps left by foreign bodies. The long *chitinous membranes (4)* are, however, pathognomonic of echinococcosis. These appear in histological sections as homogeneous, often slightly laminated red strips which show up very brightly with HE staining. This "cuticle" is a product of the echinococcus and enables the diagnosis to be made. *Scolices* are sometimes seen in the neighborhood of the cuticle, confirming the presence of the parasite itself.

The **histological picture** of **Fig. 297** shows the cystic material under **higher magnification**. One can see the empty hollow spaces of the cysts *(1)* in which the scolices must be looked for (not present in the picture). However, the wide bright red chitinous membranes *(2)* are characteristic of echinococcus. Betwcen the cysts there is loose connective tissue with a non-specific inflammatory infiltrate *(3)*.

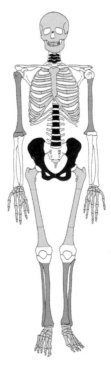

Fig. 293. Localization of bone echinococcosis. *Black,* very common; *dark gray,* common; *light gray,* rare. (After BÜRGEL and BIERLING 1973)

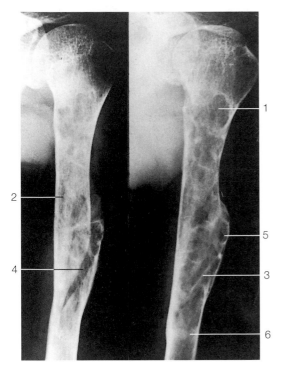

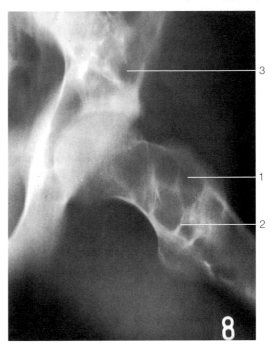

Fig. 294. Echinococcosis (proximal humerus)

Fig. 295. Echinococcosis (left femoral neck)

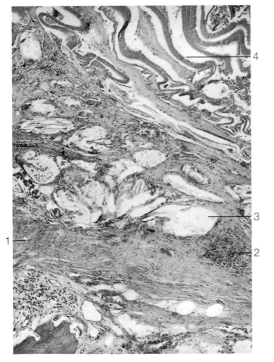

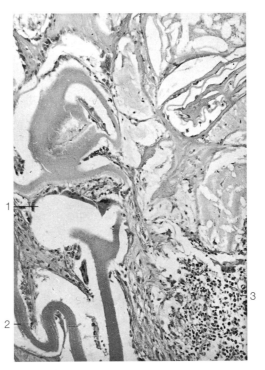

Fig. 296. Echinococcosis; HE, ×40

Fig. 297. Echinococcosis; HE, ×80

Inflammatory Periostitis Ossificans

In cases of osteomyelitis the inflammation spreads out from the bone marrow cavity through the Haversian and Volkmann canals into the periosteum. This leads to an inflammatory reaction on the part of the periosteal connective tissue, which after about ten days causes fibro-osseous trabeculae to differentiate out. The newly built trabeculae are at first orientated radially to the cortex and bound together in the form of arcades. They are finally mineralized and form a bony shell (*"sequestral cavity"*) which is attached to the bone from outside. In the **maceration specimen (Fig. 298)** we can see a greatly roughened and deeply notched bone surface. The bony thickening of the periosteum varies in degree, but extends along the entire shaft of the long bone. Its severity depends upon the intensity of the inflammation. In the **radiograph (Fig. 299)** the inflammatory periostitis ossificans is clearly shown. Within the long bone there are destructive osteolytic lesions *(1)* with reactive sclerotic zones *(2)* of osteomyelitis. The osteomyelitic bone is enclosed by a widened and darkly clouded mantle of periosteum *(3)*. The double contour of the periosteum is clearly recognizable. The first reactive periosteal changes can be observed 2 to 3 weeks after the start of the osteomyelitic process in the form of perpendicular *"spicules"*. True bony shells with radiologically reduplicated contours appear later, and can completely disappear again after the healing of the disease.

Histologically (Fig. 300) we can see many newly developed fibro-osseous trabeculae *(1)* with numerous osteocytes and deposited layers of osteoblasts *(2)* in the widened periosteum. The bony trabeculae are woven together and more or less parallel, and are aligned at right angles to the bone surface. In places they are bound together in arcades *(3)*. Between these trabeculae there is loose granulation tissue with inflammatory cells *(4)* (lymphocytes, polymorphonuclear leukocytes, plasma cells).

Traumatic Periostitis Ossificans

An inflammatory reaction can also follow traumatic damage to the bone, such as a fracture or an osteosynthetic procedure, and this can lead to the development of a more or less severe periostitis ossificans. In the **radiograph (Fig. 301)** we can see a femur in which intramedullary pinning *(1)* was employed for the treatment of a fracture. A severe periosteal reaction developed which spread throughout the whole of the bone *(2)*. The newly formed bony structures give the widened periosteum the appearance of an irregular honeycomb.

Fig. 302 shows the classical **histological** picture of periostitis ossificans. We can see many new fibro-osseous trabeculae with large osteocytes and patchy deposition *(1)*. Osteoblasts are lining the bony structures *(2)*. The trabeculae are bound together to form a dense irregular network, which differs from the appearance of an inflammatory periostitis ossificans. Between the trabeculae one can see loose fibrous or granulation tissue, in some places with deposits of hemosiderin. It can be difficult to distinguish between traumatic periostitis ossificans and callus tissue on the basis of a biopsy alone.

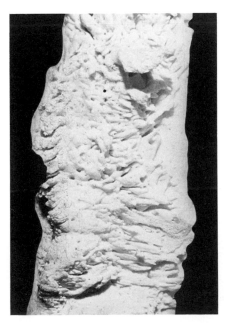

Fig. 298. Periostitis ossificans (maceration specimen)

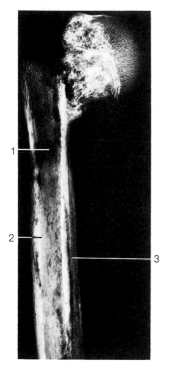

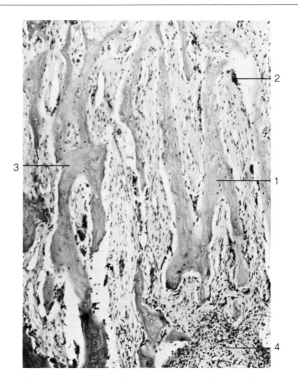

Fig. 299. Purulent inflammatory periostitis ossificans (femur)

Fig. 300. Purulent inflammatory periostitis ossificans; HE, ×25

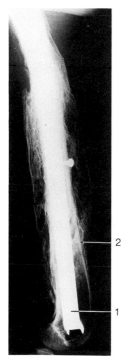

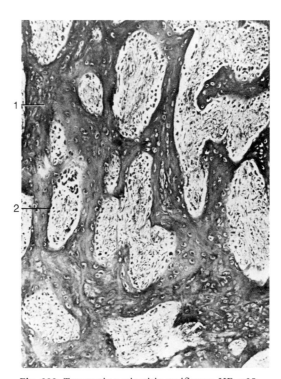

Fig. 301. Traumatic periostitis ossificans (femur)

Fig. 302. Traumatic periostitis ossificans; HE, ×25

Ossifying Periostosis Due to Impairment of the Blood Supply

Following venous stasis in the soft parts (due to varicosity, for instance) an ossifying periostosis can develop locally – usually in the tibia or femur. In **Fig. 303** one can see the **radiograph** of a normally structured femur. Clouding of the periosteum, which varies in width and has an undulating border, is apparent near the middle of the shaft *(1)*.

Tumorous Ossifying Periostosis

Bone tumors, particularly when malignant, lead to destruction of the neighboring bone and simultaneously bring about a local inflammatory reaction. Such processes penetrate the cortex and stimulate the periosteal connective tissue to lay down new bone, which can be observed radiologically. **Figure 304** shows the **radiograph** of an osteoblastic osteosarcoma of the distal femoral metaphysis in which the affected region of the bone is densely clouded *(1)*. In the periosteum there are irregular shadows which include "streaks" lying perpendicular to the surface *(2)*. These are the so-called *spicules* which provide a ray-like border to that region of the bone, and represent the periosteal reaction to the malignant growth of the tumor. **Histologically (Fig. 305)** we can see parallel-orientated patchy bone trabeculae with active osteocytes and a few deposited osteoblasts *(1)*. Between these newly formed trabeculae there is mostly only loose, highly vascular granulation tissue *(2)*. Only in rare cases can one see sparsely distributed tumor tissue which has infiltrated the region, and therefore a biopsy of the ossifying periosteal reaction would have only limited diagnostic value.

Osteoarthropathie hypertrophiante pneumique (Pierre Marie-Bamberger)

This skeletal disease represents a particular form of periostitis ossificans that can occasionally arise in the course of chronic heart or lung disease, and which can lead to extensive symmetrical thickening of the long and short tubular bones by layered periosteal bone deposition.

Such periosteal changes can appear as an early symptom of a bronchial carcinoma, and they may recede again following removal of the tumor. In the **radiograph (Fig. 306)** one can recognize the cloudy appearance of the periosteum of a femur *(1)*, where the long bone is surrounded by a sleeve-like layer of periosteal bone that is wide opposite the diaphysis and narrow near the metaphyses/epiphyses *(2)*. The ends of the bone show no periosteal thickening. The layer of periosteal bone is separated from the cortex by a narrow space. **Histologically (Fig. 307)** one sees a widened periosteum of loose connective tissue, which has been invaded by numerous capillaries *(1)*. Within this, layers of new bone trabeculae *(2)* which already show a laminated layering have differentiated. At the beginning of these changes there are fibro-osseous trabeculae which lie perpendicular to the diaphysis, but which later become bound together to form arcades, so that several layers of bone lying one upon the other can arise. The adjacent cortex *(3)* is rendered cancellous owing to smooth bone resorption from the Haversian canals outwards.

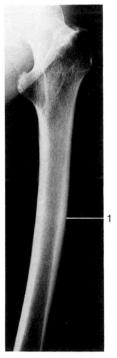

Fig. 303. Ossifying periostosis due to a circulatory disturbance (femur)

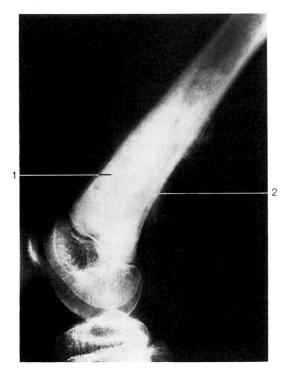

Fig. 304. Tumorous bony periostosis: osteosarcoma (distal femur)

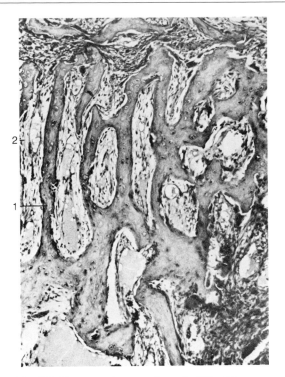

Fig. 305. Tumorous bony periostosis; HE, ×25

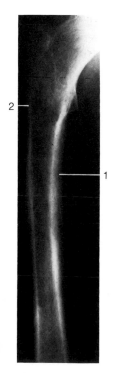

Fig. 306. Osteoarthropathie hypertrophiante pneumique (Pierre Marie-Bamberger) (femur)

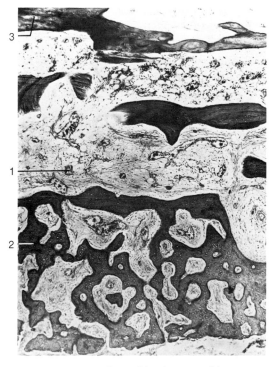

Fig. 307. Osteoarthropathie hypertrophiante pneumique (Pierre Marie-Bamberger); HE, ×20

8 Bone Necroses

General

Just as in the case of any other living tissue, bone tissue can die, and this will result in the appearance of necrotic material; in other words, a bone necrosis. Such a condition may be due to: (1) impairment of the blood supply to the bone, (2) inflammation of the bone itself (osteomyelitis, p. 129), (3) radiation damage (radioosteonecrosis), (4) trauma (e.g. fracture, p. 113) or (5) a hormonal disturbance (e.g. Cushing's disease, p. 76). Bone necrosis is distinguished histologically by the absence of osteocytes within the bone tissue. The osteocyte lacunae are empty, no nuclei are seen. The lamellar layering is lost or canceled out. In any case, however, the artifacts that may arise when preparing a histological section must be taken into account. Too lengthy or too fierce decalcification in nitric acid can itself destroy the osteocytes, leaving their lacunae empty. In the presence of bone necrosis one usually finds reactive inflammatory changes in the adjacent bone tissue.

The etiology of the various types of bone necrosis has not so far been elucidated. Only in relatively few cases can it be attributed to cutting off the blood supply. Following a fracture, a piece of bone may be deprived of its blood supply and become necrotic. The same can be caused by a surgical procedure (e.g. osteosynthesis) which damages the vessels to the bone (e.g. intramedullary pinning or abrasion of the periosteum). Emboli, a stenosing arteriosclerosis or inflammation of the wall of a nutrient artery can equally well lead to impairment of the blood supply. In this way an anemic bone infarct develops. Such bone necroses are nevertheless rather uncommon, because the bone marrow and the spongiosa are most efficiently supplied with blood via the nutrient artery, and the cortex from the periosteum. This is apparently the etiology in the case of caisson disease (p. 174). As against that, the origin of bone necroses during metabolic or hormonal disorders (e.g. Cushing's disease, p. 76) is still largely unexplained. In histological sections it is important to distinguish bone necroses with simultaneous osteomyelitic changes *(septic bone necroses)* from those that show no real indications of accompanying inflammation *(aseptic bone necroses)*. It is known that in cases of purulent osteomyelitis, necroses develop in which pieces of dead bone are extruded (formation of *sequestra*). Therapeutically this implies sequestrotomy and antibiotic treatment. Although bone is, in comparison with other tissues, relatively resistant to radiation, bone necroses do indeed appear after radiotherapy (*radioosteonecroses*). In particular, it is true that, following earlier conventional weak radiation, bone absorbs radiation more strongly, so that it may possibly be subjected in effect to two or three times the dose given. This can often lead to the development of radioosteonecroses upon which, particularly in the region of the jaws where there are so many entry ports for bacteria, infective inflammation may be superimposed. Today, with the use of modern high-voltage treatment and homogeneous radiation of the soft parts and bone tissue, the possibility of overdosage is greatly reduced and the bone tissue of adults is therefore relatively radioresistant. Furthermore, because of the thorough dental hygiene carried out before employing radiotherapy in the head and neck region, the danger of a so-called *radiation osteitis* (radioosteomyelitis) of the jaw is reduced to a minimum.

With the majority of aseptic bone necroses it is assumed that only a disturbance of the blood supply can have been the cause, without there being any real proof of this. These are the *"idiopathic ischemic bone necroses"*. In a few cases a history of local trauma can be found (*"post-traumatic ischemic bone necrosis"*). In cases of the so-called *aseptic epiphyseal necroses* ("localized osteochondritis"), the bone marrow and bone tissue in the growing regions become necrotic, while the articular cartilage – which is nourished by the synovia – remains unaffected. The continued functional loading of the part of the bone affected leads to a growth deformity and disturbance of function (e.g. arthrosis deformans). This group includes especially Perthes's disease, Osgood-Schlatter disease, Köhler's disease (of the navicular bones of the feet and metatarsal heads), Kienböck's disease (lunatomalacia), Scheuermann's disease (of the spinal column) and osteochondrosis dissecans (p. 430). A particularly frequent site for aseptic bone necrosis is the femoral head, where it always leads to a severe coxarthrosis deformans. It is especially after a medial fracture of the femoral neck in old age that a secondary aseptic necrosis of the femoral head is likely to develop. Because of this experience, it is usual to remove the head surgically immediately after the fracture and replace it with a total endoprosthesis (TEP).

Following Pörschl (1971), some 90 different bone necroses have been described which have similar radiological findings and the same histological picture, and can only be distinguished from each other by their localization and etiology. Vague pains in a joint or in the limb near a joint, or in the vertebral column in children or young people, always suggests a possible aseptic bone necrosis and should be examined radiologically. In most cases a plane radiograph, which should be bilateral in the case of the limbs, is sufficient to establish the diagnosis. These examinations can be extended to include tomograms and the imaging procedures of nuclear medicine. In the scintigram of an acute bone necrosis (for instance, following trauma or acute obliteration of a vessel) there is no activity, whereas with a slowly developing spontaneous aseptic osteonecrosis the activity is increased. This is due to the reparative remodeling of the still vital bone tissue.

In the **radiograph** of **Fig. 308** one can see, in an aseptic bone necrosis affecting the medial condyle of the left femur, only a discrete irregularity of the contour (1) that is hardly recognizable as a pathological finding. The patella (2) shows up as a large round zone of increased density. In the corresponding **scintigram** (**Fig. 309**), on the other hand, this region shows a great increase in activity (1), indicating vigorous local bone remodeling. The patella is outlined in the scintigram (2). In such a case a selective bone biopsy will establish the diagnosis of an aseptic bone necrosis histologically.

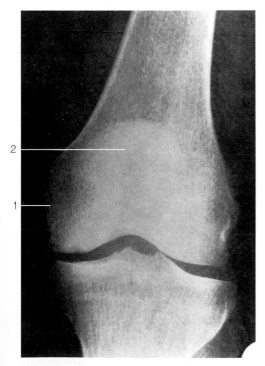

Fig. 308. Aseptic bone necrosis of medial condyle of the left femur (scarcely recognizable)

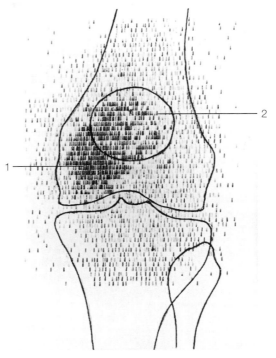

Fig. 309. Aseptic bone necrosis of medial condyle of the left femur (scintigram)

The Normal Blood Supply of Bone

Like every other living tissue, bone is dependent upon its blood supply. For this reason every bone is connected to the general circulatory system and transmits arterial and venous blood. Disturbances of the blood-flow through the tissue lead to changes in the bone, thus producing bone necrosis or a bony infarct if the blood supply is interrupted. An arterial hyperemia leads to increased local (osteoclastic) resorption, and venous stasis to increased (osteoblastic) deposition (osteosclerosis).

As can be seen from the **diagrammatic representation** in **Fig. 310**, the intraosseous circulation is extremely complicated. Small arteries and veins from the periosteum pass into the bone through the Volkmann canals and build up a rich network of vessels in the bone marrow, in the osteons and in the spongiosa. This functional vascular framework consists of a woven pattern of sinusoids and capillaries in the hematopoietic bone marrow, fatty marrow and spongiosa. It is an extensive framework and serves to provide ionic exchange between the bloodstream and the surrounding tissue. A long bone has three sources of blood supply: (1) the nutrient artery, (2) the metaphyseal arteries (which after the completion of skeletal growth join with the epiphyseal arteries) and (3) the periosteal arterioles. The bony joint ends are more strongly vascularized than the bone shafts. The efferent system consists of large effluent veins, the cortical venous system and the periosteal capillaries.

The nutrient vessels (arteries and veins) enter or leave the bone through the nutrient foramina. The number of these vessels is variable (there are several arteries in the femur, only one in the tibia). After passing obliquely through the diaphyseal cortex the vessel divides in the marrow cavity into an ascending and a descending myeloid artery. These vessels branch within the marrow to give rise to numerous arterioles which penetrate the endosteum to supply the diaphyseal cortex.

In **Fig. 310a** the blood supply of a long bone is diagrammatically illustrated in longitudinal section. The *main nutrient artery* enters the bone through its nutrient foramen, thereby passing through the dense cortical bone. The blood is then distributed through the nutrient

vasculature outwards from the diaphysis. Since the vessel passes obliquely through the cortex, hardly any contrast medium can enter the bone during peripheral angiography, which is from a diagnostic point of view very important. After entering the marrow cavity, the nutrient vessel divides into ascending and descending branches which run in a longitudinal direction within the bone. No subsidiary branches are given off within the cortex. In the marrow cavity the vessels divide into numerous arterioles, and these penetrate the endosteal surface several times on their way through the bone in order that their branches may supply the diaphyseal cortex (so-called "irregular arborization"). These are probably endarteries. The cortical capillaries are connected with those of the periosteum.

The numerous myeloid arteries drain into a dense network of metaphyseal arteries which copiously supply the ends of a long bone with blood. In addition, small arteries from the main systemic circulation run diagonally through the cortical bone and join the metaphyseal arteries within the marrow cavity. In this way the growing ends of long bones are ensured a fully adequate blood supply. The epiphyses are also provided with a good blood supply. Arterial branches from outside penetrate the cortex, enter the bone and divide, one branch running in the direction of the articular cartilage and the other supplying the epiphyseal cartilage. In fully developed bones there is a wide subdivided connection between this epiphyseal capillary system and the metaphyseal arteries.

The *venous drainage* takes place through venous sinusoids and the metaphyseal veins. In the diaphysis these enter the central venous canal which runs longitudinally through the bone. Large effluent veins take the blood once again out of the bone.

Figure 310b is a **diagram** of the blood supply shown projected onto a transverse section through a bone. The cortex is supplied by capillaries from both the marrow cavity and the periosteum. Venous drainage takes place through the marrow sinusoids and the central venous sinus.

During the period of growth the metaphyses and epiphyses have their own blood supply, which is different from that of the diaphysis.

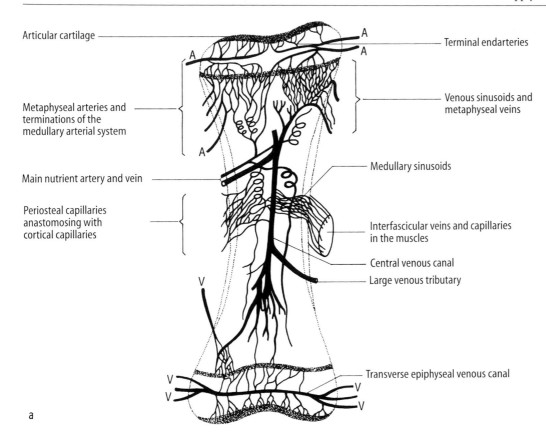

Articular cartilage ——————————— A ——————— Terminal endarteries
                                    A
                                    A

Metaphyseal arteries and ——————   ——— Venous sinusoids and
terminations of the   metaphyseal veins
medullary arterial system

                          A

Main nutrient artery and vein ————   ——— Medullary sinusoids

Periosteal capillaries
anastomosing with   ——— Interfascicular veins and capillaries
cortical capillaries   in the muscles

                                                  ——— Central venous canal
                          V   ——— Large venous tributary

                                                  ——— Transverse epiphyseal venous canal
                    V   V
                    V   V

a

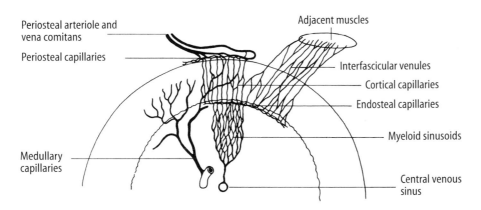

Periosteal arteriole and   Adjacent muscles
vena comitans

Periosteal capillaries   ——— Interfascicular venules
                                              ——— Cortical capillaries
                                              ——— Endosteal capillaries

                                              ——— Myeloid sinusoids

Medullary
capillaries   ——— Central venous
                                                  sinus

b

Fig. 310 a, b. Diagram illustrating blood supply of a bone. (After BROOKES 1971)

As can be seen in **Fig. 310c**, the metaphyseal and epiphyseal vessels enter the bone through numerous nutrient foramina, by which the two systems are kept apart. In the presence of complete epiphyseal cartilages there are no anastomoses between the diaphyseal blood supply and that of the epiphysis. In adults there is a subchondral circulation near the articular cartilage and a synovial circulation outside the internal synovia. The highly vascular periosteum supplies about a third of the cortex, whereas the inner third of this layer receives blood from the endosteal side through the nutrient arteries. In other words, the cortex has a dual blood supply.

This extraordinarily rich and dense system of dividing and internally communicating blood vessels in the epi-metaphyseal region of a long bone can be compared to the vasculature of the mesentery, and we can speak of the *"vascular circle of the joint"*. Band-like, it surrounds the non-articular surface of the epiphysis. Terminal capillary loops build up a vascular framework at the periphery of the articular cartilage. As in the epiphyseal region, there are several vascular loops around the shaft of the bone in the diaphyseal periosteum. The epiphyseal and metaphyseal vessels arise from this vascular circle as well as from the periarticular vascular network that supplies the joint capsule.

The epi-metaphyseal arteries are of great importance for the vitality of the bone, and they bring in approximately as much blood as does the nutrient artery. Should the nutrient artery be absent, the entire shaft of the bone may be exclusively supplied by the metaphyseal arteries and thus kept alive. Whereas the epiphyses are exclusively supplied by the epiphyseal arteries during the fetal and postnatal periods, the ends of adult bones are supplied exclusively by the metaphyseal arteries. Any disturbance of this complicated vascular system can produce a partial aseptic bone necrosis in the corresponding region (in the head of the femur, for example). No vessels are found within the epiphyseal or the articular cartilages. The growth cartilage is supplied by the epiphyseal vessels. In adults, the articular cartilage receives its nourishment partly from the subchondral metaphyseal vessels and partly from the synovial fluid. For this reason the preservation of the synovia, the joint capsule and their blood supply is of the greatest possible importance. Any reduction in the blood supply of the synovia leads to reduction of and changes in the synovial fluid, and this can cause nutritive damage to the articular cartilage.

The capillaries of the afferent system drain directly into the venules of the efferent system. The post-sinusoidal effluent stream runs through very thin-walled veins, which come together dichotomously as tributaries near the arterial divisions and drain either into the central vein in the diaphysis or into the collecting veins of the metaphyses. The venous drainage from the bone is taken away by the nutrient vein, metaphyseal veins or small perforating veins of the cortex distributed at equal intervals along the shaft. The details of this complicated vascular network with its extraordinarily large number of branches can only be demonstrated with cast specimens. Normal angiographic methods produce very incomplete results, since the contrast medium can only with difficulty reach the intraosseous vessels and does not fill all the capillaries and venules there.

Figure 311 illustrates a **normal peripheral angiogram** showing the wide caliber blood vessels of the peripheral circulation *(1)* running along the bone, and the branches entering the bone through the nutrient foramen *(2)*. It is, however, not possible to visualize the vessels within the bone by this method, although if one injects a contrast medium directly into the nutrient vessels their course within the bone can be clearly demonstrated.

Such a **normal intraosseous angiogram** is pictured in **Fig. 312**, in which a central sinus within the shaft *(1)* and an ampullary collecting vessel *(2)* are shown. The bone is traversed by a large caliber vein *(3)* that divides up at the diaphyseal-metaphyseal border *(4)* to form a vascular network. *Intraosseous angiography* makes it possible to visualize the essential components of the intraosseous vascular system. This allows one to demonstrate the gross and finer structural changes taking place in the medullary vascular system in the presence of various bone lesions (tumors, for instance, or congenital deformities), and to draw further conclusions about the nature of the lesion itself.

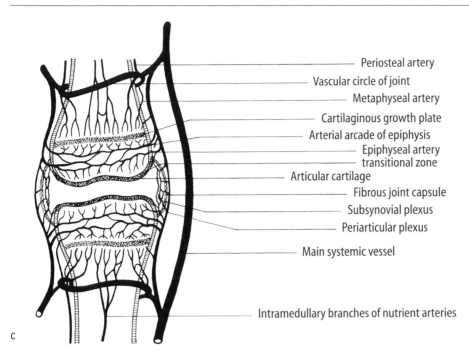

Periosteal artery
Vascular circle of joint
Metaphyseal artery
Cartilaginous growth plate
Arterial arcade of epiphysis
Epiphyseal artery
transitional zone
Articular cartilage
Fibrous joint capsule
Subsynovial plexus
Periarticular plexus
Main systemic vessel

Intramedullary branches of nutrient arteries

c

Fig. 310c. Diagram illustrating blood supply of a bone

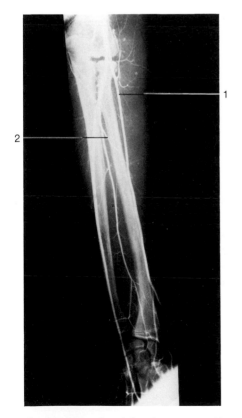

Fig. 311. Normal peripheral angiogram (forearm)

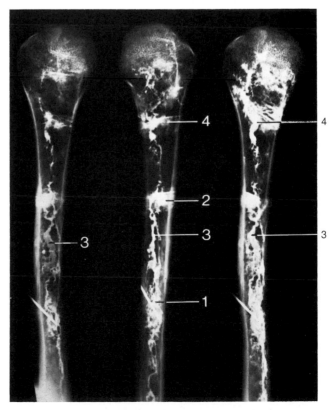

Fig. 312. Intraosseous angiogram (proximal humerus)

Idiopathic Bone Necroses

The various different bone necroses cannot be distinguished from one another in histological sections. From the nature of the marrow infiltration we can only decide whether a necrosis is septic or aseptic, or recognize a bone infarct as such. Apart from this, other clinical data (e.g. age, site of the lesion) and the radiological findings must be taken into account before the particular disease can be identified. In young people the condition announces itself with sudden pain, with or without previous bodily stress. In adults, similar pains often arise in connection with professional overwork and have a "rheumatic" character.

In **Fig. 313** one can see the **histological appearance** of an aseptic bone necrosis of the femoral head. The trabeculae of the spongiosa (1) are widened and clumsy, partly with smooth and partly with undulating borders. The lamellar layering is indistinct or absent and the osteocyte lacunae (2) are empty, which is to say that there are no osteocyte nuclei visible in the bone. This is necrotic bone tissue. Sometimes one sees deposited tabular osteons (3), which have drawn out reversal lines, and in which the osteocytes are not infrequently preserved. This is a sign of reparative bone remodeling. The marrow cavity is full of amorphous basophilic material (detritus, 4) and loose connective tissue (5) in which the occasional inflammatory cell is to be seen. The medullary connective tissue may also be necrotic, and in the necrotic zones one frequently encounters dystrophic calcification (6).

An aseptic bone necrosis can involve an entire bony element (e.g. the femoral head) or only appear in a part of it. Old or fresh necrotic changes can take over the whole of the histological picture, or reparative processes may predominate. In the **histological picture** of **Fig. 314** one can observe osteosclerotically widened trabeculae with indistinct lamellar layering (1) and empty osteocyte lacunae (2), although a few osteocytes are preserved here and there (3). Numerous osteoclasts (4) are lying in the flat resorption lacunae, and beside them there are also a few osteoblasts (5). The marrow cavity is filled with loose connective

and granulation tissue in which dilated blood vessels (6) and histiocytic elements (7) are present.

Aseptic epiphyseal necroses or **apophyseal necroses** which can be attributed to circulatory disturbances have a predilection for particular regions to each of which a corresponding name is related. Generally speaking it is only one region that is affected – an epiphysis, apophysis or a small bone. Multiple appearances are very much the exception. In **Fig. 315** the **sites** of the most frequent epiphyseal necroses are illustrated: (**a**) *Calvé's vertebra plana* attacks a vertebral body in which an aseptic bone necrosis develops and coalesces following the appearance of a fissure. The intervertebral disc remains unaltered. (**b**) *Scheuermann's disease* (adolescent kyphosis) is a condition in which microtraumas (usually in the thoracic column) produce a peripheral bone necrosis which leads to the collapse of the upper plate and the development of so-called *Schmorl's nodes* (p. 70). The resulting wedge vertebrae bring about a thoracic kyphosis. (**c**) *Perthes' disease* arises in the femoral head (coxa vara) when the avascular epiphyseal cartilage receives too little blood from the metaphysis. This leads to osteolysis of the femoral head, which becomes distorted under normal loading. (**d**) *Kienböck's disease*; a fracture following subliminal trauma leads to necrosis of the carpal lunate (lunatomalacia). (**f**) *Osgood-Schlatter disease*; chronic overloading brings about necrosis of the tibial apophysis. (**g**) *Köhler's disease I* involves necrosis of the tarsal navicula (os naviculare pedis) and *Köhler's disease II* (**h**) of the 2nd metatarsal head. *Osteochondrosis dissecans*, which belongs to the idiopathic necroses, occurs most frequently in the knee joint, less frequently in the hip, elbow and shoulder joints. *Anemic bone infarcts* are most often observed at the ends of the long bones.

Figure 316 shows the **age distribution** of the most important bone necroses. One recognizes that some idiopathic bone necroses already appear in childhood (Calvé's vertebra plana, Perthes's disease, Köhler's disease II), whereas others manifest themselves in young adults (e.g. Scheuermann's disease).

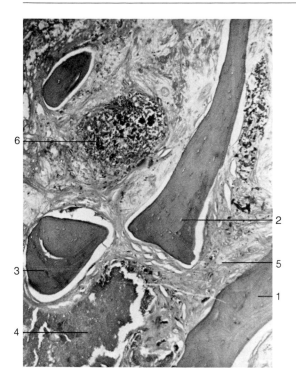

Fig. 313. Aseptic bone necrosis; HE, ×25

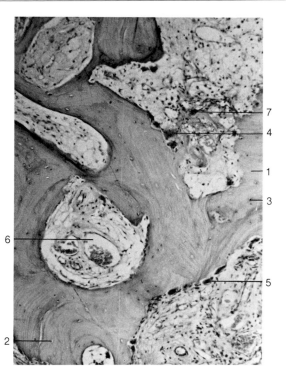

Fig. 314. Aseptic bone necrosis; HE, ×40

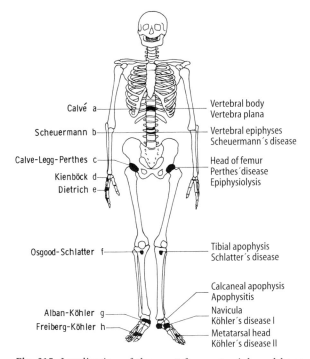

Calvé a — Vertebral body / Vertebra plana

Scheuermann b — Vertebral epiphyses / Scheuermann's disease

Calve-Legg-Perthes c — Head of femur / Perthes' disease / Epiphysiolysis

Kienböck d

Dietrich e

Osgood-Schlatter f — Tibial apophysis / Schlatter's disease

Calcaneal apophysis / Apophysitis

Alban-Köhler g — Navicula / Köhler's disease I

Freiberg-Köhler h — Metatarsal head / Köhler's disease II

Fig. 315. Localization of the most frequent epiphyseal bone necroses. (After UEHLINGER)

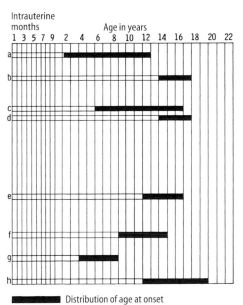

Fig. 316. Ages distribution of the most important bone necroses. (After UEHLINGER)

Femoral Head Necrosis

Necrosis of the femoral head is a relatively common condition that can develop at any age. *It is an aseptic bone necrosis caused by a disturbance of the blood supply and for which a traumatic dislocation of the hip, a medial fracture of the neck of the femur or idiopathic ischemia may be responsible.* Following injury, the vessels supplying the femoral head and neck may be torn and the blood supply cut off. In **Fig. 317** the vasculature of the head and neck of the femur is illustrated **diagrammatically**. The circumflex femoral artery arises from the deep femoral artery (arteria profunda femoris), itself a branch of the femoral artery. The circumflex artery (arteria circumflexa) forms a loop within the joint capsule above the lesser trochanter and dorsal to the femoral neck, and runs laterally into the neck, where it follows a subcortical course to the epiphysis. Between a fifth and a third of the epiphyseal blood supply comes from the acetabular artery (medial epiphyseal arteries), and the remaining four-fifths to two-thirds from the lateral epiphyseal arteries, which are branches of the obturator artery. The obturator vessels are of less importance in the adult and are often obliterated. The nearer the fracture is to the trochanter, the less danger there is of interrupting these arteries.

Necrosis of the femoral head leads to a severe arthrosis deformans (p. 424). **Figure 318** shows the **radiograph** of such a necrosis, together with coxarthrosis deformans. The head is deformed and slightly flattened. Within there is extensive osteosclerosis *(1)*, in which irregular patchy osteolysis *(2)* is to be seen. The sclerosing process reaches as far as the femoral neck *(3)*, and one can recognize peripheral osteophytes *(4)*. The joint cavity has been preserved *(5)*. There is a band-like zone of sclerosis in the joint socket *(6)*. In general, the bony structures in the neighborhood of the hip joint are indistinct.

The arthrotic deformation of a femoral head necrosis is clearly demonstrated by a **maceration specimen**. In **Fig. 319** one can see that the head is severely deformed and flattened. The cartilaginous joint surface is distorted by indentations *(1)*. Growth of the peripheral osteophytes *(2)* has caused the femoral head to bulge like a cap over the neck. The extension of the necrosis onto the femoral neck has caused the outer side of the cortex to become roughened *(3)*. On the sawn surface of the bone one can observe the irregular, partly porous, partly sclerotic framework of the spongiosa. Macroscopically one is faced with the picture of severe arthrosis deformans, radiologically there are indications that these bone changes are due to necrosis of the femoral head. It is, however, only the histological examination that can finally establish this diagnosis.

In **Fig. 320** one can see the **histological picture** of an aseptic necrosis of the femoral head. The trabeculae *(1)* have become greatly widened and obviously ill-formed as a result of the reparative processes. The lamellar layering is very indistinct and at times absent. Extensive regions of the bone tissue are free of all cells and many osteocyte cavities are empty *(2)*. This is necrotic bone tissue. Only a few scattered osteocyte nuclei are present *(3)*. A few fine drawn out reversal lines *(4)* can be clearly seen, indicating the deposition front. Here and there widened osteoid seams *(5)* are also encountered. Copious amorphous necrotic material *(6)* (stained blue by H & E) is seen lying between the trabeculae, and densely fibrous connective tissue with a few non-specific inflammatory cells. Opposite the front of the bone deposition *(7)* one can observe a wide resorption front *(8)*, where a highly cellular granulation tissue with many capillaries has forced itself up against the bone. In the bone there are numerous deep resorption lacunae which contain active multinucleated osteoclasts. In the necrotic femoral head vigorous bone remodeling is taking place, which is nevertheless unable to bring about restoration of its normal shape.

Following a medial fracture of the femoral neck the arterial blood supply to the head can be very suddenly interrupted, which will inevitably result in bone necrosis. An inadequate supply to the head may also, however, have a vascular or hematogenous origin, such as arteriosclerosis or anemia. This kind of disturbance to the arterial supply may only produce osteoporosis after three months or more, giving rise to static symptoms and pain. It is frequently associated with periostosis, and one may easily be faced with a fractured femoral neck followed by an aseptic necrosis of the head.

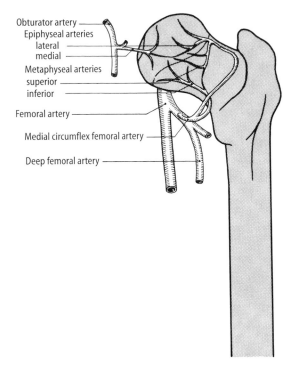

Obturator artery
Epiphyseal arteries
    lateral
    medial
Metaphyseal arteries
    superior
    inferior
Femoral artery
Medial circumflex femoral artery
Deep femoral artery

Fig. 317. Blood supply of the femoral neck and head

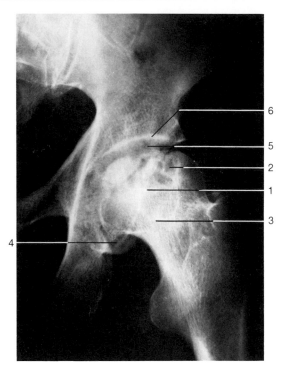

Fig. 318. Aseptic necrosis of femoral head with secondary coxarthrosis (left hip joint)

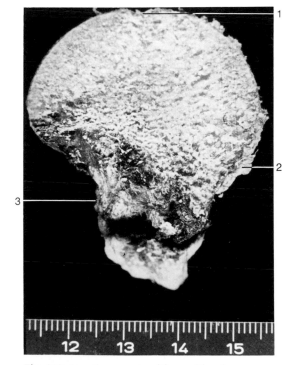

Fig. 319. Aseptic necrosis of femoral head (maceration specimen)

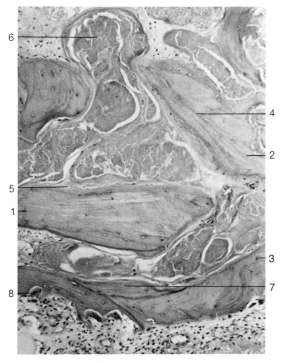

Fig. 320. Aseptic bone necrosis; HE, ×25

Anemic Bone Infarction

Aseptic necrosis within a bone may take the form of focal lesions. *Anemic bone infarcts are focal lesions of bone and bone marrow tissue that are surrounded by a hemorrhagic seam, and which are due to local disturbances of the blood supply.* At first the fatty marrow becomes necrotic; and the cancellous framework within the infarct may remain untouched for a long time, so that no pathological fractures occur. It is only secondarily that the necrosis involves the bony structures. Anemic bone infarcts are rarely the result of an interrupted blood supply (emboli, arteriosclerosis, arteritis), since this is mostly well secured for the bone by a widely distributed vascular system.

Such bone infarcts in the femur *(1)* and upper part of the tibia *(2)* are shown in the **radiograph** of **Fig. 321**. In the femur one can recognize an irregularly bordered map-like area *(3)* in the middle of the bone, with straggly, jagged regions of increased density intermingled with round areas of translucency. No fresh infarct can be seen in the radiograph, and no clinical symptoms are called forth. It is only when, because of breakdown of the neutral fat, calcium deposits build up and hydroxyapatite is precipitated in large quantities that the classical structural changes occur. The outer contours of the bone are retained.

In the **histological picture** shown in **Fig. 322** one can see a widely meshed cancellous network with a large marrow cavity that is filled with fatty tissue *(1)*. The trabeculae *(2)* are narrowed and have undulating or jagged outlines, without any osteoclasts. They contain few osteocytes, which in advanced cases may be absent altogether, indicating a cancellous osteonecrosis. The fatty marrow *(1)* is partly retained. Some areas of the fatty tissue are necrotic, as can be recognized by the eosinophilia and the homogenization of the fat cells *(3)*. In the neighborhood of the fresh fatty necroses one observes old necrotic regions *(4)*, tissue organization and scarring. Here and there fibrin is spread about and amorphous basophilic material deposited in the marrow cavity *(5)*. Dystrophic calcification also arises here and can be identified radiologically.

Caisson Disease

The etiology and pathogenesis of many of the bone infarcts which appear randomly on radiological examination are uncertain. *In cases of the so-called caisson disease (diver's disease) anemic bone infarcts are due to the sudden development of intravascular gas bubbles (nitrogen) when the diver returns too suddenly from a high atmospheric pressure to the normal level at the surface.* The infarcts are found predominantly at the upper and lower end of the femur and at the upper ends of the tibia and humerus. Should the infarct appear in an epiphysis (Ahlbäck's disease), the bony and cartilaginous structures may break up under the stress and bring about a severe arthrosis deformans.

In **Fig. 323** one can see the **radiograph** of such an infarct in a case of caisson disease, where it is indistinguishable from those with a different etiology. In the *tomogram* there is a considerable irregular increase in the density of the cancellous structures *(1)* in the distal femoral metaphysis. Between them lie coarse patchy translucent areas *(2)*. These changes reach right up to the epiphyseal cartilage *(3)*, which in this 11-year-old boy is still open. The outer contour of the bone is fully preserved.

In caisson disease the **histological** picture of a typical anemic bone infarct is also to be seen. In **Fig. 324** one can see the strongly developed trabeculae of the spongiosa *(1)* with lamellar layering and small osteocytes, as well as smooth borders. The bone tissue is therefore still vital. The fatty marrow tissue, however, contains large patchy fat cells without nuclei *(2)* and often with strikingly eosinophilic cytoplasm *(3)*. In the older regions scar tissue *(4)* has developed. For bone infarcts following long-term glucocorticoid treatment see p. 76. Such localized lesions in cases of the so-called diver's disease have been relatively seldom observed and are hardly ever subjected to histological examination. The bone damage must be analyzed after taking into account both the radiological findings and the case history. Such a radiological examination leads with sufficient certainty to the diagnosis and does not require further investigation by bone biopsy. It is a matter of one of the so-called *"leave-me-alone-lesions"*. The pathologist can only use a bone biopsy to establish the existence of a bone necrosis, it says nothing about the etiology.

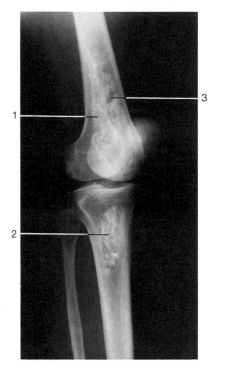

Fig. 321. Anemic bone infarct (distal femur, proximal tibia)

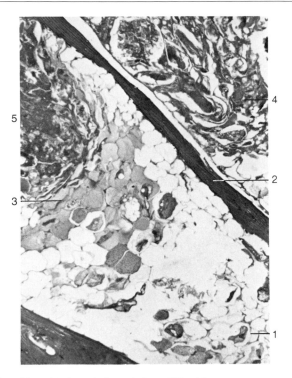

Fig. 322. Anemic bone infarct; HE, ×25

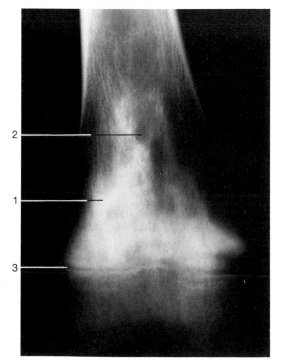

Fig. 323. Bone infarct in caisson disease (distal femur)

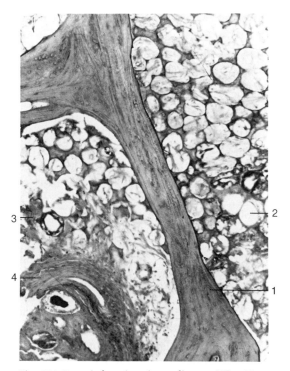

Fig. 324. Bone infarct in caisson disease; HE, ×25

Spontaneous Bone Necroses

Perthes' Disease

This condition is an aseptic epiphyseal necrosis brought about by an insufficient blood supply to the cartilaginous tissue surrounding the epiphysis. *Perthes' disease is a partial or complete aseptic necrosis of the femoral head which begins in the center of the head, and which develops in childhood if the ossification center of the epiphysis is not adequately supplied with blood from the lateral epiphyseal arteries.* Up to the 7th year of life the epiphyseal arteries are the only source of blood for the epiphyseal center of ossification (see **Fig. 317**). The disease announces itself between the 4th and 12th years of life with a slight limp and fairly trivial pain. Following adequate early treatment (relieving the load on the hip joint) the central necrotic area of the head can be revitalized and the condition cured. More severe deformation of the head leads eventually to coxarthrosis deformans.

Perthes' disease is usually diagnosed **radiologically**. In **Fig. 325** one can see such an appearance in the left hip of a 3-year-old boy. The epiphysis (1) is deformed and flattened, and inside there is an irregular sclerotic increase in density. The epiphyseal cartilage (2) is widened and unequal, and close by one can see a narrow sclerotic band. The neck of the femur (3) is shortened and widened, with osteoporotic loosening of its internal structure. The joint cavity (4) is greatly enlarged and the socket (5) very much flattened (coxa plana). One can observe a band of reactive osteosclerosis in the roof of the socket.

It is only very rarely in cases of Perthes' disease that tissue from the femoral head is subjected to histological examination. If it is, one usually finds a partial aseptic bone necrosis that is especially related to the ossification center in the epiphysis. **Figure 326** illustrates the **histological picture** of such a necrosis. The trabeculae (1) are sclerotically widened and contain several drawn out reversal lines (2). Since this is necrotic bone tissue, the osteocyte lacunae (3) are empty. The marrow cavity has been taken over by loose connective and granulation tissue (4) which contains numerous dilated blood capillaries (5). Clumps of calcium deposits are seen as dark patches (6). Advanced cases in older patients present the morphological picture of a severe coxarthrosis deformans (p. 807).

Kienböck's Disease (Lunatomalacia)

This bone lesion is not infrequently diagnosed radiologically, and the operation material thereafter assessed histologically. *It is an aseptic bone necrosis of the lunate bone which attacks men between 20 and 30 years of age. It can be traced back to previous traumatic damage to the wrist joint* (dislocation, or the conditions affecting hand workers or those who use pneumatic machinery). The disease causes pain in the wrist and leads eventually to osteoarthrosis deformans.

In the **radiograph** shown in **Fig. 327** one can see that the lunate is flattened and appears to have been compressed (1). The outer contours are blurred and unequal. Inside this wrist bone there is an osteosclerotic increase in density, mingled, however, with patchy translucencies. In general the lunate appears to be, in comparison with the other wrist bones, highly radioopaque, compressed and deformed.

In the **histological picture** of **Fig. 328** one can recognize, as the substrate of the radiological increase in density, the osteosclerotically widened trabeculae (1). These nevertheless show mostly empty osteocyte lacunae (2), although osteocytes are present in the reactive deposition fronts (3). The necrotic bone contains numerous osteoclastic resorption lacunae (4). The marrow cavity has been taken over by loose connective and granulation tissue (5).

In its early stage, lunatomalacia is characterized by a peripheral fissure, and radiologically one often sees fragments of cortex looking as though they had been blasted off the main bone. Near a fracture, circumscribed myelofibrosis and osteolysis develop. Numerous osteoclasts surround the microscopic fragments. In the 2nd stage, the fissure has been extended by increased loading until a complete fracture is present. Reparative processes with osteosclerosis and new bone deposition characterize the 3rd (late) stage.

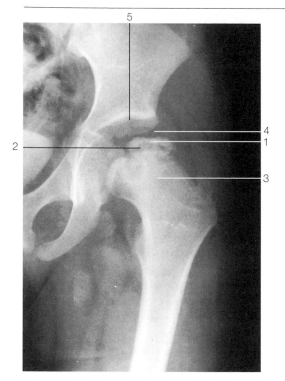

Fig. 325. Aseptic necrosis of femoral head in Perthes' disease

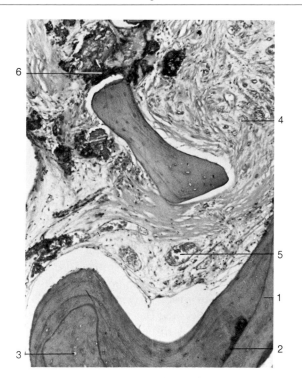

Fig. 326. Aseptic necrosis of femoral head (Perthes); HE, ×25

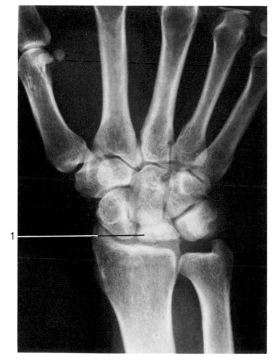

Fig. 327. Lunatomalacia (Kienböck's disease)

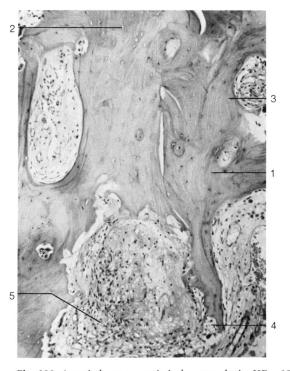

Fig. 328. Aseptic bone necrosis in lunatomalacia; HE, ×25

Causal Bone Necroses

Radiation Bone Necroses

Bone is a tissue with a population of osteocytes and a marrow cavity with a richly cellular content. These cellular structures are fairly sensitive to ionized radiation. *The radionecrosis of bone represents a local necrosis of bone and myeloid tissue within a radiation field which can secondarily respond with an inflammatory reaction (the so-called "radiation osteitis").* Particularly in the bones of the jaws we can expect secondary bacterial infection of the originally bland bone necrosis, and then we have to deal additionally with a purulent osteomyelitis. The necrotic bone tissue produces sequestra, and the secondary osteomyelitis can spread in the affected bone and become the starting point for a generalized sepsis. A threatening late complication of radiation bone necroses is a radiation osteosarcoma (p. 300).

Figure 329 shows the **radiograph** of a radionecrosis of bone in the proximal part of the right humerus. One can recognize the advanced bone remodeling in the humeral head *(1)* and in the adjacent scapula *(2)*. In the humeral head osteolytic bone destruction *(3)* predominates, in the scapula there is a sclerotic increase in density. Within these areas of osteosclerosis there are many patchy osteolytic lesions *(4)*. The outer contours of these bones – especially near the joint – are jagged, undulating and blurred.

In the **histological picture** of such a radionecrosis of bone shown in **Fig. 330** the bony structures *(1)* are necrotic. The lamellar layering is indistinct and the osteocyte lacunae are empty *(2)*. The outer contours of the trabeculae *(3)* are undulating and there is no osteoblastic or osteoclastic activity. The marrow cavity is partly filled with a loose scar tissue *(4)*, which is in places hyalinized and contains blood vessels *(5)*. In the secondarily infected inflamed marrow there is a necrotic mass *(6)*, together with a dense infiltrate of polymorphonuclear leukocytes *(7)*. Radiation damage to a bone or part of a bone is frequently seen when malignant tumors are intensively irradiated and the neighboring bone comes within the area involved. Radiotherapy is often employed against various bone lesions (a Ewing's sarcoma, for instance, or an eosinophilic granuloma). In these cases one must always be prepared for the severe complication of a radionecrosis, and this can lead to a pathological fracture, secondary radiation osteitis or osteomyelitis.

Post-traumatic Bone Necrosis

Bone necrosis can also develop after local traumatic damage to a part of a bone. *A bone necrosis following a fracture arises in the neighborhood if a section of the bone breaks loose and the blood supply is cut off.* The necrotic bone tissue here may be found together with the spongiosa and cortex to form the texture of the bone tissue near the fracture, or it may appear as a sequestrum. A pseudarthrosis usually develops here (p. 124).

Figure 331 shows the **radiograph** of a post-traumatic bone necrosis. This involved fractures of the distal end of the tibia *(1)* and the adjacent fibula *(2)* which were fixated by osteosynthesis *(3)*. One can still clearly see the transverse fracture line *(4)* of an injury that lay well back in the past, so that the appearance represents a post-traumatic pseudarthrosis. In the region of the fracture *(5)* an intraosseous, poorly delineated increase in the structural density is seen, which represents a section of necrotic bone. The true formation of sequestra in this necrotic region cannot be observed.

The **histological picture** reproduced in **Fig. 332** shows some osteosclerotically widened bony structures *(1)* and some narrow trabeculae *(2)* in which the lamellar layering has become indistinct. No nuclei can be detected in the osteocyte lacunae *(3)*. This is therefore necrotic bone tissue. Reversal lines *(4)* indicate the presence of reactive remodeling. The marrow cavity is filled with loose fibrous tissue *(5)* that has been invaded by a few blood vessels *(6)*. Here and there amorphous basophilic material *(7)* is encountered. This kind of necrotic bone tissue must be removed surgically in order to avoid consolidation of the fracture or the development of a pseudarthrosis.

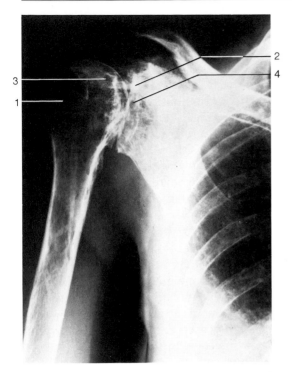

Fig. 329. Radionecrosis of bone (proximal humerus)

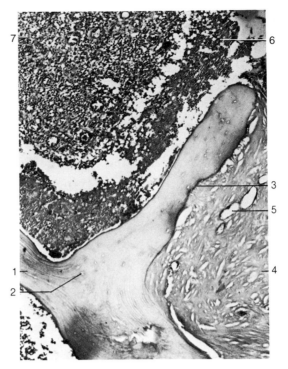

Fig. 330. Radionecrosis of bone with secondary osteomyelitis; HE, ×25

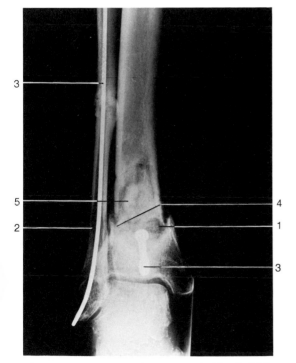

Fig. 331. Post-traumatic bone necrosis (distal tibia)

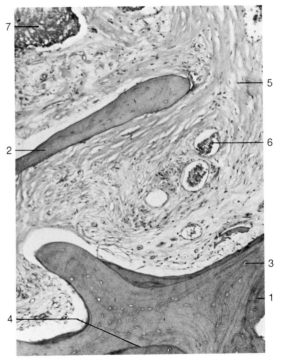

Fig. 332. Post-traumatic bone necrosis; HE, ×25

Inflammatory Bone Necrosis

Inflammation of bone (osteomyelitis, p. 129) is a frequent cause of bone necrosis. *This is a bone necrosis appearing within an osteomyelitic lesion.* If the necrotic bone tissue is separated by osteoclasts and an intervening region of granulation tissue, it is called a *sequestrum.* Such a demarcation is, however, often not present, and the inflammatory necrosis extends throughout a large section of the bone, so that both the spongiosa and the cortex may be drawn in.

In **Fig. 333** one can see the **radiograph** of an inflammatory bone necrosis in the proximal part of the right femur, which extends into the head and the whole of the neck. The femoral head *(1)* is severely deformed and shows well developed peripheral osteophytes *(2).* Within, there are very unequal straggly and coarsely flecked regions of increased density, among which patchy areas of translucency can be seen. These structures reach as far as the femoral neck *(3).* The outer contours of the bone are retained and no periosteal reaction can be seen.

The joint cavity *(4)* is severely reduced in size. Reactive bone remodeling is also taking place in the roof of the socket. Such a radiological appearance at first suggests aseptic necrosis of the femoral head (p. 172).

Histological examination of operation material, however, reveals an active inflammatory process which is either the cause or the result of this bone necrosis. In **Fig. 334** one sees ungainly trabeculae *(1)* with indistinct lamellar layering and no osteocytes. The marrow cavity is filled with leukocytes, the nuclei of which are very markedly lobed *(2),* and inflammatory granulation tissue *(3).* Here one can see large numbers of bacteria *(4).* This is therefore a very active purulent granulating osteomyelitis, with cancellous bone necroses. The bone inflammation probably caused the bone necrosis in the spongiosa; it is also possible, however, that a primarily aseptic bone necrosis became secondarily infected. In any case, it is important to diagnose the presence of the inflammatory process in such necrotic bone, so that the appropriate antibiotic treatment may be started.

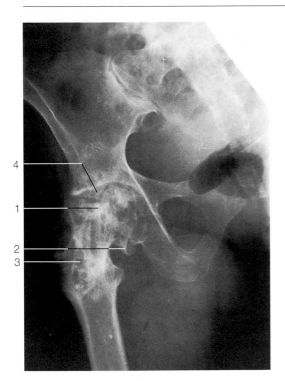

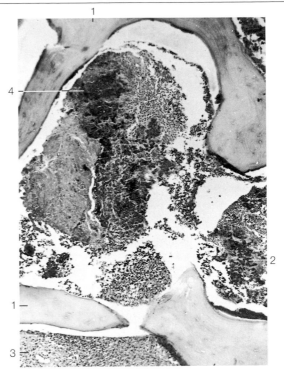

Fig. 333. Inflammatory bone necrosis
(right proximal femur)

Fig. 334. Inflammatory bone necrosis; HE, ×64

9 Metabolic and Storage Diseases

General

Disorders of metabolism, which are bound up with the storage of physiological substances, can also bring about changes in the skeleton. These substances are mostly stored in the cells of the reticulo-histiocytic system, which is significantly activated. For this reason the pathological storage foci in the bone are mostly found in the marrow cavity. Here they destroy the cancellous trabeculae, producing a reactive osteoporosis and often leading to localized bone necroses. This bone destruction is seen in the radiograph as an irregular patchy osteolysis. Since they are systemic diseases, several lesions in several different bones usually appear. Apart from the bones, other tissues and parenchymatous organs may be involved, and this can cause functional disorders.

Pathological deposits of metabolic products can, however, also appear in the joints, tendons, tendon sheaths and bursae and produce reactive inflammatory changes, which is particularly the case with gout (p. 184).

There is a whole range of metabolic disorders which can cause storage diseases and manifest themselves in bone. Very often these are inherited congenital conditions. In all these pathological storage processes the lysosomes play an important role. Together with the endoplasmic reticulum, the Golgi apparatus and the so-called vacuolar apparatus, the lysosomes make up the digestive tract of the cell, which is responsible for the digestion of exogenous and endogenous material. More substances introduced for cellular metabolism than the cell can cope with, insufficient or no lysosomal enzymes (congenital enzymatic defect) or the introduction of material that the lysosomal enzymes are in any case incapable of digesting, can cause such material to be stored. This material can then be identified in osseous storage foci.

Among the bone storage diseases the lipodoses constitute a large and important group.

In *Gaucher's disease* the cerebroside, cerasin, is electively stored in the cells of the reticulo-histiocytic system, in *Niemann-Pick* disease, the phosphatide, sphingomyelin. *Hereditary essential hypercholesterolemia* – an inherited disorder of cholesterol metabolism – produces xanthomas in the soft parts (tendons) and bones. Among the lipoid storage diseases which involve bone, one can include *lipoid granulomatosis (Erdheim-Chester disease)* and *Hand-Schüller-Christian disease*, the latter being included among the bone granulomas (p. 195) for didactic reasons. *Gargoylism (Hunter-Hurler-Pfaundler disease)* is a disorder of the mucopolysaccharide metabolism which causes disturbances of growth by damaging the zone of endochondral bone development. Disorders of protein metabolism can also occasionally affect the skeleton, and *amyloidosis* can bring about the deposition of amyloid in the marrow cavity. A disorder of phenylalanin-tyrosin metabolism is the underlying cause of *ochronosis,* and depends upon an enzymatic defect of homogentisin oxidase.

In most cases these storage diseases bring about pathological changes in the parenchymatous organs and functional disturbances which suggest the diagnosis. The bone involvement remains more in the background. For this reason the underlying metabolic disorder is usually identified by some diagnostic method other than a bone biopsy. If additional skeletal changes appear in the radiograph, then they must perhaps be clarified by a bone biopsy so that they can be allotted to the most appropriate metabolic disorder. In the majority of such cases, the histologist is already aware of the nature of the underlying metabolic or storage disease when making the histological diagnosis. Storage diseases of bone are relatively uncommon. Often the diagnosis can only be suspected, and this must prompt the clinician to undertake further methods of examination.

Gout

The deposition of monosodium urate in the connective and supporting tissues is responsible for the clinical picture of gout. *Gout is a metabolic disease of genetic origin in which a raised serum uric acid level (hyperuricemia) results in the deposition of monosodium urate in the connective and supporting tissues.* The prerequisite for the deposition of urates in these tissues is hyperuricemia (the normal serum level is 4 mg%, in gout 6–19 mg%). Urates are deposited in the joints, tendons, tendon sheaths, bursae, kidneys and skin. It has been established that an autosomal dominant hereditary factor is responsible for the *endogenous disorder of uric acid metabolism*. In highly civilized countries the morbidity is 0.1–0.5%. Gout arises mostly in middle age and is very much more common in men (95% men, 5% women). Not every hyperuricemia leads to the development of the so-called gouty tophi. *Secondary hyperuricemia* may follow an increased intake of nucleic acid in the diet or following massive destruction of cells and cell nuclei with the liberation of nucleic acid (after treatment for leukemia, for instance). The deposition of urate crystals commonly involves the periarticular tissue of the metatarsophalangeal joint of the great toe, joints of the fingers and the elbow joint; and this constitutes the clinical picture of *arthritis urica* (p. 452, Fig. 859).

The severity of an attack of gout is reflected in the radiological changes. In **Fig. 335** one can see in a **radiograph** of the hand, marked destruction of bone in the neighborhood of the joints with large defects *(1)* and severe articular damage *(2)*. A defect appears as though punched out, and is surrounded by marginal sclerosis *(3)*. These lesions have attacked the regions around the interphalangeal joints, where they lie at some distance from the joint capsule. There is no subarticular osteoporosis. This distinguishes gout from rheumatoid arthritis (p. 442), which attacks the metacarpophalangeal joints and is accompanied by osteoporosis.

The **macroscopic picture** of a predominantly chondral form of gouty joint is shown in **Fig. 336**. It involves a hip joint of which the cartilaginous surface is completely covered by a chalk white layer *(1)*. The shiny appearance of the articular cartilage has been lost. The uric acid can seep into the articular cartilage to a depth of up to 1 mm, making it hard and brittle. This can impair the lubrication, resulting in splinter formation, erosions and roughening of the surface *(2)*. These defects open up a passage for the uric acid to reach the deeper layers of the cartilage, where it can bring about further mechanical wear and tear. As a result of this joint damage the picture of arthrosis deformans finally develops. This urate deposition brings about a vigorous and painful inflammatory reaction, which has its morphological counterpart in the edematous and very reddened joint capsule *(3)*.

In its advanced stages gout can break into the subchondral spongiosa, causing local destruction. In the **histological picture** of **Fig. 337** one can recognize roundish foci of varying size within the marrow cavity of the subchondral spongiosa *(1)* which represent deposits of urate crystals. By closing down the iris diaphragm of the microscope one can make the fasciculated structure of this material stand out. Under polarized light it is birefringent. These are the so-called *gouty tophi*. In their neighborhood one can observe a rampart of histiocytes *(2)* with a few foreign body giant cells. Inside the tophus the tissue is necrotic; outside, highly cellular granulation tissue at first develops, and later a connective tissue capsule with fibrocytes and fibroblasts. One can recognize such scar tissue in the marrow cavity of the bone *(3)*, and the trabeculae *(4)* may be sclerotically widened or necrotic. The articular cartilage is undermined peripherally and attacked on both sides: from the joint cavity by the uric acid, and from below by the gouty tophi.

Figure 338 shows a gouty tophus under **higher magnification**. The fasciculated arrangement of the urate crystals, which are birefringent, is clearly seen *(1)*. In the surrounding area, one can see some large histiocytes *(2)* and a foreign body giant cell *(3)*. The inflammatory reaction in the marrow cavity causes intraosseous granulation tissue to develop, and very rapidly brings about complete destruction of the joint. Clinically this causes great pain and severe limitation of movement, which are very characteristic of gout.

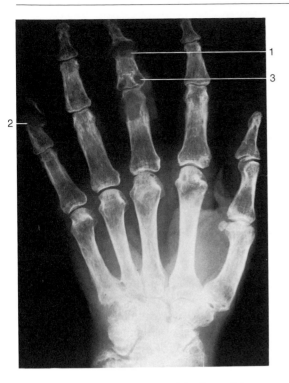

Fig. 335. Arthritis urica (gout) of the finger joints

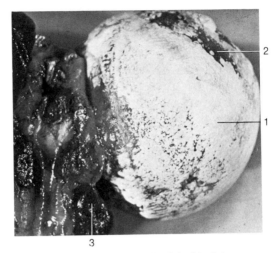

Fig. 336. Arthritis urica (gout) of the hip joint (femoral head)

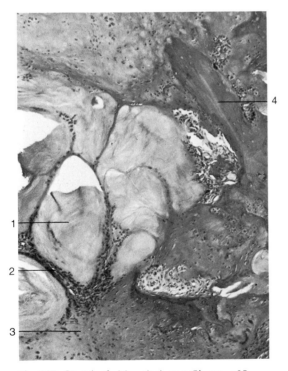

Fig. 337. Gout (arthritis urica); van Gieson, ×25

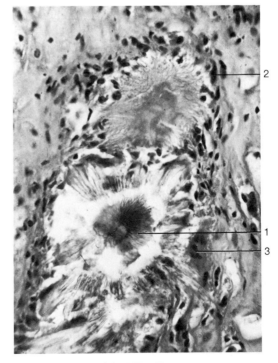

Fig. 338. Gouty tophus; HE, ×51

Amyloidosis of Bone

Amyloid is a special product of metabolism that may be deposited in various organs and tissues, leading there to morphological changes and functional disorders. Chemically it consists of protein and polypeptide (90% protein) and is similar to the immunoglobulins. *Bone amyloidosis consists of the deposition of amyloid in the marrow cavity of numerous bones, leading to a reactive bone remodeling which is in part osteolytic and in part osteosclerotic.* The causal pathogenesis of this disease is not understood. One distinguishes between *primary amyloidosis* (paramyloidosis) without any recognized previous illness and without deposition of amyloid in the lymph nodes, gastrointestinal tract or cardiovascular system, and *secondary amyloidosis,* which is preceded by a lengthy infectious disease – chronic osteomyelitis, for instance. The primary form can be the forerunner of a medullary plasmocytoma (p. 348). Skeletal amyloidosis is rare, and is especially liable to present serious difficulties with regard to radiological diagnosis.

In the **radiograph** one sees curious remodeling structures in several bones which seem to suggest a systemic disease. **Figure 339** shows such changes in the bones of the left upper part of the thoracic cage, including the shoulder joint and proximal part of the humerus. In the clavicle *(1)*, the ribs *(2)* and the head of the humerus *(3)* one is struck by the irregular cancellous framework and patchy osteolysis. The structures are indistinct. The **overall radiological exposure of the pelvis** in **Fig. 340** shows a total sclerotic increase in bone density *(1)* and fine patchy areas of osteolysis *(2)*. In the iliac wings there are large regions of translucency *(3)*. Marginally there are signs of osteoporosis *(4)*.

Histologically the demonstration of amyloid deposition in the marrow is diagnostically decisive. In **Fig. 341** one can see a sclerotically widened trabecula *(1)* which has smooth edges, without any deposited osteoclasts or osteoblasts. The marrow cavity is filled with fatty tissue and hematopoietic bone marrow *(2)*, and there is a deposition of shiny red homogeneous material, partly in clumps *(3)* and partly flattened *(4)*, that has no cellular inclusions. Even in the neighborhood of this deposition there is no reactive tissue.

Under **higher magnification** one can see in **Fig. 342** that these clumps of foreign material

(1) have sharp borders, and that no perifocal foreign body reaction is apparent. The material is a transparent red color, homogeneous and acellular. Close by there is fatty marrow *(2)* with hematopoietic cells *(3)*. With a combination of congo red staining and a polarizing microscope the substance deposited within the bone is easily identified as *amyloid*. In this way a bone biopsy (probably from the iliac crest) can, if the radiograph is inconclusive, provide the diagnosis. The finding of a generalized skeletal amyloidosis must be followed by a search for a possible underlying disease, since primary (idiopathic) amyloidosis is rare. With older patients an attempt must immediately be made to confirm or exclude a medullary plasmocytoma. Localized amyloidosis suggests other tumors (medullary carcinoma of the thyroid, pancreatic insuloma). Systemic amyloidosis arises most often in chronic cases of purulent inflammation (osteomyelitis, tuberculosis) and is not uncommon with rheumatoid arthritis (p. 442). Finally, there are other malignant tumors which can precipitate bone amyloidosis (e.g. Hodgkin's disease, carcinoma of the kidney or stomach). In other words, the diagnosis of bone amyloidosis always brings up the question of the cause of this metabolic disorder.

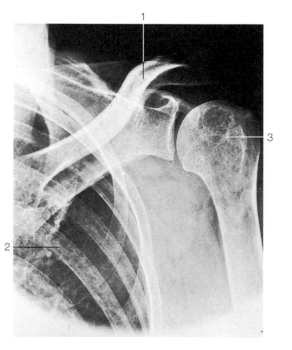

Fig. 339. Amyloidosis of bone (left shoulder joint, thorax)

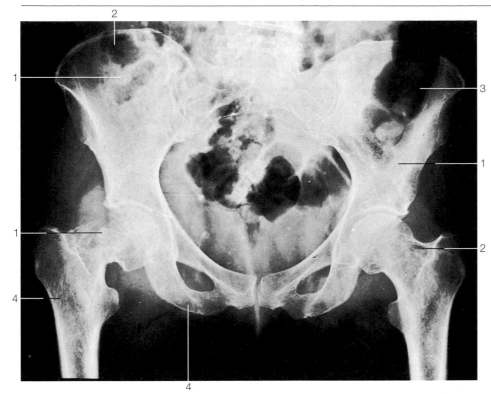

Fig. 340. Amyloidosis of bone (pelvis)

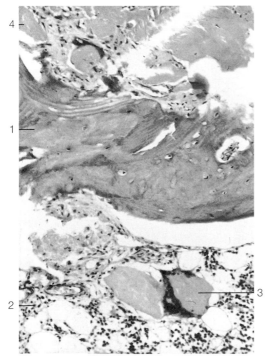

Fig. 341. Amyloidosis of bone; HE, ×64

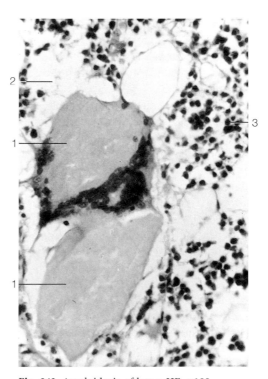

Fig. 342. Amyloidosis of bone; HE, ×100

Diabetic Osteopathy

Diabetes mellitus, the most frequent hereditary chronic metabolic disease, is due to a relative or absolute insulin deficiency. It can affect the bones and joints directly or indirectly. *Diabetic osteopathy involves structural changes in the skeleton, including the joints, which often appear in diabetes mellitus without any etiological connection being obvious.* In children and young people disorders of development and growth are seen. In adults, curious osteoporoses, hyperostoses and osteoarthropathies occur. In these cases late diabetic complications (such as osteodystrophy with chronic renal insufficiency, diabetic enteropathy, chronic pancreatitis, malabsorption, diabetic neuropathy and angiopathy) also affect the bony structures. A principal site for diabetic osteopathy is the spinal column.

In **Fig. 343** one sees several thoracic vertebral bodies in lateral view in a **maceration specimen**. The spongiosa *(1)* shows severe osteoporosis with rarefaction, particularly in the transverse trabeculae. The loss of bone has led to collapse of the lower plates *(2)*. There is hypertrophic atrophy with increased strength of the supporting trabeculae *(3)*. The anterior longitudinal ligament *(4)* is ossified, which is why the ventral cortex *(5)* appears to be markedly wider than normal.

These structural changes appear in the **radiograph**. In **Fig. 344** one can see a thoracic column in a.p. view. The vertebral bodies show osteoporotic loosening of the spongiosa *(1)* and the supporting trabeculae are emphasized. There are marked spondyloarthrotic changes with peripheral osteophytes *(2)* and lateral bony "clasps" *(3)*. In the center the ossified anterior longitudinal ligament is clearly seen *(4)*. This ossification of the anterior longitudinal ligament in the thoracic region, which is typical of diabetes mellitus, is particularly impressive in a **lateral radiograph**. In **Fig. 345** one can again discern the irregular osteoporosis of the vertebral spongiosa *(1)*. Ventrally one sees the wide and radiodense anterior longitudinal ligament *(2)* bulging across the intervertebral spaces. Such an ossifying spondylosis constitutes **Forestier's disease** and indicates in the radiograph a possible case of diabetes mellitus.

The **radiograph** of a specimen of the thoracic vertebral column of a chronic diabetic shows these skeletal changes particularly well in **Fig. 346**. We can see high grade osteoporotic vertebral bodies *(1)*, in which the supporting spongiosa is very clearly demonstrated. The upper plates *(2)* and the dorsal cortex *(3)* are rarefied. On the other hand, the wide shadow of the ossified anterior longitudinal ligament *(4)* is prominently displayed.

The local bridge-like bony fusions of this type of spondylosis are even more clearly seen in a **maceration specimen**. In **Fig. 347** one can observe osteoporosis of the vertebral spongiosa with hypertrophic bone atrophy *(1)*. The supporting spongiosa is retained throughout and prominent. The vertebrae appear to be somewhat flattened, but have preserved their general shape. The wide band-like zone of sclerosis on the ventral surface of the vertebrae *(2)* which bridges over the intervertebral spaces with bars of bone and presses forward at these points is striking. This is the ossified anterior longitudinal ligament which is pathognomonic of Forestier's disease.

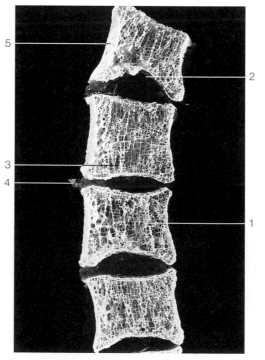

Fig. 343. Diabetic spondylopathy (thoracic column, maceration specimen)

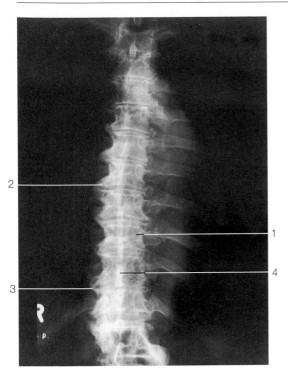

Fig. 344. Diabetic spondylopathy
(Forestier's disease, thoracic column)

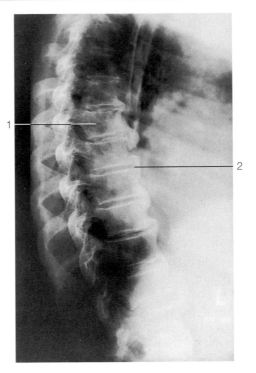

Fig. 345. Diabetic spondylopathy
(Forestier's disease, thoracic column)

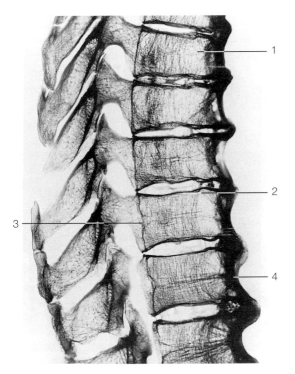

Fig. 346. Diabetic spondylopathy
(Forestier's disease, thoracic column)

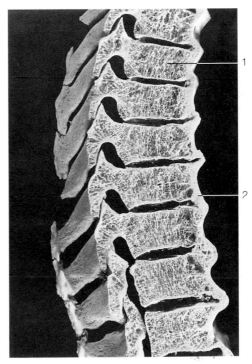

Fig. 347. Diabetic spondylopathy
(Forestier's disease, thoracic column, maceration specimen)

About 2.4% of those patients who have suffered for many years from diabetes mellitus show signs of a so-called *diabetic osteoarthropathy*. This is a neuropathic condition of metabolic origin, in which neurological disturbances (hyposensitivity, loss of motor power) play an important part. It is almost exclusively the lower extremities (anterior region of the foot) which are affected. **Figure 348** shows a **maceration specimen** of the skeleton of a diabetic foot seen from the side. The metatarsal bones *(1)* are narrowed down to a point by concentric atrophy close to the joint, and "look as if they had been sucked". The toes have taken up a clawfoot position *(2)* and a metatarsophalangeal joint is dislocated *(3)*. Fragments of bone can be forced off from the osteoporotic metatarsus *(4)*.

These skeletal changes can be recognized in the **radiograph**. In **Fig. 349** one can observe the marked porosity of the spongiosa in the neighborhood of the joint *(1)*, which at the distal end of the third metatarsal has led to a fracture *(2)*. Proximal to this, extensive reactive periostitis ossificans *(3)* can be seen. Distally, the short tubular bone has been narrowed to an arrow-like point, and the contours of the metatarsophalangeal joint *(4)* have been destroyed. The contours have been rendered indistinct by extensive swelling of the soft parts. The **maceration specimen** of the anterior part of the foot depicted in **Fig. 350** shows the severe trophic damage to the bones and joint very impressively. The metatarsal bones *(1)* taper distally. The metatarsophalangeal joints *(2)* are very narrowed and deformed, and there is osteoporosis near the joint. In the region of the great toe one can see an extensive dislocation *(3)*. All the toes *(4)* are angulated dorsally and deformed. Apart from the concentric bone atrophy there is a generalized osteoporosis of all the bones.

In the **histological picture** there are no tissue structures that are characteristic of diabetes mellitus. In **Fig. 351** the epiphyseal cartilages *(1)* of a young diabetic patient are relatively wide and the bone trabeculae *(2)* are significantly narrowed. They have smooth edges and no osteoblasts or osteoclasts have been deposited. The bone tissue is severely undermineral-

ized. The marrow cavity *(3)* is widened, and with this there is a non-specific osteoporosis, especially near the joint. In the soft parts adjacent to the bone one can recognize **histologically** the typical signs of *diabetic microangiopathy*. In **Fig. 352** the arteries show fibrotic thickening of the intima *(1)* with narrowing of the lumen. The cortex *(2)* shows deep resorption recesses *(3)* resulting from subperiosteal bone resorption.

The development in diabetics of premature arteriosclerosis does not, however, have any pathogenetic relationship to diabetic osteoarthropathy, but it is certainly true that these arteriosclerotic changes are often responsible for peripheral impairment of the circulation and therefore for the development of gangrene (mostly in the foot). This leads very easily to infection of the soft parts, and the inflammation, which is usually purulent, attacks the bone and sets up a purulent osteomyelitis (p. 134). The tissues that are submitted for morbid anatomical examination from chronic diabetics are mostly amputation specimens which show signs of *diabetic gangrene* with osteomyelitis. One can suspect the presence of diabetes mellitus histologically from the microangiopathy of the soft parts. In addition to the diabetic hyperostotic spondylosis (Forestier's disease), *hyperostosis frontalis interna* (internal frontal hyperostosis) is a typical skeletal manifestation in chronic diabetics.

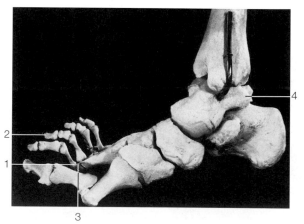

Fig. 348. Skeleton of diabetic foot (maceration specimen)

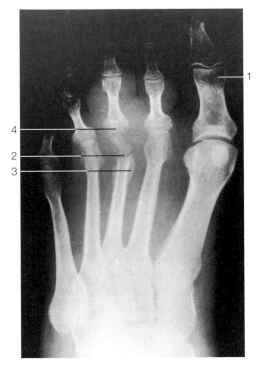

Fig. 349. Diabetic osteoarthropathy (toes)

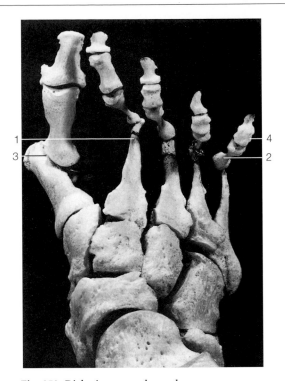

Fig. 350. Diabetic osteoarthropathy
(toes, maceration specimen)

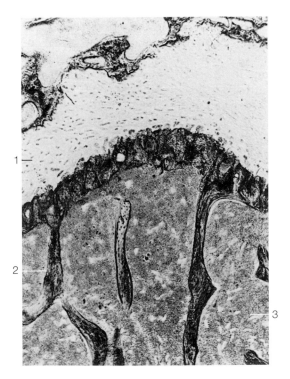

Fig. 351. Diabetic osteoarthropathy; HE, ×20

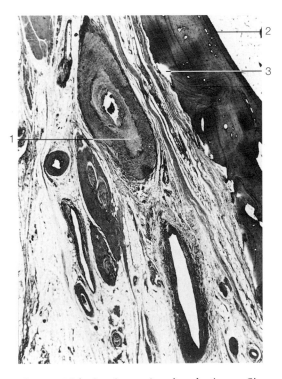

Fig. 352. Diabetic microangiopathy; elastic van Gieson, ×40

Gaucher's Disease

Sometimes tissue is removed for histological evaluation from a patchy osteolytic lesion in which a fine honeycomb of "foam cells" is found. These suggest a possible storage disease. *Gaucher's disease is the result of the storage of cerasin in cells of the reticulo-histiocytic system, with possible involvement of the cells of the bone marrow bringing about corresponding defects in the skeleton.* It depends upon an autosomal recessive enzymatic defect, which causes a disturbance of the glucocerebroside catabolism and an abnormal cerebroside deposition in early childhood, youth, or even in adult life. The patients usually manifest a severe hepatosplenomegaly and cerebral function is impaired.

Radiologically there is initially osteoporosis in the region of an affected bone lesion as a result of resorption of the bone trabeculae in the neighborhood of the Gaucher cells. In addition, the proliferation of the reticulo-histiocytic cells brings about destruction of the bony structures, leading to a patchy osteolysis. Finally, the histiocyte proliferation obstructs the intraosseous blood supply and causes bone infarcts that are mostly subarticular or diaphyseal. The femoral head and the diaphyses of the tibia and femur are most frequently affected. In **Fig. 353** one sees osteolytic lesions in the right side of the pelvis (ilium *(1)*, pubis *(2)*) and in the right femoral head *(3)* of an adult, with osteosclerotic areas of increased density in between. The hip joint is arthrotically deformed.

Figure 354 shows the typical **histological picture** of Gaucher's disease. We see a highly cellular granulation tissue with dense collections of lymphocytes *(1)* and reticular cells *(2)*. The picture is dominated by large complexes of histiocytes *(3)* that have undergone an epithelial-type transformation and show an abundantly present cytoplasm with fine honeycomb-like creases. The nuclei of these cells are eccentrically placed. These are the pathognomonic *"Gaucher cells".* Their cytoplasm contains PAS positive material and gives a positive response to Sudan staining (lipoids). If such groups of cells are present, the histological diagnosis of Gaucher's disease is sufficiently certain.

Ochronosis

It is rare for ochronosis to be seen in a biopsy specimen, and it also very seldom turns up in the autopsy room. Here the macroscopic appearance of abnormal pigmentation is striking, particularly in the articular and costal cartilages. The cartilage varies in color from yellowish-brown to black, and similar staining can even affect the tendons, ligaments and joint capsules. *Ochronosis (alkaptonuria) is a hereditary disorder of amino-acid metabolism resulting from an enzymatic defect of homogentisic oxidase, in which an abnormal quantity of homogentisic acid is both excreted in the urine and deposited in various tissues (cartilage, for instance).* This deposition in the skeleton can lead to an **ochronotic arthropathy.** In the vertebral column it reduces mobility. The laying down of ochronotic pigments in the ligaments and vertebral cartilages causes an **ochronotic spondylosis** to develop with marked degenerative changes both in the intervertebral discs and the cartilaginous plates.

In **Fig. 355** one can see a **radiograph** of the lumbar column (a.p. view) with severe degenerative changes. The intervertebral spaces *(1)* have become much narrowed because of degeneration of the disks. These are very radiodense *(2)* owing to the secondary ossification. There is a significant spondylosis deformans with peripheral osteophytes *(3)*. The spongiosa of the vertebrae *(4)* shows osteoporotic loosening.

Histologically one sees in **Fig. 356** degeneratively altered articular cartilage tissue with foci of myxoid degeneration *(1)* and deposition of a dark brown pigment *(2)*. The specimens examined are mostly autopsy material.

Arthropathia ochronotica is characterized by a combination of severe thoracic and lumbar spondylosis with a symmetrical polyarthrosis of the major joints, including the unloaded shoulder joint. The disease usually becomes manifest around the 40th year of life, when stiffening of the vertebral column is noticed. This must be distinguished from Bechterew's spondylitis ankylopoetica (p. 450). Ochronosis is indicated by the deposition of dark pigment in the sclera and auricular cartilages.

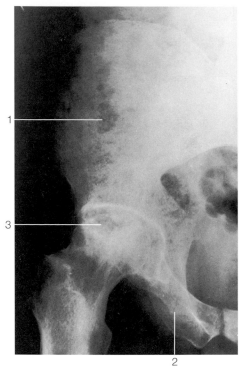

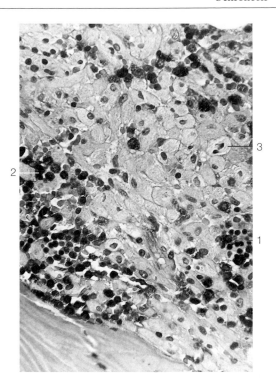

Fig. 353. Gaucher's disease (osteolytic lesions in right side of pelvis – ilium – pubis – and right femoral head)

Fig. 354. Gaucher's disease; HE, ×64

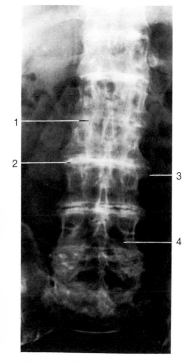

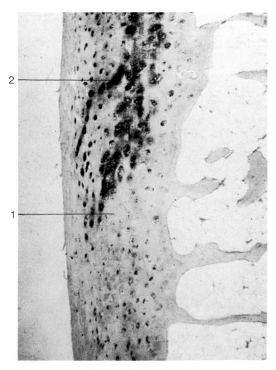

Fig. 355. Ochronosis (lumbar column)

Fig. 356. Articular cartilage in ochronosis; HE, ×20

10 Bone Granulomas

General

Granulomatous processes can develop in bone which frequently give rise to great clinical and radiological difficulties. All granulomatous lesions have in common the fact that they appear primarily in the marrow cavity. From there they extend into the cortex, bringing about an erosion of its endosteal side which can be recognized in the radiograph. Usually, a local osteolytic lesion is involved, since the cancellous trabeculae in the neighborhood of the granuloma are destroyed. This leads to the appearance of a "bony cyst". In the radiograph the peripheral reaction in the region around such an osteolytic focus provides a very important diagnostic criterion. In rare cases a circumscribed area of osteolysis in the cortex can also arise from a bone granuloma.

Some of these granulomatous processes show an *inflammatory reaction.* A dentogenous osteomyelitis of the jaw with non-specific granulation tissue may lead to the development of a cyst in the jaw (p. 132). An intraosseous "bony cyst" may also appear radiologically with plasma cell osteomyelitis (Fig. 259) or with a Brodie's abscess (Fig. 258). In the material from a curettage, non-specific inflammatory granulation tissue is always present. This spreads out more diffusely in the marrow cavity in cases of chronic osteomyelitis (Figs. 244 & 245). A specific inflammatory process must be borne in mind when examining such material histologically. Behind a bone granuloma a tuberculous lesion may lurk (Fig. 265), a Boeck's granuloma (Fig. 275) or typhoid osteomyelitis (Fig. 285). An osteomyelitis of fungal origin (Fig. 289) can present as a giant cell bone granuloma. There are also granulomatous processes in bone which can be interpreted as *tumor-like bone lesions.* The first that comes to mind is *histiocytosis X,* the etiology of which is unknown. Normally speaking the *eosinophilic granuloma,* the chronically progressive *Hand-Schüller-Christian disease* and the malignant *Letterer-Siwe* disease are grouped collectively under this heading, since radiological or histological differentiation between them is very difficult or frankly impossible. Many reactive giant cell bone granulomas show tumor-like changes. We know, for instance, that in cases of long-standing primary hyperparathyroidism that have been recognized too late, resorptive giant cell granulomas (the so-called "brown tumors", p. 84, Fig. 150) develop, which are sometimes difficult to distinguish from true osteoclastomas (p. 338. Figure 638). This type of granulomatous reaction focus with osteoclastic giant cells is found in the jaw as a "reparative giant cell granuloma" (p. 204) and in the hands or feet as a "giant cell reaction of the short tubular bones" (p. 204). Aneurysmal bony cysts (p. 412, Fig. 786) can also be counted as reactive bone granulomas. Finally, a few benign tumors, such as the benign histiocytoma (Fig. 610), the xanthofibroma (Fig. 588) and the osteoid osteoma (Fig. 479) have a granulomatous character.

A bone granuloma can sometimes ape a *malignant bone tumor.* This is particularly true of the malignant bone lymphoma (Fig. 675) and the osseous Hodgkin's lymphoma (Fig. 683), which contain true granulation tissue. A polymorphic cellular granulation tissue can also dominate the histological picture of a telangiectatic osteosarcoma (Fig. 518).

Granulomatous bone changes can also arise as the result of various internal and external actions on bone. A histiocytic granulation tissue with a foreign body reaction can arise close to implanted prosthetic material – an artificial hip, for instance. Metallosis can also develop here (Fig. 225), where the metallic particles entering the surrounding tissue can bring about an inflammatory reaction. Finally, such a reaction can be caused by a metabolic or storage disease, as in the case of gout (Fig. 335) for example.

Eosinophilic Bone Granuloma (ICD-O-DA-M-4405/0)

The eosinophilic bone granuloma belongs to a group of non-tumorous bone diseases of unknown etiology, which may be regarded as an inflammatory histiocytosis or be classified under the tumor-like bone lesions. *This is a local osteolytic bone condition, brought about by reticulo-histiocytic granulation tissue with a variable content of eosinophilic granulocytes.* The lesion is found mostly in children and young people between 5 and 10 years of age, although its appearance in adults is by no means rare. There is usually a solitary bony focus in one of the cranial bones (frontal or parietal), or in the mandible, humerus, ribs or proximal femoral metaphyses. Other bones are more rarely involved. Multiple bony lesions (up to 40) may appear. The foci can grow extraordinarily rapidly in a short time and bring about extensive bone destruction. This causes local pain and swelling of the soft tissues, and pathological fractures can sometimes arise.

In the **radiograph** there is a local osteolytic focus in the marrow cavity that can give the impression of a "bony cyst". In **Fig. 357** there is a solitary eosinophilic bone granuloma in the distal part of the left humerus (1). The focus is slightly elliptical and fairly clearly delineated. In the a.p. radiograph one can recognize that it lies almost in the center of the marrow cavity of the long bone and reaches out to the cortex. This is also clearly seen in the lateral view (2). Here the cortex is severely narrowed but not broken through. No periosteal reaction can be seen. Since there is no marginal sclerosis, the osteolytic focus looks as if it has been punched out.

In **Fig. 358** one can see an eosinophilic bone granuloma in the proximal region of the left femur. The affected region of the bone is considerably raised up in the shape of a spindle (1). In the center of this elevated region one can recognize a large irregularly delineated area of osteolysis (2) that extends through the whole diameter of the shaft. In places the cortex is included in the osteolysis (3) and appears to have been penetrated. Here one can see a slight widening of the periosteum. At another point (4) the osteolytic focus is sharply demarcated,

where it is close to a sclerotic increase in the density of the bony structures (5).

Histologically this is a highly cellular granulation tissue, characterized by vigorous proliferation of histiocytes and reticular cells. One can distinguish four distinct phases in the histological picture.

Figure 359 shows the *proliferative phase* (Phase 1) of an eosinophilic bone granuloma. One can recognize the proliferative growth of histiocytes (1). The relatively large cells have a pale, somewhat granular cytoplasm, which is also eosinophilic in places, and a round distended nucleus. In between, there are groups of lymphocytes and eosinophilic granulocytes (2), which at this phase of development may, however, be very sparsely represented. The eosinophilic granules in these cells are often only demonstrable with Giemsa staining. New bone formation is not observed in such a focus. Peripherally there may be isolated autochthonous bone trabeculae among the "granulation tissue".

The *granulomatous phase* (Phase 2) of an eosinophilic bone granuloma is shown in **Fig. 360**. This is the classical picture of an eosinophilic granuloma. One can recognize loose granulation tissue with capillaries (1) present and sprouting, and diffuse infiltrates of highly eosinophilic granulocytes (2). These have more obviously round nuclei and eosinophilic granules in the cytoplasm (well shown up with Giemsa staining). In between there are varying numbers of large histiocytes (3) with very unevenly elongated cytoplasm and round centrally placed nuclei. The eosinophils can be focally concentrated in the granulation tissue and give rise to true "eosinophilic myeloid abscesses". Multinucleated giant cells may also be present. At the periphery of the lesion, collagen fibers are being laid down (4). The granulomatous lesion is bounded by the autochthonous trabeculae (5) of the bone marrow spongiosa.

The granulomatous phase of an eosinophilic bone granuloma reflects the active phase of this bony lesion. Since there are numerous eosinophilic leukocytes in the intraosseous granulation tissue, the histological diagnosis is usually not very difficult.

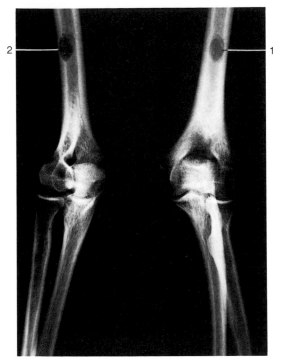

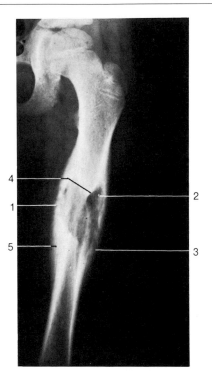

Fig. 357. Eosinophilic bone granuloma (distal humerus)

Fig. 358. Eosinophilic bone granuloma (proximal femur)

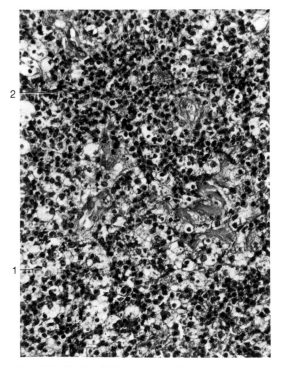

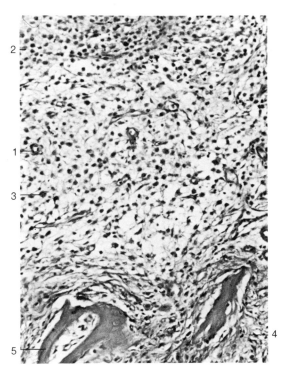

Fig. 359. Eosinophilic bone granuloma
(proliferative phase); HE, ×64

Fig. 360. Eosinophilic bone granuloma
(granulomatous phase); HE, ×64

The 3rd phase of an eosinophilic bone granuloma, the **xanthomatous** phase, reveals itself by the appearance of numerous histiocytes and foam cells. In **Fig. 361** one can recognize a highly cellular granulation tissue in which many large complexes of foam cells *(1)* predominate. These cells have a strikingly pale and extensive cytoplasm in which much lipoid has been stored. They have relatively small round isomorphic nuclei, and practically no mitoses are seen. Other histiocytic cellular elements *(2)* show a significantly eosinophilic cytoplasm where phagocytosed erythrocytes and leukocytes, hemosiderin granules or Charcot-Leyden crystals can sometimes be demonstrated. Between these histiocytes, one repeatedly sees more and more eosinophil leukocytes *(3)* either singly or in groups, and occasionally also multinucleated giant cells *(4)*. In this phase, however, the histiocytes, particularly the foam cells, predominate over other cells in the eosinophilic bone granuloma. The xanthomatous phase does not always appear during the progressive course of this type of bone granuloma.

In the regressive stage of an eosinophilic bone granuloma we find **fibrous scarring** (4th Phase) as shown in **Fig. 362**. In part of the lesion *(1)* there is highly cellular granulation tissue with capillaries present and sprouting, and with numerous eosinophils and histiocytes. There is also, however, a large area of progressive collagen fiber development, which finally brings about complete scarring of the lesion. On the right side of **Fig. 362** *(2)* one can see fibrous tissue with deposited fibroblasts and fibrocyte nuclei. In this scar tissue, fibrous bone trabeculae on which osteoblasts have been deposited finally become differentiated out *(3)*. Whereas an eosinophilic granuloma can be completely healed radiologically, insofar as its morbid anatomy is concerned, the original bone structure is only incompletely restored, although the load-bearing capacity of the bone is again fully achieved. The prognosis of an eosinophilic granuloma is good, and spontaneous healing is frequent. With a solitary lesion curettage is indicated, and radiotherapy (4–18 Gy) and the administration of corticoids is effective.

Occasionally a benign eosinophilic bone granuloma can pass over into **Hand-Schüller-Christian disease** (HSC). This is a reticulohistiocytosis which manifests itself with the classical triad of *"map-like skull, exophthalmos (often unilateral) and diabetes insipidus"*. The course of the disease tends to be chronic, and may be accompanied by hepatosplenomegaly, lymphadenopathy, anemia and loss of weight. It almost exclusively affects children and young people. It is impossible to distinguish between an eosinophilic bone granuloma and Hand-Schüller-Christian disease by radiological and histological methods alone. In **Fig. 363** one can see the tissue from this type of osteolytic bone lesion, which consists of a partly dense, partly loose assembly of large histiocytes. Many histiocytes have an extensive eosinophilic cytoplasm *(1)*, in others it is foamy and contains fat *(2)*. In general the tissue has the appearance of a lipogranuloma, where the adipose degeneration is probably a secondary phenomenon and the tumor-like character is due to the proliferation of the histiocytes. The nuclei of the histiocytes vary in size and shape. Several eosinophilic granulocytes are strewn about *(3)*. Histologically it is not possible to distinguish this sort of cell and tissue picture from the xanthomatous phase of an eosinophilic bone granuloma (**Fig. 361**). The diagnosis of Hand-Schüller-Christian disease is only possible if the clinical data are also taken into account.

The malignant form of histiocytosis X, **Abt-Letterer-Siwe disease**, is very rare and affects children under 2 years of age. Its course is acute, fulminating and usually fatal. Radiologically the bone lesions show a malignant destructive process. As can be seen in **Fig. 364**, the histiocytes have variously sized bizarre nuclei with prominent nucleoli *(1)*. Numerous multinucleated giant cells *(2)* are present. In general the histiocytic tissue shows many different and polymorphic types of cells. Nevertheless, Letter-Siwe disease can only be diagnosed from a bone biopsy if supported by the radiological and clinical picture. Histiocytosis X usually presents no clinical picture. Rapidly growing granulomas cause local pain and swelling of the soft parts, and can bring about a spontaneous fracture. A solitary bone granuloma can regress of itself within a few months.

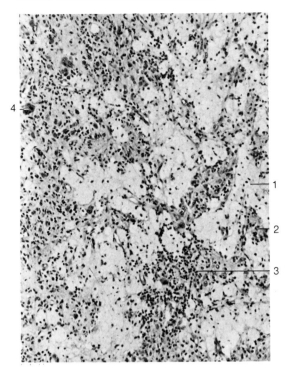

Fig. 361. Eosinophilic bone granuloma (xanthomatous phase); PAS, ×40

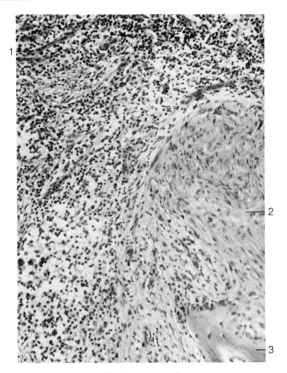

Fig. 362. Eosinophilic bone granuloma (phase of scar formation); HE, ×32

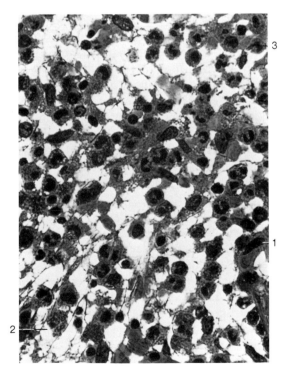

Fig. 363. Hand-Schüller-Christian disease; PAS, ×64

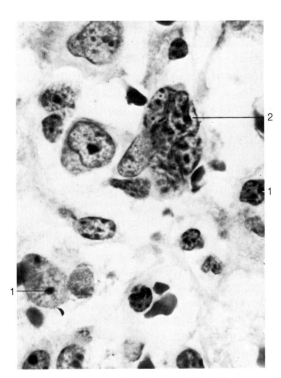

Fig. 364. Abt-Letterer-Siwe disease; HE, ×100

Lipoid Granulomatosis (Erdheim-Chester Disease)

A disorder of fat metabolism can manifest itself in the skeleton and lead to radiological changes which can only be elucidated by examination of a biopsy. *Lipoid granulomatosis (Erdheim-Chester disease) is a granulomatosis of the fatty tissue in the marrow (and in the internal organs) which results in an assemblage of cholesterol-containing foam cells and conspicuous intramedullary formation of new bone.* There is marked hyperlipemia. The serum levels of phospholipids and cholesterol are raised. This disease, which is accompanied by a particular radiological and clinical symptomatology, should be distinguished from Hand-Schüller-Christian disease (p. 198), from essential familial hypercholesterolemia and from Faber's disease. Marked hypercholesterolemia is not always present.

In Erdheimer-Chester disease, one usually sees a diffuse sclerotic increase in density of the bony structures in the **radiograph**, particularly at the ends of the long bones. In **Fig. 365** one can see such a diffuse osteosclerosis in the distal parts of the femurs *(1)* and proximal parts of the tibias *(2)*. The epiphyses *(3)* are not sclerosed. This diffuse cancellous sclerosis extends to both the metaphyses and diaphyses *(4)*. It indicates new intramedullary bone formation. In the *skeletal scintigram* these regions of bone show an intensive increase in activity. In the *computer tomogram* (CT) and *MR tomogram* (MRT) the density of the marrow cavity is markedly increased. Such an advancing osteosclerosis must be accounted for by a bone biopsy.

Histologically one sees in **Fig. 366** an intramedullary lesion consisting of a dense collection of histiocytic foam cells *(1)* which possess a pale cytoplasm containing much cholesterol. Loose collections of lymphocytes and plasma cells are strewn about *(2)*. The foam cell granuloma is interspersed with a few collagen fibers *(3)*. The trabeculae *(4)* are sclerotically widened, and their outer contour is undulating and partly frayed. The fibrotic marrow and sclerosed spongiosa can be greatly expanded by the formation of new bone, especially at the ends of the long bones, which is why only a few foam cells are found here.

Erdheimer-Chester disease is a bone condition that has so far seldom been described. Histologically it is very similar to other intraosseous foam cell granulomas in which vigorous reactive osteosclerosis is typical. In order to reach a diagnosis the clinical findings must be taken into account.

Membranous Lipodystrophy (Nasu's Disease)

This rare and curious granulomatous bone disease has been almost exclusively observed in Japan and Finland. *It is a metabolic disorder ("inborn error of metabolism") of the intraosseous and extraosseous fat cells, which brings about cystic lesions with pathological fractures in the limb bones, together with pain and difficulty in walking.* The disease is progressive in young people and leads to dementia and early death. The cause is probably a genetic defect of the lipoid metabolism.

In **Fig. 367** one can see a **radiograph** of the foot and distal part of the leg in a case of membranous lipoid dystrophy. In the talus *(1)* there is a region of osteolysis that shows no internal structure. The cortex is narrowed from within, but intact. There is no periosteal reaction. One can also see large areas of translucency in the calcaneus *(2)*, distal part of the tibia *(3)* and fibula *(4)* which are poorly delineated.

As the **histological examination** shows, the translucent intraosseous foci are filled with peculiarly altered fatty tissue. In **Fig. 368** there are large fat cells *(1)*, and between them numerous folded membranes *(2)* which are strongly eosinophilic. In many places they are surrounding hollow cystic spaces *(3)* which are in some cases filled with amorphous eosinophilic material. The membranes are PAS positive and contain fine reticulin fibers. In the fatty tissue there are some scattered infiltrates of lymphocytes and eosinophils *(4)*. These foci lack the normal cancellous trabeculae. Similar histological changes are also seen in the extraosseous fatty tissues (in the skin and abdomen) and in the liver and lungs. At the same time there is cerebral atrophy with demyelinization, gliosis and reduction in the neuronal cells, which accounts for the psychiatric symptoms. The disease is accompanied by a sudanophilic leukodystrophy of the brain. This is probably a recessive autosomal hereditary condition. In the terminal phase pathological fractures appear, and cerebral death.

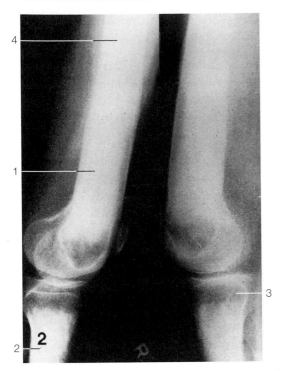

Fig. 365. Lipoid granulomatosis (Erdheim-Chester disease) (distal femurs, proximal tibias)

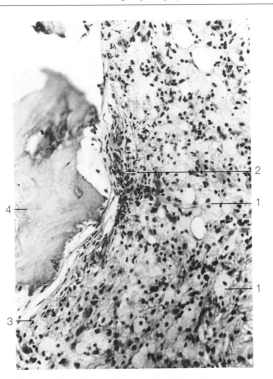

Fig. 366. Lipoid granulomatosis; HE, ×40

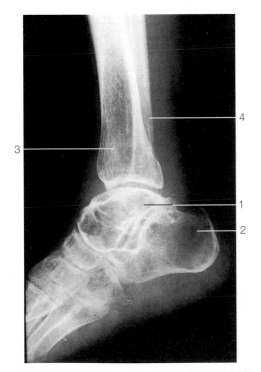

Fig. 367. Membranous lipodystrophy (Nasu's disease) (distal tibia, fibula, ankle joint)

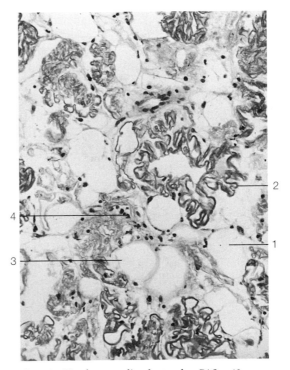

Fig. 368. Membranous lipodystrophy; PAS, ×40

Malignant Histiocytosis (ICD-O-DA-M-9720/3)

Granulomatous bone diseases can in the more rare cases undergo malignant change, and are then classified as malignant medullary reticuloses. *Malignant histiocytosis is a rare hematological disease which runs a malignant course, attended clinically by fever, cachexia, hepatosplenomegaly, lymphadenopathy and progressive pancytopenia.* In the skeleton there are multiple and disseminated foci of destruction and bone remodeling, which can lead to diagnostic difficulties.

In **Fig. 369** one can see in the **radiograph** such a focus of destruction in the right 8th rib *(1)*. The bone of the rib is eaten away by numerous osteolytic lesions *(2)* which are sometimes confluent. This process has raised up the outer contour of the bone *(3)*. Between these osteolytic lesions there are irregular sclerotic areas of increased density *(4)*. Less marked but similar changes can also be seen in the 7th ipsilateral rib *(5)*.

A **radiograph** of malignant histiocytosis with bony involvement of the proximal part of the right femur is seen in **Fig. 370**. The whole of the femoral head *(1)*, neck *(2)* and adjacent region of the shaft *(3)* show high grade osteosclerotic change. The contours of the hip joint *(4)* are unclear and partly raised up. In the marrow cavity there is a fine patchy porosity *(5)*. Such a radiological picture cannot provide a diagnosis and must be supported by a bone biopsy.

In a **histological section** the massive infiltration of the bone marrow by atypical histiocytes is striking. In **Fig. 371** one can see a normally structured trabecula *(1)* with a smooth border. It shows lamellar layering, and a few osteocytes *(2)* are present. The marrow cavity has been infiltrated by numerous histiocytes *(3)* which are loosely deposited there. They differ in size and shape, and contain nuclei *(4)* which also differ in size and shape. A few isolated fat cells *(5)* and some lymphocytic infiltrates *(6)* can also be seen.

Under **higher magnification** the structure of the tumorous histiocytes in **Fig. 372** is more clearly shown. These are tumor cells which clearly reveal their polymorphy and varying sizes *(1)*. The cells possess large vesicular nuclei *(2)* which may sometimes be kidney-shaped *(3)*. Cells with two nuclei can also be seen *(4)*. The cytoplasm *(5)* contains pale areas and is definitely basophilic with Giemsa staining. In the center of the picture one can recognize a blood vessel *(6)*, the lumen of which contains tumorous histiocytes that have entered the bloodstream. The **higher magnification** of **Fig. 373** shows histiocytes of different sizes *(1)*, often with an extensive granular cytoplasm *(2)* and polymorphic nuclei *(3)*. Here one frequently sees several moderately sized nucleoli *(4)*, and once again such a histiocyte appears in the lumen of a blood capillary *(5)*. Sometimes these cells have phagocytosed erythrocytes.

A malignant histiocytosis is a rare histiocytic lymphoma, which results in generalized swelling of the lymph nodes, hepatosplenomegaly and infiltration of the skin and lungs. With this inclusive involvement of other organs, the bone changes play a rather subordinate role in diagnosis. Histologically a malignant histiocytosis is therefore more likely to be spotted in a skin or liver biopsy or in an excised lymph node with a similar infiltrate. The tumor cells contain non-specific esterase and acid phosphatase, and immunohistochemically lysozyme positive histiocyte markers (alpha-1-antitrypsin and alpha-1-antichymotrypsin). The prognosis is poor and life expectation can only be extended by means of aggressive chemotherapy. Solitary bony histiocytic tumors have a significantly better prognosis than when the condition has become generalized. Death is usually due to a cerebral hemorrhage or pneumonia.

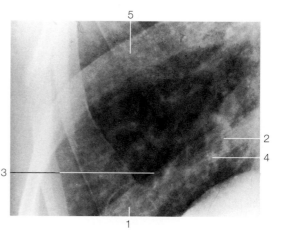

Fig. 369. Malignant histiocytosis (right 8th rib)

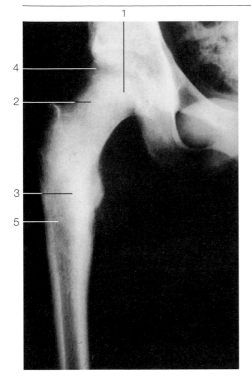

Fig. 370. Malignant histiocytosis (proximal right femur)

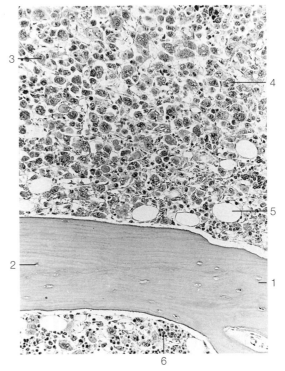

Fig. 371. Malignant histiocytosis; HE, ×64

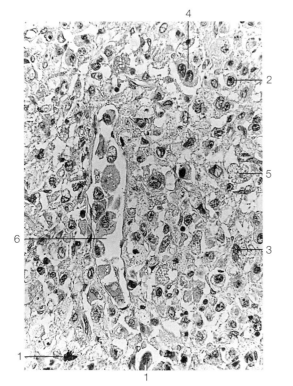

Fig. 372. Malignant histiocytosis; HE, ×120

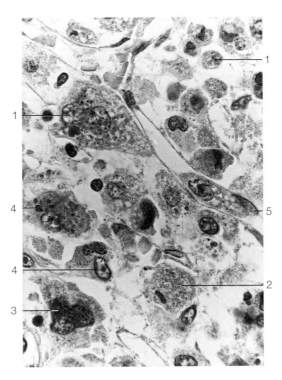

Fig. 373. Malignant histiocytosis; HE, ×180

Reparative Giant Cell Granuloma of the Jaws (ICD-O-DA-M-4413/0)

A giant cell lesion in the jaw bones is only in rare cases a true giant cell neoplasm. It is most often a reactive process in the course of an attack of hyperparathyroidism or the result of local trauma. *A reparative giant cell granuloma of the jaws is an accumulation of non-tumorous granulation tissue with osteoclastic giant cells which is to be interpreted as the reaction to and organization of traumatic bleeding into the bone.* The mandible is more often affected than the maxilla. Most of the patients are between 10 and 25 years of age.

In the **radiograph** of **Fig. 374** one can see such a bony granuloma in the right side of the mandible. It is a large slightly elliptical "bony cyst" (1) that has taken up the whole width of the jaw, and which is sharply bordered by a narrow band of marginal sclerosis. The cortex is thinned from within, but not penetrated. In the region of the neighboring tooth 47 one can see a zone of sclerosis (2). The "bony cyst" shows no internal structure.

In the **histological picture** of a reparative giant cell granuloma of the jaw the most obvious feature is the granulomatous nature of this lesion. In **Fig. 375** one sees a loose vascularized stroma in which a large number of proliferating fibroblasts and fibrocytes (1) are lying. They have rather slender drawn-out nuclei which are fully isomorphic. A few nuclei appear to be somewhat hyperchromatic (2). Mitoses are rarely encountered. This matrix can be edematously infiltrated and soaked with blood, and near the hemorrhagic extravasation, hemosiderin deposits can be seen. There are also small foci of lymphocytes, plasma cells and histiocytes (3). One is struck by the multinucleated giant cells (4) which are irregularly distributed throughout the tissue, either alone or in groups. The proliferating fibroblasts and irregularly dispersed giant cells distinguish this lesion from an osteoclastoma (p. 340 and Fig. 642). Sometimes cystic degeneration and osteoid or bone formation are observed in a reparative giant cell granuloma. Histologically this lesion is practically identical with the resorption giant cell granulomas seen in cases of hyperparathyroidism (p. 84, and Figs. 151 & 152).

Giant Cell Reaction of the Short Tubular Bones (ICD-O-DA-M-4411/0)

Osteolytic lesions of the short tubular bones of the hand or foot can arise which produce a massive local expansion and give a very strong impression of a malignant bone tumor. *In fact, this is due to benign non-tumorous granulation tissue in the marrow cavity of a short tubular bone, which consists of a fibroblastic matrix with numerous osteoclastic giant cells and which is the result of traumatic damage to the bone.* This also shows a certain resemblance to an aneurysmal bony cyst (p. 412).

In **Fig. 376** one can see the classical **radiological appearance** of such a giant cell reaction. The 2nd metatarsal of the left foot has undergone a fusiform expansion (1) which is pressing upon and displacing the neighboring bones. In the enter of the bone there is a "bony cyst" which is opaque internally, but where small pale cystic regions (2) can be distinguished. On one side the cortex shows a sclerotic increase in density (3), indicating slow benign growth. Elsewhere, however, the cortex (4) is severely narrowed, and a patchy osteolysis can be recognized. No periosteal reaction can be observed. The discrete and streaky patches of thickening which one can see inside the osteolytic zone are striking. They indicate the formation of new bone.

The **histological picture** is characterized by highly cellular granulation tissue which can be reminiscent of an aneurysmal bony cyst (p. 416 and Fig. 794). In **Fig. 377** one sees highly cellular granulation tissue with a marked fibrous stroma (1) in which isomorphic fibrocytes and fibroblasts, as well as multinucleated giant cells (2) are lying. The wide, densely packed osteoid trabeculae (3) are plain to see. These are pathognomonic of this lesion and distinguish it from giant cell neoplasms.

The appearance of a giant cell reaction in a short tubular bone is accompanied by pain and swelling of the soft tissues which, together with the expansion and local destruction of the bone, seem very much to suggest a malignant process. Nevertheless this lesion is almost always cured by local curettage.

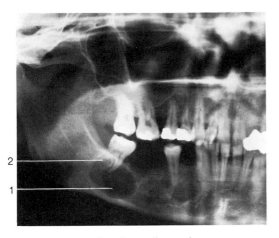

Fig. 374. Reparative giant cell granuloma (right side of mandible)

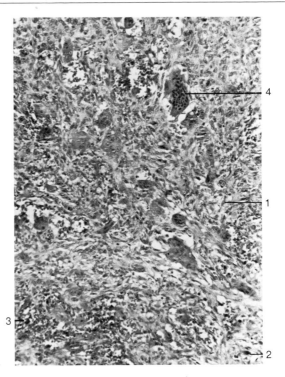

Fig. 375. Reparative giant cell granuloma; HE, ×40

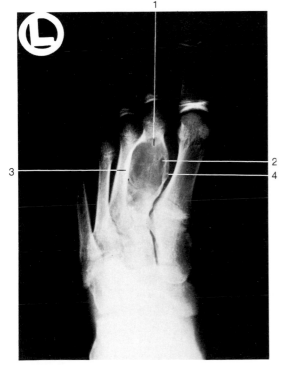

Fig. 376. Giant cell reaction of short tubular bones (left 2nd metatarsal)

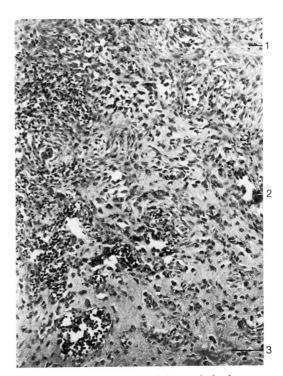

Fig. 377. Giant cell reaction of short tubular bones; HE, ×40

11 Bone Tumors

General

From many points of view neoplasms of bone occupy a peculiar position among the tumors which afflict mankind. For one thing, they are comparatively **rare**, so that the physician often does not possess the experience which is necessary for diagnosing and treating this disease. The **symptomatology** is meagre and uncharacteristic, and very often only becomes apparent when the tumor is well advanced. Arriving at the correct **diagnosis** is particularly difficult and requires a complete combination of both radiological and histological examinations. Great difficulties are also attendant upon arriving at an exact **classification** of any bone tumor, and this is essential for assessing its **prognosis**. Finally, there are **problems of treatment** which make great demands upon surgeons, and radiologists and oncologists. In the case of a bone tumor there are various individual aspects to be taken into account, so that questions of diagnosis and treatment can only be solved by the closest interdisciplinary cooperation.

Primary bone tumors are relatively rarely met with in general practice, in hospitals and in the material submitted to pathologists. Modern specific and effective therapeutic possibilities require from us more than ever before an exact differentiated diagnosis. There is hardly any other system of the body in which the nature of a neoplasm can appear in so many forms or be so difficult to interpret as in the skeleton. Even the distinction between benign and malignant neoplastic growth, or between tumors and reactive bone changes, often presents major difficulties. This alone requires great experience in interpreting both the clinical picture and the morphology of bone neoplasms. By means of extensive statistical investigations the characteristics of bone tumors may be elaborated and our knowledge of these diseases enlarged. Valuable information is already available in the USA, where a survey of a large number of cases has been obtained.

In recent years this has been supplemented by a series of European investigations. But although we have in this way acquired extensive knowledge about the clinical, radiological and morphological course and action of various therapeutic procedures, we are always meeting tumors which do not conform to any recognized pattern and bring up entirely new diagnostic and therapeutic problems. A meticulous analysis of these cases is the basis upon which the pathologist, together with the radiologist and clinician, has to seek a solution.

The pathologist, who has the task of finding the "definitive" diagnosis, must above all have precise knowledge of the macroscopic and microscopic morphology, and must be able to assign each tumor to its correct place in the generally accepted scheme of classification. Furthermore, the pathologist must have at least some knowledge and experience of morphological changes in the radiograph. The taking into account of the **radiological morphology** is an absolutely essential part of diagnosing a bone tumor. For this reason pathologists should never diagnose bone tumors without being aware of the radiological findings and assessing these personally in the radiograph. This applies most especially to malignant bone tumors, for which a mutilating operation is often necessary. The histological section alone is often insufficient to allow a bone tumor to be diagnosed with certainty. The biopsy of a proliferating fracture callus, for instance, can awake suspicion of an osteoblastic osteosarcoma. The importance of this practical experience for the clinician lies in the realization that the diagnosis of a suspected malignant tumor requires that the associated representative radiographs must always be sent to the pathologist. The radiographs (including the CT and MRI images etc.) provide the pathologist with the macroscopic appearance of the tumor.

The following rules apply to the diagnosis of all bone tumors: if the radiographic appearance, age of the patient, site and histological findings accord with classical statistical experience, then the diagnosis is probably right. Depart from this rule, and you must be prepared for an incorrect conclusion. The findings must be assessed by the clinicians, radiologists and pathologists working together.

Classification. For the presentation of modern guidelines with regard to therapy, and to make possible a fruitful discussion between many types of medical and surgical specialists coming from the various fields of expertise, it is necessary that we all use the same diagnostic terminology. The enormous variation in the appearance of bone tumors that confronts the morbid anatomist makes it difficult to produce a simple, serviceable and generally agreed arrangement of ideas which will reflect general experience in this field. It is thanks to the work of JAFFE and LICHTENSTEIN that we today possess an extensive classificatory system for bone neoplasms which makes it possible to treat each variety according to its nature. Today we recognize over 50 different bone tumors and tumor-like skeletal changes. These neoplasms are arranged in terms of a **classification system** that is based on the histogenesis of the individual tumors. The classification in general use today was published in 1962 by ACKERMANN et al. in the Atlas of the Armed Forces Institute of Pathology (AFIP) under "Tumors of bone and cartilage", and by SCHAJOWICZ et al. 1972 and 1993, and is widely accepted by the WHO. The Tumor Histology Key "International Classification of Diseases for Oncology – ICD-O-DA" (1978) is also based on this classification, and this has made a computerized codification of bone neoplasms possible. In addition there are many other classificatory schemes which have not, however, achieved worldwide acceptance.

In the international classification, 9 groups of tumors are distinguished (see **Table 3**). A distinction is made between benign and malignant growths. The **primary skeletal neoplasms** arise from *cartilaginous tissue* (chondromas, chondrosarcomas), from *bone tissue* (osteomas, osteosarcomas), from *connective tissue* (fibromas, fibrosarcomas), from *bone marrow* (plasmocytomas, Ewing's sarcoma), from *blood vessels* in bone (angiomas, angiosarcomas) or from *nerve tissue* in bone (neurinomas, neurofibromas). This system of classification has provided a solid framework for the most commonly encountered bone tumors and has

proved its worth in everyday practice. In recent years, however, it has been extended and enlarged by a further subdivision of the single groups of neoplasms. Following intensive work on bone tumors, and as the result of following up cases, new neoplastic entities have been worked out which represent separate diseases. These include, for instance, the aggressive osteoblastoma, the small-cell osteosarcoma, the peripheral fibromyxoma, neuroectodermal bone tumor and others. The types of bone tumor at present recognized are shown in the classification (see **Table 3**). It is to be expected that new varieties of bone tumor will come to be distinguished in the next few years, but these will easily be entered against the background of the system of classification at present in use.

When diagnosing bone tumors, one repeatedly comes across a specimen that cannot be allotted a place in the usual classification system. The WHO tumor key has left a space for "unclassified tumors", and the pathologist should not attempt to force every tumor into this system "at all costs", but to collect widely atypical and problematic examples under this "unclassifiable" group. In this way a more precise analysis of these cases will later become possible when the new diagnostic procedures (e.g. MRT, immunohistochemistry and the like) have become established.

The classification of bone tumors displayed in **Table 3** includes only the true primary neoplasms of the skeleton. It must nevertheless be pointed out that many of these tumors do not always meet all the criteria of genuine neoplastic growth (e.g. the non-ossifying bone fibroma, osteoid osteoma). So far no uniformity of opinion has been reached about the neoplastic nature of these lesions. On the other hand, there are many skeletal lesions which, clinically and radiologically, give the impression of bone tumors. These are collected together under the term "**tumor-like bone lesions**". Bone metastases are regarded as **secondary bone tumors** and also belong to this group. Finally, it must also be pointed out that the dividing line between benign and malignant bone tumors is not rigid. There are quite a number of neoplasms which exhibit "*semimalignant growth*", and which are locally aggressive but do not metastasize (e.g. the chondromyxoid fibroma, aggressive osteoblastoma, adamantinoma of the long bones etc.). After

Table 3. Classification of the Primary Bone Tumors

Tissue of Origin	Benign Tumors	Malignant Tumors
Cartilaginous tissue	• Osteochondroma • Enchondroma/Chondroma, periosteal (juxta-cortical, epiexostotic) chondroma • Chondroblastoma • Chondromyxoid fibroma	• Chondrosarcoma: primary/secondary • Periosteal (juxtacortical, epiexostotic) chondro-sarcoma • Malignant chondroblastoma • Dedifferentiated chondrosarcoma • Mesenchymal chondrosarcoma • Clear-cell chondrosarcoma • Extraskeletal chondrosarcoma

Bone tissue	• Osteoma
	• Osteoid osteoma
	• Osteoblastoma
		• Osteosarcoma: primary/secondary
		
		• Aggressive osteoblastoma
		• **Intraosseous osteosarcomas:**
		  – Telangiectatic osteosarcoma
		  – Small cell osteosarcoma
		  – Intraosseous well-differentiated (low malignancy) osteosarcoma
		  – Multicentric osteosarcoma
		• **Surface osteosarcomas:**
		  – Parosteal osteosarcoma
		  – Periosteal osteosarcoma
		  – Highly malignant surface osteosarcoma
		• **Secondary osteosarcomas:**
		  – Paget osteosarcoma
		  – Radiation osteosarcoma
		  – Osteosarcoma in a bone infarct

Connective Tissue	• Non-ossifying bone fibroma • Xanthofibroma • Osseous fibromyxoma • Metaphyseal fibrous cortical defect • Ossifying bone fibroma • Cortical desmoid • Osteofibrous bone dysplasia • Fibrous bone dysplasia • Desmoplastic bone fibroma • Benign fibrous histiocytoma • Osteoclastoma (grade 1)	• Osseous fibrosarcoma • Malignant mesenchymoma • Malignant fibrous histiocytoma • Osteoclastoma (grade 3)
Fatty tissue	• Osseous lipoma	• Osseous liposarcoma • Osteoliposarcoma
Bone marrow		• Medullary plasmocytoma (myeloma) • Ewing's sarcoma • Primitive neuroectodermal bone tumor (PNET) • Malignant bone lymphoma
Vascular tissue	• Bone hemangioma • Hemangioendothelioma • Hemangiopericytoma • Osseous lymphangioma	• Osseous hemangiosarcoma • Hemangioendothelioma • Hemangiopericytoma • Osseous lymphangiosarcoma • Adamantinoma of the long bones
Nerve tissue	• Neurinoma (schwannoma) • Neurofibroma • Ganglioneuroma	
Muscle tissue	• Osseous leiomyoma	• Osseous leiomyosarcoma
Notochordal tissue		• Chordoma • Chondroid chordoma

complete surgical removal of such tumors an absolute cure is to be expected.

The classificatory principle whereby bone neoplasms are related to the tissue from which they are derived is justified, if we consider the mechanism by which they grow. The enormous variety of these tumors is due to the complexity of the processes of bone growth and bone replacement. In **Fig. 378** (from JOHNSON 1953) the topographical and functional tissue differentiation in growing and adult bone from which bone tumors are derived is indicated. According to the theory of bone neoplasia put forward by JOHNSON (1953), the form and site of the neoplasm are dependent upon the prevailing bone-remodeling processes as they occur in the normal ontogenesis of the region in which the growth is located. The time of life at which a tumor appears corresponds to the ontogenetically determined greatest activity of the cells of origin. This accounts for the association of primary bone tumors with the region of most intensive growth in length, and their appearance particularly during the period of skeletal growth.

As is shown on the left side of **Fig. 378**, the most intensive bone growth occurs in the epiphyses and the adjacent metaphyses. The arrows indicate the action of the osteoblasts, which contribute to growth in length of the bone at the epiphyseal cartilages by endochondral ossification, and to growth in thickness by periosteal and endosteal new bone formation at the metaphysis. Growth of osseous neoplasms is closely bound up with the function of the local cell population. The function of the osteoblasts is to build up the organic bone matrix – the osteoid – out of collagen fibrils and mucopolysaccharides. This fundamental characteristic is also retained in tumors derived from osteoblasts, in the **sclerosing osteosarcoma**, for instance. This tumor arises in the diaphysis, close to the metaphysis, or, as a **periosteal sarcoma**, at the transition from metaphysis to diaphysis. The **osteolytic osteosarcoma**, however, is characterized by its bone resorbing function. This biological property is bound up with the action of the osteoclasts, which are seen in large numbers in the histological picture of this tumor. During skeletal development they act together with the osteoblasts to transform primary into secondary spongiosa. They are marked in **Fig. 378** with

crosses. **Osteoclastomas** also develop at the site of osteoclastic function, namely, in the epiphysis, and spread towards the metaphysis. A similar localization applies to the **chondroblastomas**, where numerous giant cells also take part. **Chondrosarcomas**, on the other hand, arise in the zone of intensive cartilage proliferation, that is to say, in the metaphyses. **Fibrosarcomas** develop from the intraosseous connective tissue of the bone, and are therefore encountered in the diaphysis, close to the metaphyses. Neoplasms that arise from the bone marrow (e.g. **Ewing's sarcoma**) spread out in the diaphysis, where the marrow is found. Since the localization of a bone tumor within a bone represents a very important diagnostic criterion, this knowledge about the tissue of origin of a neoplasm can be useful.

Localization of the Benign Bone Tumors (Fig. 379). A complete survey of all benign bone tumors makes it clear that they are especially likely to appear in the region of the knee, and it is here that 31% of such neoplasms are found. The second most frequent location is at the hip joint (including the femoral neck and pelvis) with 13.2%, and the shoulder girdle (proximal part of humerus, scapula) with 12.9%. Other frequent sites are the bones of the hand (9.3%), the spinal column (9.3%) and the skull (5.2%). In general, benign tumors can appear in any bone, but a predilection for certain regions should nevertheless be taken into account.

Age Distribution of the Benign Bone Tumors (Fig. 380). The age distribution of all benign bone tumors shows a clear association with youth, and by far the majority of these neoplasms are discovered during the 2nd decade of life. As is apparent, however, from the diagram of **Fig. 380**, these tumors can in fact appear at any age. It is therefore to be assumed that most benign tumors arise in youth, but are often only detected at a more advanced age. In this connection one is always coming across chance findings where the benign tumor has produced no symptoms, but a radiological examination for some other reason (trauma, for instance) has led to the discovery of a benign tumor the existence of which has long been unsuspected. Many of these tumorous bone lesions do not require surgical treatment.

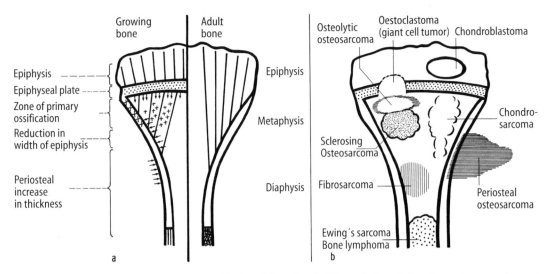

Fig. 378. a Diagram showing the topographical and functional differentiation of the tissues in normal growing bone (*left half of* **a**) and adult bone (*right half of* **a**), *Crosses*, osteoclasts; *arrows*, osteoblasts. **b** Topographical sites of a few primary bone tumors. (After JOHNSON 1953)

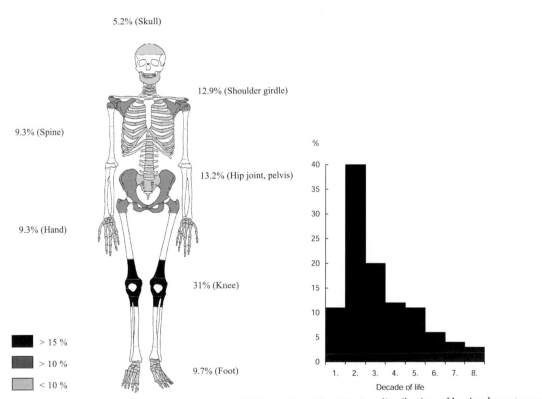

Fig. 379. Localization of benign bone tumors (5472 cases). Others: 9.4%

Fig. 380. Age distribution of benign bone tumors (5472 cases)

Localization of the Malignant Bone Tumors

(Fig. 381). Malignant tumors are also especially likely to appear in the region of the knee (24.9%), and the distal part of the femur is more likely to be affected than the proximal region of the tibia. Bone sarcomas appear relatively frequently in the bones of the pelvic girdle (19.8%). The spinal column is also a common site (17.6%). As the third most likely places to be attacked, mention should be made of the shoulder girdle (11.9%) and the skull (13.1%).

Age Distribution of the Malignant Bone Tumors

(Fig. 382). The overall survey of malignant bone tumors reveals two frequency peaks: one in the 2nd and one in the 6th decade of life. Fewer neoplasms of this kind are met with in small children (1st decade of life), extreme old age (8th and 9th decades), and in middle age (4th and 5th decades). Examining the age distribution of different types of tumor has revealed that some of them (e.g. chondrosarcomas, Fig. 431) appear with almost equal frequency at any time of life. On the other hand, some tumors have a clear predilection for childhood (e.g. Ewing's sarcoma, Fig. 661), young adult life (e.g. osteosarcomas, Fig. 509). Other tumors appears virtually only in old age (e.g. the medullary plasmocytoma, Fig. 653). Taking into account the age of the patient is an important factor when diagnosing any malignant bone tumor, and must without fail be considered.

Case History of Malignant Bone Tumors (Fig. 383).

If one compares the time which has elapsed between the onset of the symptoms of a malignant bone tumor with the patient's first visit to the physician, it appears that 77.8% of all patients do so within the first two months. On the other hand, in only 29.6% of cases is the correct diagnosis made within the first three months. The chondrosarcoma is the first to produce symptoms; osteosarcomas and plasmocytomas drive about 80% of patients to seek medical advice within the first two months, and sooner or later a lymphoma of bone will draw attention to itself. An osteosarcoma is likely to be the first to be recognized as a malignant neoplasm. At the other extreme, a fibrosarcoma of bone reveals itself as a malignant tumor, clinically and radiologically, relatively late on.

The Prognosis of the Malignant Bone Tumors

(Fig. 384). The life expectation of a patient with a malignant neoplasm of bone depends upon timely diagnosis and adequate treatment. As indicated by our earlier research (1977), the prognosis at that time had to be assessed as bad. Out of 165 patients with malignant bone tumors, 87.7% died within the first 3 years – most of them within 1 year of the diagnosis. More recently, however, we have been able to record a significantly longer survival time. This is undoubtedly the result of earlier diagnosis and the differential analysis of each neoplasm, as well as more modern methods of treatment. It is now possible to record a five year survival in more than 60%–75% of malignant bone tumors. Here the ever increasing interdisciplinary cooperation between clinicians, radiologists, oncologists, and pathologists has proved decisive.

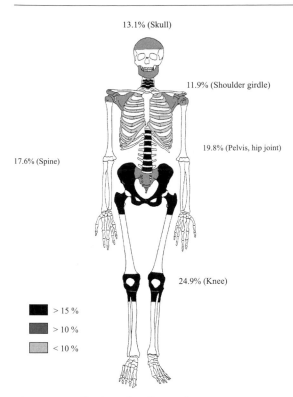

13.1% (Skull)

11.9% (Shoulder girdle)

19.8% (Pelvis, hip joint)

17.6% (Spine)

24.9% (Knee)

■ > 15 %

▨ > 10 %

▧ < 10 %

Fig. 381. Localization of malignant bones tumors (5020 cases). Others: 12.7%

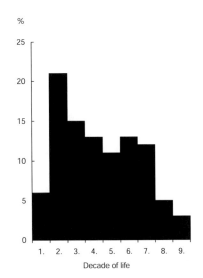

%

Fig. 382. Age distribution of malignant bone tumors (5020 cases)

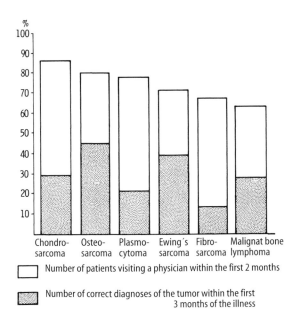

Chondro-sarcoma   Osteo-sarcoma   Plasmo-cytoma   Ewing's sarcoma   Fibro-sarcoma   Malignat bone lymphoma

☐ Number of patients visiting a physician within the first 2 months

▨ Number of correct diagnoses of the tumor within the first 3 months of the illness

Fig. 383. Comparison of the interval between the onset of symptoms and the first visit to a physician for malignant bone tumors. (ADLER 1977)

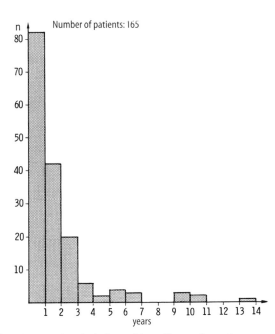

Number of patients: 165

Fig. 384. Survival time with malignant bone tumors. (ADLER 1977)

Cartilaginous Tumors

Osteochondroma (ICD-O-DA-M-9210/0)

Osteochondromas are by far the most common non-malignant bony neoplasms, constituting some 40% of the benign tumors of bone. *They consist of new bone formations which are covered by a wide cap of hyaline cartilage, and which bulge forward like a mushroom from the bone surface into the surrounding soft parts.* Since these tumors take a long time to increase in size, they frequently only make themselves noticed as swellings after a considerable time. Pain is not always present, but large tumors lead to limitation of movement. The symptoms can last for 20 years.

Localization (Fig. 385). Osteochondromas can arise in any bone in which endochondral ossification (replacement bone formation) takes place. Such "osteocartilaginous exostoses" have been observed in practically all bones. The most usual site is, however, in the long bones, where the lesion is most often found in the region of the metaphyses. In more than a third of the cases (39.2%), the distal femoral, or proximal tibial or humeral metaphysis is affected. The most frequent location of all is the distal femoral metaphysis. Other bones (skull, ribs, spine, pelvis) are much less often affected. In fact, we have found quite a large number of cases involving the short tubular bones of the hands and feet (13%).

Age Distribution (Fig. 386). Most osteochondromas develop in young people and are discovered during the 2nd and 3rd decades of life. Of the neoplasms examined by us, 41% had been removed surgically during the 2nd decade and had involved more men than women. However, as can be seen from **Fig. 386**, an osteochondroma can also turn up late in life.

Some authors regard the osteochondroma as a local failure of endochondral ossification. Its tumorous nature is, however, suggested by the frequently observed tendency to proliferate. Osteochondromas weighing more than 5 kg have been described. In fewer than 1% of solitary osteochondromas is malignant change to be expected, and in general these tumors have

a very good prognosis. After they have been removed with a chisel a recurrence rate of just 2% has been recorded. It is, however, important that all the cartilage including the periosteum is completely removed, since it is from the periosteum that the tumor can develop again. A special form of this clinical picture is represented by the appearance of *multiple osteocartilaginous exostoses,* which has a significant familial background (p. 62). Although the morphological appearance of the individual lesions is identical with that of the solitary osteochondroma, *"exostosis disease"* is a recognizable entity. The tumors accumulate in the neighborhood of the shoulder, knee and ankle. The risk of spontaneous malignant change in this condition amounts to 15%, mostly resulting in chondrosarcomas.

In the **radiograph** an osteochondroma presents as a mushroom-like bulge, attached to a bone by a broad base or a stem. It arises without any seam from the host spongiosa and usually has a connective tissue covering of periosteum. The cartilage cap lies in this outer region, and is recognizable only as a shadow, if at all. However, calcified foci may be seen in the cap. **Figure 387** shows a classical osteochondroma of the distal femoral metaphysis which is attached to the cortical bone of the femur by a strong stem *(1)*. The exostosis juts out proximally into the soft parts and is swollen like a mushroom at the end *(2)*. Here one can see irregular patchy translucencies, separated by a dense network. The outer contour is clear and relatively sharp, with a somewhat notched appearance. The stem, on the other hand, has a completely smooth border *(1)*. Fine sclerosis can be seen at the base *(3)*. The adjacent bone is unremarkable. **Figure 388** shows an osteochondroma at the proximal femoral metaphysis that has a rather feathery appearance and is attached to the bone by a broad base *(1)*. The tumor is heavily sclerosed internally, and one can again see patchy translucent areas. *Mushroom-like osteochondromas* often have a narrow stem, and most of them jut out proximally, reaching well into the soft parts (Fig. 387). The neoplasm can be more than 8 cm in size, and by pressing on the soft tissues and nerves cause pain. The stem can be recognized radiologically by the parallel structures in the spongiosa. The tumor can easily be removed with a chisel. Ses-

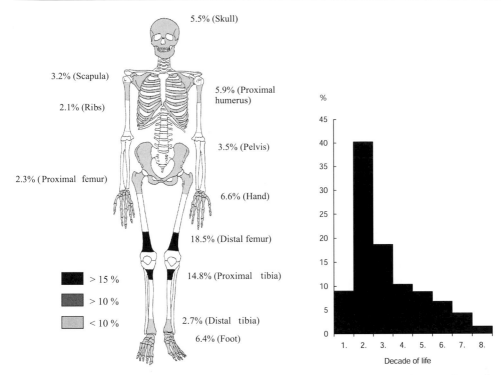

5.5% (Skull)

3.2% (Scapula)

2.1% (Ribs)

5.9% (Proximal humerus)

3.5% (Pelvis)

2.3% (Proximal femur)

6.6% (Hand)

18.5% (Distal femur)

14.8% (Proximal tibia)

> 15 %

> 10 %

< 10 %

2.7% (Distal tibia)

6.4% (Foot)

%

45

40

35

30

25

20

15

10

5

0

1. 2. 3. 4. 5. 6. 7. 8.

Decade of life

Fig. 385. Localization of osteochondromas (1952 cases). Others: 28.5%

Fig. 386. Age distribution of osteochondromas (1952 cases)

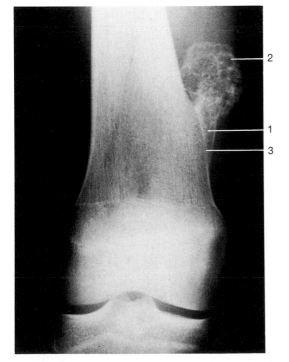

Fig. 387. Osteochondroma (distal femoral metaphysis)

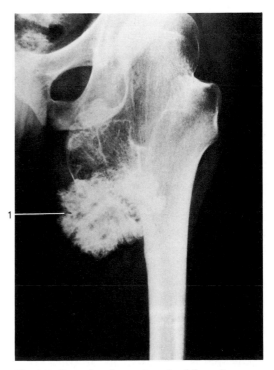

Fig. 388. Osteochondroma (proximal femur)

sile osteochondromas are attached to the cortex by a broad base.

The **macroscopic appearance** of an osteochondroma corresponds to the radiological findings. In **Fig. 389** one can see the resected specimen of an osteochondroma from the proximal region of the fibula that is attached by a broad base to the long bone, and is bulging out like a mushroom or a cauliflower. The sawn surface of the fibula *(1)* shows that the structure is unchanged. The exostosis consists of several nodular or spherical components *(2)* that are covered externally by a layer of cartilage and periosteal connective tissue. By far the larger part of this exostosis is made up of mature, fully mineralized bone tissue with a wide-meshed spongiosa. Fatty tissue has been laid down in the marrow cavity. The hemispherical surface of the osteochondroma is covered by a cap of cartilage some 0.1–3 cm thick, which can nevertheless be incomplete. In young people it is usually thicker than in adults, but if it is thicker than 3 cm the suspicion of malignancy must be entertained. At an advanced age the cartilaginous cap may become fully ossified, so that sometimes one finds only an *"osseous exostosis"* without any cartilage. A bursa often develops above an osteochondroma, and later this may also calcify or ossify.

In the **overall histological picture (Fig. 390)** of a section through an osteochondroma one can recognize the wide stem, which is directly attached to the host bone, and the internal wide-meshed and irregular cancellous framework *(1)*. The original cortex of the long bone is missing here. Throughout the cancellous framework of the exostoses one can also see fatty marrow and hematopoietic bone marrow. In the outer zone of the stem *(2)* and in the subchondral zone *(3)* one can observe the narrow cortex that gives the lesion a sharp outline in the radiograph. The wide end of the exostosis is covered by a 1.5 cm cap of cartilage *(4)* which is poorly delineated from the subchondral bone. The whole exostosis lies under a narrow periosteal mantle *(5)* of loose, richly fibrous connective tissue. With old osteochondromas, which may be encountered in advanced old age, this characteristic layer of cartilage ossify and therefore become undetectable.

Under **higher magnification (Fig. 391)** one can recognize inside an osteochondroma an irregular, partly widened, partly dense cancellous scaffolding in which the trabeculae often appear to be osteosclerotically widened *(1)*. They have smooth outer borders, and in proliferating osteochondromas rows of activated osteocytes may be deposited. The trabeculae show lamellar layering and one can see small osteocytes and sometimes a few reversal lines. This is completely mature bone tissue. The marrow cavity *(2)* is filled with fat and connective tissue, and occasionally one encounters a typical hematopoietic focus. The appearance of the external cartilage cap *(3)* suggests a faint lobular formation, which is very characteristic of all cartilaginous tumors. Within, one is struck by the numerous greatly distended chondrocytes, which differ in size and distribution. These chondrocytes can, as in a normal growing epiphysis, be arranged in rows. The subchondral cortex in **Fig. 391** is only poorly developed. It can, however, be much more stoutly built up. In the external region above the cartilaginous cap *(4)* there is a layer of loose periosteal connective tissue.

Under **higher magnification** (**Fig. 392**) the most striking object is the cap itself, which in this instance may possibly be showing signs of a malignant change. Outside one can see the covering fiber-rich periosteum *(1)*. The hyaline cartilage cap has a basophilic or eosinophilic matrix containing groups or rows of mononucleated cartilage cells, and resembles the columnar cartilage of a normal epiphyseal line. The chondrocytes are often densely packed together and are seen to be distended. The chondroblastic capsules have become widened *(2)*. In the subchondral region one can see in **Fig. 391** how the cartilaginous tissue is putting out finger-like processes into the adjacent bone tissue *(5)*. Inside the bony structures we often find islets of cartilage. This is very characteristic of an osteochondroma. The ungainly trabeculae are layered with osteoblasts *(6)*. In the marrow cavity there is loose connective tissue with many capillaries *(2)*.

Because of the microscopic structures described above, the histological diagnosis of a solitary osteochondroma is very easy, particularly when the typical radiological findings are present. Nevertheless, when such a lesion has been removed with a chisel it should be examined with the greatest possible care, so as not to overlook the possible malignant change that is especially likely to take place in multiple os-

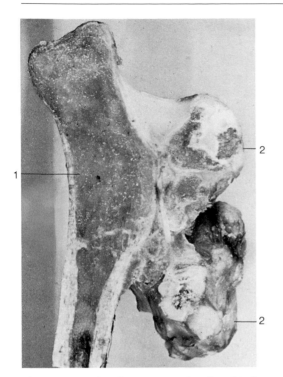

Fig. 389. Osteochondroma removed with a chisel

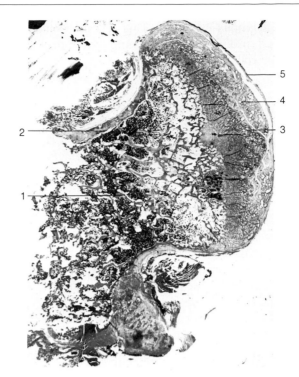

Fig. 390. Osteochondroma (overall view); HE, ×2

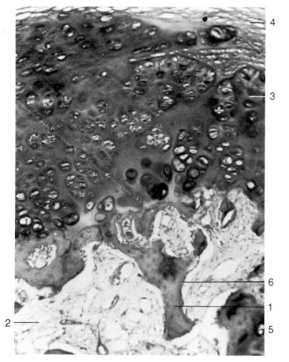

Fig. 391. Osteochondroma; HE, ×25

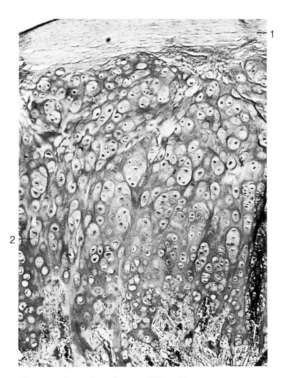

Fig. 392. Osteochondroma; HE, ×40

teocartilaginous exostoses. This reveals itself by lobulated proliferation buds and polymorphic cartilage cells.

Subungual Osteocartilaginous Exostosis

Subungual osteocartilaginous exostosis is a reactive, often exophytically growing cartilaginous proliferation at the tip of a terminal phalanx, usually that of the great toe. The radiological appearances and the histological picture can sometimes arouse the suspicion of a chondrosarcoma, from which this lesion must certainly be distinguished. In most cases there is a history of local trauma, with or without subsequent infection, which is seen as the cause. The lesion makes itself noticed by the pain.

In the **radiograph (Fig. 393)** one can see a roundish exostosis in the distal part of the terminal phalanx of the great toe which is jutting out into the soft parts around the bone *(1)*. It is less than 1 cm in size and is not very clearly distinguished from them. Inside there are cloudy regions of increased density, and also some patchy translucencies. This exostosis usually bulges forwards against the toenail, thus causing severe pain. The phalanx itself is largely undamaged *(2)*, although the cortex can show erosions on one side.

In the **histological section (Fig. 394)** one can see a bony framework within the exostosis that is mostly made up of newly formed fibrous bone trabeculae *(1)* with numerous osteocytes and deposited osteoblasts. In between one can recognize a loose, partly fiber-rich granulation tissue, with many capillaries and loose infiltrates of lymphocytes, plasma cells and histiocytes *(2)*. In the outer layer there is highly cellular cartilaginous tissue *(3)* in which multinucleated chondrocytes with hyperchromatic nuclei are found. The polymorphic nuclei must not be taken to indicate the presence of a malignant neoplasm.

A similar non-tumorous lesion is the so-called *"bizarre parosteal osteochondromatous proliferation"* ("Nora lesion"), which develops on the surface of the short tubular bones of the hand or foot and consists of a mixture of cartilage, bone and connective tissue. Whereas one sees in the radiograph a roundish, sharply delineated mass on the surface of the bone, the histological appearance is that of highly cellular cartilaginous tissue with large, bizarre nuclei, multinucleated cartilage cells and irregular bony trabeculae with a prominent deposition of osteoblasts and osteoclasts. This usually posttraumatic proliferation, with a certain tendency to recurrence after removal, should not be mistaken for a malignant bone neoplasm in spite of cell proliferation.

Enchondroma (ICD-O-DA-M-9220/0)

The enchondroma is the second most common of the benign bone tumors with a frequency of 19%. *It is a benign primary bone neoplasm, which consists of mature hyaline cartilage and is laid down in the center of the marrow cavity of a bone.* Many of these very slow growing tumors are symptomless and are discovered by chance during a radiological examination. Sometimes the tumor may announce itself by causing a pathological fracture.

Localization (Fig. 395). The principal site of the enchondromas is in the short tubular bones of the hand or foot, with the hand being more often affected, and it is here that more than 50% of these neoplasms are found. In these bones the enchondroma has a good prognosis, and malignant change is not to be anticipated. Recurrence is unlikely after complete removal of the tumorous cartilaginous tissue. From the point of view of the prognosis, however, the site of these tumors is of great importance. With enchondromas of the ribs (2.8%) there is, even with unremarkable histological findings, a possibility of malignant growth. Enchondromas – particularly giant enchondromas – of the long bones (28.4%) should be classified as semimalignant, since they often spread across the whole width of the shaft, lead to polycystic widening of the bone, and have a strong tendency to recur. It is particularly the distal part of the femur and the proximal humeral metaphysis which are affected. Enchondromas of the pelvis are in fact always malignant, even when histological examination reveals no certainly malignant structures.

Age Distribution (Fig. 396). Enchondromas are observed at all ages. The average age of our patients was 27 years – the youngest being 6 and

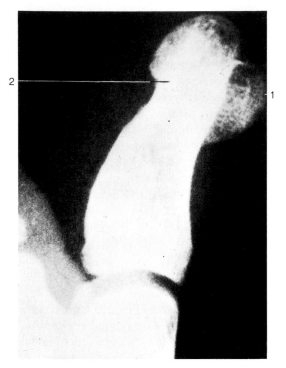

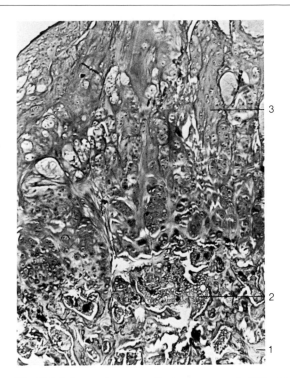

Fig. 393. Subungual osteocartilaginous exostosis (great toe)

Fig. 394. Subungual osteocartilaginous exostosis; HE, ×10

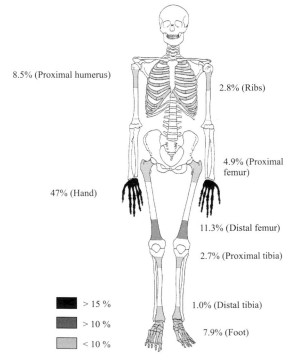

8.5% (Proximal humerus)

2.8% (Ribs)

4.9% (Proximal femur)

47% (Hand)

11.3% (Distal femur)

2.7% (Proximal tibia)

1.0% (Distal tibia)

> 15 %

> 10 %

< 10 %

7.9% (Foot)

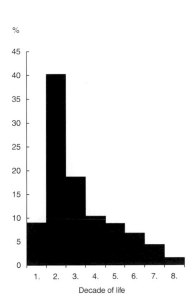

Fig. 395. Localization of enchondromas (636 cases); others 13.9%

Fig. 396. Age distribution of enchondromas (636 cases)

the oldest 78. We were able to establish a definite increase in the middle years (2nd to 6th decade). At 54.2% men are slightly more often affected than women (45.8%).

A **radiograph** is often sufficient for the diagnosis of an enchondroma of the hand or foot. A classical enchondroma of the 1st metacarpal (thumb) can be seen in **Fig. 397**. The tumor is lying in the center of the bone, which it has raised up like a bubble *(1)* so that a bulge is obscuring the original edge of the bone. One can see a sharply delineated diaphyseal "bony cyst" that has destroyed the cortex and is sharply outlined externally by a fine shell of bone. No periosteal reaction is to be seen. The inside of the "cyst" is filled out with fine irregular trabeculae, and its density is greatly increased. Sometimes patchy calcification foci can appear here, and that is very characteristic of cartilaginous neoplasms. Opposite the unaffected adjacent spongiosa the enchondroma is only partly and incompletely bordered by reactive marginal sclerosis. Since enchondromas of the fingers are frequently multiple, one should look for other foci in the radiograph.

The surgical specimens sent to the pathologist usually consist of curetted material that has been much broken up. **Figure 398** illustrates the original **macroscopic appearance** of an enchondroma of the finger. The marrow cavity has been taken over by lumpy and partly lobular cartilaginous tissue that presents a shining glassy grayish-white cut surface *(1)*. Here and there inside the tumor one can recognize hemorrhages *(2)* and calcification foci *(3)*. The tumor tissue is toughly elastic and can with further calcification become hard. These are mostly small tumors, but in **Fig. 398** a large part of the marrow cavity of the phalanx has been taken up by neoplastic tissue. The cortex *(4)* has been preserved and is in places sclerotically thickened *(5)*. With larger tumors, and if the cortex has been destroyed, the neoplasm must be carefully examined for signs of malignancy. In the soft parts *(6)* lying adjacent to such a tumor periosteal chondromas can arise (Fig. 405).

Much more serious problems than those met with in the short tubular bones of the hand and foot are presented by *enchondromas of the long bones, ribs* and *pelvis,* which on the grounds of their localization alone must be regarded as possibly semimalignant or as frankly malignant. **Figure 399** shows the **radiological** appearance *of an enchondroma of the distal part of the radius.* The bone is raised up near the tumor and shows signs of patchy destruction *(1)*. The neoplasm appears to have broken through the cortex, and one can recognize the shadow of a tumor which has reached out through the outside of the bone into the adjacent soft parts. The patches of increased density within the long bone have irregular borders, and the spongiosa in the neighborhood is much more translucent *(2)*. The increase in structural density has been brought about by deposition of calcium in the tissue of the tumor, whereas the uncalcified regions give the impression of osteolysis. With enchondromas of the long bones the radiological findings are often too uncharacteristic for an exact diagnosis to be made with sufficient certainty, and a bone infarct (Fig. 321 and p. 174) can easily be mistaken for a calcified enchondroma. Particularly in the long bones, patchy areas of calcification often appear in the region of the tumor, whereas enchondromas of the short tubular bones mostly form areas of translucency. Only after seeing a bone biopsy can an exact diagnosis be made.

With *enchondromas of the ribs* it is usual to resect the affected region of the rib completely and submit it to histological examination. **Fig 400** shows the **radiograph** of such a tumor. The affected region is markedly raised, so that this "bony cyst" is evidently limited externally by a narrow layer of bone *(1)*. Inside the tumor one sees only sparse straggly and patchy areas of increased density. This variety of neoplasm may reach a considerable size and show macroscopically a lobular formation and a glassy cut surface. Histologically, it is necessary to study the cellular picture of the individual chondrocytes precisely in order to exclude the criteria of malignancy (polymorphy of the cells and their nuclei, hyperchromatic nuclei, multinucleated cells, mitoses, infiltrating growth, invasion of a blood vessel).

The *radiological diagnosis* of enchondromas includes, as well as the conventional radiograph, tomography, computer tomography and angiography. Practically no blood vessels can be demonstrated within the neoplasm, since cartilaginous tissue is nourished by diffusion. With chondrosarcomas, on the other hand, vascular structures may appear.

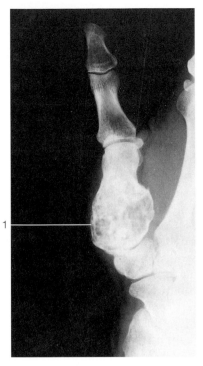

Fig. 397. Enchondroma (1st metacarpal)

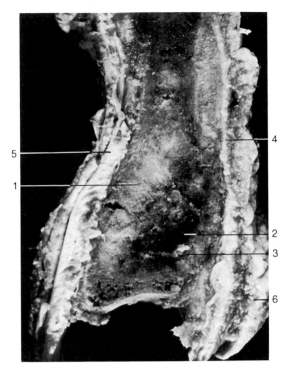

Fig. 398. Enchondroma (cut surface, little finger)

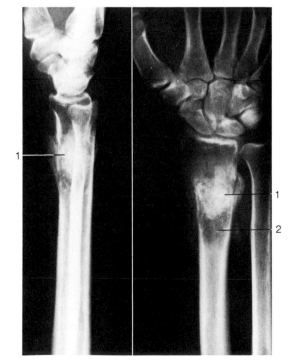

Fig. 399. Enchondroma (distal part of radius)

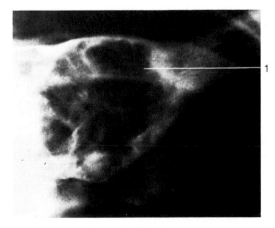

Fig. 400. Enchondroma (Rib)

In the **histological section** (**Fig. 401**) through an enchondroma one can see, in the middle of the original cancellous framework of the bone, hyaline cartilage that clearly shows the nodular and lobular formation generally typical of tumor cartilage. The regions of lobular cartilage *(1)* vary both in size and cell density. These are proliferation buds which are separated from one another by connective tissue septa or regions of bone *(2)*. These connective tissue septa contain only a few occasionally dilated blood vessels with delicate walls *(3)*. The tumor is only poorly vascularized and is forming no new vessels or arteriovenous shunts, which is why no diseased vessels appear in the angiogram. In the outer zones of an enchondroma one often observes osteosclerotically widened trabeculae *(4)*, or a cortex that has similarly increased in density and which will show up radiologically. This is a reactive osteosclerosis, suggesting slow and usually benign tumor growth.

Under **higher magnification** (**Fig. 402**) one can recognize that the lobular formation of the tumor is also to be found within the areas of hyaline cartilage. Again and again one observes proliferation buds *(1)* in which the chondrocytes are smaller and more closely packed. The nuclei of these cartilage cells appear to be pyknotic and elongated, and have a dense chromatin content. These are mononuclear cartilage cells with poorly defined borders. Nearby one can recognize chondrocytes *(2)* lying close together in groups in the cartilaginous tissue in enlarged chondroblastic capsules. Double nucleated lacunae are present, but only occasionally. No mitoses can be seen in the chondrocytes. A basophilic cartilaginous framework *(3)*, which with greater degeneration may in parts become eosinophilic, surrounds groups of distended cartilage cells with roundish isomorphic nuclei. Isolated spaces resembling blood vessels can be seen *(4)*. It should be noted that the cell density within the tumor varies, and this must not be used as a criterion for judging the degree of malignancy. Enchondromas of the short bones of the foot in particular are often highly cellular, whereas chondrosarcomas can be poor in cell content. Especially at the periphery of the lobes one often finds groups of greatly distended chondrocytes which nevertheless contain only one monomorphic nucleus.

In **Fig. 403** one can see under **higher magnification** the peripheral regions of the lobes of two proliferation buds *(1)*. They are separated from each other by loose connective tissue *(2)*. Inside, there are isomorphic fibrocytes with isomorphic nuclei. There is no sarcomatous stroma and few blood vessels are found within the intervening connective tissue. The nodular cartilaginous foci have fairly sharp borders. Inside there are numerous isomorphic chondrocytes with roundish or elongated nuclei which have a dense chromatin content. They are lying in cell nests of varying width. Only very occasionally are two nuclei seen within one cell nest *(3)*. The basic framework is basophilic; it can, however, sometimes show a myxoid porosity or eosinophilic degeneration, which offers no clue to the degree of malignancy. Mitoses are practically never seen in benign enchondromas. Such a tranquil picture allows one – always taking into account the site and the radiological findings – to diagnose a benign enchondroma.

Foci of calcification are frequently encountered in enchondromas, and these appear in the radiograph as more or less well-marked shadows. One can see such a focus in an enchondroma in **Fig. 404** *(1)*. In the histological section these foci are mostly very ragged. The calcium deposits are found in clumps or dark, spear-like deposits. Kossa staining is not necessary to show up the calcium salts. Focal deposits of calcium are characteristic of all cartilaginous neoplasms. The surrounding tumorous tissue remains unreactive *(2)*. There is a dystrophic calcification.

It can be extremely difficult to distinguish between benign and malignant cartilaginous neoplasms from a histological section alone, and serial sections of a single region of cartilage must be precisely analyzed. Large chondrocytes with large dark nuclei and giant cells do not belong to a benign chondroma. One must also remember that a secondary malignant change within a chondroma that is at first benign can appear in certain sections of the tumor without involving the whole of it.

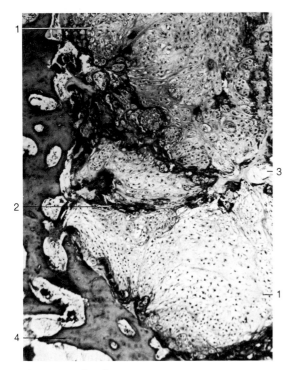

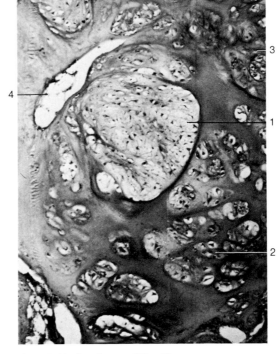

Fig. 401. Enchondroma; HE, ×10

Fig. 402. Enchondroma; HE, ×25

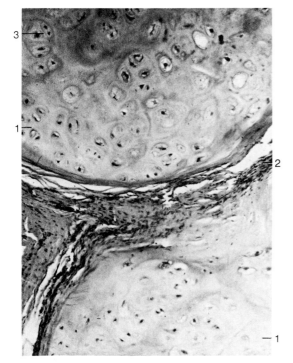

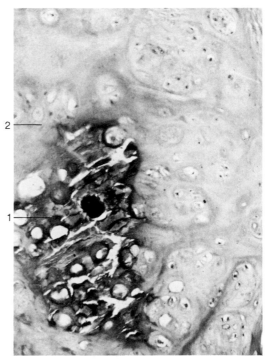

Fig. 403. Enchondroma; HE, ×40

Fig. 404. Enchondroma; HE, ×40

Periosteal (Juxtacortical) Chondroma (ICD-O-DA-M-9221/0)

Benign cartilaginous neoplasms can also develop outside bone itself, and especially in the periosteal connective tissue. These are the so-called juxtacortical or periosteal chondromas. They can erode the underlying cortex without actually breaking into the marrow cavity. Such tumors are much less common than the central enchondromas. They are mostly found in the short tubular bones of the hand or foot, more rarely in the long bones or ribs. They have no topographical relationship to the cartilaginous epiphyseal plate, since the cartilaginous proliferation comes from the periosteum. In this way growth can continue even after the skeleton is mature. This does not indicate malignancy.

In the **radiograph** of **Fig. 405** one can see a periosteal enchondroma of the intermediate phalanx of the left index finger *(1)*. One sees a large swelling of the soft tissues in which patchy calcification foci *(2)* are deposited. These changes reach out to cross the neighboring joint *(3)*. The short tubular bones of the middle and proximal phalanges have been eroded from outside *(4)*, but they show no radiological changes within. The adjacent bone erosion can lead to changes in the intraosseous structure, with straggly regions of increased density. The radiological findings, however, do show that the actual pathological process is confined to the periosteum, and that the bony changes are only reactive in nature. Even increase in activity shown on the scintigram does not allow one to assume an intraosseous process here.

The **histological picture** of this tumor is very similar to that of a central chondroma. In **Fig. 406** one can recognize the lobular formation typical of a cartilaginous neoplasm. There is often no connective tissue laid down between the nodular areas of cartilage *(1)*. There are generally more cells than in a central chondroma. The chondrocytes show greater pleomorphy and their nuclei are more hyperchromatic. More cells with two nuclei are present *(2)*. This suggests a certain tendency towards proliferation, without actually indicating malignancy. Clinically, these periosteal chondromas are painful (periosteal pain).

Proliferating Chondroma

When assessing the diagnosis of cartilaginous neoplasms, one is always coming across tumors that, because of their localization, should be evaluated as potentially malignant, and the chondrocytes of which show a certain degree of nuclear polymorphy in histological sections. UEHLINGER has described these neoplasms as "proliferating chondromas" and placed them among the semimalignant tumors. This applies particularly to large chondromas of the pelvis, femoral neck, proximal humeral metaphysis and vertebral column, which may well be chondrosarcomas. These include the multiple osteocartilaginous exostoses (p. 62) and the multiple enchondromas of Ollier's disease (p. 60). In *Ollier's disease* the enchondromas usually appear on one side of the skeleton (in the metaphyses and diaphyses of various bones). They are neither inherited nor familial. In 50% of cases a chondrosarcoma develops. The simultaneous appearance of multiple enchondromas and hemangiomas constitutes *Maffucci's syndrome.*

In the **radiograph** of **Fig. 407** one can see a large chondroma that has involved the left femoral neck *(1)* and trochanteric plane *(2)*. The cortex has been penetrated and the tumor is spreading out into the soft parts *(3)*, and the outer contour is nodular and poorly defined. The tumor is patchy, with dark areas, and shows regions of increased density interspersed with translucent areas.

In the **histological section** (**Fig. 408**) one can see the typical lobular formation of a chondroma with the clear borders shown by such cartilaginous nodules *(1)*. The individual lobes vary in their tissue maturity, so that quiescent regions with a copious chondroid background and loosely distributed isomorphic chondrocytes alternate with other regions showing increased polymorphy of cells and nuclei *(2)* and a sparse chondromyxomatous intermediate tissue. These changes, together with the disposition of the cartilage cells to form rows, chains and cell nests, are histologically an indication of a certain tendency to proliferate. This semimalignant type of growth is to some extent confirmed by its locally destructive quality and the increased likelihood of recurrence.

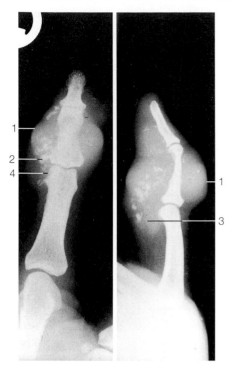

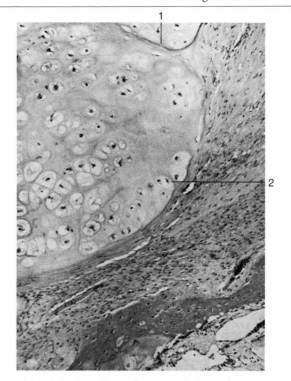

Fig. 405. Periosteal chondroma (left index finger)

Fig. 406. Periosteal chondroma; HE, ×25

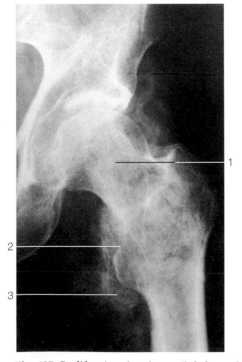

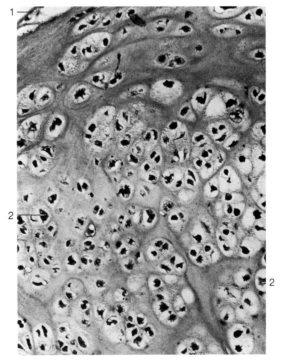

Fig. 407. Proliferating chondroma (left femoral neck)

Fig. 408. Proliferating chondroma; HE, ×64

Chondroblastoma ("Codman's Tumor") (ICD-O-DA-M-9230/0)

The chondroblastoma is a rare benign tumor of cartilage, making up less than 1% of all bone neoplasms. *It is normally a benign primary cartilaginous neoplasm consisting of foci with polygonal chondroblasts and deposited osteoclastic multinucleated giant cells, which arises in the epiphyses.* Men are more usually (60%) affected than women. In the majority of cases the first symptom is pain, and the tumor may have been present for some time (up to two years) before it is discovered. The pain is often projected to a neighboring joint. Swelling is mostly not very noticeable, since chondroblastomas are usually small. Because of the peripheral site of the tumor a pathological fracture is uncommon.

Localization (Fig. 409). A chondroblastoma usually arises in a long bone, more rarely it has been described in the axial skeleton (pelvis, spinal column, ribs, sternum) and in the bones of the skull. The tumor almost always attacks an epiphysis and can spread into the adjacent metaphysis. Chondroblastomas outside the region of the epiphysis are unusual and extremely difficult to evaluate.

Age Distribution (Fig. 410). This tumor is most often encountered in young people, one third appearing in the 2nd decade of life. As shown in **Fig. 410**, however, a chondroblastoma can also be observed in extreme old age, and also in early childhood.

On radiological examination the predilection of the tumor for an epiphysis is striking, and it usually involves extensive destruction of the region of the bone affected. **Figure 411** is a **radiograph** showing a chondroblastoma of the proximal humeral epiphysis. In the humeral head one can recognize a somewhat eccentrically displaced osteolytic cyst, which has slightly elevated this region of the bone. The roundish osteolytic zone is in part sharply divided from the neighboring tissue by a narrow band of marginal sclerosis *(1)* which is in places absent *(2)*. The cortex *(3)* is greatly narrowed, but fully intact. Within the "bony cyst" there is an irregular increase in the density of the trabecu-

lae *(4)*, which can give the tumor a multicystic appearance. In a chondroblastoma such as this, patchy foci of calcification can be seen in the radiograph. These are, however, never so pronounced as in a calcifying enchondroma of the long bones. If the narrowing of the cortex is very far advanced a slight bony periosteal reaction can arise, but this is rare. Invasion of the neighboring joint is more likely. With such changes one must not conclude that the growth is malignant. From the point of view of differential diagnosis, a chondroblastoma must be distinguished from an osteoclastoma (p. 337). At a similar site, the reactive osteosclerotic changes and calcium shadows of a chondroblastoma would be unusual in an osteoclastoma.

Chondroblastomas are usually curetted, so that the pathologist only receives tissue fragments. Sometimes, however, the tumor is excised as a block and sent in accordingly. The **macroscopic picture** of a chondroblastoma of the proximal humeral epiphysis (as it appears in the radiograph of Fig. 411) can be seen in **Fig. 412**. One can recognize a fairly sharply delineated tumor lying somewhat eccentrically in the epiphysis. The suggestion of its lobular formation is unmistakable. The actual tissue of the tumor *(1)* has a grayish-blue, partly yellowish and slightly shining cut surface of a tough elastic consistency. The greater part of it is set through with hemorrhages *(2)*. In a few places there are tiny deposits of calcium *(3)*, and foci of cystic degeneration *(4)* are also to be seen. The tumor also shows an incomplete band of sclerosis which varies in width *(5)*. In one place *(6)* the cortex has been penetrated by tissue from the tumor, and here one can see a marked periosteal reaction. The advanced local destruction of the bone tissue and occasional penetration of the cortex are not be taken as signs of malignancy.

The growth of a chondroblastoma is usually slow and not very aggressive. There are, however, cases in which very severe destruction is seen on the radiograph. Nevertheless, after bioptic examination a radical operation is found to be unnecessary. Generally speaking a thorough curettage suffices to bring about healing of the tumor. Recurrence is rare, and radiotherapy is not indicated.

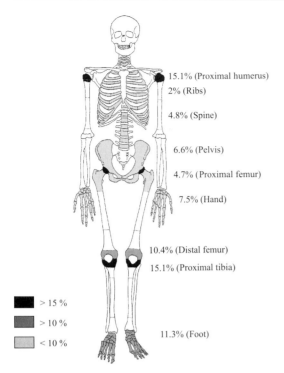

15.1% (Proximal humerus)

2% (Ribs)

4.8% (Spine)

6.6% (Pelvis)

4.7% (Proximal femur)

7.5% (Hand)

10.4% (Distal femur)

15.1% (Proximal tibia)

11.3% (Foot)

■ > 15 %

■ > 10 %

□ < 10 %

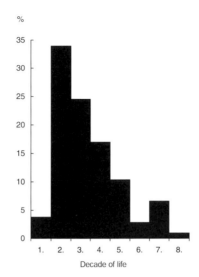

Fig. 409. Localization of chondroblastomas (106 cases); others: 22.5%

Fig. 410. Age distribution of chondroblastomas (106 cases)

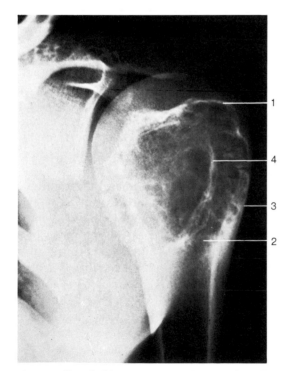

Fig. 411. Chondroblastoma (proximal humeral epiphysis)

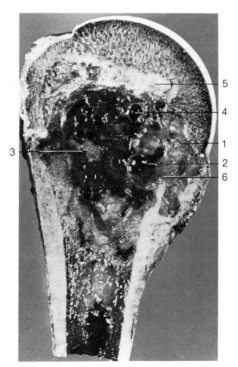

Fig. 412. Chondroblastoma (cut surface, proximal humeral epiphysis)

In the **radiograph** of **Fig. 413** one can recognize a classical chondroblastoma of the left femoral neck. This tumor also started in the proximal femoral epiphysis *(1)*, but has extended well into the femoral neck, where it is sharply separated from the normal bone by a fine region of sclerosis *(2)*. In this case the entire diameter of the bone has been taken up by the tumor. The cortex *(3)* is severely narrowed, but complete. There is no recognizable periosteal reaction. The effect of the tumor has mostly been to bring about local osteolysis, without the bone having become expanded. Its outer contour is mostly normal, and inside the osteolytic zone one can see only discrete straggly and patchy shadowing.

In the **overall histological picture** (**Fig. 414**) one recognizes very highly cellular neoplastic tissue, with unequally sized roundish nodular and lobular areas of chondroid tissue *(1)*. This illustrates the lobular formation of the tumor that is characteristic for all cartilaginous neoplasms. These chondroid foci have fairly sharply defined borders, and peripherally one can recognize within them varying numbers of giant cells. Between the islets of cartilage there is a highly cellular stroma *(2)* containing only a few blood vessels. The focal deposits of calcium within the tumor tissue are very characteristic of a chondroblastoma. Near these calcified areas necroses are only seldom encountered, but sometimes there is reactive osteoid formation here.

Under **higher magnification** (**Fig. 415**) there are essentially two different tissue structures to distinguish. On one side there is a large region of chondroid *(1)*, and nearby one can see highly cellular granulation tissue *(2)*. Here and near to the border a large number of multinucleated giant cells can be observed *(3)*. The irregularly distributed cells within the chondroid field may be described as chondroblasts. These cells are roundish or polygonal and have oval or round nuclei. In highly cellular regions spindle-shaped cells may be present. The nuclei are often hyperchromatic and have one or two nucleoli. Mitoses are likewise present, and the nuclei have multiple notches. A very important diagnostic feature is the strikingly sharp border formed by the outer cell membrane, although this is not always visible. The dark nuclei are mostly surrounded by a light halo, closely resembling the cell nests of chondrocytes. Between these chondroblasts there is a chondroid matrix that is usually basophilic, but occasionally eosinophilic. It is here that foci of mucoid degeneration or large foci of calcification may appear. The peculiarity of the histological structure of this neoplasm is the presence of numerous multinucleated giant cells that can lead to it being confused with an osteoclastoma. On the one hand, there are small multinucleated giant cells in close relationship to the field of chondroblasts *(3)*, on the other hand, there are large multinucleated giant cells among hemorrhages and blood sinuses. In this way both tumor giant cells and multinucleated macrophages may be encountered. In the regions of stroma between the chondroid fields *(2)* there are many spindle-shaped cells with isomorphic drawn-out nuclei. Here also hyperchromatic and polymorphic nuclei may be seen, as well as single mitoses, and multinucleated giant cells are scattered about. This agitation of the cellular picture must not be equated with malignant neoplastic growth. The relationship between the chondroid foci and the highly cellular stroma varies in individual chondroblastomas. In a bone biopsy the stroma may predominate throughout, which can make the diagnosis a great deal more difficult. This means that the analysis of a chondroblastoma requires examination of the most highly cellular parts of the tumor, and the taking into account of every available radiograph.

In 17% of chondroblastomas the additional components of an aneurysmal bony cyst (p. 412) can be demonstrated. In **Fig. 416** these structures *(1)* are visible, as well as those of a chondroblastoma *(2)*. This is due to reactive change, which must be taken into account when judging the radiograph and the bone biopsy. A bone biopsy from a osteolytic bone lesion may contain nothing but the tissue of an aneurysmal bony cyst. However, whereas aneurysmal bony cysts lie at the metaphysis, a chondroblastoma is a lesion of the epiphysis.

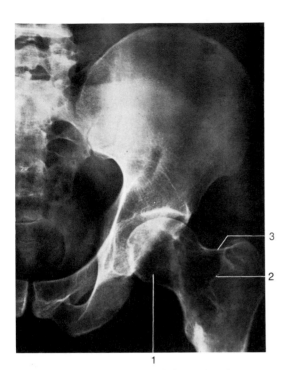

Fig. 413. Chondroblastoma (left femoral neck)

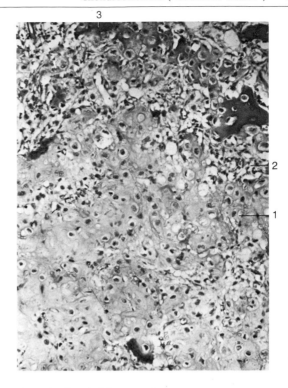

Fig. 414. Chondroblastoma; HE, ×30

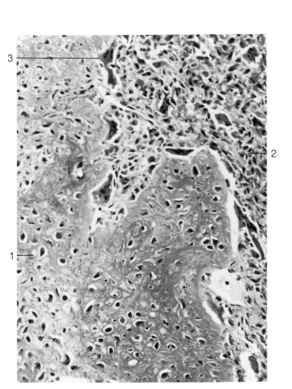

Fig. 415. Chondroblastoma; HE, ×64

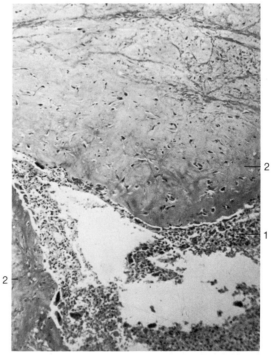

Fig. 416. Chondroblastoma with aneurysmal bony cyst; HE, ×40

Chondromyxoid Fibroma (ICD-O-DA-M-9241/0)

This is a very rare neoplasm of bone which makes up just 0.5% of all bone tumors. *The chondromyxoid fibroma represents a circumscribed benign neoplasm which is composed partly of chondroid and partly of myxoid tissue, and which is sometimes capable of local invasive growth.* This tumor was originally regarded as a chondrosarcoma, since the tissue shows highly immature tumor cells. Today it is classified as semimalignant, since it does display destructive local growth and has a definite tendency to recur, but it does not produce metastases. The presenting symptom is a dragging pain, and sometimes a local swelling may appear. Chondromyxoid fibromas can also be discovered by chance in the course of a routine radiological examination.

Localization (Fig. 417). Typical chondromyxoid fibromas are found in the metaphyses, with the most common site being the proximal metaphyses of the long bones of the lower limb, particularly the tibia. Occasionally they appear in the ulna, radius, scapula, sternum, calcaneus, phalanges of the fingers and toes, vertebrae, ribs or pelvis. We found 16% of these tumors in the short tubular bones, whereas all investigators have recorded their presence in the long bones in two thirds of cases. Sometimes both the metaphysis and epiphysis are taken up by the tumor.

Age Distribution (Fig. 418). The most likely time for the condition to arise is, according to the literature, during the 2nd and 3rd decades of life, the average age given being 23 years. In a sample of 80 chondromyxoid fibromas we found a second peak in the 6th decade, with a significantly greater number in women. In other words, it may be accepted that this rare bone neoplasm can appear at any age.

The radiograph of a chondromyxoid fibroma of a long bone shows – according to its projection – a central ovoid metaphyseal cyst, which is attached by its base to the epiphyseal cartilage and sends a pointed projection toward the diaphysis. The sharply bordered eccentric region of osteolysis which can lead to elevation of the bone is characteristic. In **Fig. 419** one can see a chondromyxoid fibroma of the right tibial head that shows up as an eccentrically placed ovoid bony cyst. It is clearly delineated by a narrow band of marginal sclerosis *(1)*. The internal contours of the neoplastic defect are smooth, and usually there is no internal trabecular structure. Areas of calcification or ossification capable of casting shadows are not seen. These characteristics give the chondromyxoid fibroma a very typical radiological appearance. The tumor is situated in the tibial metaphysis, but has crossed the epiphyseal line and has partly invaded the epiphysis *(2)*. The immediately adjacent cortex is partly narrowed and partly widened by reactive osteosclerosis. It remains, however, fully intact and no periosteal reaction can be seen. This is in general a radiological picture which suggests a benign lesion. In considering the differential diagnosis, it is particularly a chondrosarcoma (p. 236) which must be considered and excluded. Chondromyxoid fibromas of the short and flat bones usually involve the whole of the diameter and bring about a nodular elevation with trabecular inclusions.

In **Fig. 420** one can see the **radiograph** of a chondromyxoid fibroma of the proximal tibial metaphysis which is lying in a highly eccentric position. It appears to show a periosteal process which has led to an erosion of the cortex *(1)* from without. The suggestion of peripheral lobulation and marginal sclerosis is not pronounced, and in this exposure one cannot distinguish between the tumor and the surrounding soft parts. Such a chondromyxoid fibroma as this, with an extraosseous component, is not typical. They are, however, sometimes seen and have been described in the literature. The character of such a tumorous bone lesion can only be established by a bone biopsy. An eccentric localization practically always appears on the radiograph as an hourglass bulge of the cortex, which is paper thin and sometimes hardly still visible. It is often shaped like a grape. There is usually no periosteal reaction. Untreated chondromyxofibromas may penetrate the cortex and bring about pressure erosion of the neighboring bone. In the short tubular bones, a spindle-shaped elevation is typical.

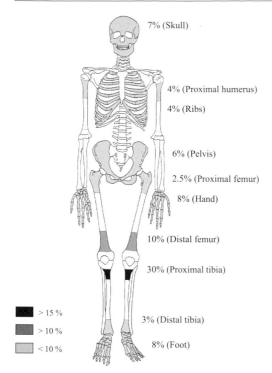

7% (Skull)

4% (Proximal humerus)

4% (Ribs)

6% (Pelvis)

2.5% (Proximal femur)

8% (Hand)

10% (Distal femur)

30% (Proximal tibia)

3% (Distal tibia)

8% (Foot)

■ > 15 %
▨ > 10 %
▢ < 10 %

Fig. 417. Localization of chondromyxoid fibroma (80 cases); others: 17.5%

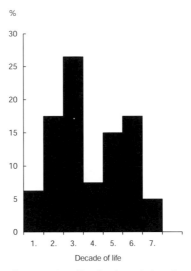

Fig. 418. Age distribution of chondromyxoid fibromas (80 cases)

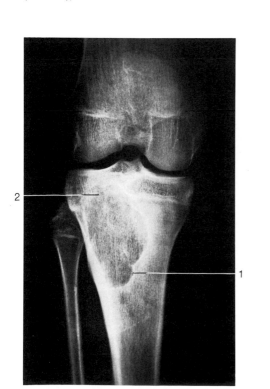

Fig. 419. Chondromyxoid fibroma (right tibial head)

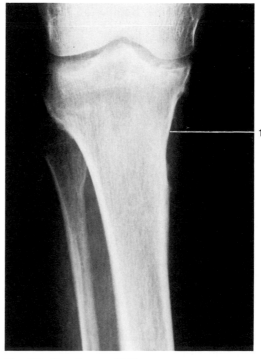

Fig. 420. Chondromyxoid fibroma (proximal tibial metaphysis)

The **radiograph** of **Fig. 421** shows a chondromyxoid fibroma of the 1st right metatarsal *(1)*. The affected proximal part of the bone is raised up all round to give it a spindle-like appearance, and the cortex on both sides is severely narrowed from within, but still intact. Distally, the tumor is sharply bordered by marginal sclerosis *(2)*. Within, there is diffuse shadowing with small patchy areas of translucency. No calcium inclusions can be seen. The tumor lies in the proximal metaphysis and appears to have penetrated the epiphyseal plate *(3)* and invaded the epiphysis itself.

A very typical **radiological picture** of a chondromyxoid fibroma can be seen in **Fig. 422**. In the left distal femoral metaphysis one can see a strikingly eccentrically situated cystic lesion *(1)*, which is sharply bordered on the inside by a marked area of garland-shaped marginal sclerosis *(2)*. The cortex is greatly narrowed and notched from without *(3)*. Inside the lesion there are a few dense trabeculae, but no patchy shadows of calcification. The eccentric position and the cyst-like appearance of the neoplasm are clearly seen in the **lateral radiograph** of **Fig. 423**. A narrow region of marginal sclerosis *(1)* sharply defines the outline of the lesion. The whole tumorous region is bulging dorsally and outwards *(2)*, and is here polycystic. Within, the increase in density of the trabeculae has given the lesion a grape-like appearance, and this can be seen in about 40% of chondromyxoid fibromas. This is in general the radiological appearance of a benign lesion.

Figure 424 is a **radiograph** of a chondromyxoid fibroma of the distal part of the humerus. Once again there is a sharply bordered "bony cyst" *(1)* lying in the bone. The cortex is irregularly narrowed from within *(2)* but still intact. This part of the bone is slightly raised up. There is no periosteal reaction. Inside, there is a diffuse increase in density, but there are no calcification shadows. Penetration of the cortex is not a feature of an uncomplicated chondromyxoid fibroma. In these tumors an aneurysmal bony cyst (p. 412) sometimes develops as a secondary phenomenon and can penetrate the cortex on one side. In the radiograph this may easily awake suspicion of malignancy, a problem which must be resolved by bone biopsy.

Histologically the lobulated formation of the tumor tissue in these cartilaginous neoplasms is characteristic. In **Fig. 425** one can see a large porous myxomatous area *(1)* in which cells with ill-defined boundaries and bizarre nuclei lie loosely bound together. The nuclei are in part drawn out into a spindle shape *(2)*, in part roundish and uneven *(3)*. They vary in size and contain much chromatin. No mitoses are seen. Adjacent to the cartilaginous lobules there is a highly cellular connective tissue stroma *(4)* with fibrocytes, fibroblasts and lymphoid cells. Many blood vessels *(5)* can be seen within it. The sometimes considerable polymorphy and hyperchromasia of the nuclei seen inside the myxomatous area must not be regarded as indicating the presence of a malignant neoplasm (e.g. a chondrosarcoma, p. 236). In general the tumor presents a very characteristic histological picture, and with the help of the radiological findings the correct diagnosis is usually made. There are, however, also cases with an atypical histological appearance in which the pattern of a chondroblastoma (p. 226) or an aneurysmal bony cyst (p. 412) predominates in the biopsy material, or which give the impression of a myxosarcoma. Regressive changes of the tumor tissue with hyalinization can also cause diagnostic difficulties.

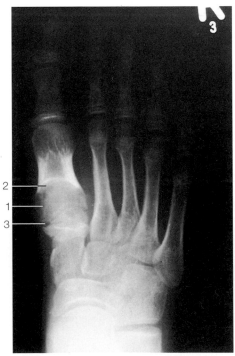

Fig. 421. Chondromyxoid fibroma (1st right metatarsal)

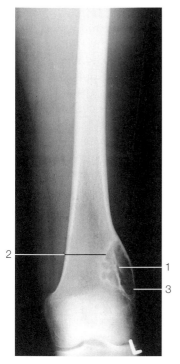

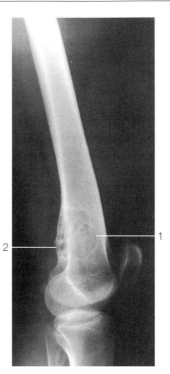

Fig. 422. Chondromyxoid fibroma
(left distal femoral metaphysis, a.p. radiograph)

Fig. 423. Chondromyxoid fibroma
(left distal femoral metaphysis, lateral radiograph)

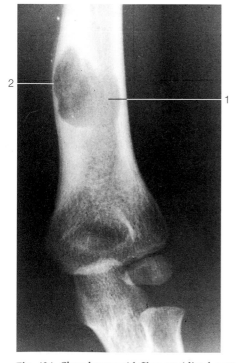

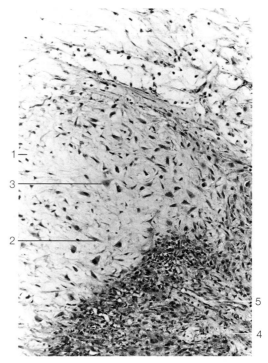

Fig. 424. Chondromyxoid fibroma (distal part of humerus)

Fig. 425. Chondromyxoid fibroma; HE, ×82

With a chondromyxoid fibroma it can be difficult histologically to decide between benign and malignant growth. As is apparent in the **overall histological view** shown in **Fig. 426**, the picture is that of a very clearly defined lobular formation with roundish nodules of varying size *(1)*. It is characterized by the mixture of highly cellular immature areas *(2)* with differentiated myxomatous and chondroid regions *(3)*. The histological structures seen within one chondromyxoid fibroma can differ greatly, and can also vary markedly from tumor to tumor. The myxomatous, fibrous and chondroid zones and areas may show very different degrees of emphasis; the chondroid elements can sometimes only appear in small foci, but can sometimes also determine the histological picture and lead to confusion with a chondrosarcoma.

Even under **higher magnification (Fig. 427)** the lobular and nodular formation of the neoplasm is obvious. The lobular centers of the chondroid areas *(1)* consist of a loose wide-meshed network of bipolar spindle-shaped or multipolar star-shaped cells which are thickly concentrated at the periphery of the lobules. This dense, mantle-like cramming together of the tumor cells around the edges of the lobules and nodules is an important histological characteristic of the chondromyxoid fibroma. All the same, this kind of distribution of the tumor cells can sometimes be found in a chondrosarcoma, which must be borne in mind when a diagnosis is being made. Even with **moderate enlargement (Fig. 427)** one can recognize that the densely packed tumor cells have a pale cytoplasm and a rather sharp cell membrane, and therefore resemble the cartilage cells of a chondroblastoma (p. 229). The matrix of the chondroid regions is partly mucoid, partly chondroid. In the myxomatous regions the intercellular substance is generally PAS negative, since the proteoglycans have probably been replaced by water. Between the chondroid nodules there are dense regions of stroma *(2)* consisting of spindle cells and several vascular loops *(3)*. If the vascularization is more pronounced, the impression of an aneurysmal bony cyst (p. 412) may arise. The spindle cells have isomorphic nuclei. Mitoses are very rare. Sometimes osteoid or fibro-osseous tissue may differentiate within the interlobular stroma. In a few places collections of round lymphoid cells *(4)* can be observed.

Under **higher magnification (Fig. 428)** it is clear that the nodular chondroid areas are fairly sharply delineated *(1)*. Within the nodules there is a loose network of chondroid cells which now and then reveal multipolar cell borders with cytoplasmic processes. The nuclei are sometimes slightly elliptical, sometimes elongated. They are mostly small and stain intensely, and are often pyknotic. There is no striking nuclear polymorphy, and mitoses are not seen. The interstitial tissue is sometimes porous, with myxomatous foci *(2)*, so that this region is PAS negative. Alcian blue staining is here mostly positive. Between the lobules there is a band of loose stroma with spindle cells *(3)* within which one can recognize blood vessels, and in one place fibrous bone *(4)* has differentiated. Numerous multinucleated giant cells are often found in the interstitial tissue in the immediate neighborhood of the chondroid lobules. During the course of maturation of a chondromyxoid fibroma the matrix and collagen fibers undergo an increase. In the periphery of the tumor the tissue is sometimes sharply separated from the bone by a connective tissue capsule. During the slow growth of the neoplasm reactive bone formation is often seen. This is responsible for the marginal sclerosis and is usually visible in the radiograph (Fig. 419).

In **Fig. 429** one can see under **higher magnification** a section through a chondroid focus within a chondromyxoid fibroma. The pronounced myxoid loosening of the tissue *(1)* is striking. The tumor cells have nuclei which are sometimes roundish, sometimes elongated, and an eosinophilic cytoplasm. In one place one can recognize a multinucleated giant cell *(2)*. It can be extraordinarily difficult to classify a chondromyxoid fibroma precisely from the radiological and histological appearance. Mixed forms of chondromyxoid fibromas, chondroblastomas and chondromatous giant cell neoplasms have been described. Sometimes the tumor can penetrate into the marrow cavity far beyond the radiologically identifiable borders. Within the tissue of the tumor, calcification foci are only sparsely encountered. In addition to collagen fibers, the presence of numerous reticular fibers can be histochemically established.

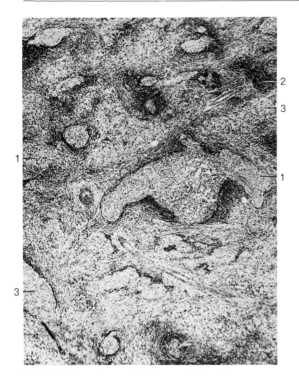

Fig. 426. Chondromyxoid fibroma; HE, ×20

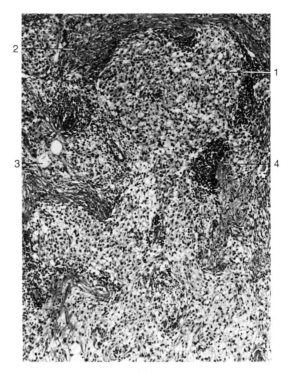

Fig. 427. Chondromyxoid fibroma; HE, ×40

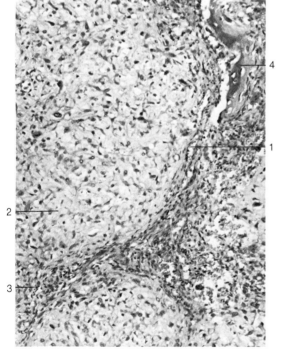

Fig. 428. Chondromyxoid fibroma; HE, ×64

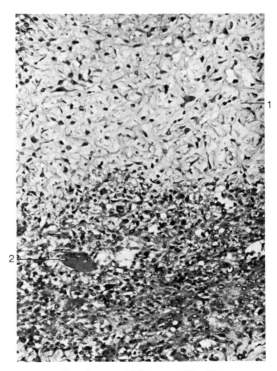

Fig. 429. Chondromyxoid fibroma; HE, ×82

Chondrosarcoma (ICD-O-DA-M-9220/3)

The chondrosarcoma is a malignant bone tumor which originates from the cartilaginous tissue of the skeleton and which is composed of abnormal cartilage and a little connective tissue. This malignant form of cartilaginous neoplasm can develop spontaneously from local cartilage (**primary chondrosarcoma**) or from a cartilaginous neoplasm that was previously benign (**secondary chondrosarcoma**). It is a slow-growing tumor, which is why the patient usually presents with a long history in which the only symptoms are often only pain and local swelling. Because of the non-specific symptomatology, chondrosarcomas are often wrongly treated for a long time and diagnosed late. This neoplasm has a tendency to invade blood vessels and to form long intravascular tentacles. Metastases appear late and are most likely to attack the lung. Involvement of the regional lymph nodes is rare. After incomplete removal of the tumor there is a strong likelihood of recurrence. Even with a tumor biopsy metastases can be implanted in the path of its removal.

Localization (Fig. 430). Most primary chondrosarcomas develop in the center of the epiphysis of a long bone and spread out into the metaphysis. The main site is the axial skeleton, including the shoulder girdle, proximal regions of the femur or humerus (44.3%), the pelvis being most often affected (14.2%). These neoplasms are also relatively often found in the ribs or proximal part of the femur. A further common site is around the knee, but only rarely are they encountered in the short tubular bones of the hand or foot. It is remarkable that the proximal ends of the long bones are much more frequently attacked than the distal ends. In rare cases a chondrosarcoma can develop outside the skeleton (in the soft tissue, larynx, joint capsules etc.).

Age Distribution (Fig. 431). Chondrosarcomas appear at any age with equal probability, the average being 46 years. In children and young people they are relatively less common. As against this, secondary chondrosarcomas are found more frequently in the young than the old. We found a peak in the 6th decade of life. Men are somewhat more frequently affected than women.

Among all bone tumors the chondrosarcoma, at 16%, comes third after the plasmocytoma and the osteosarcoma. Its prognosis is significantly better than that of the osteosarcoma. The five-year survival period is reported as being between 21%–76%, the degree of differentiation being an important factor. Adequate treatment involves complete removal of the tumor, either by block resection, amputation or disarticulation. Radiotherapy is ineffective and therefore not indicated, and chemotherapy has so far also been unsuccessful.

In the **radiograph** the majority of chondrosarcomas show evidence of malignant growth. With a central chondrosarcoma the most impressive feature is a moth-eaten osteolysis, and lumpy neoplastic nodes grow quickly through the borders of the bone. **Figure 432** depicts a chondrosarcoma of the proximal metaphysis of the right humerus in a 13-year-old boy. The entire region of the bone is taken up by dark, cloudy shadows, which are not clearly separated from the shaft *(1)*. The tumor appears to have broken through the epiphyseal cartilage and invaded the epiphysis *(2)*. It has also penetrated the cortex and produced a bony periosteal reaction in the form of so-called *spicules (3)*. A clear tumorous shadow can be seen in the soft tissues *(4)*. In the peripheral region of the tumor a so-called *Codman's triangle (5)* is visible, which is highly characteristic of expansively growing malignant bone tumors. It consists of a region of reactive new bone formation in which no tumor tissue is present. A biopsy in this region would therefore be useless.

The **macroscopic picture** of the cut surface of this tumor (**Fig. 433**) shows that the entire bone is occupied by nodular, glassy tumor tissue, which is set through with necroses and hemorrhages *(1)*. A large area of the cortex *(2)* has been destroyed, and large tumorous nodes are jutting out extensively into surrounding regions *(3)*. The tumor has sent an intraosseous process into the diaphysis *(4)*. In one place a Codman's triangle *(5)* can be seen. This chondrosarcoma has thus destroyed the whole proximal part of the humerus, so that a pathological fracture could arise here very easily.

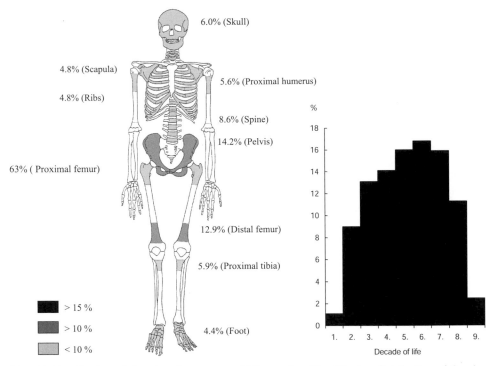

6.0% (Skull)
4.8% (Scapula)
5.6% (Proximal humerus)
4.8% (Ribs)
8.6% (Spine)
14.2% (Pelvis)
63% (Proximal femur)
12.9% (Distal femur)
5.9% (Proximal tibia)
> 15 %
> 10 %
< 10 %
4.4% (Foot)

Fig. 430. Localization of the chondrosarcomas (558 cases); others 26.5%

%
18
16
14
12
10
8
6
4
2
0
1. 2. 3. 4. 5. 6. 7. 8. 9.
Decade of life

Fig. 431. Age distribution of the chondrosarcomas (558 cases)

2
3
4
5
1

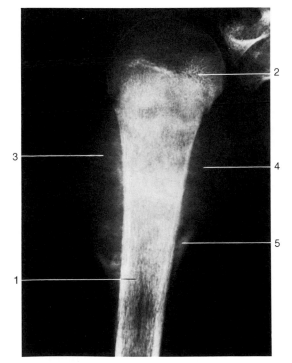

Fig. 432. Chondrosarcoma (proximal humerus)

1
2
3
1
5
4

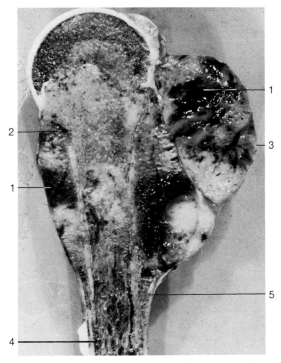

Fig. 433. Chondrosarcoma (cut surface, proximal humerus)

Figure 434 shows the **radiograph** of a chondrosarcoma in the right distal femoral metaphysis of a 57-year-old woman. In the lateral exposure one can recognize very dark shadowing of the whole of the metaphysis which reaches out into the epiphysis. The peripheral part of the epiphysis *(1)* is free from neoplastic tissue, and there is no sign that the tumor has invaded the nearby knee joint *(2)*. In children malignant bone tumors do not break through the epiphyseal cartilage until an advanced stage, and only force their way late into the neighboring joint. The cortex of the femur has been invaded by the tumor and cannot be distinguished from the marrow cavity. It has already infiltrated the adjacent soft parts, as can be recognized by the dense shadow it projects *(3)*. The tumorous bony reaction of the periosteum is clearly seen in the form of the dense periosteal layers *(4)* and spicules *(5)*. In one place *(6)* a Codman's triangle can be seen.

The **macroscopic appearance** of such a central chondrosarcoma in the distal femoral epiphysis is to be seen in **Fig. 435**. On the sawn surface of the distal part of the femur one can see the glassy gray shining tissue of the tumor, which is lying in the center of the bone and taking up the entire marrow cavity. Most of it is set through with hemorrhages *(1)* and in places one can see patchy calcification *(2)*. The tumor has pushed its way distally into the epiphysis *(3)*, but the cartilaginous joint surface *(4)* is completely intact. Proximally it reaches out a long way into the diaphysis *(5)*, and here the characteristic lobular formation of a chondrosarcoma is apparent. The cortex is partly eroded from within, and partly thickened. In one place *(6)* one can clearly see how the tumor has penetrated into the periosteum. Nearby a Codman's triangle *(7)* is recognizable. On the whole the periosteum is considerably thickened by reactive new bone formation. This appearance of the cut surface of a central chondrosarcoma and the elastic but firm consistency of the tumor tissue are quite characteristic of this neoplasm.

The **radiograph** of **Fig. 436** shows a chondrosarcoma in the ala of the right iliac bone in a 58-year-old woman, One can see an irregular sclerotic increase in density that reaches right into the true pelvis *(1)*. The original border of the bone has in this case, however, not been penetrated. Nevertheless, the opposite side of the zone of sclerosis is not sharply defined. One recognizes patchy areas with irregular translucent foci of destruction in the periphery of the tumor which extend up to the border of the ala *(2)*. There is no evidence that the tumor has invaded the soft tissues. The joint space of the right hip joint *(3)* is completely preserved, and one cannot detect any invasion of the joint by the tumor. With radiological findings such as these, additional special exposures (lateral radiograph, tomograph, angiograph etc.) should be undertaken in order to obtain further information about the size and extent of the tumor. Furthermore, one should these days also employ computer and MR-tomography, since these can supply additional useful diagnostic information. Determining the degree of density and the signal changes can thereby help to assess the amount of calcification and ossification in such a neoplasm. The final diagnosis is then made possible by a planned biopsy and histological examination of the tissue itself.

Figure 437 shows a **maceration specimen** of the pelvis in which a large, deeply fissured tumor *(1)* of the left iliac bone can be seen, which has involved the ischium. This is a chondrosarcoma which probably arose in an osteocartilaginous exostosis. The tumor tissue was heavily calcified and has therefore survived maceration. The neoplasm has broken a long way through the edges of the bone and a large part of it has pushed its way far into the surrounding soft tissues. One can clearly recognize the nodular and lumpy formation of the tumor, which has brought about extensive destruction of the pelvic bone.

Without doubt the chondrosarcoma belongs among those bone tumors which are extremely difficult to diagnose histologically. If the radiograph reveals signs of a very destructive tumor growth, and marked anaplasia of the cells and their nuclei shows up histologically, the diagnosis of a malignant cartilaginous neoplasm is relatively easy. However, distinguishing histologically between a proliferating chondroma (p. 224) and a highly differentiated chondrosarcoma can be extremely difficult. A cartilaginous neoplasm must be regarded as malignant when on the one hand its position makes it possible to suspect at least potential malignancy, and on

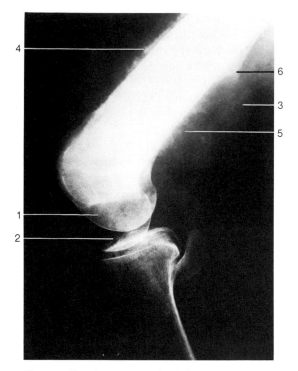

Fig. 434. Chondrosarcoma (distal femur)

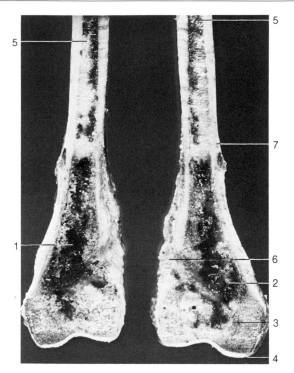

Fig. 435. Chondrosarcoma (cut surface, distal femur)

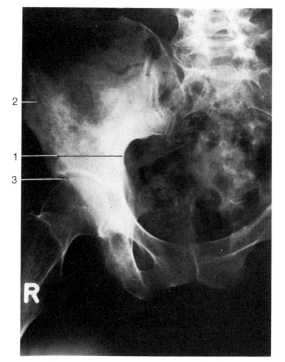

Fig. 436. Chondrosarcoma (right iliac bone)

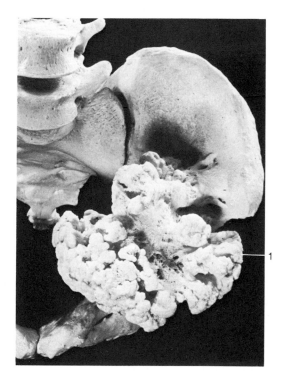

Fig. 437. Chondrosarcoma
(maceration specimen, left iliac bone)

the other hand it contains numerous ill-shaped nuclei with dark clumps of chromatin, many multinucleated chondrocytes and cartilage giant cells. It is frequently necessary to take several tissue samples from different regions of such a tumor in order to make a reliable histological analysis possible.

In the **overall histological view** shown in **Fig. 438** one is immediately struck by the pronounced lobular formation of the cartilaginous neoplasm. One recognizes differently sized nodes *(1)* of hyaline cartilage, which vary in cell density. These nodules are fairly sharply delineated by narrow connective tissue septa *(2)*. There are also some blood vessels *(3)* which are nevertheless not numerous within the neoplasm itself. At the periphery of the nodules the cell density is greater than in the center.

In dealing with chondrosarcomas three different grades of differentiation are recognized, and this is highly relevant for the prognosis. The tumorous cartilaginous tissue must be very precisely examined microscopically if an accurate diagnosis is to be reached. **Figure 439** depicts a *grade 1 chondrosarcoma* under **higher magnification.** The chondrocytes are closely packed together but somewhat irregularly distributed. Within the hyaline matrix, which here and there may reveal myxomatous change, one can see tumorous chondrocytes which mostly have distinct cell boundaries *(1)*. They contain nuclei that vary somewhat in size and show a moderate degree of polymorphy *(2)*. Mitoses are practically never seen, and the lobular architecture of the cartilaginous tissue is preserved.

Figure 440 depicts a *grade 2 chondrosarcoma*. One recognizes the greater irregularity in the distribution of the tumorous chondrocytes, which may often be found packed closely together in groups. The cell boundaries are very indistinct and often no longer identifiable at all. There are greater and smaller areas in which no nuclei or only small nuclear fragments can be seen *(1)*. There are numerous foci of myxomatous degeneration. The most noticeable feature is the greater degree of polymorphy of the nuclei in comparison with grade 1. Some of the nuclei of the tumor cells are roundish and isomorphic *(2)*, some are unevenly elongated *(3)*, and some are more distended *(4)*. Large numbers of giant nuclei *(5)*

and multinucleated tumor cells are present. One also comes across nuclei in the form of hyperchromatic plaques *(6)*. The background tissue is weakly basophilic or eosinophilic and contains roundish vacuoles *(7)* that remind one of empty chondroblastic capsules. Mitoses are only rarely demonstrable within the chondrocytes of such a tumor as this.

Figure 441 depicts a *grade 3 chondrosarcoma*. Here the most striking feature is the pronounced polymorphy of the tumor cells and their nuclei. One can again recognize the nodular formation, the nodules being sharply bordered by a loose connective tissue with a few blood vessels *(1)*. The tumor cells are irregularly distributed within the connective tissue, and appear to be blown out into large cell nests *(2)*. The nuclei vary in size, and one often sees giant nuclei *(3)* with a very dense chromatin content. The very pronounced polymorphy of the nuclei is striking, and they may display many bizarre ramifications. Pathological mitoses may be seen in such neoplasms, even though they are relatively infrequent in comparison with the number of polymorphic cells and nuclei. In a neoplasm of this kind it is not difficult to recognize its malignant character.

From the histological point of view, cartilaginous tumors are extraordinarily difficult neoplasms to diagnose. This applies particularly to the *border-line* cases, where it must be decided from the histological appearance whether one is still dealing with a proliferating chondroma or whether it is already a highly differentiated chondrosarcoma. In order to reach a precise diagnosis – upon which a choice of one of the very different types of treatment available will depend – a great deal of histopathological experience is required. Taking into account the clinical and radiological findings, which provide some suggestion as to whether the tumor growth is benign or malignant, tissue samples must whenever possible be taken from several parts of the tumor.

The criteria for malignancy are (1) many cells with distorted nuclei, (2) several chondrocytes with two nuclei and (3) cartilaginous giant cells with one or more nuclei containing clumps of chromatin. Necrotic foci in the tumor tissue also suggest malignancy. The number of cells is an uncertain criterion, since this can also be high in chondromas.

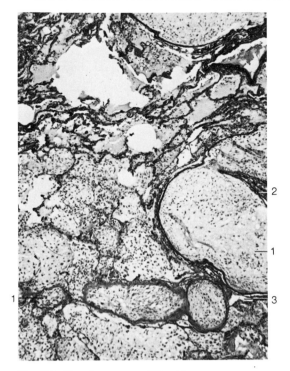

Fig. 438. Chondrosarcoma; HE, ×25

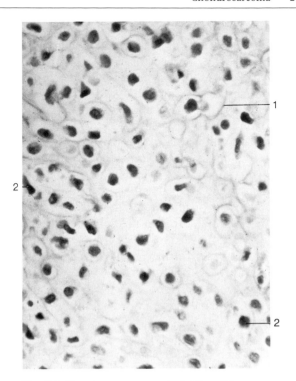

Fig. 439. Chondrosarcoma grade 1; HE, ×100

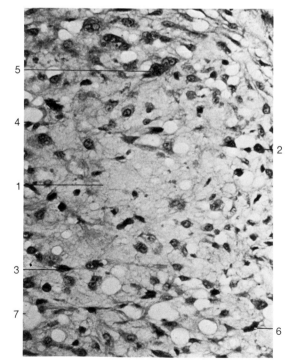

Fig. 440. Chondrosarcoma grade 2; HE, ×100

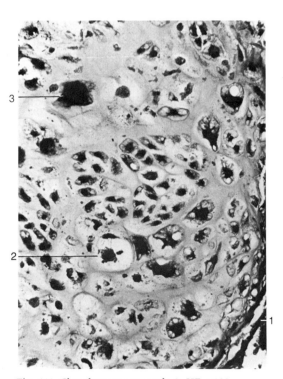

Fig. 441. Chondrosarcoma grade 3; HE, ×100

In **Fig. 442** one can see the **radiograph** of a cartilaginous neoplasm in the proximal part of the humerus of a 36-year-old man. The entire proximal metaphysis reveals a patchy osteolysis with flattish and straggly increases in density which reach down into the adjacent diaphysis. The tumor is centrally placed in the bone and has taken up the whole of the marrow cavity at this level. One can recognize large irregular patches of translucency *(1)*, and between them the areas of increased density just described. A few patchy densifications *(2)* indicate calcified foci. The proximal humeral metaphysis is somewhat distended upward by the central tumor, and the cortex appears to have been partly invaded *(3)*; it is, however, still intact and even appears to have become thickened *(4)*. Outwardly it has for the most part a smooth border, and no reactive periosteal changes can be seen. Proximally, the tumor reaches as far as the epiphyseal cartilage *(5)*, which here forms a sharp border. The epiphysis itself is free from tumor tissue. With a radiological appearance such as this one must consider, apart from a calcified enchondroma or a chondrosarcoma, the possibility of a bone infarct (p. 174). Only examination of a bone biopsy could provide the correct diagnosis of this bone lesion. In this case, it revealed the presence of a highly differentiated chondrosarcoma.

Figure 443 shows the **histological picture** of just such a highly differentiated chondrosarcoma, which on radiological examination could easily be taken at first for an enchondroma. With this sort of cartilaginous neoplasm appearing in a long bone, however, the pathologist must always be particularly critical, and always keep in mind the possibility of a chondrosarcoma among his differential diagnoses. One can recognize the indications of lobulated cartilaginous tumor tissue in which the tumor cells are unequally distributed. The chondrocytes are lying in cell nests which are sometimes large and expanded *(1)* and sometimes small *(2)*. The nuclei are almost all hyperchromatic and polymorphic. One observes large polymorphic nuclei *(3)* next to others which are small, roundish and isomorphic *(4)*. Mitoses are very rarely present and cannot usually be detected. The cartilaginous matrix may be weakly basophilic or eosinophilic.

In **Fig. 444** one can see the **radiological picture** of a moderately highly differentiated chondrosarcoma (grade 2). The lobulated and nodular formation of the tumor tissue is obvious, and the nodes relatively sharply delineated *(1)*. In this case there is a fairly equal distribution of the tumorous chondrocytes within the area of cartilage. These nevertheless display a significant degree of nuclear polymorphy, their shape being sometimes elongated *(2)* and sometimes more nearly round *(3)*. A few chondrocytes with two nuclei are also seen *(4)*. No mitoses are visible. The cartilaginous matrix is partly eosinophilic and partly porous and weakly basophilic. In one place one can recognize a trabecula of varying width *(5)*. The adjacent stromal connective tissue is porous and penetrated by a few blood vessels *(6)*.

Fig 445 is also the **picture of a histological section** through a moderately differentiated chondrosarcoma. One recognizes two cancellous trabeculae *(1)* in which no osteocytes remain to be seen, and the lamellar layering is also invisible. These are necrotic bone trabeculae as seen in the neighborhood of a chondrosarcoma. Between these trabeculae there is tumorous cartilaginous tissue which displays its clearly nodular formation.

The nodule is fairly sharply delineated by loose connective tissue with a few blood vessels *(2)*. The marked myxomatous porosity of the tumor tissue is striking, and this suggests that it is highly undifferentiated. It is of course true that no PAS positive substances have to be demonstrable in myxomatous tissue, but in most cases the acid mucopolysaccharides (proteoglycans) can be specifically stained with safranin O. Whereas morphologically highly differentiated tumors of cartilage produce large amounts of acid mucopolysaccharides with a high content of sulfaton ions, proteoglycans are only sparsely present in undifferentiated chondrosarcomas. When assessing the degree of differentiation the form of the nuclei must always be most carefully observed, and here the significant presence of polymorphy can be recognized. Malignant neoplasia is also revealed by the destruction of the autochthonous cancellous trabeculae, which are eroded or necrotic. Extensive necroses within a cartilaginous tumor are rare. As against this, the vessels both inside and outside the tumor ought to be carefully examined so that a possible invasion of the blood vessels by neoplastic tissue does not go undetected.

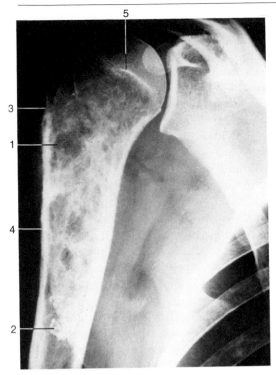

Fig. 442. Chondrosarcoma (proximal humerus)

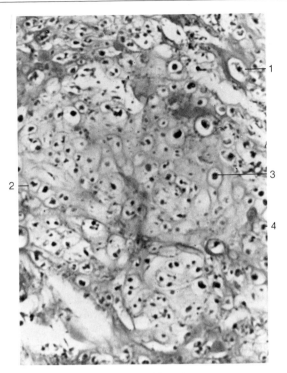

Fig. 443. Chondrosarcoma; HE, ×40

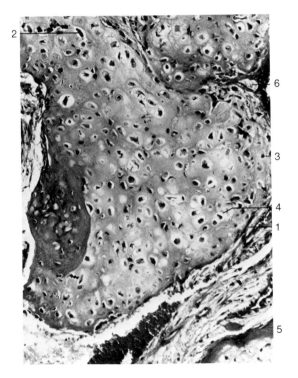

Fig. 444. Chondrosarcoma; HE, ×25

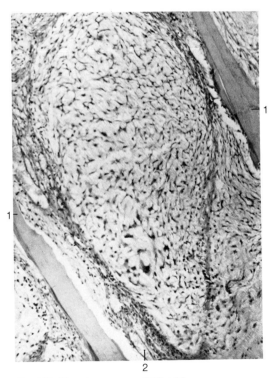

Fig. 445. Chondrosarcoma; PAS, ×25

In the **vertebral column** chondrosarcomas usually develop very slowly and are often late in being discovered. They often attain a considerable size. In **Fig. 447** one can see on a lateral **radiograph** of the thoracic column of a 73-year-old woman an irregular area of sclerosis with patchy translucencies and an indistinct border at the ventral side of the 7th thoracic vertebral body *(1)*. This shadow extends in a ventral direction *(2)* and is projected also onto the 8th thoracic vertebral body *(3)*. The space between the 7th and 8th vertebrae *(4)* is, however, maintained. In the sclerotic region there are several striking patches of calcification *(5)*. This finding strongly suggests a cartilaginous neoplasm, and its expansive growth makes one think from the radiological appearance alone of a possible chondrosarcoma. As can be seen in **Fig. 446**, the **myelogram** reveals an extradural block below the body of Th 7 *(1)*. An indistinctly bordered focus with fine sclerotic patches is seen on the side of the 7th thoracic vertebra *(2)*. This has invaded the cortex and at this point destroyed it and entered the adjacent extra-osseous tissue. *(3)*. The intervertebral spaces on either side of the 7th thoracic vertebral body *(4)* have been maintained.

Recurring chondrosarcomas of the vertebral column can eventually reach a considerable size. In **Fig. 448** one can see a **macroscopic specimen** of a chondrosarcoma of the spinal column. The tumor has developed in 7th thoracic vertebral body *(1)* and enlarged itself into the thoracic cavity. The spongiosa of the vertebra has been extensively destroyed and replaced by the whitish glassy tissue of the tumor. It is remarkable that the tumor has remained limited to the vertebra and has not penetrated the neighboring intervertebral spaces or their disks, and both the adjacent vertebrae *(2)* are free of any tumor. This is typical of malignant tumors of the vertebra, and can also be confirmed from the radiograph. Instead, the tumor has broken out ventrally from the bone to form a massive neoplastic node *(3)* which is lying in front of the column. It extends over a region occupied by 10 vertebrae without having infiltrated any of them. The cut surface reveals a glassy gray tumor tissue which is elastic in consistency and nodular. Inside the tumor one can see blood-soaked necroses *(4)* and numerous white foci of calcification *(5)*.

The outside of the neoplastic mass has a fairly distinct border *(6)* and is partly covered by a connective tissue capsule. Obviously the tumor has invaded the spinal canal *(7)* and has here brought about destruction of the cord.

Histologically one recognizes the classical morphology of a chondrosarcoma. In the overall view shown in **Fig. 449** highly cellular cartilaginous tissue is found in which several nodules *(1)* stand out. These contain some small isomorphic chondrocytes *(2)* and some distended cartilage cells *(3)* with polymorphic and hyperchromatic nuclei. Foci of calcium deposition are often encountered. The tissue must be carefully examined under **higher magnification** for the presence of atypical forms of cell and nuclei. In **Fig. 450** one recognizes that the cartilaginous tumor cells are lying in large chondroblastic capsules *(1)*. They contain highly polymorphic nuclei, some roundish, some more elongated, which are often unevenly drawn-out *(2)*. All the nuclei are dark and reveal an irregular distribution of chromatin. Some of the cells contain two nuclei *(3)*. On the other hand, no mitoses are found.

Chondrosarcomas, especially in the vertebral column, have a tendency to break into blood vessels and form extensive tumorous thrombi. In the venous system such a neoplastic plug can further proliferate continually until it even reaches the right side of the heart, and then continue on as

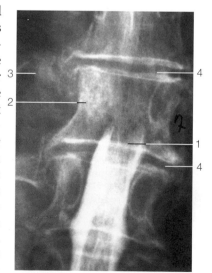

Fig. 446. Chondrosarcoma (body of Th 7, myelogram)

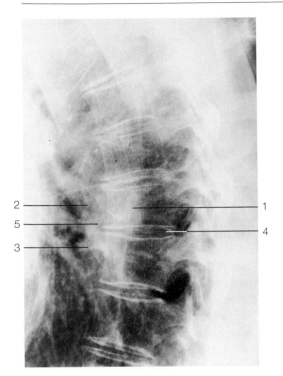

Fig. 447. Chondrosarcoma (body of Th 7)

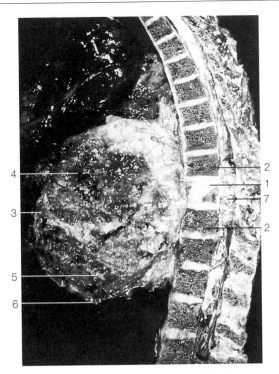

Fig. 448. Chondrosarcoma (thoracic column)

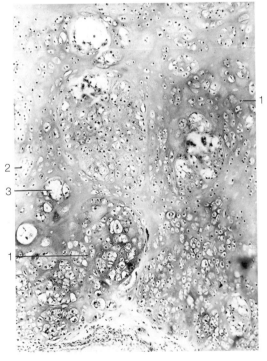

Fig. 449. Chondrosarcoma; HE, ×64

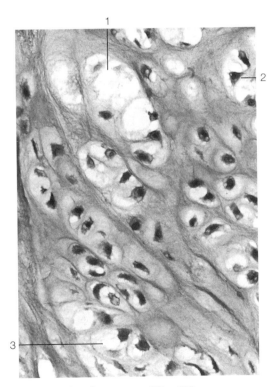

Fig. 450. Chondrosarcoma; HE, ×120

far as the bifurcation of the pulmonary artery. Angiographic examination makes it possible to demonstrate this type of tumorous growth, which is typical of the chondrosarcoma.

Dedifferentiated Chondrosarcoma

Chondrosarcomas can be classified in terms of their morphological structure and the appearance of their cells and their nuclei into various grades of malignancy. On this basis, the prognosis can to a certain extent be assessed (p. 240). There are also cartilaginous tumors which show a particularly high degree of malignancy. *These dedifferentiated chondrosarcomas represent a type of highly malignant cartilaginous neoplasm which frequently derives from an ordinary chondrosarcoma, and which under histological examination reveals, in addition to the tumorous cartilaginous structures, some of the tissue components of a fibrosarcoma or an osteosarcoma.* A bone biopsy may show only the tissue of a fibrosarcoma or an osteosarcoma, and even the picture of the related metastases can conceal the original cartilaginous character of the primary neoplasm. Analysis of the cartilaginous tissue of the tumor usually indicates a chondrosarcoma of grade 3. Sometimes, however, it presents with highly differentiated cartilaginous tissue, which can only with difficulty be recognized as malignant ("borderline for malignancy"). This tumor is today an accepted entity among the neoplasms of bone. Dedifferentiated chondrosarcomas can be derived from primary as well as from secondary chondrosarcomas.

In **Fig. 451** the **radiograph** shows a dedifferentiated chondrosarcoma in the proximal part of the right femur of a 63-year-old man. One observes an irregular shadowy increase in the density of the proximal femoral metaphysis which reaches out into the trochanters and the femoral neck. In a few places the clearly lobular and nodular structure of the tumor *(1)* can be seen. The bony spongiosa has been extensively destroyed by the tumor, which has in places penetrated the cortex *(2)* and invaded the adjacent soft parts *(3)*. One can recognize a tumorous soft tissue shadow *(4)* which shows patchy areas of calcification.

In **Fig. 452** a dedifferentiated chondrosarcoma in the proximal part of the right humerus can be recognized. In the **macroscopic picture** one can see from the sawn surfaces of the long bone that the spongiosa has been extensively destroyed by the tumor. The neoplastic tissue has partly invaded the epiphysis *(1)*, and part of the tumor has been soaked with blood. Inside the tumor one can observe the gray glassy tissue of the tumor *(2)*, which has a tough elastic consistency. On one side *(3)* the cortex has been preserved, and on the other *(4)* it has been occupied along a wide front by neoplastic tissue and destroyed. The tumor reaches out into the neighboring diaphysis *(5)* where glassy neoplastic nodes can be seen.

The **histological picture** of a dedifferentiated chondrosarcoma is shown in **Fig. 453**. The most striking feature is the large number of cells. One can see, on the one hand, tumorous cartilaginous tissue *(1)* with distended chondrocytes of various sizes, which possess polymorphic nuclei. On the other hand, there is highly cellular sarcomatous connective tissue *(2)* with small densely loaded hyperchromatic nuclei which are markedly polymorphic. The abrupt transition from neoplastic cartilage to spindle-cell sarcomatous tissue is very characteristic *(3)*. In this intermediate zone the neoplastic tissue is often loosely formed and granulomatous.

Under **higher magnification** one can clearly recognize the highly undifferentiated formation of the tumor. In **Fig 454a** the tumor cartilage with its large numbers of chondrocytes is apparent. The cartilage cells vary in size and are often greatly distended. They have hyperchromatic and highly polymorphic nuclei *(1)* that are often drawn into star shapes, and multinucleated cells are also present. Irregular areas of calcification *(2)* are seen again and again in the matrix. Such cartilaginous tissue shows all the morphological signs of a high degree of malignancy.

In **Fig. 454b** one can see a section of spindle-cell tumor tissue which is almost identical with a polymorphocellular fibrosarcoma. The nuclei are drawn out into spindle shapes, hyperchromatic and highly polymorphic. There are also ungainly giant cells present, and frequent mitoses. In many dedifferentiated chondrosarcomas the characteristic structures of an osteosarcoma (p. 279) may be seen.

In many cases a dedifferentiated chondrosarcoma may appear following incomplete curettage of an ordinary chondrosarcoma, and this must be regarded as a recurrence accompanied by an increase in malignancy. A differentiated chondrosarcoma may further dedifferentiate into a purely osteoblastic osteosarcoma. The only possible treatment for this is radical removal of the tumor, although even then the prognosis remains poor.

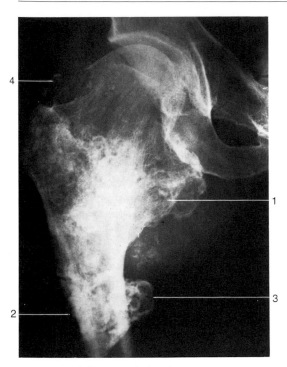

Fig. 451. Dedifferentiated chondrosarcoma (right proximal femur)

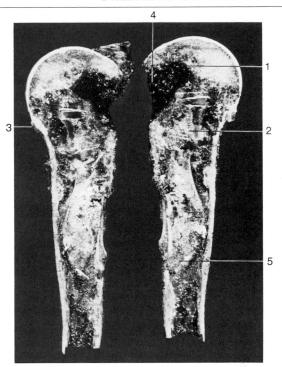

Fig. 452. Dedifferentiated chondrosarcoma (cut surface, proximal humerus)

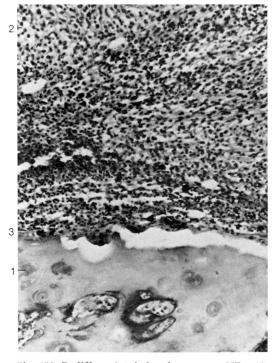

Fig. 453. Dedifferentiated chondrosarcoma; HE, ×40

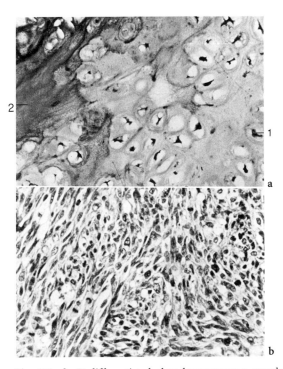

Fig. 454a,b. Dedifferentiated chondrosarcoma: **a** anaplastic tumorous cartilage; HE, ×64; **b** spindle-cell sarcomatous tumorous tissue; HE, ×64

Clear-Cell Chondrosarcoma

Among 470 chondrosarcomas, DAHLIN found 9 cases which showed a close histological resemblance to an osteoblastoma (p. 264) or a chondroblastoma (p. 226). *This is a malignant tumor of cartilage which is found predominantly in the femur and which is characterized by benign giant cells and chondrocytes with a strikingly pale cytoplasm and sharply defined cell boundaries.* This special form of chondrosarcoma makes up just 2% of this group of neoplasms. Because it is so often mistaken for a benign bone tumor, however, knowledge and awareness of this growth is therefore important. It is found predominantly among males. The tumor can appear at any age and, apart from the femur, such neoplasms have been described in the humerus, vertebral column and pelvis. Because of the slow growth of this tumor, the clinical symptoms – usually local swelling – only appear very late.

Figure 455 shows the **radiograph** of a clear-cell chondrosarcoma. In the proximal region of the left femur, osteolytic destruction of bone (1) has led to a marked elevation of the bone. The destructive lesions show large and small foci of osteolysis, set through with septum-like zones of sclerosis (2). In this case the cortex (3) is also involved in the osteolytic process, although normally it remains intact and is only slightly expanded. Within the osteolytic zones one can recognize fine patches of calcification (4), although these may also be absent. The tumor has taken in the whole of the femoral neck and the proximal femoral metaphysis, and is also reaching out into the femoral head (5).

The **histological picture** of this tumor shows unambiguous cartilaginous structures that make one think of a benign chondroblastoma (p. 229). As can be observed in **Fig. 456**, there is a highly cellular tissue present that shows no clearly lobulated form such as is found in other cartilaginous tumors, and nodular areas are only vaguely distinguishable. The most striking feature is the dense packing together of large tumor cells with a very pale cytoplasm and well-defined cell borders (1). They mostly have a central roundish nucleus. In the tumor tissue there are small calcified foci (2) and sometimes, as in chondroblastomas, fine bands of calcification. There are always benign multinucleated giants cells (3) of the same type as the osteoclast – either alone or in groups. In the periphery there are misshaped trabeculae (4), which are often necrotic, and have layers of lamellar osteons (5) with many osteocytes. Rows of osteocytes (6) lie deposited along them. These represent reactive autochthonous bone changes. In the neighborhood of these bony structures one can see many filled blood vessels in the connective tissue stroma (7).

In **Fig. 457** one can see another region of the tumor. This is again dominated by dense layers of tumor cells with strikingly pale cytoplasm and well-defined cell borders (1). They mostly possess a single small roundish, hyperchromatic nucleus. There are no mitoses, although many large chondroblastic cells contain large, bizarre nuclei (2). The most striking feature of this picture is, however, the irregular deposition of osteoid (3), which shows varying degrees of calcification. Fibro-osseous trabeculae (4) and bony trabeculae (5) arranged in laminated layers are seen within the tumor. These structures are found either centrally in the lobules or diffusely distributed throughout the tissue. They give the neoplasm an appearance very similar to that of an osteoblastoma. Finally, the structures of an aneurysmic bony cyst (p. 417) may appear in the tumor.

Under **higher magnification** as in **Fig. 458** the whole cytological picture comes into view. The tumor cells are large and have a voluminous, very pale cytoplasm (1), and are sharply delineated by a prominent cell border. The nuclei are roundish or oval and hyperchromatic, but fairly isomorphic. Multinucleated chondroblasts are rare and there are no mitoses. This quiescent cellular picture can easily lead to the diagnosis of a benign tumor. However, as has already been apparent, we are dealing with a malignant tumor that has a tendency to metastasize and therefore needs to be treated by radical surgical resection. Radiotherapy is useless. The cases of clear-cell chondrosarcomas so far described have indicated that the survival time is short, which may, however, be attributed to the late recognition of the malignant character of the growth and the subsequent therapeutic delay and inadequacy. The prognosis of these cases can surely be improved.

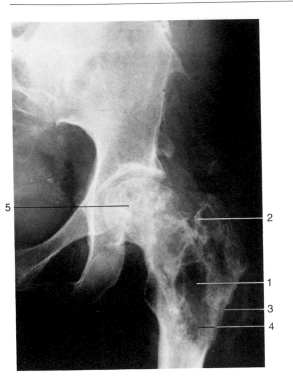

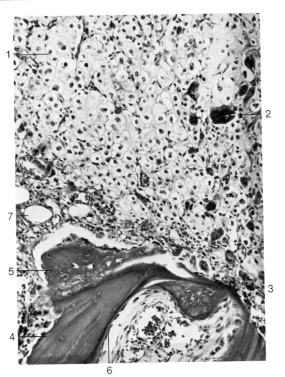

Fig. 455. Clear-cell chondrosarcoma (left proximal femur)

Fig. 456. Clear-cell chondrosarcoma; HE, ×40

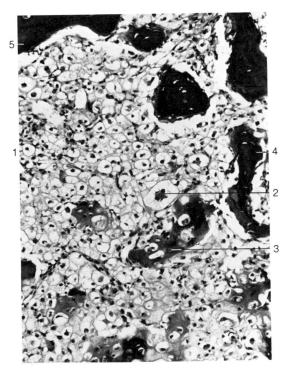

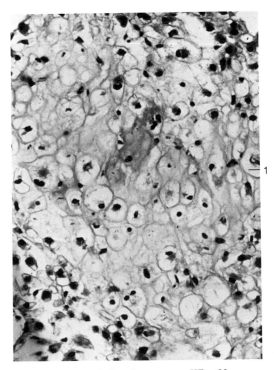

Fig. 457. Clear-cell chondrosarcoma; HE, ×64

Fig. 458. Clear-cell chondrosarcoma; HE, ×82

Mesenchymal Chondrosarcoma (ICD-O-DA-M-9240/3)

This neoplasm is very rare, accounting for 0.3% at the most of the malignant tumors of bone. *It is a malignant bone tumor that is composed histologically of malignant cartilaginous tissue and an undifferentiated stroma of small round cells.* A third of them appear in the soft tissues. Pain and swelling are the principal symptoms. These tumors appear in the skull, spinal column, ribs, pelvis and long bones, but show no special predilection for any one site. The age of the patient lies between 20 and 60 years, with an average at 33 years. The prognosis is significantly worse than for mature chondrosarcomas. The tumor has a strong tendency toward local recurrence and the formation of metastases. Only rarely does a patient survive for longer than 5 years. The only effective therapy is radical surgical removal of the entire growth. The bone biopsy from a mesenchymal chondrosarcoma can be confused histologically with a Ewing sarcoma (p. 352), a reticular-cell sarcoma (p. 358) or with a hemangiopericytoma, p. 374).

In the **radiograph** it is mostly the osteolytic destruction of bone that is observed. In **Fig. 459** one can see a mesenchymal chondrosarcoma of the left femoral neck. In the bone there is a large eccentrically placed osteolytic area *(1)* that extends almost as far as the cortex. This layer is clearly narrowed at that point and appears to have been partly destroyed from within. No periosteal reaction can, however, be perceived. The lesion has an indistinct and irregular border, and there is no marginal sclerosis. Inside one can see patchy shadows, representing foci of calcification. The radiological impression is that of a malignant bony neoplasm, although it is not possible to distinguish it from a typical chondrosarcoma.

In representative regions of the tumor, which unfortunately are sometimes not included in the biopsy, the **histological picture** of a mesenchymal chondrosarcoma is very characteristic. In **Fig. 460** we can see an **overall view** of this tumor. One can recognize the very clear lobular and nodular formation, with nodules of varying size. They are fairly sharply separated by narrow connective tissue septa *(1)* which contain blood vessels. Inside the nodules *(2)* there is a relatively benign looking cartilaginous tissue, whereas a very highly cellular mesenchymal tissue of small undifferentiated cells is lying in the periphery of the lobules *(3)*. This biphasic pattern of the tissue is very characteristic of a mesenchymal chondrosarcoma, in which the amount of the two types of tissue structure can vary greatly.

Under magnification (**Fig. 461**) one can again recognize the lobular formation that is typical of all cartilaginous tumors. The nodules *(1)* consist of cartilaginous tissue. The chondrocytes are small, and have small dark nuclei in which no mitoses can be detected. There is, however, significant nuclear polymorphy, with some nuclei being roundish in shape *(2)* and others more elongated *(3)*. There is a sharp border between the cartilaginous tissue and the highly cellular stromal tissue *(4)*. The latter consists of small densely packed undifferentiated round cells with dark nuclei, very much resembling those of a Ewing sarcoma (p. 352). The nuclei of these cells are hyperchromatic and sometimes spindle-shaped, with hardly any recognizable cytoplasm. These therefore show a close resemblance to reticular cellular elements.

Under **higher magnification** (**Fig. 462**) one recognizes that the highly cellular mesenchymal tumor tissue surrounding the cartilaginous nodules is fully undifferentiated. There are densely packed, partly round-celled, partly spindle-celled components without any differentiated structure. Mitoses are only rarely detectable. A loose fibrous framework between the tumor cells can awake the impression of a reticulum cell sarcoma (malignant lymphoma of bone – p. 358). The tissue has been invaded by a few fine-walled capillaries. The organization of the tumor cells in the environment of these blood vessels can in places give the impression of a hemangiopericytoma (p. 374). Both the structural elements of this tumor must be present in the biopsy before the diagnosis of mesenchymal chondrosarcoma can be made.

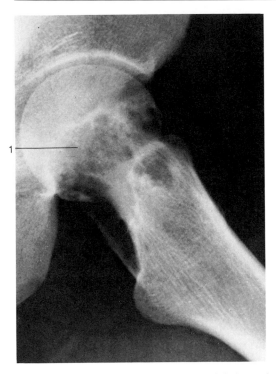

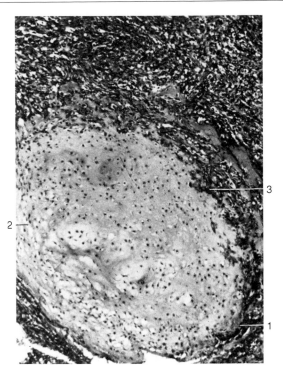

Fig. 459. Mesenchymal chondrosarcoma (left femoral neck)

Fig. 460. Mesenchymal chondrosarcoma; HE, ×30

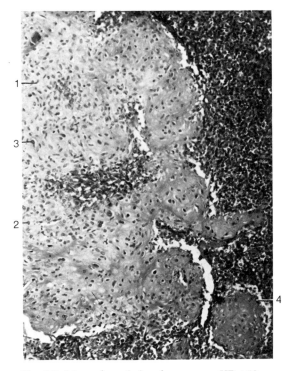

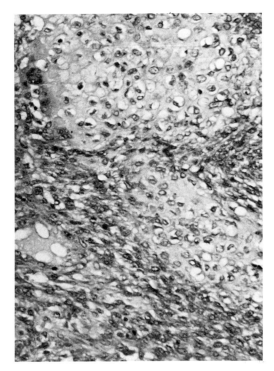

Fig. 461. Mesenchymal chondrosarcoma; HE, ×40

Fig. 462. Mesenchymal chondrosarcoma; HE, ×64

Periosteal and Extraskeletal Chondrosarcoma (ICD-O-DA-M-9221/3)

A malignant cartilaginous neoplasm can develop in the periosteal connective tissue or elsewhere in the soft parts. This type of tumor has been described in, amongst other places, the larynx and the lungs.

A periosteal chondrosarcoma is a malignant cartilaginous neoplasm that develops in the periosteal connective tissue of a bone, and which may then penetrate into the bone from outside. **Figure 463** shows a **maceration** specimen of such a periosteal chondrosarcoma. One can recognize an enormous tumor that reaches out from the periosteum deeply into the soft tissues. The external configuration of this neoplasm clearly reveals its nodular formation *(1)*. Inside, there are irregular gaps between the tumorous nodes *(2)* which were probably occupied by mucous foci. The cut surface shows a few places with a glassy appearance *(3)*, through which the tumor tissue reached into the adjacent cortex of the femoral bone. The tumor encloses the whole of the proximal femoral epiphysis like a shell. The marrow cavity is free from tumor tissue *(4)*, but the cortex nevertheless shows signs of irregular reactive thickening.

The **histological appearance** of the periosteal chondrosarcoma cannot be distinguished from an intraosseous chondrosarcoma. In **Fig. 464** one can recognize lobulated cartilaginous tissue in which the chondrocytes are irregularly distributed. They mostly have a single nucleus and lie within large cell nests *(1)*, or else the nests cannot be identified *(2)*. The nuclei are often only sketchily polymorphic, sometimes roundish *(3)* and sometimes drawn out or indented *(4)*. No mitoses are to be seen. The cartilaginous matrix is weakly basophilic or eosinophilic. It may in places be porous and myxomatous, and calcification foci are present which are usually also apparent in the radiograph. Outside *(5)*, one can see the loose periosteal connective tissue in which this neoplasm arose. Sometimes it is impossible to decide whether a periosteal chondrosarcoma has developed out of an osteochondroma. Treatment consists of complete surgical removal of the growth. So long as the tumor has not broken into the adjacent bone, enucleation of the neoplastic mass may be attempted in order, if possible, to save the limb.

An extraskeletal chondrosarcoma is a malignant cartilaginous neoplasm that has no topographical relationship to a bone. Such growths can arise in any tissue, and they are not all that uncommon in teratomas (of the ovary, for instance). Specific sites include the neighborhood of the larynx, the soft tissues, the tongue, the urinary bladder, the pulmonary artery and the intercostal muscles.

Figure 465 shows the **macroscopic appearance** of a chondrosarcoma from the urinary bladder of a 54-year-old woman. The tumor had in part a bone-hard consistency and could only be divided with a saw. On the cut surface in the center of the tumor one can see a glassy gray tissue that is elastic, taut and distended. The lobular formation of the growth is just recognizable. Particularly in its outer regions there are signs of irregular calcification. The tumor is sharply separated from the surrounding structures.

In the **histological section** (**Fig. 466**) of the cartilaginous part of the tumor the characteristic picture of a moderately highly differentiated chondrosarcoma can be recognized. In the middle of a markedly porous and partly myxomatous stroma one can observe cartilage cells with small, partly pyknotic nuclei. There are many chondrocytes with 2 or 3 nuclei. The tumor shows signs of severely regressive changes, including also large calcification foci in the peripheral parts. The biological behavior of this growth is largely dependent upon its position. Metastases appear relative late. Timely and complete removal may achieve a complete cure.

Tumors of cartilage make up a truly large group among the primary bone tumors, and have their own particular diagnostic and therapeutic aspects. There is a total of 14 entities among the cartilaginous tumors, some of which are not true tumors, but rather tumor-like lesions (the "subungual osteocartilaginous exostosis", p. 218, for instance, or "bizarre parosteal osteochondromatous proliferation" = "Nora lesion", p. 218). Many true cartilaginous tumors can be classified as forms of skeletal dysplasia (e.g. enchondromatosis = Ollier's disease, p. 60; osteochondromatosis = multiple osteocartilaginous exostoses, p. 62). In this connection the familial constitution and heredity must be taken into account. It is necessary to distinguish between reactive cartilaginous pro-

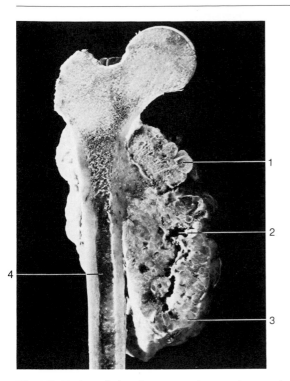

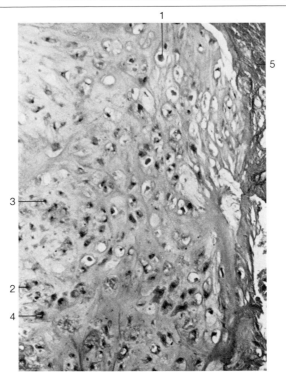

Fig. 463. Periosteal chondrosarcoma (maceration specimen, proximal femur)

Fig. 464. Periosteal chondrosarcoma; HE, ×40

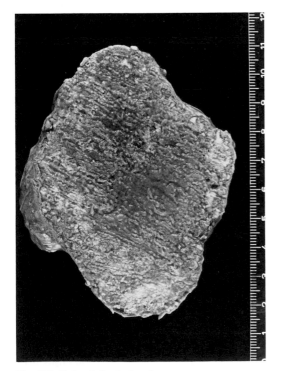

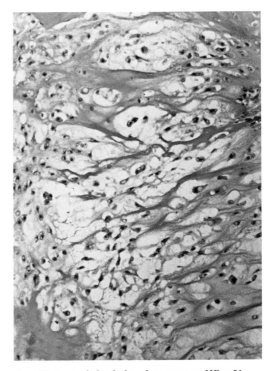

Fig. 465. Extraskeletal chondrosarcoma

Fig. 466. Extraskeletal chondrosarcoma; HE, ×51

liferates and true cartilaginous tumors, as well as dysontogenetic tumors.

Curiously enough, the majority of cartilaginous tumors do not develop in the regions of autochthonous cartilage (articular cartilages, intervertebral disks etc.). It is much more a matter of true bone tumors which have developed during ontogenesis in the place where bone remodeling is most active; namely, the metaphyses. It is here that most cartilaginous tumors are localized (e.g. osteochondromas, p. 214; chondroblastomas, p. 226; chondromyxoid fibromas, p. 230, chondrosarcomas, p. 236). Not only this, but cartilaginous tumors can also arise within a bone where there is normally no cartilaginous tissue, namely, in the diaphyses (e.g. enchondromas, p. 218; proliferating chondromas, p. 224;), in the periosteum (e.g. periosteal, juxtacortical chondromas, p. 224; periosteal chondrosarcomas, p. 252) or in the joint capsule (articular chondromatosis, p. 458). These tumors are therefore distributed all over the skeleton, but not randomly. Each cartilaginous tumor has its typical localization, a fact which must be taken into account when making a diagnosis. Finally, cartilaginous tumors can arise in various tissues and organs outside the skeleton altogether (extraskeletal chondromas, extraskeletal chondrosarcomas. p. 252).

Radiologically the majority of cartilaginous tumors show signs of osteolysis, since the autochthonous mineralized bone tissue is destroyed. Characteristically, focal areas of dystrophic calcification are found in the tumorous tissue. These usually appear in the radiograph as fine patchy regions of increased density indicating the presence of a cartilaginous tumor. With very advanced calcification the tumor may appear as a compact "calcium-dense mass" within the ruined spongiosa. The radiological findings (including CT and MRT) will show whether the tumor is intraosseous (e.g. an enchondroma, p. 218) or whether it is lying outside the bone (e.g. an osteochondroma (ecchondroma) p. 214; periosteal juxtacortical chondroma, p. 224). In the case of an osteochondroma, the cartilaginous cap which covers the bony stem represents the actual tumor tissue. It must be completely removed surgically in order to prevent recurrence. With the help of scintigraphy it is possible to determine whether proliferation is taking place within the growth.

Histologically the cartilaginous tumors are among the most difficult of all bone tumors to diagnose. They all reveal a nodular and lobulated formation of the tissue, which can thus be identified as actual tumor tissue, in contrast to reactive cartilaginous tissue (e.g. in cartilaginous callus, p. 118, or in cases of post-traumatic myositis ossificans, p. 478). Tumorous cartilaginous tissue is also often a component of a different variety of tumor (e.g. a chondroblastic osteosarcoma, p. 274). The problem with diagnosing cartilaginous tumors histologically lies in the monomorphic nature of cartilaginous tumor tissue. Particularly with enchondromas of the long bones (p. 218), it can be extraordinarily difficult to distinguish between a benign cartilaginous tumor and a low-grade malignant chondrosarcoma. These are the so-called "border line cases". In connection with histological diagnosis, one frequently hears the phrase "tumors of questionable malignancy", which may be recurrent and can undergo secondary degeneration into malignancy. Such a neoplastic development may well be based on a false primary classification of the tumor tissue, since tumorous cartilaginous tissue, with only slight nuclear polymorphy and few multinucleated chondrocytes, is usually found in a low-grade malignant chondrosarcoma. There are no mitoses. When making the diagnosis, all clinical data – and most particularly the radiological examination (including scintigraphy) – must be taken into account in order to obtain as reliable an identification of the tumor as possible.

The localization of a chondrosarcoma is of decisive diagnostic significance to an extent which is true of hardly any other bone tumor. In the short tubular bones of the hand and foot a tumor – in spite of a certain amount of nuclear polymorphy and hyperchromasia in the cartilage cells – is usually a benign enchondroma. Chondrosarcomas are rare in these bones, although they can arise here in older patients, where they carry a good prognosis after surgical removal. On the other hand, enchondromas do not occur in the pelvis, where the tumor is practically always a chondrosarcoma. Also, in the vertebral column and ribs, cartilaginous tumors are nearly always malignant. This means that the histological diagnosis of these tumors is strictly limited, and, in addition to the radiological findings, the facts gained from experience must be taken into account. Finally, the type of treatment must be chosen with these known biological facts in mind.

Osseous Bone Tumors

Introductory Remarks

Bone neoplasms in the strict sense arise from bone tissue and, in general, manifest themselves by their high content of bone substance. The essential tumor-producing cells are osteoblasts, which in these circumstance also have the capacity for producing osteoid. A few of these neoplasms contain more or less extensive osteoid structures in the form of flat or lattice-like deposits, or they form true osteoid trabeculae. These latter make up an irregular network on which, for the most part, osteoblasts are laid down (e.g. in an osteoid osteoma, p. 260, or osteoblastoma, p. 264; osteosarcoma, p. 274). In other osseous bone tumors there is more or less complete mineralization of the osteoid, so that true tumorous bone develops. Here it is a matter either of partially mineralized woven bone trabeculae (e.g. in an ossifying bone fibroma, p. 316, or osteosarcoma, p. 274) or of mature laminated bone trabeculae (e.g. in an osteoma spongiosum, p. 256). It is even possible for very dense bone tissue with Haversian canals to develop, which closely resembles the bone tissue of the cortex (e.g. in an osteoma eburneum, p. 256). In such highly mature bone tumors it is often the case that no more osteoblasts are found, since they have been enclosed in the bone substance again as osteocytes which do not in any way differ from normal osteocytes.

With the mature bone tumors it is not possible to distinguish the cellular and histological structures from those found in normal bone tissue, except for the numbers present, which must be taken into account when making a diagnosis. In less mature neoplasms (osteoid osteomas and osteoblastomas) the osteoid structures are of great diagnostic significance. It requires a certain amount of experience to be able to recognize these for what they are with HE staining, and in this connection special stains (van Gieson, Azan, PAS and Goldner) can be helpful. In osteosarcomas the osteoid trabeculae have a peculiarly characteristic appearance which allows them to be recognized as "tumor osteoid". This structure owes its origin to disorganization in the course of the collagen fibers. The fibro-osseous trabeculae also have a particular structure in osteosarcomas, so that we speak of "tumorous bone" as a product of tumorous osteoblasts. Against the background of a disorganized organic matrix the calcification of these bone trabeculae becomes irregular, and this is easily recognizable histologically. In addition to the actual bony structures, the interstitial tissue in these neoplasms should also be looked at, since this may consist of fatty tissue (e.g. in osteomas) or connective tissue (e.g. in ossifying bone fibromas). In malignant neoplasms there is a sarcomatous stroma that is distinguishable by a marked polymorphy of the cells (e.g. in osteosarcomas).

The formation of new bone in bone neoplasms produces in the radiograph a more or less marked shadowing, the diagnostic significance of which is of paramount importance. Completely mineralized bony structures produce a very dense radiographic shadow (e.g. with an osteoma eburneum or an osteoblastic osteosarcoma). Cancellous bony tissue appears in the radiograph as a porous, net-like or trabecular structure (e.g. in an osteoma spongiosum). Osteoid trabeculae produce only a weak and rather pale shadow, depending on the degree of mineralization (e.g. in the nidus of an osteoid osteoma or in an osteoblastoma).

Uncalcified osteoid structures (in an osteolytic osteosarcoma, for instance) show up on the radiograph largely as patches of osteolysis. Finally, the new bone formation in a reactively altered periosteum should be considered. In the radiograph this appears in the form of so-called spicules or bony shells and is an indication of the underlying bone process.

Bone tumors of osteoblastic origin are represented in their own group in the classification table (p. 209), and include both benign and malignant neoplasms. Distinguishing between a benign and a malignant bone tumor – whether radiologically, or histologically in biopsy material – can be quite extraordinarily difficult. A proliferating fracture callus, for instance, can present with irregular osteoid and fibro-osseous trabeculae surrounded by a highly cellular stroma, and look very like an osteosarcoma.

Osteoma (ICD-O-DA-M-9180/0)

Osteomas are absolutely benign bone lesions and are included among the benign bone tumors, although it is also not uncommon for them to appear reactively (e. g. in the neighborhood of a meningeoma). *They are circumscribed new formations of compact or cancellous lamellar bone with included fibrous or fatty marrow which undergo a very slow expansive growth.* Osteomas develop almost exclusively in the preformed membranous bone of the skull, where they are found particularly frequently in the paranasal sinuses, more rarely in the skull cap and the bones of the jaws. They are very seldom found in other bones, and arise mostly in the periosteum (periosteal osteoma), although they may also appear in the cortex or spongiosa. Very often it is a matter of ossification in some other bone lesion already present (e.g an osteochondroma or fibrous dysplasia). Osteomas may appear at any age, although they are more frequent in middle and late adulthood. Men are twice as commonly affected as women.

Osteomas are seen on the **radiograph** as slightly elliptical, very radiodense, sharply delineated foci. In **Fig. 467** one can see such an appearance in the proximal part of the left humerus. The local ossification has included the adjacent cortex *(1)*, which in this region is nevertheless outwardly smooth, and without any thickening of the periosteum. The tumor is separated from the spongiosa by a distinct and somewhat undulating border *(2)*. No internal structure can be recognized.

Figure 468 shows the **radiograph** of an osteoma of the skull lying in the left frontal sinus *(1)*. The tumor shows up as a very dense shadow with a well-defined border. The surrounding bone is unremarkable. In **Fig. 469** one can see the **macroscopic appearance** of a osteoma in a vertebral body. In the middle of the spongiosa one can recognize a roundish focus of very dense bone *(1)*, the border of which is somewhat indented but sharply delineated. It contains bone tissue like ivory, in which only a few small pores can be seen.

Histologically an *osteoma eburneum* contains a dense, mature and fully mineralized bone tissue in which true Haversian osteons have developed. In **Fig. 470** one can discern several Haversian canals with narrow lumens *(1)* that have smooth borders and appear to be empty. The lamellar layering of the bone tissue can be seen *(2)*, and numerous small osteocytes have been deposited there. In this way the tumor tissue resembles a sclerotic increase in density of the cortex, but without reversal lines.

In **Fig. 471** a **histological section** through an *osteoma spongiosum* is depicted. This is also fully mature bone tissue of layered lamellae that includes osteons *(1)*. Because of the often necessarily strong decalcification the majority of the osteocyte lacunae are empty. In the outer layer *(2)* one can see a wide zone of lamellar bone. Inside, there are irregular and ungainly bone trabeculae *(3)* with smooth borders and no layers of osteoblasts. These thickened trabeculae are laminated and fully mineralized. In the marrow cavity one can recognize fatty tissue *(4)* which has been penetrated by a few blood vessels *(5)*.

Very often an osteoma produces no symptoms and is only discovered by chance. It is characterized by a slow increase in size as a result of constant new bone formation. In *Gardner's syndrome* osteomas in the skull are found together with intestinal polyps, epidermal cysts and other changes in the connective tissue.

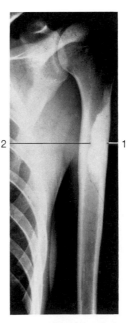

Fig. 467. Osteoma (left proximal humerus)

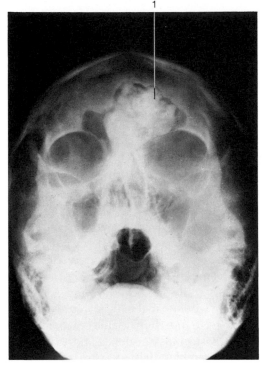

Fig. 468. Osteoma (frontal sinus)

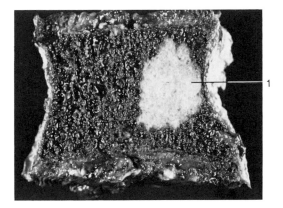

Fig. 469. Osteoma (vertebral body, cut surface)

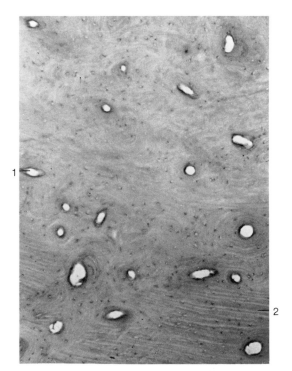

Fig. 470. Osteoma eburneum; HE, ×20

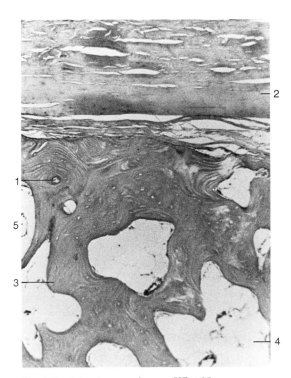

Fig. 471. Osteoma spongiosum; HE, ×25

In the peripheral parts of the skeleton osteomas are mostly without symptoms, and are only discovered radiologically and by chance. In **Fig. 472** such an osteoma can be seen in the proximal part of the right tibia. In the a.p. **radiograph** there is a sharply bordered focus of dense shadow in the middle of the bone *(1)* that shows regions of translucency within. In the lateral view one can see that this focus is lying eccentrically in the dorsal part of the bone *(2)*. With such a radiological finding one should use scintigraphy to determine whether an increase in activity indicates a proliferative process. Apart from this, no bioptic procedure (and certainly no operative interference) is necessary (the so-called *"leave-me-alone lesion"*).

Figure 473 shows a coronal exposure of the skull in which one can recognize **radiologically** a round, sharply bordered focus of increased density *(1)* in the frontal bone. It caused no pain, but was remarkable for its constant increase in size.

In the **computer tomogram** of **Fig. 474** one clearly recognizes the dense, oval, sharply bordered shadow *(1)* in the frontal bone. This is an expanding space-occupying lesion that has caused a slight indentation in the brain *(2)* on the inside, and appears to be bulging outwards externally *(3)*. In this way such an osteoma can be recognized and even cause slight discomfort. The radiological diagnosis is easy.

In the **radiograph** of **Fig. 475** the skull lesion shows up more distinctly. In the a.p. view one can see a circular sclerotic focus *(1)* that appears to have a somewhat vague external border. In the lateral view the skull cap has been raised up to give a fusiform outline *(2)*, and the density is greatly increased.

Histologically, the structures seen within a proliferating osteoma may vary considerably. In **Fig. 476** one can see a wide layer of cancellous bone tissue *(1)* in which the trabeculae are mature and fully mineralized, with fatty tissue lying in between *(2)*. In the center, on the other hand, there is a fibrous stroma, many disorganized fibro-osseous trabeculae *(3)* and deposits of osteoid. Here the bone trabeculae may be layered with osteoblasts. Such a morphological appearance resembles that of an osteoid osteoma (p. 263) that has been slowly ossified from without. This benign lesion has a distinct far outer border, and is covered by a connective tissue capsule *(4)*.

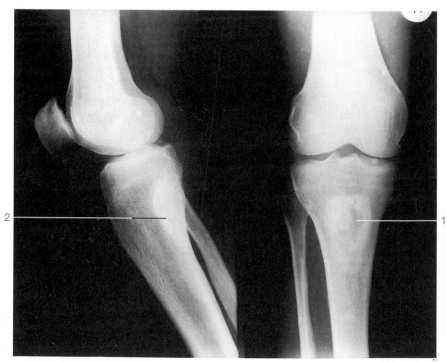

Fig. 472. Osteoma (right proximal tibia)

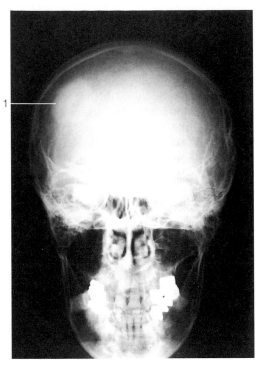

Fig. 473. Osteoma (right frontal bone)

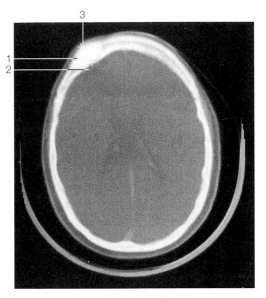

Fig. 474. Osteoma (frontal bone, computer tomogram)

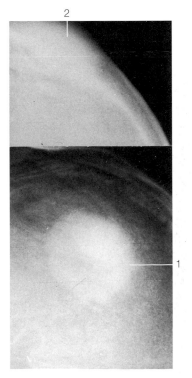

Fig. 475. Osteoma (skull cap)

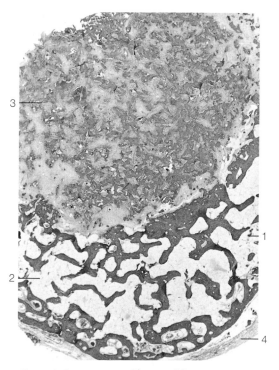

Fig. 476. Osteoma, van Gieson, ×10

Osteoid Osteoma (ICD-O-DA-M-9191/0)

These peculiar bone lesions are today generally regarded as benign bone tumors, although some authors see them as inflammatory foci. *The osteoid osteoma is a small benign osteoblastic bony neoplasm that is characterized by a central region of translucency of up to 3 cm (the so-called "nidus") and a prominent perifocal sclerotic zone, and which can give rise to severe pain.* The pain occurs mostly at night, but can be controlled by analgesics (aspirin). This nocturnal pain, which is very typical of an osteoid osteoma, is an important diagnostic feature and may be confirmed by the so-called "aspirin test". The lesion was first described in 1935 by JAFFE as an independent benign bony neoplasm and separate from inflammatory processes occurring in bone. It makes up about 10% of the benign bone tumors, although it is a matter of experience that it often cannot be identified histologically in surgically material because the "nidus" has not been bioptically encountered. The diagnosis is therefore based upon a combination of the clinical symptoms (nocturnal pain), the radiological findings (nidus with perifocal sclerosis) and the result of the histological examination. If the latter alone is taken as the basis for diagnosis the frequency of the osteoid osteoma falls to under 3% of benign bony neoplasms.

Localization (Fig. 477). This neoplasm is most often found in the long and short tubular bones, about half of them occurring in the femur or tibia (50.6%) and especially in the diaphysis near the end of the shaft. Osteoid osteomas can appear in either the spongiosa or the cortex (the so-called cortical osteoid osteoma). Their presence in the periosteum or outside the bone is extremely rare. A relatively common site is the spinal column, where the neural arches or transverse processes are most often affected. They are almost unknown in the sternum and clavicle: a fact of diagnostic importance. The mandible is also very rarely affected. Otherwise almost any part of the skeleton may be involved.

Age Distribution (Fig. 478). The osteoid osteoma is a neoplasm of youth, and about 51% of cases appear between the ages of 5 and 24 years, with a peak in the second decade. After 40 years its occurrence may be virtually discounted. Males are four times more often affected than females.

It is invariably a benign neoplasm, and so far no malignant change has ever been observed. Indeed, there have been reports of spontaneous cures, with an osteoma-like ossification of the "nidus". Naturally the question arises as to whether this is a true tumor or an inflammatory focus. In any case, bacteria have never been demonstrated within the "nidus". Treatment consists of complete surgical removal of the "nidus" by curettage or *en bloc* excision which can, because of the pronounced perifocal sclerosis, be often very difficult. After incomplete removal of the nidus recurrence is possible. It should be mentioned that multifocal osteoid osteomas may sometimes appear.

Figure 479 illustrates the classical **radiograph** of an osteoid osteoma of the distal femoral metaphysis. This is a tomogram, in which the nidus can most easily be located. The nidus *(1)* appears as a roundish translucent focus of about 1–3 cm in diameter with a tiny sclerotic patch inside. The tumor is lying in the cortex, which is here considerably thickened and sclerotically very dense *(2)*. The osteosclerosis is often so pronounced that the small nidus cannot be identified. In these cases an angiogram may be helpful in bringing the venous side of the circulation within the nidus into view. With an osteoid osteoma within the spongiosa the reactive osteosclerosis is much less obvious.

Figure 480 shows the **radiograph** of an osteoid osteoma in the spongiosa of the right side of the mandible. The nidus reveals a large central shadow *(1)* that is surrounded by a pale mantling zone of sclerosis *(2)*. Externally only a narrow sclerotic cover is seen.

Whereas osteoid osteomas in the bones of the ankle or wrist, or in the long bones, have a characteristic radiographic appearance that established the diagnosis, if they occur in the spinal column the diagnosis may be extremely difficult. There is usually a painful scoliosis, and when this appears in childhood or adolescence the possibility of an osteoid osteoma should always be borne in mind.

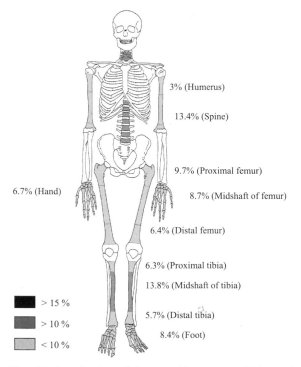

3% (Humerus)

13.4% (Spine)

9.7% (Proximal femur)

8.7% (Midshaft of femur)

6.7% (Hand)

6.4% (Distal femur)

6.3% (Proximal tibia)

13.8% (Midshaft of tibia)

5.7% (Distal tibia)

8.4% (Foot)

■ > 15 %

■ > 10 %

☐ < 10 %

Fig. 477. Localization of the osteoid osteomas (298 cases); others: 17.9%

%

Fig. 478. Age distribution of the osteoid osteomas (298 cases)

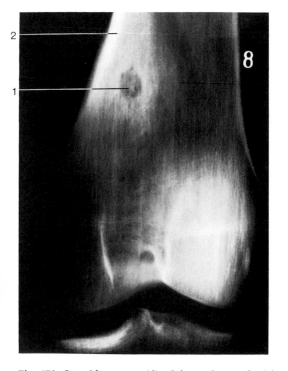
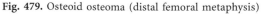

Fig. 479. Osteoid osteoma (distal femoral metaphysis)

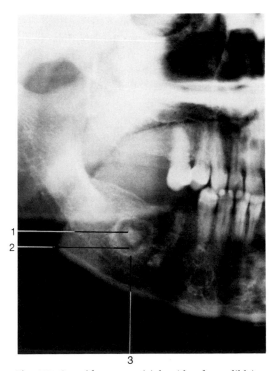

Fig. 480. Osteoid osteoma (right side of mandible)

The radiograph in **Fig. 481** shows a spindle-shaped enlargement *(1)* of the long bone in the middle of the shaft of the right tibia, which is caused by the marked thickening of the cortex in this region. Such a radiological appearance is very typical of a cortical osteoid osteoma. The osteosclerosis is very prominent and extends almost throughout the whole of the diaphysis. It has brought about severe narrowing of the marrow cavity. Within this zone of sclerosis a small nidus *(2)* is only seen with difficulty. There is no periosteal reaction. Surgical removal of this nidus is sufficient to relieve the pain.

Only the tissue from the nidus is available for the histological diagnosis, since the marginal sclerosis only contains osteosclerotic bone tissue from which no diagnostic conclusions can be drawn. **Figure 482** shows the typical **histological picture** of an osteoid osteoma. The nidus consists of highly cellular tissue in which one is struck by the numerous irregular osteoid trabeculae *(1)*. In the HE section these appear as homogeneous eosinophilic bands which are almost completely free of cells. They are variously thick and ungainly; some are short, others long and curved. These osteoid trabeculae stand out clearly from the surrounding osteosclerotic bone tissue, from which they have moved away in a radial formation. They carry numerous deposits of active osteoblasts *(2)*. Between the disorganized osteoid trabeculae there is a stroma *(3)* containing cells and an enormous number of vessels. One can make out many dilated fine-walled capillaries *(4)* which may be distended with blood. This abundant vascularity of the nidus makes it possible to display the vessels of an osteoid osteoma in an angiogram. In the stroma one can identify many fibrocyte and fibroblast nuclei which may be somewhat hyperchromatic, but which are monomorphic. No mitoses are present. Numerous osteoclastic giant cells *(5)* can be recognized which display fewer nuclei than would be present in an osteoclastoma (p. 341). In the stroma there are often fresh hemorrhages, deposits of hemosiderin and a few lymphoplasmatic cellular infiltrates.

In **Fig. 483** one can see the **histological picture** of another osteoid osteoma, which appears to be more compact and to contain more fibers. The stroma consists of collagenous connective tissue with numerous densely packed fi-

brocyte nuclei *(1)*. Here also one sees many dilated fine-walled blood vessels *(2)*. The shapeless, sometimes wide, sometimes narrow osteoid trabeculae *(3)*, which are irregularly distributed and often bound together to form a poorly organized network, are striking. Rows of active osteoblasts are also present *(4)*. The osteoid trabeculae are partly mineralized and here and there show reversal lines. This kind of calcification in a more long-standing osteoid osteoma is most pronounced in the center of the nidus, and only slight or even absent peripherally. This is also reflected in the radiograph, where the center of the nidus is a dense shadow surrounded by a translucent zone (see Fig. 480). Fibro-osseous trabeculae may also develop in an osteoid osteoma, but the tumor is free from cartilaginous tissue.

Under **higher magnification** the variegated cellular appearance of the tumor is clearly seen. In **Fig. 484** one can see extensive irregular deposits of osteoid *(1)* which only seldom show included cell nuclei. The trabeculae do not have smooth edges, and the loose borders contain osteoblasts *(2)* and multinucleated osteoclasts *(3)*. The nuclei are highly hyperchromatic and polymorphic, but there are no mitoses. The stroma is penetrated by wide capillaries *(4)*, and also displays a fine network of osteoid deposits *(5)*. Such a picture of cells and tissues must not be confused with that of an osteosarcoma, and this can be avoided by also taking into account all aspects of the tumor, including the radiological appearance.

The painful symptoms of an osteoid osteoma can be explained by the different degrees to which the tumor is filled with blood, since this presses on the nerves within it. Nerve fibers, however, have hardly ever been demonstrated within the nidus. The average duration of painful symptoms found in the history of patients with osteoid osteomas has been reported as 1.3 years. The pain increases in intensity in the course of weeks or months, and it can lead to impairment of movement due to painful reflex disturbance. When the lesion is in the vertebral column there is a characteristic painful reflex disturbance of posture and limitation of function. The local vertebral and root pain constitute a main symptom. The pain sends the patient in search of medical advice, and surgical removal of the nidus relieves the symptoms.

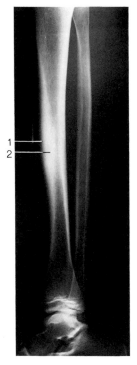

Fig. 481. Osteoid osteoma (tibial shaft)

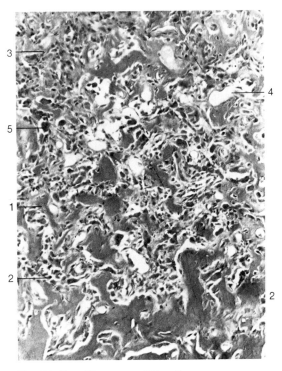

Fig. 482. Osteoid osteoma; HE, ×40

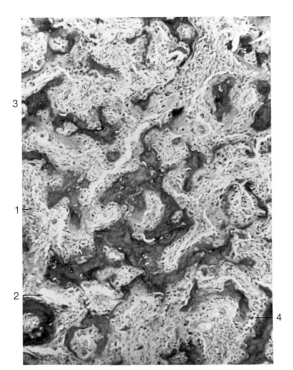

Fig. 483. Osteoid osteoma; HE, ×51

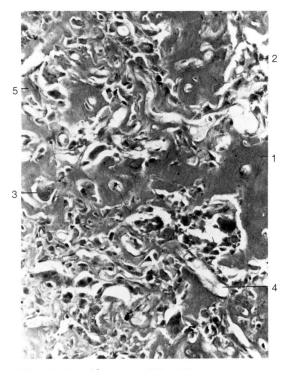

Fig. 484. Osteoid osteoma; HE, ×100

Osteoblastoma (ICD-O-DA-M-9200/0)

This tumor is morphologically very similar to the osteoid osteoma (p. 260), from which it is sometimes histologically indistinguishable. Indeed, it is questionable whether it in fact a separate neoplastic entity and not merely a variant of the osteoid osteoma. However, because of its differences in size, localization, radiological appearance and clinical symptoms, the osteoblastoma is recognized by the WHO as a separate neoplasm of bone. *It is a benign osteoblastic bony tumor which develops in the spongiosa of a bone, and consists of osteoid structures and osteoblasts within a richly vascular stroma.* In comparison with osteoid osteomas, osteoblastomas are mostly much larger, and can reach a size of 2–10 cm (the "giant osteoid osteoma" of DAHLIN). The perifocal sclerosis characteristic of an osteoid osteoma is either absent or only weakly developed. There is slight inconstant pain, not especially at night. These symptoms can last for anything from a few weeks to 5 years. If it is situated in the vertebral column, slow growth of the tumor can lead to neurological impairment or even to a paraplegia. Osteoblastomas are comparatively rare neoplasms, making up less than 1% of primary bone tumors. Men are three times as often affected as women.

Localization (Fig. 485). The most frequent site for osteoblastomas is the vertebral column, where 27.9% of these tumors are found. They may appear in a vertebral body, but usually appear in the neural arch or transverse process. The second most frequent sites are the long bones (26.6% in femur or tibia) and the short tubular bones of the hand or foot (18.5%). Other bones (ribs, pelvis) are less frequently affected. In the tubular bones the tumor is found mostly in the metaphyses or diaphyses, and in the hand and foot the epiphyses may also be attacked. Multicentric osteoblastomas have been described, but they are very rare.

Age Distribution (Fig. 486). Osteoblastomas are found mostly in young people, the most susceptible age extending from the 10th to the 25th year of life, with an average at 17 years. Of these tumors, 60% are discovered during the 2nd and 3rd decades.

These benign bone tumors should be treated conservatively by curettage or en bloc excision, and cures have been seen even after incomplete removal. The value of radiotherapy is – particularly in view of the accompanying dangers – extremely doubtful. Malignant transformation into an osteosarcoma has been reported, but here doubts have arisen concerning the primary diagnosis. The differential diagnosis of an osteoblastoma involves above all the distinction between it and an osteosarcoma.

Figure 487 shows the **radiograph** of an osteoblastoma in the left side of the lower jaw. One can recognize a large opaque bony cyst *(1)* taking up the total width of the mandibular bone, which itself appears to be somewhat raised up. The "bony cyst" has no internal structure, and there is no nidus present. The tumor, which has a relatively distinct border, is surrounded outside only by a discrete layer of marginal sclerosis *(2)*. Such a bony focus cannot be diagnosed radiologically as an osteoblastoma, it must be distinguished, amongst other lesions, from an aneurysmal cyst of bone (p. 412) or an osteoclastoma (p. 337). On the other hand, however, the **radiological appearance** of an osteoblastoma of the vertebral column is very typical. In **Fig. 488** one can recognize a tumor in the left side of the posterior arch of the atlas (C. 1), which is considerably elevated. The outer contour, however, is intact and well defined. Within, there are cystic translucent areas of unequal size. One of these shows a slight increase in structural density in the center which could remind one of a "nidus". Between the translucent zones one can see bands of increased density. In the angiogram the greater vascularization of such a lesion can usually be seen. As a general rule it can be stated that an unusual bony focus found in the vertebral column of a young person, and showing unusual signs of destruction or sclerosis but with a benign appearance radiologically, may be regarded as a benign osteoblastoma until this diagnosis can be confirmed or refuted histologically.

Recently cases of osteoblastomas have been described, the clinical course of which did not fulfil expectations. These are the so-called *"aggressive osteoblastomas"*, which have a strong tendency to recur.

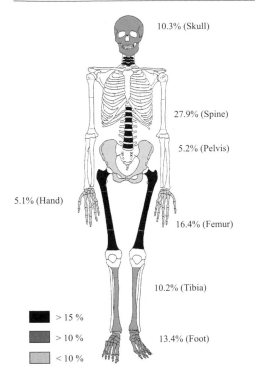

10.3% (Skull)
27.9% (Spine)
5.2% (Pelvis)
5.1% (Hand)
16.4% (Femur)
10.2% (Tibia)
13.4% (Foot)
> 15 %
> 10 %
< 10 %

Fig. 485. Localization of the osteoblastomas (97 cases); others: 11.5%

%
35
30
25
20
15
10
5
0
1. 2. 3. 4. 5. 6. 7. 8.
Decade of life

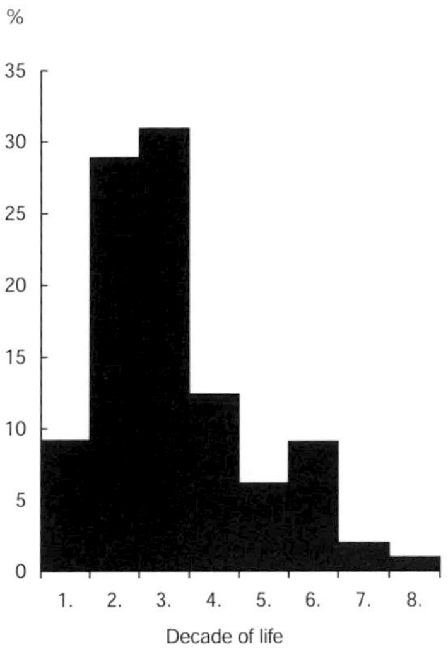

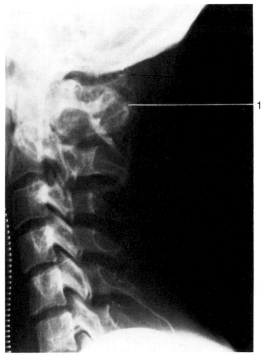

Fig. 486. Age distribution of the osteoblastomas (97 cases)

1
2

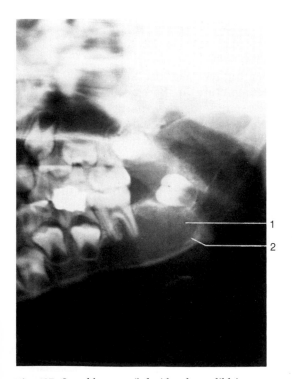

Fig. 487. Osteoblastoma (left side of mandible)

1

Fig. 488. Osteoblastoma (cervical column, arch of atlas)

A **macroscopic picture** of an osteoblastoma can be seen in **Fig. 489.** The section and sawn surface of the 3rd toe shows marked deformity and expansion of the middle phalanx, the outer contours of which are indistinct *(1)*. In the marrow cavity there is a large round focus about 2 cm in diameter and with a fairly sharp border *(2)*. The center of this tumor is porous and filled with blood, so that it appears grayish red. Here the tissue is brittle and crumbling. The periphery of the tumor is more markedly ossified and calcified, so that the tissue appears dense. These structures show up as shadows of varying density in the radiograph. A true nidus, such as one sees in an osteoid osteoma (p. 261), is not typically present in an osteoblastoma, and the prominent marginal sclerosis is usually absent. In this case, however, the spongiosa of the short tubular bone is generally dense and sclerotic *(3)*, which shows up clearly in contrast to that of the terminal phalanx *(4)*. The connective tissue of the periosteum is also thickened.

The **histological appearance** of osteoblastomas is very variable. In the center of the neoplasm one finds highly cellular tissue in which the variation in the number and density of the osteoid trabeculae is striking. These are significantly wider and longer than those seen in an osteoid osteoma. In **Fig. 490** one recognizes the very numerous osteoid trabeculae *(1)* with their irregular outer contours. In some places they are narrow and have a smooth outline, in others the outline is undulating, with jagged indentations. They are sometimes lined with rows of active osteoblasts *(2)*. In the neighborhood one can see numerous multinucleated osteoclastic giant cells *(3)*. Osteocytes with large irregular nuclei are enclosed within the osteoid trabeculae. Between the osteoid structures there is a highly cellular stroma of loose connective tissue, which is penetrated by large numbers of dilated capillaries *(4)*. In many cases osteoblastomas are seen to contain hemorrhages and hemosiderin deposits. The stroma cells are mostly osteoblasts, which are the basic cells of this tumor. They vary in size, and so do their nuclei, which are sometimes ovoid, and sometimes abnormally elongated and showing many indentations and uneven extensions. The chromatin content of the nuclei is quite variable, and the nuclei may be hyperchromatic. Many osteoblastomas present a truly monomorphic pattern of the cells and nuclei, so that the benign character of the neoplasm is easily recognized. Usually there are no mitoses present. However, in a few osteoblastomas a more or less marked polymorphy may be seen, and a few mitoses may be found. In such cases the differential diagnosis from an osteosarcoma may be difficult, and this can only be established histologically if the clinical and radiological findings are also taken into account. A sarcomatous stroma, pronounced cellular polymorphy and atypical mitoses are not signs of a benign osteoblastoma.

The calcium content of osteoblastomas is variable. In **Fig. 491** a dense irregular network of shapeless osteoid trabeculae which have many indentations can be seen **histologically.** They are often layered with osteoblasts *(1)* with long drawn-out nuclei. Within the osteoid trabeculae there are large osteoblasts with dark nuclei. The osteoid structures are irregularly and incompletely calcified, and there are pale areas of unmineralized osteoid *(2)*. In between, one can recognize dark, calcified osteoid foci *(3)*. These tumors may also produce fibro-osseous trabeculae. The extent of the ossification is correlated with the age of the neoplasm. The loose connective tissue stroma contains isomorphic fibroblasts, a few osteoclasts *(4)* and many fine-walled capillaries *(5)*.

Under **higher magnification** (**Fig. 492**) there is a clear picture of the osteoblasts, which are often clustered together in dense groups *(1)*. Between these tumor cells there are net-like osteoid deposits *(2)*. The scattered osteoclasts *(3)* are much smaller than in an osteoclastoma and contain fewer isomorphic nuclei.

SCHAJOWICS (1994), depending on the radiological appearances, distinguished various types of osteoblastoma. The *medullary* and *cortical osteoblastomas* show an osteolytic focus of more than 2 cm diameter in the marrow or cortex of a bone, without any real marginal sclerosis. The *peripheral (periosteal) osteoblastoma* lies on the bone surface and appears to be derived from the periosteum. The *multifocal sclerosing osteoblastoma* can appear either in the marrow cavity (central or endosteal) and also in the region of the periosteum (peripheral or juxtacortical) and is delineated by a region of marginal sclerosis. It is somewhat similar to an osteoid osteoma, although here the presence of several translucent foci ("nidus") is remarkable.

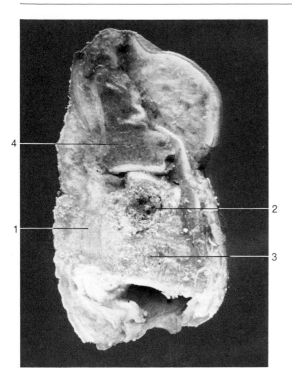

Fig. 489. Osteoblastoma (3rd toe, cut surface)

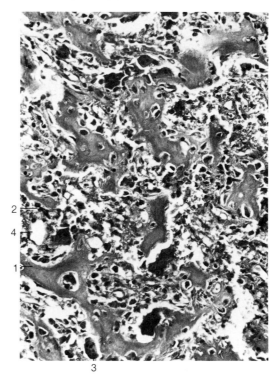

Fig. 490. Osteoblastoma; HE, ×30

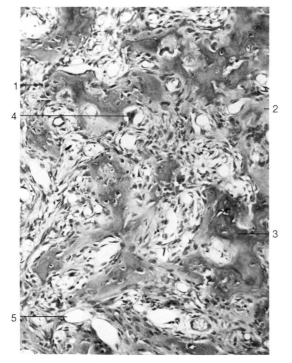

Fig. 491. Osteoblastoma; HE, ×51

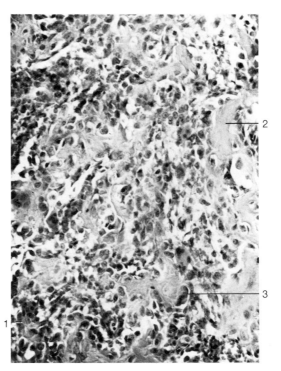

Fig. 492. Osteoblastoma; HE, ×84

Osteoblastomas can often produce confusing radiological findings which are difficult to interpret. They can reach an unusual size or appear in an unusual site. Extensive destruction of bone can arouse suspicion of a malignant bone tumor, so that a bioptic investigation is necessary.

In **Fig. 493** one can see in the **radiograph** a large focus of destruction in the left lesser trochanter of a 19-year-old man *(1)*. This region of the bone is set through with numerous patchy osteolytic foci, between which lie straggly bands of dense sclerosis. The outer contour of the trochanter is raised up in places *(2)*. The lesion is separated from the inside of the bone by a wide, band-like zone of osteosclerosis *(3)*. No reactive change was observed in the periosteum. In the scintigram, the focus showed a strong increase in activity. The differential diagnosis of a honeycomb-like lesion such as this could include a benign bone tumor (e.g hemangioma, lipoma), a malignant bone tumor (e. g. Ewing's sarcoma, osteosarcoma, bone metastasis) or even a local osteomyelitis. The actual diagnosis of a benign osteoblastoma can only be made from a bone biopsy. The localization is extremely unusual for this type of tumor.

An osteoblastoma of the right tibial head can be seen in **Fig. 494**. In the a.p **radiograph** there is a slightly oval zone of osteolysis *(1)* in the proximal tibial metaphysis below the former site of the epiphyseal cartilage *(2)*. This focus is sharply bordered by a narrow region of peripheral osteosclerosis. Inside, one can see discrete areas of increased density. A **lateral radiograph** is necessary in order to make a precise diagnosis. In **Fig. 495** it can be seen that the lesion is lying in a dorsal position *(1)*. It is a *cortical osteoblastoma*. The cortex is here obviously thickened. It bulges outwards slightly, but is clearly delineated. There is no periosteal reaction. In the neighborhood there is an area of slight osteosclerosis that also reaches into the spongiosa *(2)*. Radiologically this is a benign lesion. In the **computer tomogram** of **Fig. 496** the tumor is seen as a cystic area of translucency *(1)* situated in the dorsilateral region of the cortex. Inside, there is a larger focus of increased density. The surrounding bone is markedly sclerotic and dense *(2)*. The spongiosa of the tibial head at some distance from the tumor *(3)* also shows signs of a sclerotic increase in density.

Histologically the lesion presents a very mixed picture with numerous cells that can often give the impression of a malignant bone tumor. In **Fig. 497** one can see a loose connective tissue stroma infiltrated with lymphocytes and plasma cells *(1)* and shot through with many dilated and fine-walled capillaries *(2)*. Nevertheless, the stroma cells show no polymorphic nuclei or mitoses. Numerous shapeless osteoid trabeculae *(3)* are irregularly distributed, on which rows of active osteoblasts *(4)* have been deposited. Here and there these rows show more than one layer *(5)*. In addition, there are a few multinucleated osteoclasts *(6)*. The histological picture is that of a very actively proliferative tumor, which is also usually confirmed by the increased activity in the scintigram. There is, however, no sarcomatous stroma, i.e. the cellular and nuclear polymorphy and pathological mitoses that would indicate a malignant tumor are absent. The osteoid trabeculae do not have the appearance of tumorous osteoid such as is seen in an osteosarcoma (p. 279). A combination of radiological and histological findings should provide sufficient and secure grounds for diagnosing this tumor as benign.

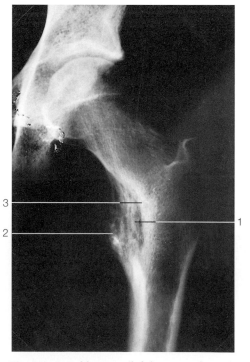

Fig. 493. Osteoblastoma (left lesser trochanter)

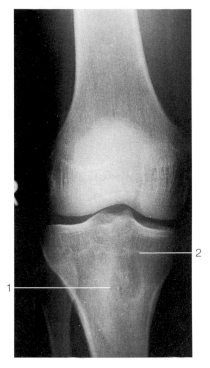

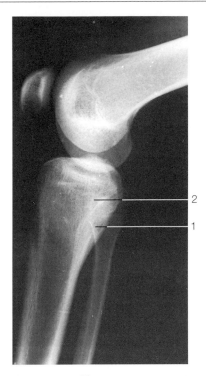

Fig. 494. Osteoblastoma
(right proximal tibia, a.p. radiograph)

Fig. 495. Osteoblastoma
(right proximal tibia, lateral radiograph)

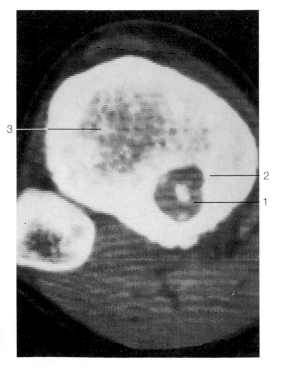

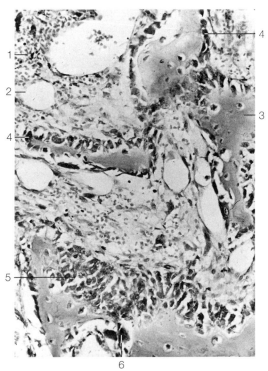

Fig. 496. Osteoblastoma
(right proximal tibia, computer tomogram)

Fig. 497. Osteoblastoma; HE, ×100

Aggressive Osteoblastoma

After incomplete removal, a fair number of osteoblastomas may recur, and even develop into osteosarcomas. Distinguishing histologically between a proliferating osteoblastoma and a highly differentiated osteosarcoma can be extremely difficult. In 95% of cases, recurrence of an osteoblastoma takes place more than 2 years after the first operation – the majority after 5 or more years. Early recurrence gives rise to suspicion of malignancy. *An "aggressive osteoblastoma" is a primary bone tumor that produces a large amount of osteoid and which is very similar to the typical osteoblastoma. Its clinical course is, however, characterized by numerous recurrences where the radiograph reveals malignant destruction and the histological picture shows many polymorphic osteoblasts with pathological mitoses.* This neoplasm shows only a local aggressive and destructive growth, and has a strong tendency to recur, but does not produce metastases. For this reason an "aggressive osteoblastoma" has a better prognosis than an osteosarcoma.

This tumor was first described in 1976 by SCHAJOWICZ and LEMOS. The neoplasm is rare, and so far only a few cases have been seen. Its **main localization** is in the femur, tibia or fibula, although it has also been described in the spinal column, pelvis and metatarsal bones. The **age distribution** ranges from 6 to 67 years, with an average age of 34 years. The patient usually complains of local pain after about 3–5 months, without any swelling being palpable. Radiological examination very soon reveals a destructively growing bone tumor.

In **Fig. 498** one can see the **radiological picture** of an "aggressive osteoblastoma" in the proximal part of the left femur. The tumor has developed in the femoral neck *(1)*. Here there is an indistinctly delineated zone of osteolysis with coarse patchy regions of increased density, which has brought about narrowing of the cortex from within. The tumor has grown on one side into the intertrochanteric region *(2)* and, on the other side, through the edge of the bone and into the acetabulum of the left hip joint as far as the pelvic wall *(3)*. Here one can see a large neoplastic mass which is in part sclerotically dense, in part patchy and in part highly osteolytic *(4)*, and which has in particular ex-

tensively destroyed the bone of the pelvis. Such a far-reaching and destructive tumorous growth suggests radiologically the presence of a malignant neoplasm and is in no sense typical of a benign osteoblastoma. Furthermore, the tumor has spread into the adjacent soft parts.

The **radiograph** of another "aggressive osteoblastoma" can be seen in **Fig. 499**. Here there is a large patchy zone of destruction *(1)* in the transitional region between the metaphysis and diaphysis in the proximal part of the fibula of a 15-year-old boy. One can see patchy osteolyses of unequal size, and partly patchy, partly straggly regions of increased density in between them. On one side the cortex has become included in the process of destruction and is partly obliterated *(2)*. The focus has an indistinct border and reveals no marginal sclerosis. The other side of the cortex has been preserved and is somewhat sclerotically thickened. Periosteal thickening is absent. In the a.p **radiograph** in **Fig. 500** one can again see the focus of destruction in the proximal part of the right fibula *(1)*. This part of the bone has been pushed up into a bulge. The lateral cortex is to a large extent raised up, without any recognizable infiltration of the soft parts. This is a predominantly osteolytic defect in which a few sclerotic increases in density can be seen. The lesion has no distinct border and shows no marginal sclerosis. Radiologically it might well be a malignant lesion that could only be identified by a bone biopsy. The radiologically demonstrable structures are not typical of a benign osteoblastoma.

The **bone scintigram** of this tumorous bone lesion seen in **Fig. 501** shows a significant increase in activity *(1)* involving the entire focus. The center of the tumor is more marked than the periphery. This suggests a strong tendency to proliferate. Furthermore, the growing regions of the proximal parts of the fibula *(2)* and tibia *(3)*, and the distal part of the femur *(4)* are strongly activated, which is physiologically normal for a fifteen-year-old boy. As with a benign osteoblastoma, an "aggressive osteoma" can also appear in the radiograph as a sharply delineated focus of osteolysis with slight marginal sclerosis. In such cases the diagnosis depends exclusively on the histological pattern.

Macroscopically the tumor tissue of an "aggressive osteoblastoma" is uncharacteristic. It is

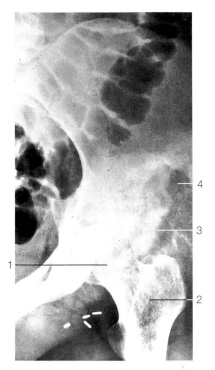

Fig. 498. Aggressive osteoblastoma (left femoral neck)

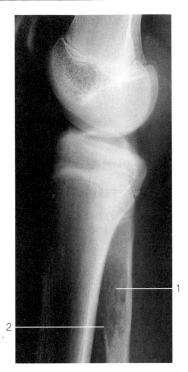

Fig. 499. Aggressive osteoblastoma (right proximal fibula)

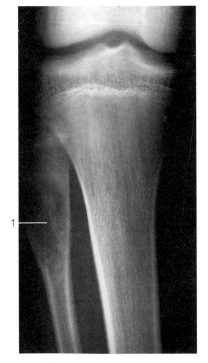

Fig. 500. Aggressive osteoblastoma (right proximal fibula)

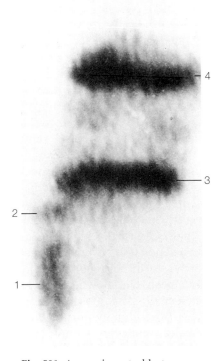

Fig. 501. Aggressive osteoblastoma
(right proximal fibula, scintigram)

grayish-red or grayish-brown with a variable number of calcium deposits. Unlike many osteosarcomas, it contains no hard sclerotic zones.

Figure 502 shows what is basically the **histological appearance** of an "aggressive osteoblastoma". One can see an irregularly dense network of osteoid trabeculae (1) on which rows of active osteoblasts (2) have been deposited. The osteoblasts appear prominent because of their hyperchromatic and polymorphic nuclei, and in some places they form several rows (3). A loose connective tissue stroma (4) lies between the osteoid trabeculae, and this is set through with fine-walled blood capillaries (5) that are often dilated. The stroma cells (fibroblasts, fibrocytes) are also frequently striking because of their shapeless, hyperchromatic and sometimes polymorphic nuclei. From time to time pathological mitoses can also be seen here.

Under **higher magnification** the tumor cells in **Fig. 503** can be more clearly recognized. The loose connective tissue stroma (1) contains numerous dilated fine-walled capillaries (2). There are stout osteoid trabeculae (3) on which rows of active osteoblasts (4) have been laid down. These have markedly hyperchromatic and polymorphic nuclei in which pathological mitoses can be seen. Some of these cells are osteoclasts as can be demonstrated by testing for tartrate-resistant acid phosphatase (TRAP). The osteoid deposits are in part more highly calcified (5): the so-called *"spiculated blue bone"* which is characteristic of the "aggressive osteoblastoma". The polymorphic osteoblasts with their dark, polymorphic nuclei – which may also show atypical mitoses – are decisive for the diagnosis. There is here a great similarity to an osteosarcoma (p. 274) although the distinct sarcomatous stroma is absent.

Figure 504 shows the **histological picture** of a part of the tumor that is unusually highly cellular. There are a few deposits of osteoid (1) on which extraordinarily sturdy and polymorphic osteoblasts (2) have been laid down, often as more than a single layer (3). The unusually large number of fibroblasts (4) with polymorphic and hyperchromatic nuclei showing pathological mitoses is striking. In between there are small collections of lymphocytes (5). All this presents the picture of a highly cellular tissue with a large number of polymorphic cells, thus giving a strong impression of a malignant tumor.

As can be seen **histologically** in **Fig. 505**, the tumorous osteoid laid down in the form of trabeculae is completely absent from some areas of the picture. One finds here a stroma with polymorphic cells and deposits of osteoid, which only appears as a narrow band (1) between the exceedingly vigorous polymorphic osteoblasts (2). In a few places there is patchy osteoid (3) with calcifications that show up as "spiculated blue bone". In this illustration the size of the tumor cells (osteoblasts), and the size, shape and hyperchromasia of the nuclei – together with the strikingly disorganized formation of the tissue – present a picture which is certainly compatible with that of a malignant growth. Furthermore, patchy extensions of osteoid and calcified osteoid in the form of unequal, hardly recognizable trabeculae ("spiculated blue bone") and regions of densely deposited osteoclasts are often described in "aggressive osteoblastomas". It is also said that these osteoblasts have a clearly "epithelioid" appearance. They have abundant cytoplasm and shapeless hyperchromatic nuclei.

There are many reasons for asking whether "aggressive osteoblastomas" actually exist. The radiological appearance of these tumors has, in all the case histories hitherto published, shown signs of malignancy. The criteria of malignancy are likewise met in the histological picture (highly cellular tumorous tissue with polymorphic tumor cells; polymorphic hyperchromatic nuclei, sometimes with atypical mitoses; the production of classical tumorous osteoid). The clinical course too, with its frequent recurrences and increasing destruction of bone, as well as the invasion of the adjacent soft parts by the tumor (Fig. 498), also suggest malignancy. In addition, our cytophotometric DNA measurements of the tumor cells have indicated malignant growth. This would seem to imply that the so-called "aggressive osteoblastoma" is really an osteosarcoma of low malignancy, which manifests only local aggressive growth over a long period, thus leading to local destruction of bone. Metastases only occur in late-discovered cases or in those where the treatment has been inadequate. The diagnosis of a "malignant osteoblastoma" which is sometimes made is misleading and should not be used. The treatment of choice is a wide en bloc excision reaching well into the healthy tissue.

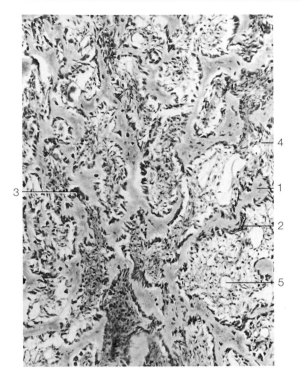

Fig. 502. Aggressive osteoblastoma; HE, ×40

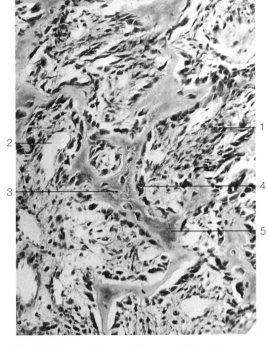

Fig. 503. Aggressive osteoblastoma; HE, ×64

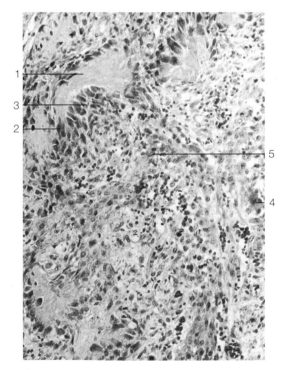

Fig. 504. Aggressive osteoblastoma; HE, ×51

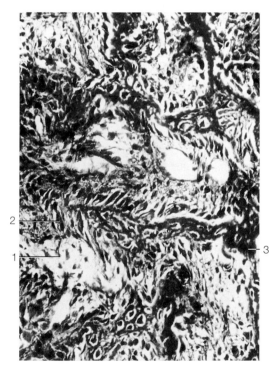

Fig. 505. Aggressive osteoblastoma, PAS, ×84

Bone Island (Compact Island)

Sometimes during the course of a radiological examination one comes across, quite by chance, a circumscribed roundish region of high density in a bone – in the pelvis, for instance, or in a long bone. *This is a circumscribed focus of sclerotic ossification in the spongiosa of a bone. It produces no symptoms and requires no treatment.* If this radiological finding is recognized, no bioptic investigation is necessary (the so-called *"leave-me-alone lesion"*). Such a focus usually remains static, but it may undergo spontaneous remission. In rare cases an increase in size has been observed. With older patients it is sometimes necessary to exclude an osteoblastic bone metastasis.

Macroscopically one can see in the *maceration specimen* of **Fig. 506**, in the middle of completely normal spongiosa *(1)*, a very dense sclerotic focus *(2)* with a sharp, slightly undulating outer contour. One has the impression as of a stone having been deposited into the spongiosa. The inside of this focus consists of very compact, fully mineralized bone tissue. In a few places one can see small cavities that are filled with cancellous bone and fatty marrow. The immediately adjacent spongiosa is not sclerotically increased in density, which is why the focus stands out sharply from its surroundings in the radiograph.

Histologically the focus consists of compact, sclerotically dense bone tissue which contains a few small osteocytes and which is fully mineralized. **Figure 507** shows the tissue from a porous region of a bone island. One can see here very wide, mature bony structures in which true osteons with narrow Haversian canals *(1)* have developed. These bony structures have smooth borders and show no signs of osteoblastic or osteoclastic activity. In between them there is fatty tissue *(2)*. Blood capillaries with delicate walls can be recognized within the Haversian canals. To this extent the tissue is very similar to an osteoma eburneum (p. 257). A bone island can be distinguished from an osteoma because it usually has no tendency to grow and does not produce any deformity of the bone. Originally it was assumed to be a harmless congenital variant of cancellous bone structure. A few authors see in it a minimal manifestation of osteopoikilosis (p. 108).

Osteosarcoma (ICD-O-DA-M-9180/3)

The osteosarcoma is the true malignant neoplasm of bone, in which malignant osteoblasts differentiate from the sarcomatous stroma and tumorous osteoid and tumorous bone (sometimes even tumorous cartilage) develop. In this tumor the many potential varieties of differentiation of the osteoblast in terms both of osteogenesis and osteolysis are realized. The most characteristic feature of the osteosarcoma is the production of tumorous osteoid, which is nevertheless not always recognizable because it has no specific staining reaction. The tumor is highly malignant and usually metastasizes early. After the medullary plasmocytoma (p. 348), the osteosarcoma is the second most frequently encountered malignant neoplasm of bone, making up more than 20% of the bone sarcomas. Nevertheless, it is a relatively rare disease. In a population of a million people, only 4 or 5 osteosarcomas are to be expected. Men are more frequently affected than women.

Localization (Fig. 508). Osteosarcomas can appear in any bone, but over 50% are observed in the long bones. The principal site is the metaphysis. Over 40% of these tumors arise in the distal metaphysis of the femur or the proximal metaphysis of the tibia, making the neighborhood of the knee joint the overall most frequently affected site. However, osteosarcomas in the pelvis or proximal part of the femur are also quite common.

Age Distribution (Fig. 509). The neoplasm appears very much more frequently in young people, the peak – including 44% of cases – in the second decade of life. For tumors of the jaw the age is somewhat higher. In elderly or aged patients it is usually a secondary osteosarcoma, arising as the result of irradiation or in the presence of Paget's osteitis deformans (p. 102). Local trauma cannot be made responsible for the appearance of an osteosarcoma, but it may be the cause of one being discovered. The tumor develops below the cortex or in the center of the bone, and produces local destruction. All regions of the bone (spongiosa, marrow cavity, cortex, periosteum, and the surrounding soft parts) are affected. In the periosteum a peculiar kind of bone deposition takes place.

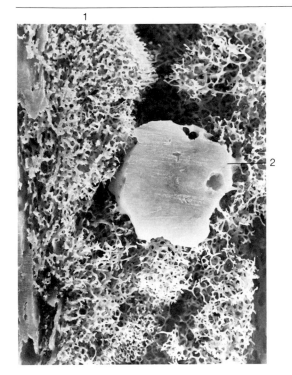

Fig. 506. "Bone island", (maceration specimen)

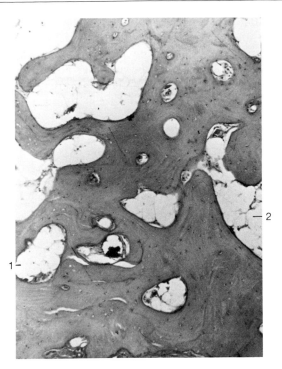

Fig. 507. "Bone island"; HE, ×25

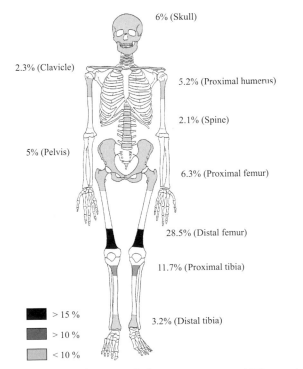

6% (Skull)

2.3% (Clavicle)

5.2% (Proximal humerus)

2.1% (Spine)

5% (Pelvis)

6.3% (Proximal femur)

28.5% (Distal femur)

11.7% (Proximal tibia)

3.2% (Distal tibia)

> 15 %
> 10 %
< 10 %

Fig. 508. Localization of the osteosarcomas (656 cases); others: 29.7%

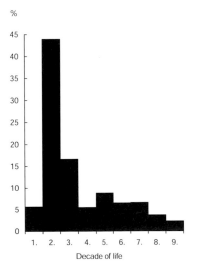

Fig. 509. Age distribution of the osteosarcomas (656 cases)

Radiologically we distinguish between osteoblastic and osteolytic osteosarcomas, in one of which new bone deposition predominates, and in the other bone destruction. The radiograph is nevertheless not pathognomonic, even if it is practically always possible to guess that malignant tumor growth is present. In about 64% of cases the radiograph allows one to assume that it is probably an osteosarcoma. **Figure 510** shows a **radiograph** (tomogram) of an *osteoblastic osteosarcoma* of the distal femoral metaphysis. One can recognize an extensive increase in sclerotic density in the marrow cavity of the metaphysis that reaches as far as the adjacent diaphysis, without the proximal border of the tumor being restrained. In the distal direction the tumor extends as far as the cartilaginous epiphyseal plate *(1)*, which has, however, not been penetrated. This is entirely typical; the epiphyseal plate seems to form a barrier against the extension of the neoplasm from the metaphysis into the epiphysis, which cannot be passed until an advanced late stage of the tumor growth has been reached. In the metaphysis *(2)* the sclerosis is at its most dense; more proximally, irregular coarse patches of osteolysis are very marked in the tumor *(3)*. The cortex has been included in the tumor and has been broken through in a number of places *(4)*. The periosteum is here and there greatly thickened *(5)*, and radially orientated so-called *spicules* can be recognized. Here we have reactive periosteal bone deposition which is often to be seen in the neighborhood of an osteosarcoma (p. 163). In one place a so-called *Codman's triangle (6)* is observable, in which reactive periosteal new bone that contains no tumor tissue is being laid down. A biopsy taken from this region would therefore be useless.

Figure 511 is a **macroscopic example** of an osteoblastic osteosarcoma. The distal femoral metaphysis has been completely taken up by very densely ossified tumor tissue *(1)* which reaches right up as far as the cartilaginous epiphyseal plate *(2)*. The epiphysis is free from tumor tissue *(3)*. The tumor extends through the medullary cavity a long way in a proximal direction, as far as the edge of the amputation *(4)*. In the metadiaphyseal region there are osteolytic foci with hemorrhages *(5)* in the tumor. The neoplasm has broken through the cortex in a number of places. The periosteum is greatly thickened and in parts ossified. With regard to the amputation, which, together with chemotherapy, is the only effective treatment for such an osteosarcoma, the level of the amputation (which must be above the end of the intramedullary extension) is one factor which must be taken into account, the other factor being the exclusion of so-called **skip metastases**. These are early intramedullary metastases in the marrow cavity of the shaft which are said to occur in one out of every four long bone osteosarcomas. Tomograms and, in particular, scintigraphy, can locate skip lesions.

With *osteolytic osteosarcomas* the local bone destruction is the most prominent feature, as against which only a small amount of tumorous bone is formed. As can be seen in the **radiograph** of such a tumor in the head of the fibula (**Fig. 512**), the bone is widely destroyed. There are moth-eaten osteolytic foci in the spongiosa and cortex *(1)*. Indistinctly seen, the epiphysis *(2)* is separated from the diaphysis *(3)*. There is a pathological fracture running through the bone *(4)*, the ends of which are displaced. The tumor has broken through the cortex and invaded the adjacent soft parts, in which patches of cloudy shadowing can be seen. The spreading of the tumor distally within the narrow cavity can only with difficulty be assessed in the radiograph.

The resected specimen from the fibula appears **macroscopically** in **Fig. 513** as a large fleshy tumor that has destroyed the proximal metaphysis and greatly expanded the bone. The tumor tissue has largely fallen to pieces, and is soaked in blood. There are very soft, slightly crushed tumorous masses in which no ossification can be detected. The cortex is destroyed in several places *(1)*, and the tumor has grown out into the adjacent soft parts *(2)*. Macroscopically it is not possible to recognize any tumor tissue in the nearby marrow cavity *(3)*.

A **histological characteristic** of an osteosarcoma is the chessboard-like distribution of tumorous osteoid, bone and cartilage (sometimes together with the structures typical of a hemangiopericytoma, an osteoclastoma, a Ewing sarcoma or an aneurysmal bony cyst) in the middle of a sarcomatous stroma. To this are added multinucleated giant cells, collagen fibrils, fibrous bone, areas of mucinous degeneration, hemorrhages and irregular calcification. The morphological picture is thus extremely variable and can cause

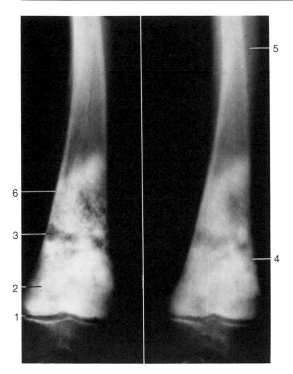

Fig. 510. Osteoblastic osteosarcoma
(distal femoral metaphysis, tomogram)

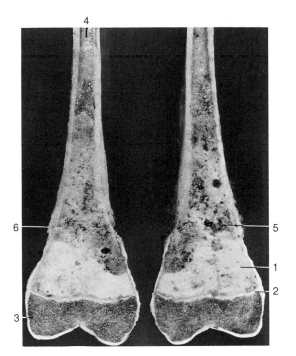

Fig. 511. Osteoblastic osteosarcoma
(distal femoral metaphysis, cut surface)

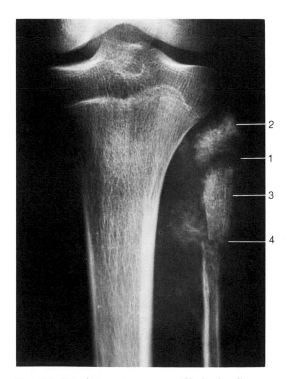

Fig. 512. Osteolytic osteosarcoma (fibular head)

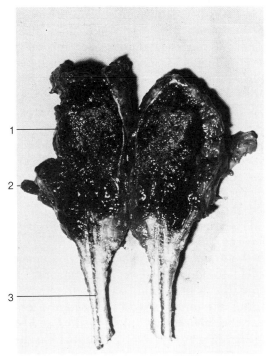

Fig. 513. Osteolytic osteosarcoma (fibular head, cut surface)

great diagnostic difficulty. The tumorous osteoid and tumorous bone arise directly in the sarcomatous connective tissue. The development of osteoid distinguishes an osteosarcoma histologically from a chondrosarcoma.

Figure 514 shows the typical **histological picture** of an *osteoblastic sarcoma*. One can recognize several autochthonous bone trabeculae *(1)* with their laminated layering. The osteocytes are small and some of the osteocyte lacunae are empty. In the marrow cavity between these trabeculae lies the malignant neoplastic tissue. One can recognize a sarcomatous stroma *(2)* with numerous spindle cells and their polymorphic and hyperchromatic nuclei. Many bizarre mitoses can also be seen here. The stroma is penetrated by a few fine-walled dilated capillaries *(3)*. In addition, one recognizes numerous osteoid *(4)* and tumorous bone trabeculae *(5)* which have very bizarre shapes and contain polymorphic osteocytes. In one place one can see a focus of tumorous cartilage *(6)*. The tumor osteoid, which is characteristic of an osteosarcoma, shows various degrees of calcification, and this is reflected in the radiograph.

As can be seen in the **histological picture** of **Fig. 515**, the osteoid structures can predominate in the tumor, while the sarcomatous stroma *(1)* is only sparsely present. For the most part it is a matter of uncalcified osteoid *(2)*, which in section shows a homogeneous pinkish-red color. In part, however, the osteoid is irregularly calcified and thus builds up a disorganized network *(3)*. Once again one is struck by the many deposited cells with their hyperchromatic and polymorphic nuclei *(4)*. In places, irregular tumorous bone trabeculae have been formed *(5)*. The tumorous tissue has been threaded through by several fine-walled capillaries *(6)*. Occasionally, isolated giant cells appear between the osteoid structures.

With the *osteolytic sarcoma* the development of calcified tumorous osteoid and bone rather fades into the background, so that the radiograph gives the impression of a destructive osteolysis. The **histological picture** in **Fig. 516** shows a highly cellular tumor tissue that has almost completely destroyed the original spongiosa. In one place there is still an autochthonous bone trabecula *(1)* that is laminated and contains a few small osteocytes. Nevertheless, this trabecula has a jagged and undulating border,

which indicates the destructive activity of the tumor. The tumor tissue displays an uneven network of tumorous osteoid *(2)* within the sarcomatous stroma with its numerous polymorphic nucleated and hyperchromatic osteoblasts – the true tumor cells. The tumorous osteoid sometimes forms coarse homogeneous plaques *(3)*. The tumor is penetrated by many blood capillaries *(4)*, and hemorrhages, hemosiderin deposits and necroses can be observed. The tumor cells frequently reveal pathological mitosis.

Under **higher magnification** (**Fig. 517**) one can see that there are fully undifferentiated tumor cells in the osteolytic osteosarcoma. In one place there is a calcified autochthonous bone trabecula *(1)*. The marrow cavity is filled up with tumorous tissue in which unequal groups of irregularly distributed small tumor cells are present. These have polymorphic and strongly hyperchromatic nuclei *(2)*. Between these loosely deposited tumor cells there is a fine network of collagenous connective tissue. One can, however, recognize broad-surfaced deposits of osteoid *(3)*, which are a product of the tumor cells. It can sometimes be very difficult to identify these osteoid structures in a highly cellular osteolytic osteosarcoma, and here Goldner staining can be helpful. Included in the osteoid areas there are many large "osteocytes" *(4)* with shapeless nuclei.

In very rare cases **multicentric osteosarcomas** have been reported, with several foci appearing simultaneously in different parts of the skeleton, without there being any evidence of lung metastases. In the *synchronous form* (Type I of AMSTUTZ) the osteosarcomatous foci lie symmetrically in the metaphyses of the long bones; they are radiodense and histologically of the osteoblastic type. Children and young people are affected. With the *metachronic form* (Type III of AMSTUTZ), foci of varying size lie asymmetrically in the skeleton and are osteolytic. Young people and adults are affected. With a multifocal osteosarcoma the question arises as to whether this is a peculiar form of the tumor or whether we are dealing with metastases.

The effective *treatment* of osteosarcomas consists of radical surgical removal of the growth (amputation, disarticulation). Radiotherapy alone is not effective and is only indicated as a palliative measure. Early irradiation can severely hinder the bioptic diagnosis.

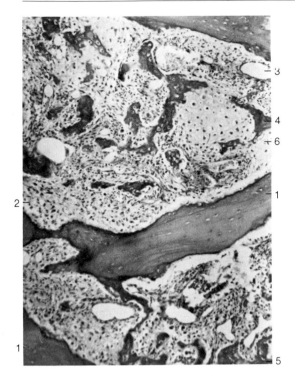

Fig. 514. Osteoblastic osteosarcoma; HE, ×25

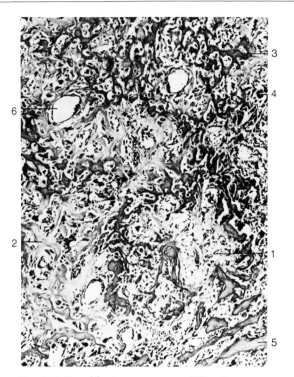

Fig. 515. Osteoblastic osteosarcoma HE, ×40

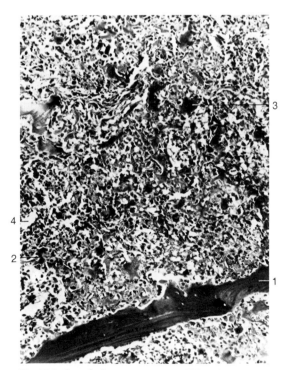

Fig. 516. Osteolytic osteosarcoma; HE, ×40

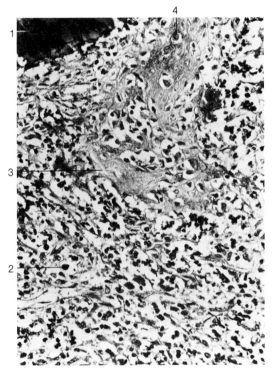

Fig. 517. Osteolytic osteosarcoma; HE, ×64

Nowadays osteosarcomas are treated in accordance with the so-called *COSS Protocol* ("cooperative osteosarcoma study") with chemotherapy (p. 306).

Telangiectatic Osteosarcoma (ICD-O-DA-M-9183/3)

Depending on the predominant structures found histologically in the tumor tissue, osteosarcomas can be subdivided into particular types. *Fibroblastic osteomas* have a relatively good prognosis – better than that of the *chondroblastic osteosarcomas*. The worst prognosis is that of the *osteoblastic osteosarcoma*. The above characterization indicates the broad morphological spectrum covered by these neoplasms. *The telangiectatic osteosarcoma is a destructive primary osteolytic bone neoplasm that contains numerous distended blood vessels and aneurysmic spaces, but only a little tumorous osteoid and bone. It is in the highest degree malignant.* Aneurysmal bony cyst structures (p. 412), numerous osteoclastic giant cells and extensive necroses can make the diagnosis very difficult. Cells with polymorphic nuclei and many pathological mitoses reveal the highly malignant character of this neoplasm, the prognosis of which is indeed extremely bad.

In **Fig. 518** one can see the **radiograph** (angiogram) of a telangiectatic osteosarcoma in the distal femoral metaphysis. In the lateral view one can observe in the anterior part of the tubular bone a roundish osteolytic zone *(1)* that is joined on to a wide sclerotic layer in the marrow cavity. The cortex is locally completely destroyed *(2)* and the tumor has pushed itself out into the adjacent soft parts like a hernia *(3)*, the boundaries of which are only with difficulty distinguishable. This radiological appearance is very similar to that of an aneurysmal bony cyst (p. 413). In the periphery of the angiogram the vessels are not only displaced by the extraosseous parts of the tumor, there are also vessels following an abnormal course with bends and bifurcations *(4)* which suggest the growth of a malignant neoplasm.

In **Fig. 519** one can see a **macroscopic picture** of the stump of a femur with a telangiectatic osteosarcoma. This tumor had developed in the distal femoral epiphysis and was removed by thigh amputation. However, the neoplasm had extended proximally through the marrow cavity above the level of the saw cut into apparently healthy tissue, and had therefore been incompletely extirpated. At the end of the stump one can see spongy blood-soaked tumorous tissue *(1)* that has broken away from the bone. It

has bulged forward below the periosteum *(2)*, resulting in a large parosteal tumor *(3)*. The cut surface reveals a spongy tissue with numerous blood-filled cavities which can give rise to uncontrollable hemorrhage. At the sawn surface of the bone one can see that the entire marrow cavity is infiltrated with partially compact pieces of tumor. The periosteum is elevated over a wide area *(4)*.

Histologically one can recognize very highly cellular tumorous tissue (**Fig. 520**), in which the large blood-filled cavities *(1)* are striking. It is highly reminiscent of an aneurysmal bone cyst (p. 417). Numerous osteoclastic giant cells *(2)* lie in the loose, mostly blood-soaked connective tissue walls of the cyst. The nuclei are markedly hyperchromatic and polymorphic *(3)* and many abnormal mitoses can also be observed. Extensive necroses can make the histological diagnosis much more difficult, but they nevertheless suggest malignancy.

In the greater part of this neoplasm there are no osteoid structures to be seen, nor indeed any tumorous bone, so that here the diagnosis of an osteosarcoma cannot be made. **Figure 521** shows a **histological section** from a telangiectatic osteosarcoma, where with Azan staining osteoid deposits can be recognized within the highly cellular tumorous tissue *(1)*. The true tumorous tissue consists of a sponge with collections of densely packed vessels *(2)* that are stuffed full of blood. Extravasation is frequent. Unequally distributed osteoclastic giant cells *(3)* are strewn about the tumorous tissue in large numbers. The hyperchromasia of the nuclei is very clear. If no osteoid structures can be identified, a telangiectatic osteosarcoma is often misdiagnosed as an aggressive aneurysmal bony cyst. Delayed diagnosis does indeed contribute to the poor prognosis of this tumor.

Previously existing observations and reports show that the telangiectatic osteosarcoma presents as a peculiar form of neoplasm. Radiologically it suggests rapidly growing osteolysis, which could signify an aneurysmal bony cyst or an osteoclastoma. Clinically, the uncontrollable hemorrhage which follows curettage is striking. The histological picture is often difficult to interpret. The prognosis is very bad and the patient's survival frequently less than a year.

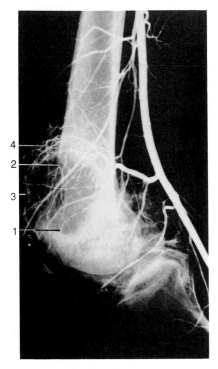

Fig. 518. Telangiectatic osteosarcoma (distal femoral metaphysis, angiogram)

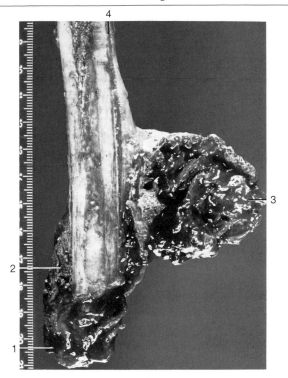

Fig. 519. Telangiectatic osteosarcoma (femoral stump, cut surface)

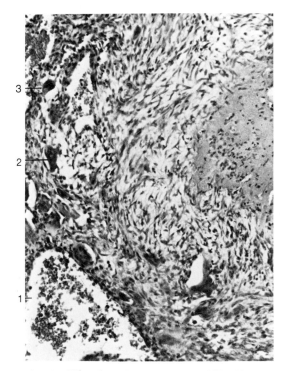

Fig. 520. Telangiectatic osteosarcoma; HE, ×40

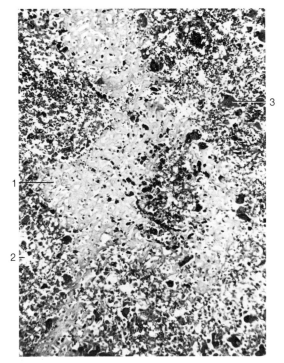

Fig. 521. Telangiectatic osteosarcoma, Azan, ×30

The **radiological findings** of a typical telangiectatic osteosarcoma in the proximal part of the left humerus is shown in **Fig. 522.** Inside the bone there are numerous patchy areas of osteolysis *(1)* which have involved both spongiosa and cortex. The changed area is not clearly delineated. The periosteum *(2)* is raised up from within, thickened and dark. The radiological findings indicate malignancy. The region resected en bloc is shown **macroscopically** in **Fig. 523.** It consists of blood-soaked sponge-like tumorous tissue *(1)* lying within the bone, and it has also involved and destroyed the cortex *(2)*. The tumor can be seen reaching down to the cut edge of the specimen *(3)*.

Figure 524 is a **radiograph** of the left knee seen in lateral view. The marked balloon-like elevation of the patella *(1)* with its unclear outer contour is striking. This bone has extended proximally far beyond the distal part of the femur *(2)* and is in general considerably expanded. Within the patella there are a few trabecular septa *(3)* which give a polycystic appearance to the lesion. **Macroscopically** the patella is seen to be enlarged. In the section shown in **Fig. 525** one can see internally a large zone of osteolysis *(1)* with is filled with blood clots *(2)*. The surrounding but still intact cancellous bone tissue *(3)* is soaked with blood. The patella is surrounded by connective tissue *(4)* which varies in thickness. The appearance of a malignant bone tumor in the patella is extremely rare, since such lesions in this region are quite exceptional. However, as the following histological pictures show, this is indeed a telangiectatic osteosarcoma.

We can observe in **Fig. 526** a very highly cellular and mixed **histological picture** that is threaded through with dilated blood-filled vessels *(1)*. There is a loose sarcomatous stroma *(2)* that contains spindle-cells, the nuclei of which are polymorphic with abnormal mitoses. There are wide, delicate tumorous osteoid trabeculae *(3)* where very many osteoblasts with giant nuclei *(4)* and osteoclasts have been deposited. Under **higher magnification** the picture with its polymorphic cells shown in **Fig. 527** is more clearly observed. Here one can see in the sarcomatous stroma the polymorphic spindle cells *(1)*, the irregular deposition of tumorous osteoid *(2)* and the many multinucleated giant cells *(3)*. The numerous dilated blood vessels *(4)* penetrating the sarcomatous stroma are also characteristic of this tumor.

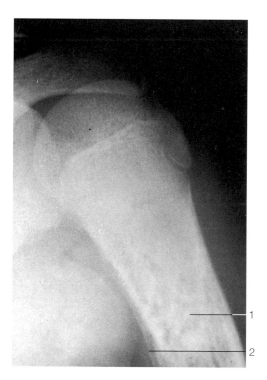

Fig. 522. Telangiectatic osteosarcoma (left proximal humerus)

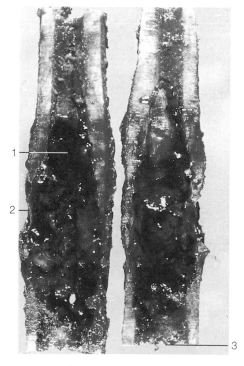

Fig. 523. Telangiectatic osteosarcoma (humerus, cut surface)

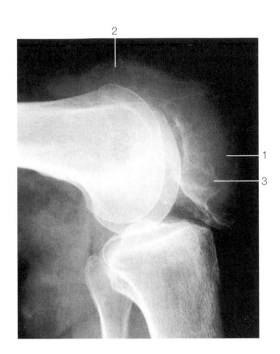

Fig. 524. Telangiectatic osteosarcoma (left patella)

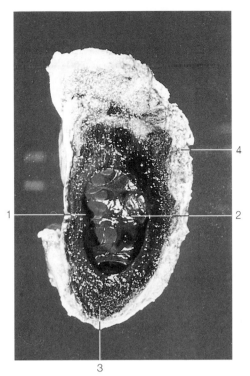

Fig. 525. Telangiectatic osteosarcoma (patella, cut surface)

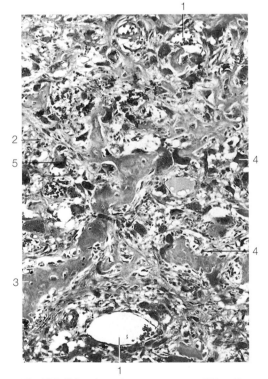

Fig. 526. Telangiectatic osteosarcoma; HE, ×40

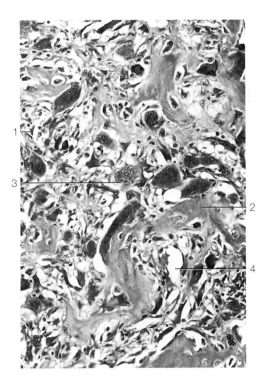

Fig. 527. Telangiectatic osteosarcoma; HE, ×64

Small Cell Osteosarcoma

In rare cases the histological picture of an osteosarcoma may present with a dense accumulation of small roundish tumor cells, which is at first glance reminiscent of a Ewing's sarcoma (p. 352). *This is a neoplasm consisting predominantly of small polymorphic tumor cells with round nuclei. Only scanty deposits of tomorous osteoid are present.* Histologically the tumor also looks like a chondroblastoma (p. 226), a reticular cell sarcoma (p. 358) or a bone metastasis (p. 399). Decisive for the diagnosis of a small cell osteosarcoma is the presence of tumorous osteoid. In **Fig. 529** one can see the **radiograph** of such a tumor in the distal part of the left femur. In the lateral view one sees a large central zone of osteolysis *(1)* which is lying in the transitional region between the diaphysis and metaphysis. The lesion is sharply delineated and contains streaky areas of increased density *(2)*.

Histologically the tissue of the tumor consists almost exclusively of a loose accumulation of round cells. In **Fig. 530** one can see such tumorous tissue with round cells which possess small, highly polymorphic and hyperchromatic nuclei *(1)*. With PAS staining these cells are seen to be rich in glycogen, making one think of a Ewing's sarcoma (p. 357). However, within the tumor there are also deposits of osteoid *(2)* to be seen, which is not the case with a Ewing's sarcoma. These structures lead to the diagnosis of a small cell osteosarcoma. The stroma, throughout which small tumor cells are strewn, is threaded through with dilated blood capillaries *(3)*. This tumor can appear in sites not typical for sarcomas (e.g. in the diaphysis of a long bone). It has a worse prognosis than the ordinary osteosarcoma.

Epithelioid Osteosarcoma

Osteosarcomas present a very mixed histological picture that is bioptically difficult to interpret. This tumor has an enormously wide spectrum of tissue differentiation. *An epithelioid osteosarcoma is characterized by a pseudoepithelial differentiation of the tumor cells and is highly malignant.* It has so far only been observed in children. One can see the **radiograph** of such a tumor in **Fig. 528**. In the distal part of the radius there is a large area of patchy osteolysis *(1)* that is not sharply delineated and reaches up into the diaphysis. The cortex *(2)* is also porotic and osteolytic. Here and there one can see dense sclerotic regions *(3)* within the tumor that are set through with small patches of osteolysis.

In the **histological picture** there are only a few areas of sarcomatous stroma with deposits of tumorous osteoid and bone, which indicate the presence of an osteosarcoma. As is shown in **Fig. 531**, there are large complexes of differentiated epithelioid cells *(1)* present. These groups of cells are packed right up against dilated blood vessels *(2)*. Sometimes invasion of the tumor cells into these vessels can be observed. A sarcomatous stroma *(3)* with polymorphic spindle-cells is only poorly developed. It contains nothing but discrete deposits of tumorous osteoid. Under **higher magnification** the epithelioid nature of the tumor cells is obvious. In **Fig. 532** one can see large groups of tumor cells with polymorphic and hyperchromatic nuclei *(1)*. Abnormal mitoses can also be observed here. The cell borders are indistinct. Penetrating capillaries *(2)* are present in large numbers. Tumorous osteoid, on the other hand, is extremely sparsely represented.

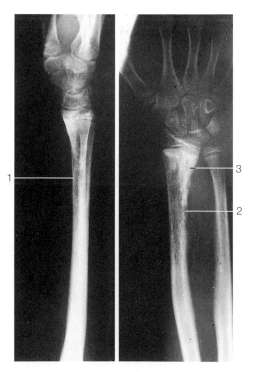

Fig. 528. Epithelioid osteosarcoma (distal radius)

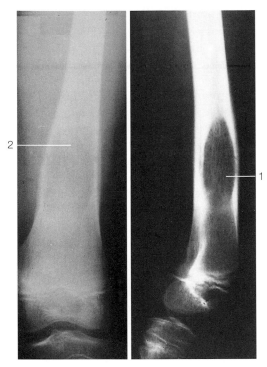

Fig. 529. Small cell osteosarcoma (left distal femur)

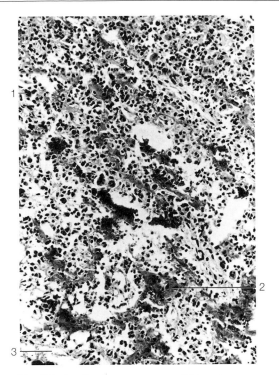

Fig. 530. Small cell osteosarcoma; PAS, ×40

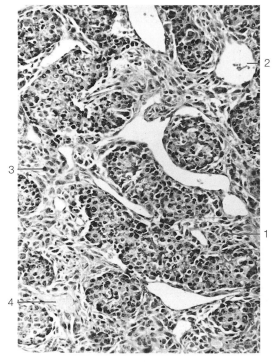

Fig. 531. Epithelioid osteosarcoma; HE, ×64

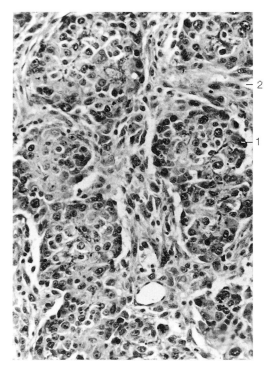

Fig. 532. Epithelioid osteosarcoma; HE, ×100

Intraosseous Well-Differentiated Osteosarcoma

The intraosseous well-differentiated osteosarcoma is a primary bone tumor of connective and bony tissue with only minimally abnormal cells and sometimes highly differentiated tumorous cartilage that nevertheless undergoes malignant growth. As in the case of the parosteal osteosarcoma (p. 288), the diagnosis can only be made in combination with the radiographic appearance. The tumor can appear in children and young people, but also at greater ages (age: 10–65 years). There is a peak in the third decade of life. Clinically there is a painful swelling that develops over the course of years. Most of these tumors are found in the proximal part of the tibia or the distal part of the femur.

The **radiograph** shows tumorous destruction of bone. In **Fig. 533** one can see such a lesion in the proximal part of the tibia. There are irregular regions of dense sclerosis *(1)*, and between them fine and coarse osteolytic areas *(2)*. The cortex is narrowed from within *(3)* and frequently destroyed. When the cortex is penetrated, reactive periostitis ossificans may develop, and the tumor may give rise to shadows outside the bone. In children, the epiphysis is not involved, but in adults it is infiltrated by the tumor as far as the articular surface.

Macroscopically the tumor is sharply marked off from the adjacent bone and soft parts. In **Fig. 534** one can see such a growth in the distal part of the femur. On the cut surface there is an ivory-hard grayish-white tumorous tissue within the bone *(1)*. Plug-like *(2)*, widely spread *(3)* infiltrations have invaded the epiphysis. The cortex has been broken through *(4)*, and broad masses of tumor are reaching out into the adjacent soft parts *(5)*. Dark necroses and grayish-white osteoblastic areas are visible.

Histologically the tumor consists predominantly of an irregular dense network of shapeless woven bony trabeculae *(1)* on which massive osteocytes have been deposited, but no osteoblasts or osteoclasts. In **Fig. 535** one can see a loose connective tissue stroma *(2)* between the trabeculae, throughout which small cells with hyperchromatic nuclei are sparsely distributed. Foci and patches of hyalinization are found in the stroma *(3)*. In general we have here the picture of a monomorphic tissue that does not at first sight appear to be malignant.

However, within the stroma there are deposits of tumorous osteoid *(4)*. In **Fig. 536** one can see on the one hand the loose connective tissue stroma *(1)* with a few polymorphs and cells with dark nuclei, while on the other, there are deposits of tumorous osteoid *(2)* and bone *(3)*.

Under higher magnification one can see in **Fig. 537** the connective tissue stroma *(1)* between the tumorous bone trabeculae *(2)*. This shows narrow spindle-shaped cells that only occasionally possess hyperchromatic nuclei *(3)*. There is moderate nuclear polymorphy, and mitoses are infrequent or even absent. However, one finds partly trabecular, partly patchy deposits of osteoid *(4)*, and this is tumorous osteoid. In rare cases cartilaginous foci can be encountered in such a tumor, the cells of which show only minimal abnormality.

In making a **differential diagnosis,** it is first necessary to distinguish between fibrous bone dysplasia (p. 318) and an intraosseous well-differentiated osteosarcoma. In a desmoplastic fibroma (p. 322) no deposits of tumorous osteoid are found. A typical osteoblastoma (p. 264) shows a marked proliferation of osteoblasts, which is not the case with an intraosseous well-differentiated osteosarcoma. Since this tumor has a low grade of malignancy, an en bloc resection through the healthy tissue is sufficient, but with incomplete extirpation of the growth, recurrence may be expected. However, this tumor does not usually metastasize.

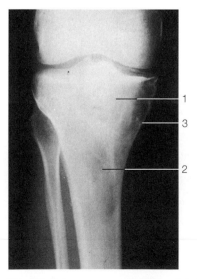

Fig. 533. Intraosseous well-differentiated osteosarcoma (proximal tibia)

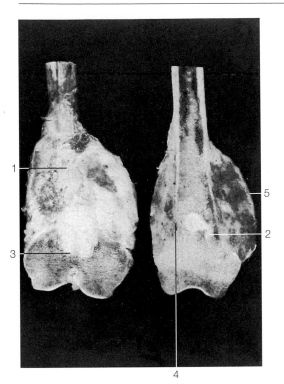

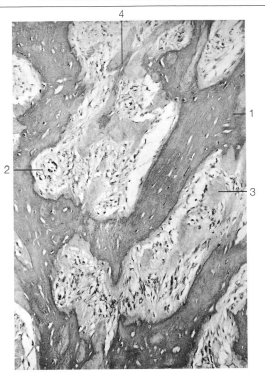

Fig. 534. Intraosseous well-differentiated osteosarcoma (distal femur, cut surface)

Fig. 535. Intraosseous well-differentiated osteosarcoma; HE, ×40

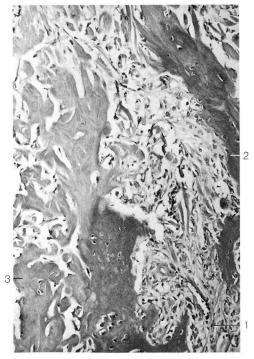

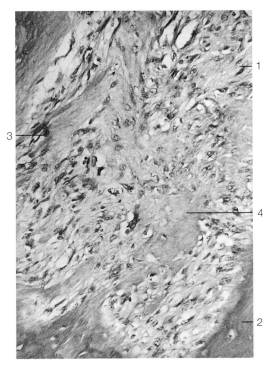

Fig. 536. Intraosseous well-differentiated osteosarcoma; HE, ×84

Fig. 537. Intraosseous well-differentiated osteosarcoma; HE, ×84

Parosteal Osteosarcoma (ICD-O-DA-M-9190/3)

The parosteal or juxtacortical osteosarcoma is a malignant bone tumor that develops in the periosteal or parosteal soft parts, and which contains fibroblastic, osteoblastic or even chondroblastic structures. It is a very rare neoplasm, making up less than 1% of all bone sarcomas. Its main localization is in the popliteal fossa, where large masses of dense tumorous tissue usually grip the distal part of the femur closely from behind. Unlike the intraosseous osteosarcomas, it is a neoplasm with a low grade of malignancy, although it is true that there is a strong tendency towards local recurrence. However, distant blood-borne metastases are rare and late in appearing. In **Fig. 538** the **course of growth** of a parosteal osteosarcoma is followed for a period of 18 years. The primary neoplasm was at first removed. Three years later there was a serious recurrence, and it was again excised. A second recurrence was shelled out 5 years later. When it recurred for the third time 18 years after its first appearance, amputation was undertaken, and this achieved a cure which lasted for more than 10 years. This tumor attacks predominantly the distal part of the femur and the proximal parts of the tibia and humerus.

The diagnosis is based essentially on the **radiological picture**, and less on the histological or anatomical findings. In **Fig. 539** one can see a parosteal osteosarcoma of the distal femoral metaphysis. In the lateral view, the solid, very dense shadow of a bony mass appears to clasp the femur from outside and from behind *(1)*. The tumor reaches from the epiphysis to the diaphysis, leaving a narrow space *(2)* between it

and the cortex. In one place, however, the tumor appears to have broken into the marrow cavity *(3)*. Its outer contour is lobulated and nodular, and reveals a few trabecular structures *(1)*. There is no Codman's triangle.

In the sawn femur depicted in **Fig. 540** one can see the mass of the tumor **macroscopically**, where it has pushed its way out of the periosteum *(1)* and has encased the tubular bone. The periosteum *(2)* is intact and acts as a partition between the tumor and the cortex. Outside, bone trabeculae can be recognized within the tumor *(3)*. There is no tumorous tissue in the marrow cavity.

As can be seen in the **histological picture** shown in **Fig. 541**, parosteal osteosarcomas usually consist of a highly differentiated tissue formed from bone trabeculae with loose connective tissue between them. This does not immediately suggest the malignant character of this neoplasm. We can see an irregular network of shapeless bone trabeculae *(1)* with many extensive reversal lines *(2)*, osteocyte lacunae *(3)* and osteocytes. The intraosseous connective tissue *(4)* contains small isomorphic fibroblasts and fibrocytes.

The newly developed bone trabeculae *(1)* are arranged in arcades, sometimes with seams of osteoblasts *(2)* (**Fig. 542**). Even under **higher magnification** the intermediate stroma is seen to contain few polymorphic cells, or none at all. One recognizes spindle-shaped, somewhat hyperchromatic connective tissue nuclei *(3)* which show no mitoses. A few dilated capillaries *(4)* are present. In the recurrent tumor there is mostly a more marked polymorphy of cells and nuclei, which does then suggest malignancy.

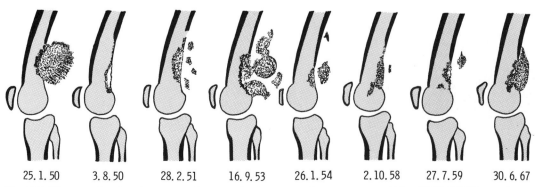

25. 1. 50   3. 8. 50   28. 2. 51   16. 9. 53   26. 1. 54   2. 10. 58   27. 7. 59   30. 6. 67

Fig. 538. Diagram showing the progressive growth of a parosteal osteosarcoma. (After UEHLINGER 1977)

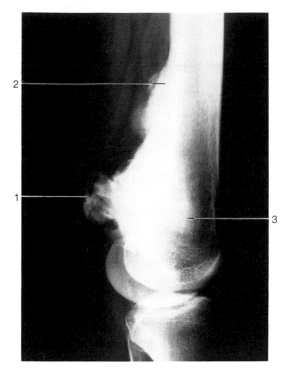

Fig. 539. Parosteal osteosarcoma
(distal femoral metaphysis)

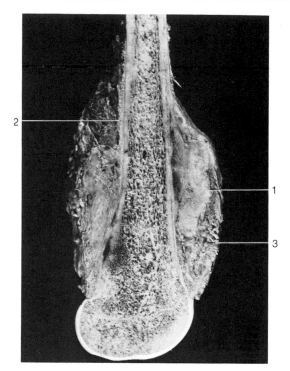

Fig. 540. Parosteal osteosarcoma (distal femur, cut surface)

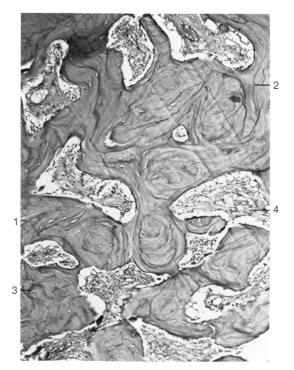

Fig. 541. Parosteal osteosarcoma; HE, ×25

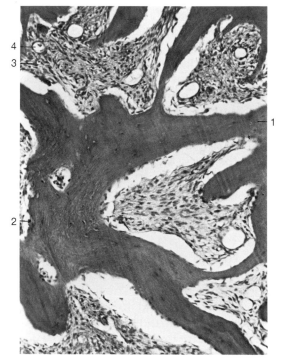

Fig. 542. Parosteal osteosarcoma; HE, ×40

Figure 543 shows a lateral **radiograph** of a parosteal osteosarcoma. A wide, mass of tumor is lying against the dorsal surface of the distal part of the femur *(1)*. The outer layer of the tumorous tissue is markedly lobulated *(2)*. The tumor is radiologically very dense, with a few irregular translucent areas. The shadow of the tumor reaches diffusely into the femur itself *(3)*, without, however, showing any signs of true invasion of the bone. The parosteal osteosarcoma is wrapped around the long bone from outside, so that part of it is projected onto the radiograph as if it lay inside the bone. Between the parosteal mass of the tumor and the cortex of the femur *(4)* it is possible to recognize a narrow, indistinct translucent strip *(5)* that is highly characteristic of a parosteal osteosarcoma. Invasion of the bone by the tumor can only be confirmed by computer tomographic radiography (CT) or magnetic resonance tomography (MRT). This kind of radiological imaging should without exception be carried out in the case of such a tumor, since the prognosis gets worse once it has invaded the bone. In this case radical treatment (possibly amputation) becomes necessary. There is no periosteal reaction, and a Codman's triangle has not appeared. With such radiological findings it must be established whether there is an intraosseous osteosarcoma that has broken outwards into the soft parts, or whether the tumor arose outside the bone and has now secondarily invaded it. Both the treatment and prognosis depend upon this knowledge.

Histologically it is mostly not possible to establish the diagnosis of a parosteal osteosarcoma with sufficient certainty if the radiographs are not available. As can be seen in **Fig. 544**, the biopsy material shows only unevenly developed bony tissue with shapeless bone trabeculae that vary in width *(1)*, and which reveal no lamellar layering, although small isomorphic osteocytes are present. They are covered with loose rows of osteoblasts *(2)*. The bone trabeculae are plaited together to form an irregular network. In between them lies a connective tissue stroma, where sparsely cellular areas *(3)* coexist with those having a rich cellular content *(4)*. These cells are fibroblasts which show no particular signs of polymorphy. Calcified focal deposits *(5)* are sometimes seen in the stroma, but typical tumorous osteoid (as found in os-

teosarcomas) is not, however, present. Even the bone trabeculae, which with their varying density appear as more or less dark shadows in the radiograph, look more like regenerating bone than tumorous bone. Only their irregular organization, at least in parts of the tumor, suggest that this is a parosteal osteosarcoma.

Under **higher magnification** one can see in **Fig. 545** that the tumorous bone trabeculae *(1)* often run parallel to one another. The typical network of tumorous bone trabeculae such as are found in an intraosseous osteosarcoma are not present. The trabeculae are extremely heavily calcified, so that the lamellar layering is no longer be recognizable. Only occasional osteoblasts *(2)* have been deposited. Between the trabeculae there is a loose connective tissue stroma, set through with granulation tissue *(3)*, where cells with round nuclei predominate, and a few spindle cells are present. There is no sarcomatous stroma. Such tissue as this could equally well conform diagnostically to a case of periostitis ossificans.

Occasional undifferentiated spindle-cells can be seen in the tumor under **higher magnification**. In **Fig. 546** the connective tissue stroma between the trabeculae *(1)* is striking in that it consists of spindle cells, and here one finds occasional spindle-cells with hyperchromatic and suspiciously polymorphic nuclei *(2)*. Mitoses are rare or completely absent. The trabeculae *(3)* are awkwardly shaped and are covered by only a few osteoblasts *(4)*. This means that a parosteal osteosarcoma can only be diagnosed histologically if the radiograph is also taken into account.

We are dealing here with an osteosarcoma of very low malignancy, with a 5 year survival rate of 80%. A 10 year survival rate of 55% has been reported. With small tumors it is sufficient to carry out a local en bloc excision through healthy tissue. With large tumors, and particularly if they have invaded the bone, amputation is necessary. In either case, complete surgical extirpation of the tumor can lead to a cure. If the removal is incomplete, recurrences appear again and again and can finally lead to lung metastases and death. The radiological differential diagnosis of such a tumor must take into account an osteochondroma (p. 214), proliferating myositis ossificans (p. 478) and an extraosseous osteosarcoma (p. 482).

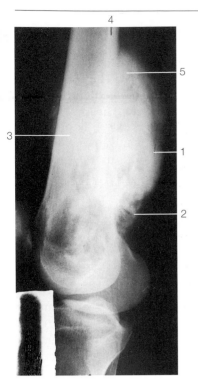

Fig. 543. Parosteal osteosarcoma (distal femur)

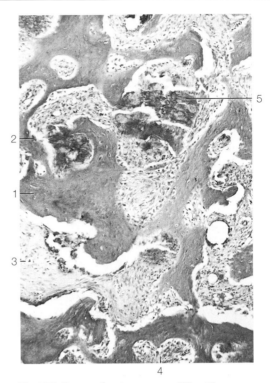

Fig. 544. Parosteal osteosarcoma; HE, ×40

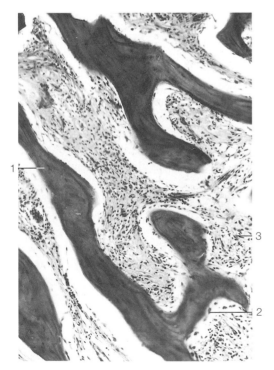

Fig. 545. Parosteal osteosarcoma; HE, ×64

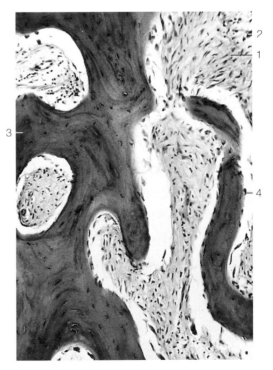

Fig. 546. Parosteal osteosarcoma; HE, ×84

Periosteal Osteosarcoma

Osteosarcomas that arise in the parosteal tissue and are therefore extraosseous in origin are frequently described as "juxtacortical osteosarcomas". The parosteal osteosarcoma (p. 288), for instance, belongs to this category. In addition to these, however, there are other malignant osteogenic tumors that run a variable course, have a variable prognosis and present a variable histological picture. Since each of these tumors requires a different therapeutic approach, it follows that they must be distinguished one from the other with particular care. *The periosteal osteosarcoma is a malignant bone tumor which obviously arises in the periosteum. As well as osteosarcomatous structures it develops predominantly chondrosarcomatous structures and infiltrates the cortex from without, thus indicating a high grade of malignancy.* This osteosarcoma differs therefore from the parosteal osteosarcoma (p. 288). It is a rare bone tumor, making up less than 1% of all osteosarcomas. The main localization is in the tibia or femur, where it mostly appears above or below the region of the metaphyses or even in the middle of the shaft. Very rarely it may be found in the proximal part of the humerus or in the iliac bone. Men are rather more frequently affected than women. The patients are somewhat older than those with conventional osteosarcomas.

Figure 547 depicts the **radiograph** of a periosteal osteosarcoma of the tibial shaft. A focus of osteolytic destruction (1) is in contact with the outside of the bone. It shows coarse patchy areas of densification and appears to have disintegrated into clumps. The lesion extends beyond the border of the bone into the soft parts on one side, while on the other side it has created wide inlets into the cortex (2). Distally a Codman's triangle (3) can be clearly seen. However, the tumor has not invaded the marrow cavity.

The growth process of a periosteal osteosarcoma is clearly discernible in the **macroscopic specimen.** Such a tumor in the distal part of the femoral shaft can be seen in **Fig. 548.** The femur and the tumor have been sawn through, and one is looking at the cut surface. The tumor (1) is lying up against the outside of the bone and bulging into the soft parts. The cut surface (2) has a glassy grayish appearance and looks like cartilage. The tumorous tissue is suspiciously nodular, and small white foci of calcification (3) can be recognized. The tissue in the center of the tumor (4) is necrotic and loosely cystic. The cortex of the femur (5) is completely intact, and no tumorous tissue is detectable in the marrow cavity (6). Outwardly the tumor is sharply demarcated. No infiltrating growth of the tumor into the neighboring tissues can be confirmed.

Histologically a periosteal osteosarcoma consists of tissue that has undergone relatively little differentiation. It is composed of tumorous cartilage, tumorous osteoid and sarcomatous stroma, all of which may vary in both amount and extent. Usually it is the tumorous cartilage which predominates. In **Fig. 549** one can see shallow, widespread cartilaginous tumor tissue (1), containing highly polymorphic cartilage cells, some with small (2) and some with large dark (3) nuclei. The nuclei are highly hyperchromatic, but mitoses are rare. Within the tumorous cartilage one often finds foci of calcification (4). In the neighborhood one can see a highly cellular sarcomatous stroma (5) that has been penetrated by a few blood capillaries (6). Here, discrete deposits of osteoid are also recognizable (7). Such tumorous osteoid is mostly to be found in the center of the cartilaginous tumorous nodes.

In **Fig. 550** the tumorous cartilage from a periosteal osteosarcoma is depicted **histologically** under higher magnification. In the middle of a loose basophilic myxoid matrix one can see cartilage cells of varying sizes with polymorphic nuclei. A few nuclei (1) are large, angular and hyperchromatic. They lie in swollen cells. Usually there are no mitoses present. In the tumorous cartilage there are large and small foci of calcification (2) that have been broken open by the sectioning. If this kind of malignant cartilaginous tissue is exclusively present in a juxtacortical tumor without any signs of osteoid, we must classify the tumor as a periosteal chondrosarcoma (p. 252). Here the prognosis is significantly better than that of a periosteal osteosarcoma. An exact and reliable classification is only possible after comprehensive reappraisal and histological examination of the whole of the tumor material.

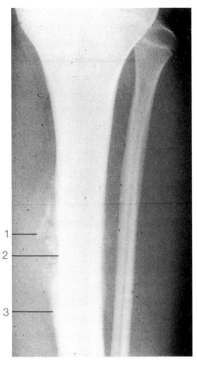

Fig. 547. Periosteal osteosarcoma (tibial shaft)

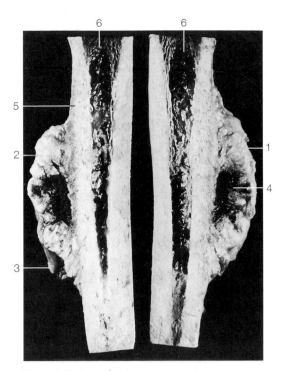

Fig. 548. Periosteal osteosarcoma
(femoral shaft, cut surface)

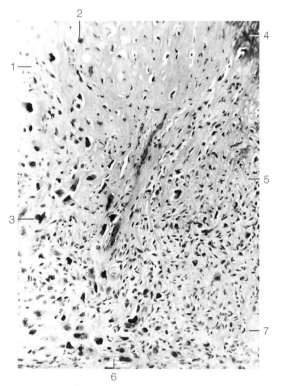

Fig. 549. Periosteal osteosarcoma; HE, ×64

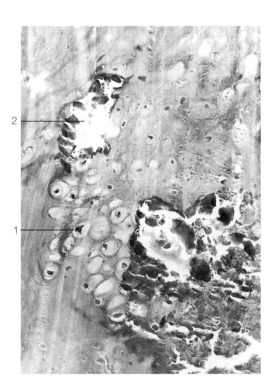

Fig. 550. Periosteal osteosarcoma; HE, ×100

Figure 551 shows a **radiograph** of the proximal part of the leg with a tumorous layer spread widely over the anterior surface of the tibial shaft *(1)* where spicules *(2)* are clearly discernible in the periosteum. A Codman's triangle *(3)* is also present. Within this periosteal shadow there are patchy regions of translucency. The cortex is intact and there is no invasion of the marrow cavity *(4)* by the tumor.

A **maceration specimen** of a periosteal osteosarcoma can be seen in **Fig. 552**. In the proximal part of the humerus there is a wide mass of deeply fissured tumor tissue *(1)* surrounding the bone like a mantle *(2)*. Externally it is lobulated and jagged and it is partly fused with the cortex *(3)*. The cortex *(4)* is, however, intact, and the tumor has not broken into the marrow cavity.

As can be seen in the **histological picture** in **Fig. 553**, the greater part of the tumor consists of cartilaginous tissue which is lobulated in form. One can recognize nests of polymorphic cartilage cells *(1)* with dark polymorphic nuclei. Cells with two nuclei are often present *(2)*. This cartilaginous tissue is identical with that of a chondrosarcoma (p. 241). It sends out tongue-shaped processes into the neighborhood *(3)*. In between there is a sarcomatous stroma *(4)* with dark polymorphic spindle-cells, in which pathological mitoses may be present.

In other parts of a periosteal osteosarcoma one may, however, see the classical **histological**

structure of an osteosarcoma. In **Fig. 554** there is a sarcomatous stroma *(1)* with polymorphic spindle-cells, penetrated by a few vessels *(2)*. Inside one can see a tangled network of osteoid deposits *(3)*. This tumorous osteoid is enclosed by tumorous osteoblasts *(4)* with dark polymorphic nuclei. Such structures in a juxtacortical sarcoma indicate the diagnosis of a periosteal osteosarcoma. In contradistinction to the parosteal sarcoma (p. 291) there is a very definite cellular and nuclear polymorphy with a morphological picture already suggesting a high degree of malignancy.

As shown in the **histological picture** of **Fig. 555**, other regions of the tumor show a malignant fibrous stroma *(1)* in which lie numerous polymorphic and hyperchromatic spindle-cells *(2)* which may show mitoses. Under **higher magnification** one can see in **Fig. 556** the very pronounced polymorphy. The nuclei are exceedingly hyperchromatic *(1)*, and there are many giant nuclei *(2)* and even multinucleate giant cells *(3)* present. Between these tumor cells there is a network of tumorous osteoid *(4)*.

With regard to treatment, the tumor must without question be completely extirpated, together with some healthy tissue. With small lesions this may be achieved by a local en bloc excision, but with larger tumors amputation is necessary. Adjuvant chemotherapy is to be recommended. The prognosis is better than with

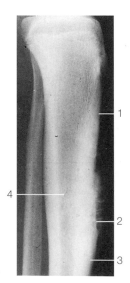

Fig. 551. Periosteal osteosarcoma (proximal tibia)

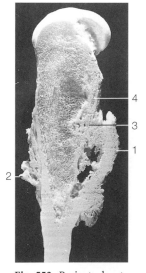

Fig. 552. Periosteal osteosarcoma (proximal humerus, maceration specimen)

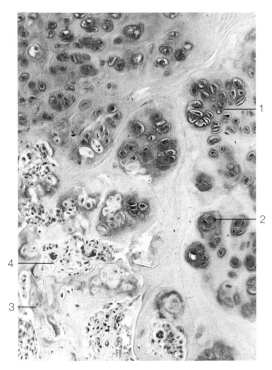

Fig. 553. Periosteal osteosarcoma; HE, ×64

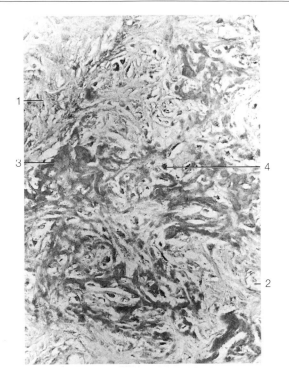

Fig. 554. Periosteal osteosarcoma; van Gieson, ×64

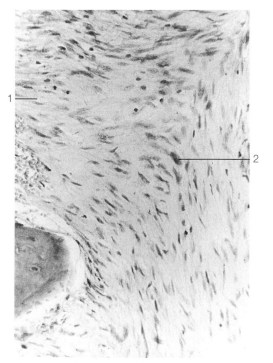

Fig. 555. Periosteal osteosarcoma; HE, ×84

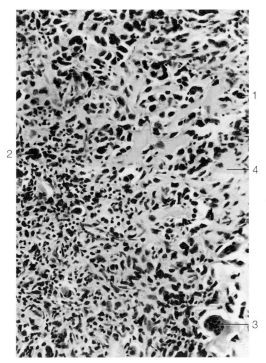

Fig. 556. Periosteal osteosarcoma; PAS, ×84

intraosseous sarcomas, although significantly worse than that of the parosteal osteosarcoma. For these reasons the different varieties of osteosarcoma must be diagnostically identified.

High-Grade Surface Osteosarcoma

This malignant bone tumor arises on the surface of a bone and is characterized by its extremely high degree of malignancy. It is a rare malignant bone neoplasm, making up less than 1% of the osteosarcomas, and has only recently been described as a separate entity. It appears predominantly in the distal part of the femur, and can show great radiological similarity to a parosteal (p. 288) or periosteal (p. 292) osteosarcoma. It can, however, also attack other bones.

In **Fig. 558** one can see the **radiograph** of a high-grade surface osteosarcoma in the proximal part of the right fibula. The periosteum *(1)* is irregular thickened over a considerable distance, and has an undulating outer contour. The underlying bone shows a discrete sclerotic increase in density *(2)*. Such a radiological picture makes one think more of chronic osteomyelitis (p. 138) with reactive periostitis ossificans than of a highly malignant bone tumor, especially since no bone destruction can be seen. In the **detailed radiograph** of such a tumor on the shaft of the humerus – shown in **Fig. 557** – one can see the destructive growth more clearly. The periosteum *(1)* is markedly thickened and contains straggly, spicule-like *(2)* densifications. The Codman's triangle is obvious *(3)*. The adjacent long bone *(4)* appears to be lightly eroded from outside. In the neighboring soft parts numerous dense patchy regions can be seen *(5)*. This proliferatively active tumor expands in all directions and even infiltrates the cortex of the nearby bone. As **Fig. 559** makes clear, the tumorous growth can be easily recognized **macroscopically**. Here we are looking at such a surface osteosarcoma on the frontal face of the distal part of the femur *(1)*. It has bulged far into the soft tissues and appears to be sharply demarcated. The cut surface consists of grayish-white, bone-hard tumorous tissue which has infiltrated the entire cortex *(2)*. The density of the spongiosa *(3)* in this region seems to have sclerotically increased, although there is no actual macroscopic indication that the tumor has invaded the inside of the bone. In this case only a histological examination can provide further information.

Histologically highly undifferentiated tumorous tissue can be seen. In **Fig. 560** one recognizes numerous tumor cells with dark nuclei that vary greatly in size *(1)* and which show a high degree of polymorphy. Many of them have large dark nucleoli *(2)*, and frequent pathological mitoses can also be seen. Between these undifferentiated spindle-cells there lies a disorganized network of tumorous osteoid *(3)*. Necrotic foci are also often encountered, and the polymorphic-cellular tumorous tissue is penetrated by a few capillaries *(4)*. The fibro-osseous trabeculae seen in a parosteal osteosarcoma (p. 291) are absent, and hardly any tumorous bone trabeculae have differentiated out. Even the tumorous cartilaginous tissue found in periosteal osteosarcomas (p. 295) is not present. In this way the tumor fundamentally differs histologically from other juxtacortical osteosarcomas.

Under **higher magnification** one can recognize in **Fig. 561** the extensive deposits of tumorous osteoid *(1)*. Between these there are abundant polymorphic spindle-cells *(2)* with shapeless dark nuclei *(3)*. The prognosis of a high-grade surface osteosarcoma is the same as that of a highly malignant intramedullary osteosarcoma. For this reason, amputation with supplementary chemotherapy is indicated. According to the reports so far available, the average life expectation is only about 1–2 years.

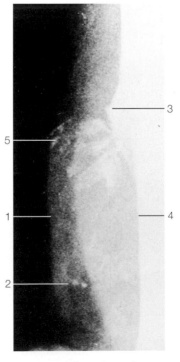

Fig. 557. High-grade surface osteosarcoma (humeral shaft)

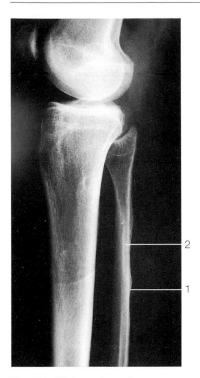

Fig. 558. High-grade surface osteosarcoma (proximal fibula)

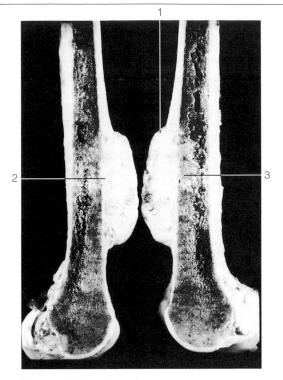

Fig. 559. High-grade surface osteosarcoma (distal femur, cut surface)

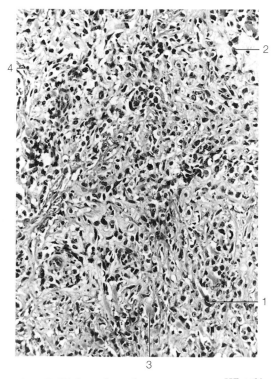

Fig. 560. High-grade surface osteosarcoma; HE, ×64

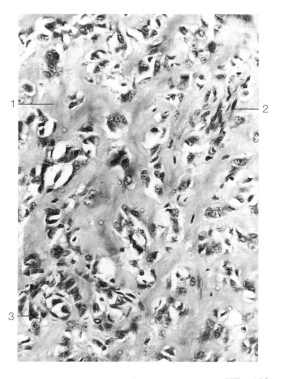

Fig. 561. High-grade surface osteosarcoma; HE, ×100

Paget's Osteosarcoma (ICD-O-DA-M-9184/3)

About 2% of cases of Paget's osteitis deformans (p. 102) develop into an osteosarcoma. This is an osteoblastic osteosarcoma that arises from the underlying condition, mostly during the 6th or 7th decade of life and more commonly in men than in women. The tumor is most often seen in the pelvis, humerus or femur, or in the spinal column or skull cap. Those bones are involved in which Paget's disease is most likely to occur. The continual remodeling must be regarded as preneoplastic. The latent period between the beginning of Paget's disease and the outbreak of the sarcoma lies between 8 and 10 years. An osteosarcoma, fibrosarcoma, chondrosarcoma or a giant cell sarcoma may develop. A Paget's osteosarcoma has an extremely bad prognosis, and a life expectation of 5 years is hardly to be expected.

In the **radiograph** the sarcomatous change is for a long time masked by the existing Paget transformation. In **Fig. 562** one can see the typical spongy bone remodeling of Paget's osteitis deformans, with the lamellar exfoliation of the cortex, in the olecranon (1), the adjacent part of the ulna (2) and in the distal part of the humerus (3). In the olecranon there is a striking zone of osteolysis (4) that has attacked the cortex. This kind of additional destruction gives rise to the suspicion of sarcomatous change, and must be investigated bioptically.

In **Fig. 563** one can see in the **radiograph** an enormous Paget remodeling of the distal part of the humerus (1), with honeycomb-like structures in the spongiosa and cortex. Following a pathological fracture a plate (2) had been inserted for stabilization. Later, a tumorous elevation of the bone developed at the original fracture site (3), which has brought about severe osteolytic destruction of the bone. Spongiosa and cortex have been completely destroyed. One can see a few straggly patches of densification which extend far into the adjacent soft parts. This is an indication of a malignant tumor.

The amputation specimen shown in **Fig. 564** shows a large tumor that has **macroscopically** taken in the whole of the distal part of the humerus and extended deep into the surrounding parts (1). In some places this is covered over by connective tissue (2), in others it has broken through this barrier and one can see tumorous

tissue flakes like fish flesh (3) with hemorrhages and necroses.

The **histological picture** of a Paget's osteosarcoma is practically identical to that of an osteosarcoma that is unrelated to a "Paget bone", although one can also recognize the bone remodeling of Paget's disease. In **Fig. 565** a Paget's osteosarcoma is again depicted. The very distorted bone trabeculae with their irregular undulating borders are striking (1). They show the mosaic structure of the reversal lines (2) which is characteristic of Paget's osteitis deformans. Osteoblasts and osteoclasts that are still active are seldom found in a Paget's osteosarcoma. The connective tissue between the bony structures contains fewer blood vessels; it consists of a sarcomatous stroma in which numerous irregular trabeculae of tumorous osteoid (3) have developed. Osteoid structures of this sort do not belong in the picture of a "Paget bone" and must awake the suspicion of a malignant change. Under **higher magnification** one can see in **Fig. 566** a few autochthonous trabeculae (1) which show the mosaic structure of Paget's disease. In the stroma there is a tangled framework of osteoid trabeculae (2) upon which osteoblasts have been deposited.

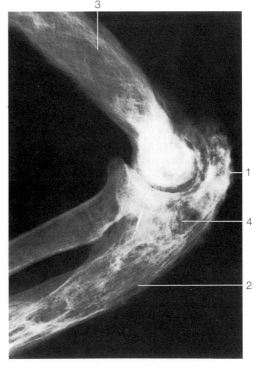

Fig. 562. Paget osteosarcoma (olecranon)

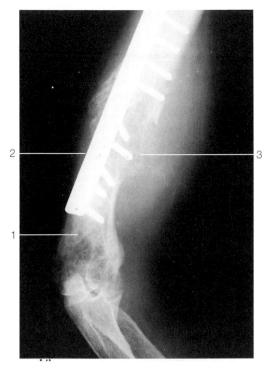

Fig. 563. Paget osteosarcoma
(following pathological fracture, distal humerus)

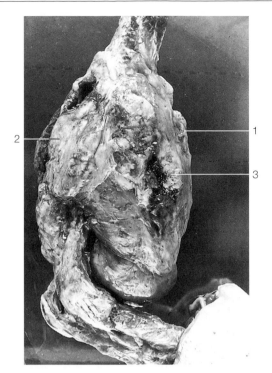

Fig. 564. Paget osteosarcoma (distal humerus)

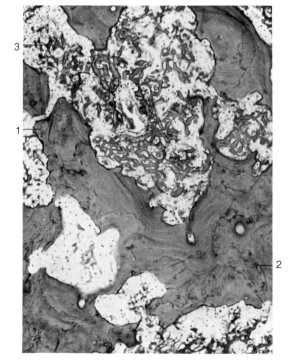

Fig. 565. Paget osteosarcoma; HE, ×40

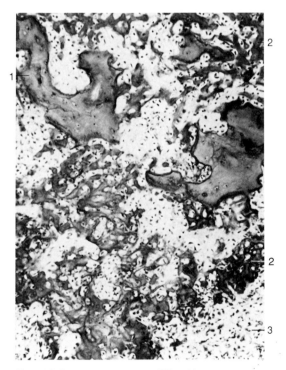

Fig. 566. Paget osteosarcoma; HE, ×64

Postradiation Osteosarcoma (ICD-O-DA-M-9180/3)

When one takes into account the frequency with which bones and soft tissues are irradiated, postradiation osteosarcomas are comparatively rare. The frequency is about 0.03% of all previously irradiated cases. In 60% of the sarcomas it is an osteosarcoma which develops, but fibrosarcomas (30%), chondrosarcomas (10%) and other malignant bony neoplasms can also arise. *Mostly it is a predominantly osteoblastic osteosarcoma that develops somewhere in a bone that has been subjected to at least 30 Gy.* The time-span between the exposure to radiation and the appearance of the tumor is variable, and can be anything between 4 and 43 years. However, even shorter latent periods have also been described.

A typical **radiological** finding can be seen in **Fig. 567**. Eight years after the irradiation of a gynecological carcinoma, a 55-year-old woman complained of pain in the left side of the pelvis. The radiograph shows a very dense sclerotic area *(1)* in the left iliac bone, close to the sacrum. The left sacroiliac suture *(2)* is intact. The dense shadow of the tumor has extended over the iliac crest into the left paravertebral soft tissues *(3)*. In **Fig. 568** it is **radiologically** clear that the highly osteosclerotic tumor has occupied a large part of the ala of the left iliac bone *(1)*, and that its borders are indistinct. The upper part of the iliac crest *(2)* is feathery and has been penetrated by the tumor. Here the left sacroiliac suture *(3)* is no longer visible, and the tumor seems to have invaded the vertebral column *(4)*.

In the **radiograph** (tomogram) shown in **Fig. 569** one can see that the sternal end of the left *(1)* clavicle is very densely osteosclerotic. In the tomogram the outer contours of this part of the bone are undulating and irregular. The articular surface of the left sternoclavicular joint is intact and can be seen. This is the case of a 16-year-old girl who had been irradiated in this region 6 years earlier because of Hodgkin's disease.

The **histological picture** of a postradiation osteosarcoma cannot be distinguished from that of a genuine osteosarcoma, although extensive radioosteonecroses (p. 178) can sometimes be confirmed many years after radiotherapy. In **Fig. 570** one can see a sarcomatous stroma *(1)* in which the nuclei are clearly hyperchromatic

and show a considerable degree of polymorphy *(2)*. Numerous pathological mitoses can be observed. Flattish and trabecular osteoid structures have been deposited *(3)* which are characteristic of osteosarcomas. Within these osteoid structures there are also polymorphic cells with shapeless hyperchromatic nuclei. One can also recognize foci of tumorous cartilage *(4)*, which are also polymorphic and have hyperchromatic nuclei. From this sort of histological picture alone it is not possible to conclude that the lesion is due to previous irradiation. This can only be obtained from the case history.

Under **higher magnification** the highly polymorphic nature of the tumorous tissue is more clearly seen. In **Fig. 571** the tumor cells show a high degree of polymorphy and have dark nuclei *(1)*. In between, one can discern a network of tumorous osteoid *(2)* that is calcified in places *(3)*. A few dilated capillaries *(4)* are running through the tumorous tissue. Postradiation osteosarcomas grow quickly, their local growth is rapid and hematogenous metastases appear early. They have a strong tendency to recur. A strong indication is therefore required to justify either the direct or indirect irradiation of a

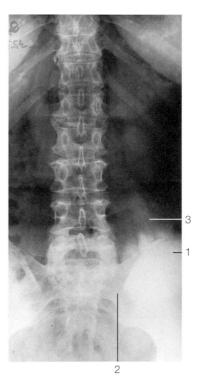

Fig. 567. Postradiation osteosarcoma (left iliac ala)

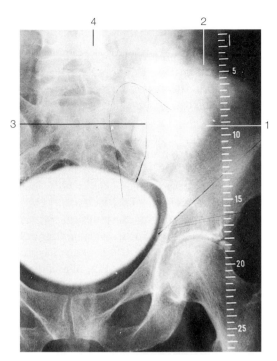

Fig. 568. Postradiation osteosarcoma (left iliac ala)

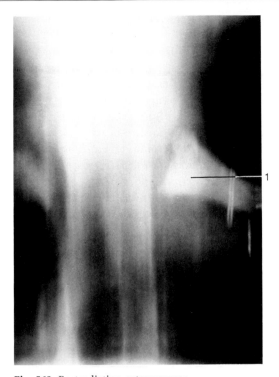

Fig. 569. Postradiation osteosarcoma
(left clavicle, tomogram)

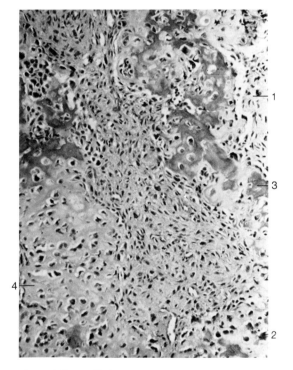

Fig. 570. Postradiation osteosarcoma; HE, ×40

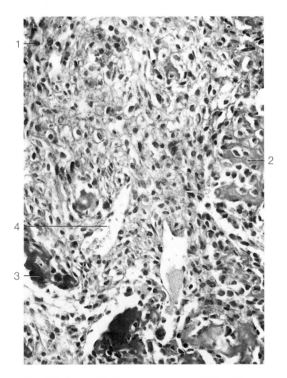

Fig. 571. Postradiation osteosarcoma; HE, ×64

bone, and it must be carried out with great care and with modern techniques, in order to avoid irradiation damage and the possible appearance of a postradiation osteosarcoma.

Bone Sarcomas in Bone Infarcts

A particularly serious complication of an anemic bone infarct (p. 174) is the secondary development of a malignant bone tumor. It can be imagined that the lengthy process of reparation which takes place in a bone infarct is an important factor in the pathogenesis of this kind of sarcoma. *This is a secondary malignant bony neoplasm that arises at the site of an existing anemic bone infarct.* Malignant fibrous histiocytomas, fibrosarcomas and osteosarcomas have all been observed in association with this condition. The risk of a sarcoma developing is greatest with those bone infarcts that have a large medullary component. Local pain, enlargement of the area of the infarct and an increase of activity in the scintigram suggest that a sarcoma may be developing.

In **Fig. 572** one can see the **histological picture** of a typical anemic bone infarct without any malignant tumorous tissue. The fatty marrow has been replaced by loose connective tissue *(1)*, in which hardly any intact nuclei are present. One area *(2)* is more strongly fibrosed and lightly calcified outside. There is an adjacent necrotic bone trabecula *(3)* without any osteocytes. These calcified structures appear on the radiograph as patchy densifications in a circumscribed infarct.

In the **radiograph** of the distal part of the right femur shown in **Fig. 573**, one can recognize uneven bone remodeling in the distal metaphysis. There is a large, dense intramedullary focus *(1)* which corresponds to a bone infarct. This focus is indistinctly demarcated. The surrounding bony tissue shows extensive patchy destruction with coarse regions of increased density *(2)* and coarse areas of osteolysis *(3)*. This process has also involved the cortex *(4)*. Such a radiological picture suggests the presence of a malignant tumor.

The **histological picture** of a bone biopsy reveals the classical appearance of a fibrosarcoma. In **Fig. 574** one can see highly cellular tumorous tissue with polymorphic spindle-cells that have dark, polymorphic nuclei *(1)*. In addition to the roundish nuclei *(2)* there are some that are elongated *(3)* and also often dark giant nuclei *(4)*. Markedly abnormal mitoses are also usually present. There is a comb-like pattern of tissue with longitudinally orientated spindle-cells *(5)* that have produced collagen fibers, and in the immediate neighborhood *(6)* other spindle-cells run in a different direction (the so-called "herring-bone pattern").

The **radiograph** in **Fig. 575** shows a large destructive lesion in the proximal part of the femur. In the center there is a large area of osteolysis *(1)* which is patchy in appearance and indistinctly bordered. In the distal part there is a more loosely sclerotic area *(2)* which is part of the original infarct. The lesion is bordered by a wide region of osteosclerosis *(3)*, which has also involved the cortex. This sclerotic zone also shows signs of patchy destruction *(4)*. A radiograph like this indicates malignant growth.

Histologically the lesion in **Fig. 576** shows both the morphology of the original bony infarct *(1)* and that of a sarcoma *(2)*. In the marrow cavity one can see necrotic fatty tissue *(1)* without any cells. The bone trabeculae *(3)* are also necrotic and no longer contain osteocytes. In the center there is a sarcomatous stroma *(2)* with polymorphic spindle-cells. Peripherally, there is a tangled network of tumorous osteoid trabeculae *(4)*, indicating a secondary osteosar-

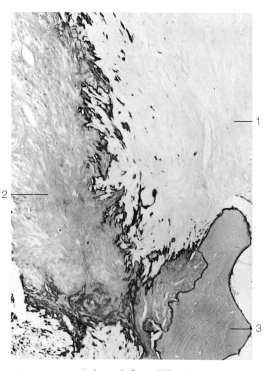

Fig. 572. Anemic bone infarct; HE, ×64

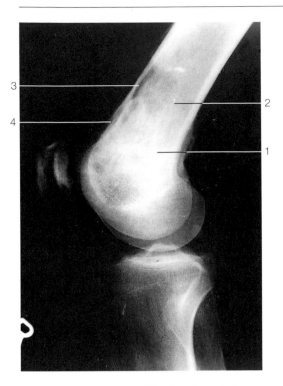

Fig. 573. Bone sarcoma arising in a bone infarct (right distal femur)

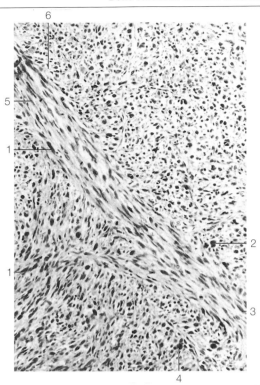

Fig. 574. Secondary fibrosarcoma in a previous bone infarct; HE, ×64

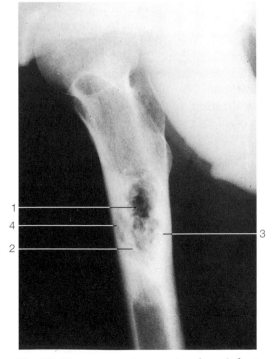

Fig. 575. Bone sarcoma in a previous bone infarct (proximal femur)

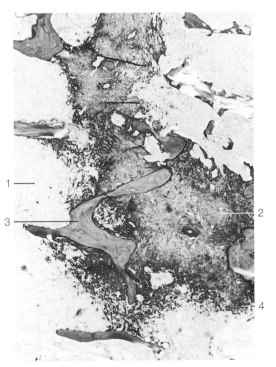

Fig. 576. Secondary osteosarcoma in a previous bone infarct; HE, ×40

coma. A bone sarcoma like this develops after about 10–15 years, particularly in patients with multiple bone infarcts. One has to say, however, that the development of such a sarcoma in these cases is somewhat uncommon.

The secondary sarcoma which arises at the site of a bone infarct is most usually a **malignant fibrous histiocytoma**. Of these tumors, 0.6% develop in the region of a bone infarct. In **Fig. 577** one can see the **macroscopic appearance** of one of these tumors in the distal part of the femur. On the sawn surface one can see a grayish-white map-like area *(1)* which represents the old anemic bone infarct. The spongiosa in the surrounding tissue is locally grayish-red and rather faded *(2)*. This is tumorous tissue, which reaches proximally into the shaft of the femur *(3)*. In one place the cortex has been infiltrated and broken through *(4)*. The malignant tumorous tissue has spread out into the parosteal soft tissue *(5)* and come to rest as a large neoplastic mass *(5)*. At the site of the original biopsy *(6)* an intraosseous hematoma has appeared.

In the **histological picture** there is highly cellular, obviously malignant tumorous tissue. In **Fig. 578** this tissue consists exclusively of densely packed histiocytes *(1)* with dark, variously sized, polymorphic nuclei *(2)*. The cells have an extensive cytoplasm which is in places pale, in places eosinophilic, and in which phagocytosed particles can sometimes be stored. There are focal deposits of infiltrating lymphocytes *(3)*. A few dilated capillaries *(4)* have also penetrated the tumorous tissue. Within this tissue, only isolated collagen fibers are visible, whereas other histiocytomas have a dense concentration of collagen fibers forming a storiform pattern (p. 329). Pathological mitoses may also be observed in the tumor cells. Around the edges there are a few newly developed fibrous bone trabeculae *(5)*. Tumorous bony trabeculae or tumorous osteoid which might suggest an osteosarcoma are absent. This kind of morphological picture seen in a bone biopsy would suggest the diagnosis of a malignant fibrous histiocytoma. In an amputation specimen the histological structures seen in a bone infarct must be present in order to confirm the origin of the sarcoma in such a lesion. The prognosis of a malignant fibrous histiocytoma is not influenced by the antecedent infarct. Bone sarco-

mas with this etiology can appear at any age, though mostly in older patients. The main localization is in the region of the knee, and particularly in the distal part of the femur. Those patients with a sickle-cell anemia, who often have several bone infarcts, are particularly predisposed towards secondary sarcomas. Treatment must be directed against each individual bone sarcoma. Amputation is usually necessary, or at least complete extirpation of the tumor. With a secondary osteosarcoma supplementary chemotherapy is also indicated.

Osseous bone tumors arise directly from the bone tissue, and are characterized by mature and immature bone and also by osteoid. Immature bone tissue consists of fibro-osseous trabeculae (as found, for instance, in an ossifying bone fibroma, p. 316), in which the connective tissue stroma predominates and justifies our classifying this tumor as a connective tissue bone tumor. In an osteoma (p. 256) there is practically only fully mature and mineralized bone tissue present: either cortical (osteoma eburneum) or cancellous (osteoma spongiosum). Trabecular or even more extensive deposition of tumorous osteoid is characteristic of an osteoid osteoma (p. 260) or an osteoblastoma (p. 264). Altogether there are 16 different varieties of osseous bone tumors, some of which (e.g. the bone island, p. 274) are either "tumor-like lesions" or could be classified under "local skeletal dysplasia".

The **localization** of these tumors inside the bone is completely variable and arbitrary. Osteomas, osteoid osteomas and osteoblastomas can appear in diaphyses, metaphyses or epiphyses. The osteoid frequently develops in the cortex ("cortical" osteoid osteoma, p. 260). Most primary osteosarcomas, however, are situated in the metaphysis. An ordinary osteosarcoma develops within the bone and infiltrates with destruction of the cortex into the surrounding parts. A particular group of osteosarcomas comprises the so-called **surface osteosarcomas**, which develop on the outer surface of a bone (e.g. the high-grade surface osteosarcomas, p. 296), or take their origin from the periosteum or parosteal soft tissues (periosteal osteosarcoma, p. 292; parosteal osteosarcoma, p. 288). The prognosis of these varies greatly from tumor to tumor (high-grade surface osteosarcoma, relatively "benign" parosteal osteo-

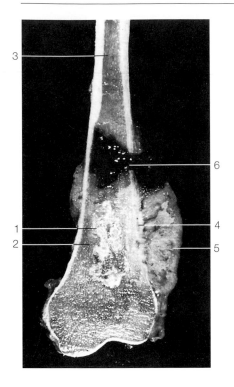

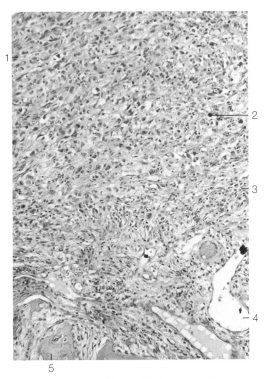

Fig. 577. Malignant fibrous histiocytoma in a bone infarct (distal femur, cut surface)

Fig. 578. Malignant fibrous histiocytoma; HE, ×40

sarcoma) and must be precisely distinguished from one another since the subsequent treatment also differs greatly.

Radiologically we are aware of both osteolytic and osteosclerotic (osteoblastic) tumors, depending on the degree of mineralization. An osteoma eburneum, for instance, presents itself as a very dense focus of bone tissue; an osteoid osteoma (p. 260) and even more so an osteoblastoma (p. 264) shows a central region of translucency. Here, the radiographic density of the tumorous osteoid depends upon the degree of mineralization. Very variable pictures are presented by the different types of osteosarcoma. In osteolytic sarcomas (p. 274) the sarcomatous stroma of the tumorous tissue predominates, and activated osteoclasts have destroyed and broken up the autochthonous bony tissue. In osteoblastic osteosarcomas, on the other hand, massive amounts of osteoid are produced by the osteoblasts, and these are heavily mineralized and strongly absorb radiation. The tumorous cartilage in a chondroblastic osteosarcoma shows fine patchy calcification radiologically, like a chondrosarcoma (p. 236).

Histologically an osteosarcoma can contain extraordinarily variable tumorous tissue, which may be composed of completely different kinds of tissue. In the middle of a sarcomatous stroma with polymorphic nucleated spindle-cells and many pathological mitoses, tissue resembling that of a chondrosarcoma (p. 236), a fibrosarcoma (p. 330), a malignant fibrous histiocytoma (p. 324), an osteoclastoma (p. 337), a hemangiosarcoma (p. 376), a hemangiopericytoma (p. 374), an aneurysmal bone cyst (p. 412) or a Ewing sarcoma (p. 352) can arise. The decisive diagnostic criterion for an osteosarcoma is the presence of tumorous osteoid. This variable and mixed neoplastic picture in an osteosarcoma naturally brings serious diagnostic problems in its wake. If only one kind of tissue is found in a biopsy this leads inevitably to an incorrect histological diagnosis. If, for example, only the structures peculiar to an aneurysmal bone cyst (without unambiguous tumorous osteoid) is found in the biopsy material, the pathologist can do nothing but diagnose an aneurysmal bone cyst. Similarly, if he sees only the structures of a giant cell tumor, the diagnosis is "osteoclastoma". Here it is absolutely essential that he takes empirical factors (e. g. the patient's age in the case of an osteoclastoma is about 30 years, with an osteosarcoma about 20–25 years) and, most important of all, the radiological findings into account (in an osteoclastoma, for instance, there may be extensive osteolysis in the epiphysis; in an osteosarcoma, destruction in the metaphysis).

It can be extremely difficult, even when examining the material removed at operation, to diagnose this kind of tumor correctly. The pathognomonic criteria for the recognition of tumorous osteoid may be minimal (this is often the case in a telangiectatic osteosarcoma, for instance, p. 280). Or else one finds the classical histological picture of an osteoclastoma, with tiny focal deposits of osteoid which may be entirely of a reactive nature. In such cases the pathologist must decide upon one diagnosis or the other, and he may be completely wrong. What is more, the distinction between the various types of osteosarcoma is of great importance for the treatment, which nowadays follows the so-called COSS protocol.

Under the **COSS protocol** ("co-operative osteosarcoma study") the patient, following the diagnosis by biopsy of an osteosarcoma, at first receives chemotherapy (for about 3 months) and then undergoes surgical removal of the tumor (excision or amputation). After that, the specimen removed at operation is histologically examined for the amount of necrotic tumor tissue produced under the influence of the chemotherapy employed (determination of the degree of necrosis). This is to decide whether the tumor tissue has reacted as a "responder" or a "non-responder". If it is a "responder", the same chemotherapy is continued postoperatively as a prophylactic measure against recurrence and possible metastases. In the case of a "non-responder" it is varied in order to avoid metastases.

Fibrous Tissue Bone Tumors

Introductory Remarks

The skeletal system, which develops from mesenchymal tissue, is characterized principally by bone and cartilaginous tissue. In addition, however, there are other differentiated tissues from which neoplasms can also develop. This includes the connective tissue which lies between the trabeculae and lines the Haversian canals. The essential tumor-forming cells are the fibroblasts, which have the ability to produce collagen fibers, that is to say connective tissue, within these tumors. For this reason a connective tissue framework is characteristic of the components of this group of neoplasms. Such tumors predominantly arise in those parts of a bone where the fibromatous elements are ontogenetically differentiated; namely, in the marrow cavity or in the region of the periosteum (see also Fig. 378 and p. 210).

In the classification of bone tumors (Table 3, p. 209) this group of neoplasms present a particular problem, since it is often not possible to decide with any certainty whether one is dealing with a true bone tumor or a reactive bony lesion. The tissue reacts locally or systemically to every conceivable bone lesion with proliferation of the local connective tissue. In the case of a fracture (p. 114) or in the presence of osteomyelitis (p. 129), fiber-rich scar tissue develops during the healing phase, and this can easily give the impression radiologically of a growing tumor. In a case of primary hyperparathyroidism, fibrous tissue is formed in the marrow cavity (p. 80) and a so-called "brown tumor" (Figs. 150–152 and p. 85) may develop. Local malformations of the skeleton be associated with an increase in the connective tissue or of a connective tissue replacement of the local bony tissue. This applies particularly to fibrous bone dysplasia (p. 56). Some of these local connective tissue proliferations are unambiguously reactive in character (e.g. connective tissue fracture callus, osteomyelitic scarring); others can be identified as true neoplasms (a desmoplastic fibroma, p. 322; or a fibrosarcoma, p. 330). The true tumorous nature of a whole range of benign connective tissue bone lesions is, however, controversial and open to question,

particularly as some of them can undergo spontaneous remission. Because of their radiological appearance and their clinical course some of them are included among the "tumor-like bone lesions" (p. 407).

The classical neoplastic type of this group is the "osseous fibroma", of which the fibrosarcoma of bone (p. 330) is the malignant variant. Whereas the latter is undisputably neoplastic in nature, the term "osseous fibroma" covers structurally different variants. If the lesion consists exclusively of a local increase in connective tissue, we speak of a "non-ossifying fibroma" (p. 308); but if many foam cells are also present, it is a "xanthofibroma" (p. 312). With lesions of this kind it is important to determine whether the process arose within the bone, or whether it developed in the periosteal connective tissue and eroded the bone from without. Inside the proliferating connective tissue large numbers of bone trabeculae can differentiate, built up by osteoblasts. We refer then to an "ossifying osseous fibroma" (p. 316). With fibrous bone dysplasia (p. 318) numerous fibro-osseous trabeculae take origin directly from the connective tissue stroma, without any contribution from osteoblasts. It is therefore necessary when confronted by a connective tissue neoplasm of bone to observe what additional products of differentiation are present in order to be able to classify the lesion precisely.

This variable morphological picture is also reflected in the radiological changes projected by the bone. With proliferation of the connective tissue alone, there is an intraosseous osteolytic focus that is often referred to in general as a "bony cyst". With benign lesions it is often surrounded by a reactive marginal sclerosis. The differentiation of mineralized bone trabeculae gives the radiographic representation of the lesion a shadowy internal structure. This may be an almost homogeneous appearance as of frosted glass, involving the whole of the lesion. There may, however, even be fine and coarse patches of densification within the tumor, brought into existence by tumorous bone formation or the deposition of calcium. Finally, we frequently also see trabecular changes in structure which make the lesion appear to be multicamerate.

Non-ossifying Bone Fibroma (ICD-O-DA-M-7494/0)

One of the most frequently occurring bone neoplasms in young people is the non-ossifying bone fibroma. *This is a sharply circumscribed osteolytic defect, which is usually eccentrically situated in the metaphysis of a long bone and which follows an absolutely benign course.* It is frequently recognized by chance, or reveals itself by causing a pathological fracture. The true neoplastic nature of this defect is disputed, since spontaneous remissions are often observed, and surgical treatment is not necessarily indicated. Probably it is more a matter of local disturbance of ossification in the growing region of a bone than a true neoplasm. Histologically the tumor shows a fibro-histiocytic or histiocytic-granulomatous formation, and is therefore often classified under the osseous histiocytomas.

Although the proportion of non-ossifying bone fibromas is about 5% of those benign bone neoplasms seen on the operating table, the true frequency rate is considerably higher and may be nearer 30%, since many cases are not discovered or only observed radiologically, and are therefore not treated.

Localization (Fig. 579). The principle site is in the long bones of the lower limb (femur, tibia, fibula), with far the greater number of neoplasms appearing in the distal femoral metaphysis. The tumor arises immediately adjacent to the epiphyseal plate and shifts with the growth of the skeleton slowly into the metaphysis and neighboring region of the diaphysis. We have also frequently found these tumors in the bones of the jaw and occasionally in the short tubular bones.

Age Distribution (Fig. 580). This lesion is confined almost entirely to the first 3 decades of life, 70% of them appearing during the 2nd decade. Cases detected later than this have probably been there a long time.

The **radiograph** of **Fig. 581** shows a classical non-ossifying bone fibroma in the distal femoral metaphysis. At some distance from the epiphyseal plate *(1)* a cystic zone of osteolysis is lying eccentrically in the metaphysis *(2)*, aligned along the long axis of the bone and with one side adjacent to the cortex. Internally

this focus is sharply bordered by an undulating band of marginal sclerosis *(3)*, so that a typical grape-like configuration is seen. The cortex is narrowed but intact, and there is no periosteal reaction.

Multiple non-ossifying bone fibromas can arise in different bones of the skeleton or even in the same bone. In **Fig. 582** one can see several osteolytic foci in a **radiograph** of the distal part of the femur, both in the region of the metaphysis *(1)* and in the adjacent diaphysis *(2)*. These foci are eccentrically situated in the bone and are sharply bordered by an undulating strip of marginal sclerosis. The cortex in this region is narrowed from within *(3)* and in places the bone is expanded externally *(4)*. The cortex is, however, fully intact and there is no visible periosteal reaction. Within these grape-like osteolytic foci there is some increase in the density of the trabeculae. In the distal part of the femur there is a confluence of several such foci. Such a confluence can be recognized distally *(5)* and similar foci are visible proximally *(6)*. Radiologically one receives the general impression of a benign osteolytic process that can be recognized as a multifocal non-ossifying bone fibroma. With a radiological picture such as this no bioptical investigation or surgical treatment is necessary. There is, however, the danger of a pathological fracture which will require surgical stabilization. During the operation it is usual to remove tumorous tissue for histological examination. The defect is filled up with spongiosa. Spontaneous healing can, however, gradually take place. In rare cases very large non-ossifying bone fibromas can develop which take up the entire width of the shaft and significantly elevate this segment of the long bone. A pathological fracture may even produce a local reactive periostitis ossificans, and the lesion may be demarcated by a broad area of irregular osteosclerosis. Such a radiological appearance may easily give the impression of a malignant bone tumor which must then be investigated by means of an extensive bone biopsy. The usually very characteristic histological appearance of the morphology of this lesion then points almost immediately to the diagnosis of an absolutely benign non-ossifying bone fibroma.

Most expanding cystic lesions of a rib are cases of monostotic fibrous bone dysplasia

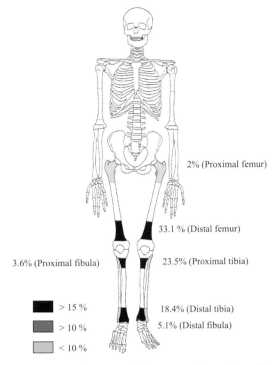

2% (Proximal femur)

33.1 % (Distal femur)

3.6% (Proximal fibula)

23.5% (Proximal tibia)

18.4% (Distal tibia)

5.1% (Distal fibula)

> 15 %

> 10 %

< 10 %

Fig. 579. Localization of the non-ossifying bone fibromas (468 cases); others: 14.3%

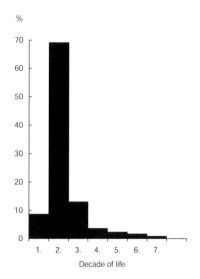

Fig. 580. Age distribution of the non-ossifying bone fibromas (468 cases)

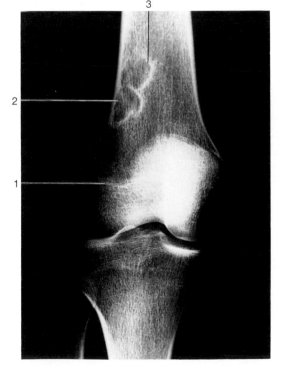

Fig. 581. Non-ossifying bone fibroma (distal femoral metaphysis)

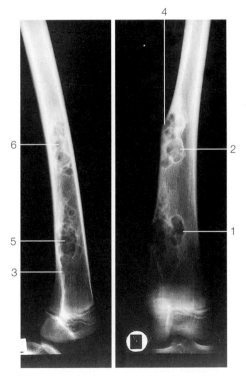

Fig. 582. Multiple non-ossifying bone fibromas (distal femur, lateral and a.p. views)

(p. 318), and only rarely is there an underlying non-ossifying bone fibroma. Such a lesion is resected en bloc. **Figure 583** shows such a resection of the 10th left rib. **Macroscopically** one can see grayish-white frayed tissue within the section of the rib *(1)*, which encloses several hollow cystic spaces *(2)*. A pathological fracture runs through the center *(3)*. The periosteum here is widened and bulges considerably *(4)*, and the cut surface reveals a glassy grayish connective tissue that also suggests tumorous tissue.

Some non-ossifying bone fibromas announce their presence with a pathological fracture. In **Fig. 584** one can see **radiologically** a wide gaping fracture line *(1)* in the distal part of the tibia. This runs through an intraosseous osteolytic focus *(2)* which is bordered by a narrow grape-like band of marginal sclerosis *(3)*. The position and form of this lesion on the radiograph makes it possible to recognize a non-ossifying bone fibroma. The pathological fracture has produced slight widening and darkening of the adjacent periosteum (i.e. reactive periostitis ossificans) *(4)*. The youth of this patient (16 years) is revealed by the continued presence of epiphyseal cartilage *(5)*. During the osteosynthetic treatment of the fracture one would take the opportunity in such a case to curette the fibromatous tissue of the tumor and submit it to histological examination.

As can be seen in the **histological picture** of **Fig. 585**, the defect has been filled up with a highly fibrous connective tissue in which no bony structures are present. The collagen fibers form whorls which are plaited together with one another. Only a few fine-walled blood vessels *(1)* are encountered. The numerous small giant cells *(2)* that lie scattered irregularly throughout the tumorous tissue are striking. Foam cells may also be present. The fibrous tissue of the tumor lies immediately adjacent to the sclerotically densified bone tissue *(3)*. There are reactive newly formed fibro-osseous trabeculae with layers of deposited osteoblasts which are responsible for the characteristic marginal sclerosis of this lesion.

The typical **histological picture** of a non-ossifying bone fibroma is shown in **Fig. 586**. One can observe the loose connective tissue deposited in plaited whorls *(1)* which contains numerous sturdy fibroblast nuclei *(2)*. Many of these cells are seen to be histiocytes. In the

neighborhood there is a large complex of foam cells *(3)*. All the nuclei are isomorphic and contain no mitoses. At the edge one can recognize a sclerotically thickened trabecula *(4)* on which rows of osteoblasts *(5)* and a few osteoclasts *(6)* have been deposited. This shows signs of reactive bone remodeling in the surroundings of the non-ossifying bone fibroma, which may produce an increase of activity in the scintigram, revealing progressive proliferation.

Under **higher magnification** one can see in **Fig. 587** many collagen fibers with isomorphic elongated oval nuclei, in which mitoses are only rarely present *(1)*. In between, a few small giant cells with up to 10 nuclei are lying *(2)*. In one place a small blood capillary has been sectioned *(3)*. Lymphocytes and histiocytic cellular elements are present. Older non-ossifying bone fibromas are poor in cells and can be largely hyalinized. In some tumors, foci of giant cells with many nuclei may be present, so that one could assume histologically that this is an osseous giant cell tumor. The latter, however, develops in the epiphyses (p. 337), whereas the non-ossifying bone fibroma arises in the metaphysis. The combined examination of radiograph and histological section should here lead to the correct diagnosis.

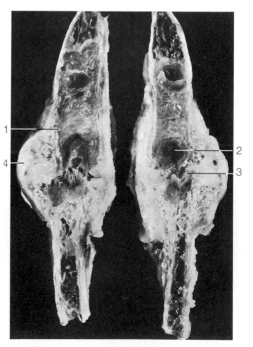

Fig. 583. Non-ossifying bone fibroma (rib, cut surface)

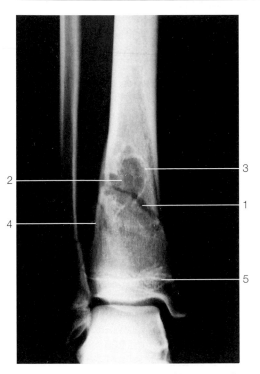

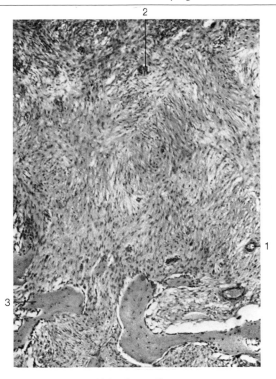

Fig. 584. Non-ossifying bone fibroma with pathological fracture (distal tibial metaphysis)

Fig. 585. Non-ossifying bone fibroma; HE, ×20

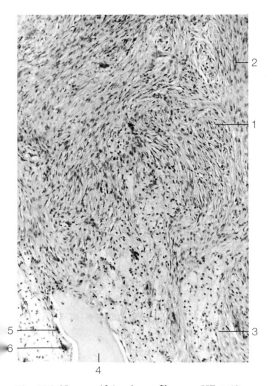

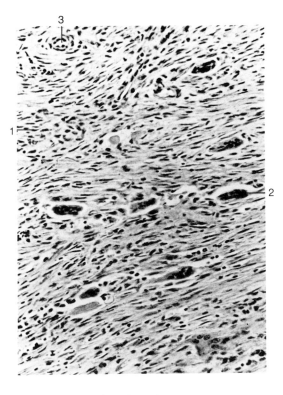

Fig. 586. Non-ossifying bone fibroma; HE, ×40

Fig. 587. Non-ossifying bone fibroma; HE, ×51

Xanthofibroma of Bone (ICD-O-DA-M-8831/0)

This is an absolutely benign tumorous bone lesion that is closely related clinically and morphologically to the non-ossifying bone fibroma, and can only be distinguished radiologically by a more nearly circular area of osteolysis, and histologically by the predominance of foam cell complexes. It is therefore solely a variant of the non-ossifying bone fibroma. The appearance of histiocytic cellular elements confirms its close relationship to the benign histiocytoma (p. 322). This benign tumor is found mostly in young adults.

In the **radiograph** of **Fig. 588** one can see a roundish osteolytic focus *(1)* in the distal tibial metaphysis lying eccentrically in the bone. It is sharply demarcated on all sides by a band of marginal sclerosis which is broader near the inside of the bone *(2)* than close to the cortex. The surrounding cancellous framework *(3)* is unaltered. Within the defect one can recognize the internal irregular trabecular structure. The bone of the tibia is slightly elevated in this region. The outer contour is, however, completely intact and there is no periosteal reaction.

As is shown in **Fig. 589**, extensive complexes of foam cells make up the **histological picture**. These foam cells *(1)* have an abundant, very pale cytoplasm which contains lipids and small round centrally-placed nuclei. These are histiocytic cells, and other histiocytes are also present *(2)*. Collagen fibers *(3)* run between the foam cells, giving the tissue a swirling appearance. They have narrow elongated connective tissue nuclei. In such a lesion one often finds foci of highly cellular granulation tissue with infiltrates of lymphocytes and plasma cells.

Fibromyxoma of Bone (ICD-O-DA-M-8811/0)

This is a primary bone neoplasm often found in the jaw bones but seldom seen elsewhere. *As in other sites (heart or skeletal muscles) it is a true bone neoplasm which is benign, and which consists of star-shaped cells in the middle of a* mucoid stroma with a few reticulin fibers running in various directions. There are no specific cellular elements (e.g. chondroblasts, lipoblasts, rhabdomyoblasts). The tumor is weakly vascularized, and the few capillaries do not show the plexiform arrangement found in embryonic lipoblastic tissue. Clinically the neoplasm manifests a slow growth that brings about circumscribed osteolysis in the bone. Although it can give the impression radiologically of an aggressively growing tumor, it is a benign lesion for which conservative surgical treatment is sufficient. In this, the bony myxoma distinguishes itself from the myxomas of the jaw bones which appear in young adult life (2nd and 3rd decades) and have a tendency to recur.

In the **radiograph** shown in **Fig. 590** one can see a fibromyxoma of the femoral neck. One recognizes a zone of osteolysis which has at one point eroded the cortex *(1)* lying eccentrically within the bone. The cortex has not, however, been penetrated and there is no periosteal reaction. The osteolytic focus has an indistinct border and stretches right into the femoral neck and greater trochanter. Within the focus one can see irregular patchy and straggly densifications, and around this a patchy osteosclerosis predominates. The whole of the neck is expanded by the destructive osteolytic process.

Histologically one can see in **Fig. 591** that the tumorous tissue consists of a very loose myxoid matrix *(1)* which is poor in cellular content. A considerable distance apart from each other there are isomorphic elongated or stellate connective tissue cells with small isomorphic nuclei. There are no mitoses. Other cellular elements, particularly chondroblasts, are not present. In some places there is the suggestion of a lobular formation, where areas of connective tissue with loose collagen fibers *(2)* form a border to the myxomatous zones. They contain narrow isomorphic fibrocyte nuclei and narrow capillaries. Whereas myxoid degenerative foci are also present in other tumors (e.g. chondromyxoid fibromas, p. 230; fibrosarcomas, p. 330), the fibromyxomas consist exclusively of such structures.

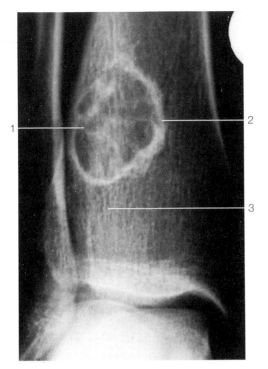

Fig. 588. Osseous xanthofibroma (distal tibial metaphysis)

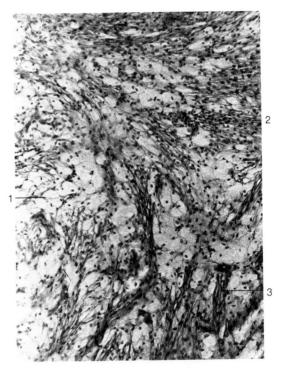

Fig. 589. Osseous xanthofibroma; HE, ×40

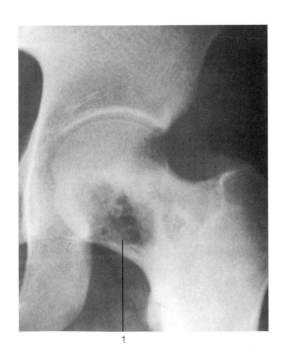

Fig. 590. Osseous fibromyxoma (left femoral neck)

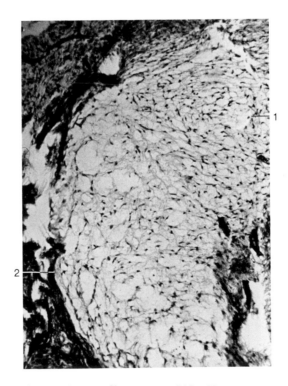

Fig. 591. Osseous fibromyxoma; PAS, ×25

Metaphyseal Fibrous Cortical Defect
(ICD-O-DA-M-7491/0)

A fibrous bone tumor can develop within a bone (non-ossifying bone fibroma, p. 308), or it can arise in the periosteum and then force its way into the bone from outside. *The metaphyseal fibrous cortical defect is a relatively small osteolytic lesion of the cortex in the region of the metaphysis of a long bone that is brought into being by a local proliferation of the periosteal connective tissue.* As a rule the lesion causes no symptoms and shows exactly the same histological tissue pattern as an intraosseously situated non-ossifying bone fibroma (p. 311). It is probably no true bone neoplasm, but rather a local developmental disorder of the growing bone. This type of lesion is almost always found in children and young people and, being harmless, is usually encountered by chance.

In the **radiograph** one can see such a metaphyseal cortical defect (**Fig. 592**) in the distal femoral metaphysis. At one place *(1)* the cortex appears to have been eroded from without, forming an indentation that is enclosed inside the bone by osteosclerosis. Within this indentation a discrete soft tissue shadow can be seen. The lesion is limited to the cortex and does not extend into the cancellous region of the bone. It is relatively small. The bony structure of the adjacent cortex and spongiosa is unremarkable.

Histologically one can see in **Fig. 593** how the proliferating tissue presses up against the cortex *(1)*. The latter displays lamellar layering and small osteocytes; it has an undulating border at which osteoblasts have been deposited. The proliferating tissue consists of highly cellular connective tissue, which is in part straggly *(2)* and in part formed into whorls *(3)*, with elongated isomorphic fibrocytes and fibroblasts. There are no mitoses. Noteworthy are a few small scattered multinucleate giant cells *(4)*. Histiocytes and foam cells may also be present.

Fibroblastic Periosteal Reaction
(ICD-O-DA-M-4900/0)

Connective tissue proliferation is by no means the inevitable sign of a bone tumor, even when it appears to be so on the radiograph. *A fibroblastic periosteal reaction is a non-tumorous proliferation of the periosteal connective tissue – mostly in the region of the distal femoral metaphysis of young people – which leads to roughening of the cortex.* This type of lesion, which can lead to considerable difficulty in interpreting the radiograph, is also known as *"periosteal desmoid"*. No sort of osteoblastic periosteal reaction is present. The cortex is neither eroded nor penetrated, it is only considerable loosened on the outer surface, so that it gives the impression of spicules. This is a harmless alteration which is often seen in this region in adolescents, particularly when they go in for sport (cycling, football). If one is familiar with its radiological appearance no bioptic investigation is necessary (so-called "leave-me-alone lesion").

In the **radiograph** one sees in lateral view (**Fig. 594**) the distal femoral metaphysis of a young person (epiphyseal plate still present, *1)* where a thickening of the periosteum *(2)* is visible extending over the surface of the cortex *(3)*. The cortex in this region is sclerotically densified and appears on the outer side to be slightly roughened. A minor degree of cancellous sclerosis *(4)* is also recognizable here. Unlike the fibrous cortical defect (p. 314) the cortex itself has not been eroded. Radiologically there are no signs of the bony structures of periostitis ossificans in this region.

Histologically the cortex is often significantly thickened and sometimes splintered. In **Fig. 595** it shows an undulating outer border *(1)*. One recognizes a loose, closely adjacent connective tissue *(2)* formed from parallel bundles of collagen fibers together with thin-walled vessels *(3)*. Very regularly shaped fibrocytes with spindle-shaped nuclei *(4)* and fibroblasts have been laid down. There is no inflammatory infiltration.

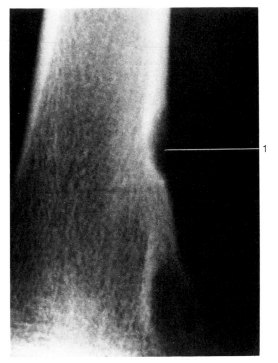

Fig. 592. Fibrous cortical defect (distal femoral metaphysis)

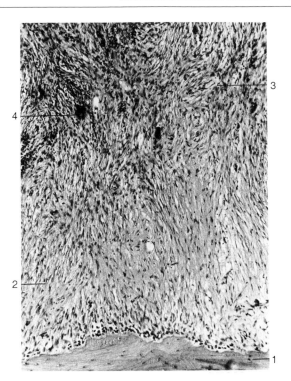

Fig. 593. Fibrous cortical defect; HE, ×25

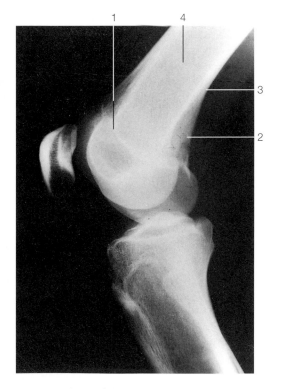

Fig. 594. Fibroblastic periosteal reaction
(distal femoral metaphysis)

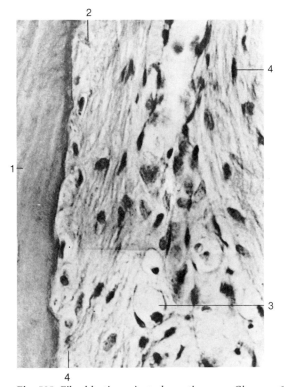

Fig. 595. Fibroblastic periosteal reaction; van Gieson, ×64

Ossifying Bone Fibroma (ICD-O-DA-M-9262/0)

In many connective tissue bone tumors there is a more or less vigorous differentiation of bone trabeculae which represent a product of the tumor. *An ossifying bone fibroma is a benign tumor which presents as a central fibro-osseous lesion principally in the jaw bones. It undergoes slow and expansive growth and can reach a large size, thus causing facial deformity.* About 90% of these benign neoplasms develop in adults in the mandible. They often remain without symptoms for a long time, but must. because of their continuous growth, be removed surgically. This tumor is only very rarely found in other parts of the skeleton. It has been described in the tibia, but that is probably more likely to be osteofibrous dysplasia (p. 316). The maturation of fibrous bone dysplasia (p. 318) into an ossifying bone fibroma and finally into an osteoma (p. 256) has been discussed.

In the **radiograph** of **Fig. 596** an ossifying bone fibroma can be recognized in the left side of the mandible *(1)*. There is a sharply demarcated slightly elliptical shadow lying in the center of the bone. In the middle of this shadowy zone, faint flaky translucencies prevent the picture from being homogeneous. During the first stage of the growth of the tumor, an osteolytic focus may even be present. The surrounding bone *(2)* is osteoporotic and porous, and in one place *(3)* the marginal sclerosis reaches into the cortex. There is no periosteal reaction.

Figure 597 shows the typical **histological picture** of an ossifying bone fibroma. One can recognize the fibromatous stroma *(1)* with numerous thin, isomorphic fibrocyte nuclei in which no mitoses can be seen. The highly cellular connective tissue is threaded through by a few fine-walled dilated capillaries *(2)*. There are deposits of fibro-osseous trabeculae *(3)* of varying widths and lengths which make up a coarse uneven network. Unlike the situation in fibrous dysplasia (p. 321), the bone trabeculae are covered with dense rows of activated osteoblasts *(4)*. They contain many osteocytes and are mineralized to varying extents. In the mature tumor, mature lamellar bone trabeculae are present.

Osteofibrous Bone Dysplasia (Campanacci)

There are structural transitions between fibrous bone dysplasia and an ossifying bone fibroma. *Osteofibrous bone dysplasia is a slow growing osteofibrous bone lesion of the long bones, which most often attacks the tibia in children under 10 years and shows great histological similarity to an ossifying bone fibroma.* The lesion develops in the shaft of a long bone and leads to a progressive deformity. Very often there is destruction of the cortex and a bony periosteal reaction. In some cases it may coincide with an adamantinoma of the long bones (p. 378). When examining such a lesion histologically one should therefore always look for that kind of tumorous structure.

In **Fig. 598** one can see the **radiograph** of an osteofibrous bone dysplasia. The middle of the shaft of a child's tibia is raised up into a curve *(1)*, over which the outer cortex is preserved and has a smooth border. No periosteal reaction can be seen. Inside the lesion one can recognize straggly irregular densifications enclosing cyst-like osteolytic foci *(2)* which give it a honeycomb-like appearance. These types of osteolytic foci also lie in the cortex.

The **histological picture** shows either a great similarity to fibrous dysplasia (p. 321) or to an ossifying bone fibroma. In **Fig. 599** one can recognize a gnarled network of both broad and narrow fibro-osseous trabeculae *(1)* which are plaited together and contain numerous osteocytes. They support rows of osteoblasts of varying density *(2)*, which may also, however, often be absent. Between these bony structures there is loose connective tissue *(3)* with numerous small, narrow fibrocyte nuclei which are isomorphic and free from mitoses. Many small capillaries *(4)* are running through this stroma. Sometimes infiltrates of lymphocytes and plasma cells are encountered. This benign bone lesion which is found predominantly in the cortex should be completely removed by en bloc resection which passes through healthy tissue. If there are remnants left behind one should be prepared for a recurrence. Malignant change is not to be expected, but a malignant second tumor must nevertheless be excluded.

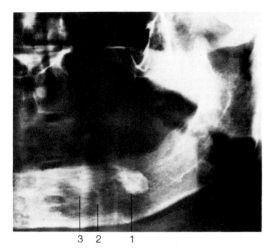

Fig. 596. Ossifying bone fibroma (left side of lower jaw)

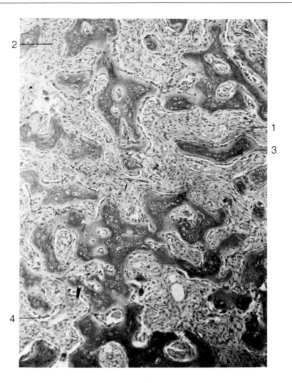

Fig. 597. Ossifying bone fibroma; HE, ×30

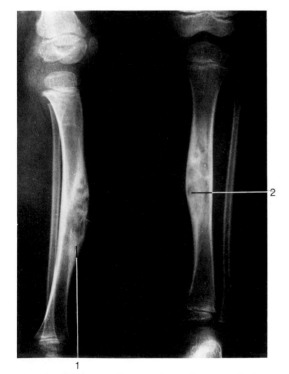

Fig. 598. Campanacci's osteofibrous bone dysplasia
(tibial shaft)

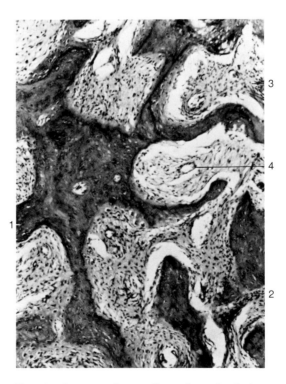

Fig. 599. Campanacci's osteofibrous bone dysplasia;
HE, ×51

Fibrous Bone Dysplasia (Jaffe-Lichtenstein) (ICD-O-DA-M-7491/0)

This quite common connective tissue bone lesion was known earlier as "ostitis fibrosa" and classified under hyperparathyroidism (p. 80). It has, however, been shown that it has nothing to do with parathyroid function. *Fibrous bone dysplasia is a relatively common malformation of the bone-building mesenchyme in which the bone marrow is replaced by fibrous marrow and the fibrous bone trabeculae remain, owing to their failure to be transformed into lamellar bone.* It is a separate bone disease which gives the impression radiologically of "bony cysts" and which, because of its clinical appearance, is classified as a "tumor-like bone lesion". The lesion is often found only by chance, and apart from slight dragging pain, or pain following exertion, and slight swelling it usually appears without symptoms. In the lower limb it leads to coxa vara. It can announce its presence with a pathological fracture. The lesion begins in the metaphyses if the long bones are affected, and encroaches upon the diaphysis. The cortex is eroded from within and bowed outwards. The periosteum remains intact, and subperiosteal new bone deposition takes place. With continued growth of the lesion there is marked expansion of the affected bone segment, which is unstable and bends under the weight of the body.

Localization (Fig. 600). The bony foci may be monostotic or polyostotic, in which case they show a certain systemic distribution throughout the skeleton. We distinguish between a diffuse monostotic type, a monomelic type, a unilateral type and a bilateral type. Fibrous bone dysplasia is one of the commonest tumorous lesions of the ribs, where there is usually a single focus. The monostotic form is to be found especially in the ribs, skull, jaw or proximal parts of the femur and tibia. The polyostotic form appears mostly in the scapula, humerus, femur or tibia. Sometimes more than 50 foci can appear simultaneously.

Age Distribution (Fig. 601). This is always a disease of the child's skeleton, and most cases are observed between 5 and 15 years of age, girls being the more frequently affected. Some cases are asymptomatic and are not observed during childhood or youth; they then appear later as chance findings in adults.

In the long bones, fibrous dysplasia leads to serious deformities of the skeleton (shepherd's crook curvature of the femoral neck and shaft with coxa vara) and in 85% of the cases to a pathological fracture. The serum calcium and serum phosphate levels are normal; the serum alkaline phosphatase may be slightly raised. Sometimes fibrous bone dysplasia is combined – especially in girls – with patchy pigmentation of the skin, neurological involvement and the precocious onset of puberty (*pubertas praecox* – the so-called *Albright's syndrome*). So far as life is concerned, the prognosis is *quoad vitam* good. Before the completion of skeletal growth the disease advances in bursts, with the bony foci growing larger and others possibly appearing. At puberty, growth of the monostotic form usually ceases, but the polyostotic form can also progress after puberty.

A radiograph and the corresponding macroscopic specimen of monostotic bone dysplasia in a rib can be seen in Figs. 95 and 96 respectively (p. 56).

In **Fig. 602** one can see the typical **radiological findings** with fibrous dysplasia of the femoral neck. One can discern a cyst *(1)* lying in the center of the bone. It is sharply bordered by marginal sclerosis *(2)*. In this region the cortex has been narrowed from within, but remains intact. The inside of the lesion is bright and is set through with narrow trabecular structures. It extends into the marrow cavity at the proximal part of the femur *(3)*, which is clearly elevated. Here the internal structure shows a pale, cloudy ("frosted glass") densification.

In the **radiograph** of **Fig. 603** one can see fibrous dysplasia in the proximal part of the radius *(1)*, which has cause the region to bulge outwards. The inside of this lesion is a diffuse shadow, the cortex has been eroded from within and greatly narrowed. The lesion has extended itself widely and taken up almost the whole proximal half of the radius. No periosteal reaction can be seen, and the cortex has a smooth outer border, indicating the benign nature of the growth.

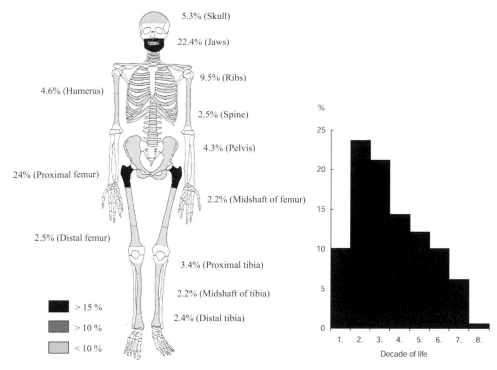

5.3% (Skull)

22.4% (Jaws)

9.5% (Ribs)

4.6% (Humerus)

2.5% (Spine)

4.3% (Pelvis)

24% (Proximal femur)

2.2% (Midshaft of femur)

2.5% (Distal femur)

3.4% (Proximal tibia)

2.2% (Midshaft of tibia)

2.4% (Distal tibia)

> 15 %

> 10 %

< 10 %

Fig. 600. Localization of the fibrous bone dysplasias
(325 cases); others: 14.7%

Fig. 601. Age distribution of the fibrous bone dysplasias
(325 cases)

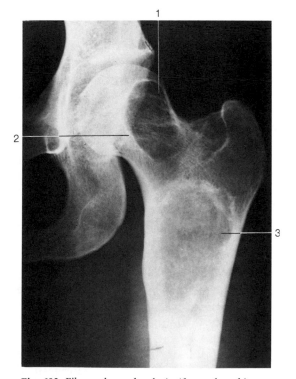

Fig. 602. Fibrous bone dysplasia (femoral neck)

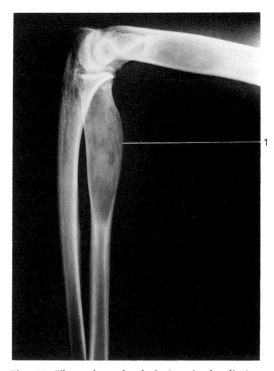

Fig. 603. Fibrous bone dysplasia (proximal radius)

The cystic destruction of bone by fibrous bone dysplasia appearing as an intraosseous osteolytic focus can take place in a long bone, usually in the metaphysis or more rarely in the diaphysis. It is, however, particularly in the femur that the destruction process can spread violently and sometimes involve two thirds of the bone. In **Fig. 604** this kind of fibrous bone dysplasia is shown in a **radiograph** of the proximal part of the femur. This is from a 7-year-old child, in whom the condition was progressive. It has brought about an ungainly expansion of the neck of the femur *(1)* and the adjacent shaft *(2)*. The femoral angle appears flattened *(3)*. Inside the bone one can discern a diffuse cloudy shadowing with translucent areas, where trabecular and septum-like densifications *(4)* have given the lesion a polycystic appearance. One refers to the "frosted glass" look of the bone focus. In some places the cortex has been eroded from within and narrowed, in others it is reactively thickened and sclerosed. It is nevertheless completely intact, and one can see outside the sharp demarcation line without thickening of the periosteum or any bony periosteal reaction.

In the **histological picture** of **Fig. 605**, one can see the inside of such a focus where, instead of the normal lamellar layering of the cancellous bone, there is a fiber-rich collagenous connective tissue *(1)*, consisting of cords and whorls. The connective tissue is relatively poor in cellular content and often forms a network. In a few places there is a storiform or cartwheel arrangement such as one meets with in fibrous histiocytomas (p. 323). The connective tissue is penetrated by only a few capillaries *(2)*. In overview the numerous, very thin bone trabeculae are striking. They are equidistantly spaced throughout the connective tissue. There is a woven formation of fibro-osseous trabeculae *(3)* which are mostly uncalcified, or only very slightly so. They are often bent, hook-shaped or horseshoe-shaped – or else they form true circles. This produces a highly decorative appearance, rather like an ornamental wallpaper. Unlike the ossifying osteofibroma (p. 316), these fibro-osseous trabeculae carry no osteoblasts. The bony structures run directly out from the stromal connective tissue. Occasionally giant cells, foci of myxoid degeneration and metaplastic cartilaginous foci are present.

In **Fig. 606** one can see the **histological picture** of a fibrous bone dysplasia under higher magnification. The background tissue consists of a spindle-cell connective tissue, with some densely and some loosely deposited collagen fibers *(1)* that always form small whorls. There is also a completely irregular arrangement of fibro-osseous trabeculae *(2)* which contain many small osteocytes. Occasionally one can see in the connective tissue a few multinucleate giant cells *(3)*. As a whole the tissue is only poorly vascularized. The clefts *(4)* in the tissue near the bone trabeculae are artefacts which have arisen during the preparation of the slide. The rows of small cells with dark roundish nuclei *(5)* are striking; these are probably small inactive osteoblasts. Such structures are occasionally found in fibrous dysplasia, which may make the distinction between it and the ossifying osteofibroma (p. 317) difficult. In general, however, the fibro-osseous trabeculae of fibrous dysplasia lack the layers of activated osteoblasts. Moreover, the bone trabeculae usually have no osteoid seams.

The characteristic **histological picture** of fibrous bone dysplasia is shown in **Fig. 607**. One can observe a richly fibrous background tissue *(1)* in which lie variously dense collections of fibrocytes and fibroblasts. These have narrow oval isomorphic nuclei, with no mitoses. Only occasionally can one observe the passage of a capillary *(2)*. The fibro-osseous trabeculae are for the most part narrow and curved *(3)*, although sometimes broad and shapeless *(4)*. The few short roundish bony structures *(5)* are transverse sections through sagittally placed trabeculae. There are no rows of osteoblasts, and the connective tissue passes directly over into the fibro-osseous trabeculae. In rare cases one can see metaplastic foci of cartilage in fibrous bone dysplasia, which may occasionally be very much stretched out. Here the question arises as to whether a primary cartilaginous tumor is also present as a second lesion. The significance of this chondromatous fibrous bone dysplasia has not so far been explained. Normally fibrous dysplasia has a good prognosis; malignant change following irradiation has been described, but for such a change to take place spontaneously is unusual.

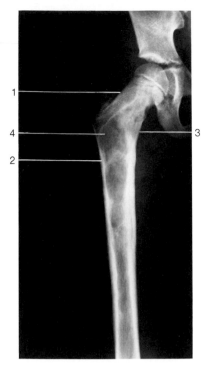

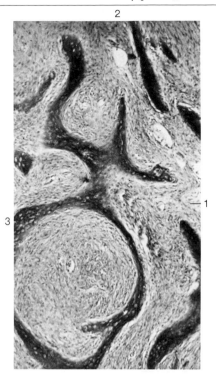

Fig. 604. Fibrous bone dysplasia (proximal femur)

Fig. 605. Fibrous bone dysplasia, van Gieson, ×25

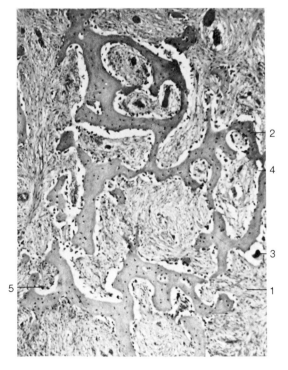

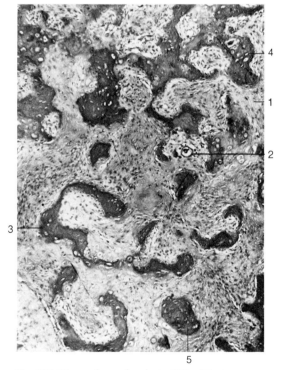

Fig. 606. Fibrous bone dysplasia; HE, ×30

Fig. 607. Fibrous bone dysplasia; HE, ×25

Desmoplastic Bone Fibroma (ICD-O-DA-M-8823/1)

In rare cases a fibromatous bone neoplasm can undergo local aggressive growth without giving rise to metastases. This is one example of a semimalignant bone tumor. *A desmoplastic bone fibroma is a very rare benign or semimalignant bone tumor consisting of connective tissue which is rich in collagen fibers and poor in cells. It displays local destructive and invasive growth, together with a tendency to recur, but does not produce metastases.* This tumor can appear in any age group, but predominantly afflicts the young. The principal localization is in the long bones, but other bones can also be affected. The symptoms are usually confined to slight pain and local swelling. Only 90 cases have so far found their way into the literature.

The **radiological changes** consist mostly of large, frequently aggressive osteolytic zones with endosteal erosion and cortical expansion, often accompanied by a pathological fracture. In **Fig. 608** one can see one of these large destructive foci in the sacrum *(1)*. The normal structure of the bone in this area has been completely lost, and the cortex cannot be seen. On the inner side of the lesion there is a discrete marginal sclerosis *(2)* that seems to be indented. The osteolytic focus is subdivided into cyst-like spaces by narrow trabeculae.

Histologically a rich collagenous connective tissue dominates the picture. In **Fig. 609** one can recognize the tumorous connective tissue in which there are many fibroblasts with small roundish or oval isomorphic nuclei. They show no hyperchromasia and mitoses are rare. The tissue of the tumor is penetrated by only a few vessels *(1)*. One can sometimes see shapeless bone trabeculae *(2)* that have been largely wrecked. These are part of the original local bone which has been destroyed by the tumor. No tumorous bone formation has taken place. Lesions with small tumor cell nuclei are said to recur more often than those with larger nuclei. In general there is a great similarity to proliferative fibromatosis or to a desmoid. When hyperchromasia and polymorphic nuclei are present the distinction between this and a fibrosarcoma of bone (p. 333) may be difficult or even impossible.

Benign Fibrous Histiocytoma (ICD-O-DA-M-8832/0)

Histiocytic cellular elements can turn up not only in fibrous bone lesions (non-ossifying bone fibromas, p. 308; xanthofibroma, p. 312) but also in bone granulomas (eosinophilic bone granulomas, histiocytosis X, p. 196). *A benign fibrous histiocytoma is a primary bone neoplasm that arises in the marrow cavity, and in which the histiocytes are capable not only of storing substances, but can also produce collagen fibers displaying a storiform arrangement.* Whereas these neoplasms appear relatively often in the soft parts they are rare in bone. Their main localization is in the femur or tibia, although they may affect any other bones, where they mostly arise in the diaphyses.

Figure 610 shows the **radiograph** of a benign fibrous histiocytoma in the shaft of the humerus *(1)*. One can discern an irregular osteolytic destructive focus that has arisen in the marrow cavity and forced its way into the cortex from within. The latter is, however, still intact, and there is no periosteal reaction. The osteolytic focus is clearly demarcated in the tomogram, even when no marginal sclerosis can be seen here. This can, however, be present.

In the **histological picture** of **Fig. 611** one can see highly cellular tumorous tissue with collagenous fibers that have built up a storiform pattern. In addition to fibrocytes *(1)* and fibroblasts *(2)*, histiocytes *(3)* dominate the picture. They have large slightly elliptical or indented nuclei, and a pale cytoplasm in which lipids can often be stored (foam cells). The cell nuclei are completely isomorphic and usually possess a single nucleus. Mitoses are practically never present. Inside the tumorous tissue only a few fine-walled capillaries are seen. In a number of histiocytomas, unevenly distributed benign giant cells may be observed.

Up to now there has been no indication that a benign fibrous histiocytoma can change into the malignant form of the same tumor, although a few cases have been described in which the appearance of an osteosarcoma within a benign fibrous histiocytoma has been observed. Apart from these extraordinarily rare exceptions, however, this is a completely benign tumor which usually heals after surgical extirpation.

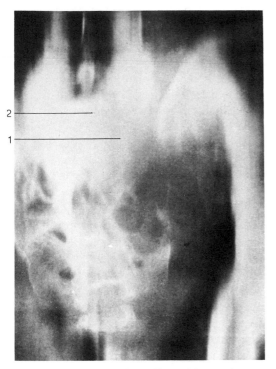

Fig. 608. Desmoplastic bone fibroma (sacrum)

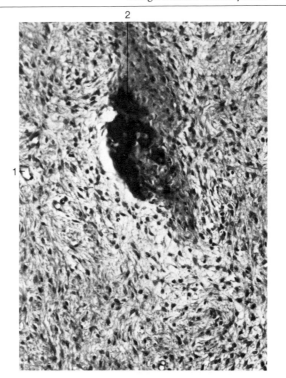

Fig. 609. Desmoplastic bone fibroma; HE, ×64

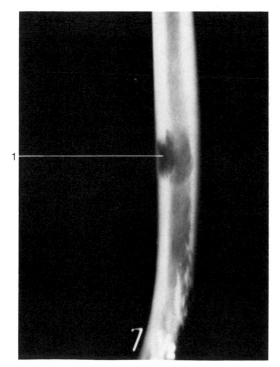

Fig. 610. Benign fibrous histiocytoma
(humeral shaft, tomogram)

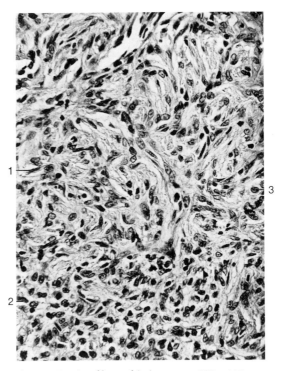

Fig. 611. Benign fibrous histiocytoma; HE, ×100

Malignant Fibrous Histiocytoma
(ICD-O-DA-M-8830/3)

The malignant fibrous histiocytoma was first recognized in 1972 as a separate independent bone tumor. Most histiocytomas were worked out from retrospective histological studies, so that they were originally classified as undifferentiated fibrosarcomas or osteosarcomas. *This is a primary malignant bone tumor where a concurrent differentiation of both fibroblasts and histiocytes occurs. It arises in the connective tissue of the bone marrow and grows less aggressively than an osteosarcoma or a fibrosarcoma.* A similar tumor in the soft tissues has long been known. So far over 500 malignant fibrous histiocytomas have been described, several of them in old bone infarcts (p. 174). Isolated cases have arisen in the neighborhood of a prosthesis.

Localization (Fig. 612). Malignant fibrous histiocytomas have been observed in a great variety of bones. The most frequent localization is in the region of the knee, i.e. in the proximal part of the tibia, the distal part of the femur and the proximal part of the fibula. The tumor has also, however, been described in the humerus, radius, ulna, pelvis, spine, and jaw and other skull bones. It is usually solitary, but on occasion several lesions may be present together. Multicentric lesions have been described in the femur + spine, femur + spine + rib, as well as in the ilium + ribs.

Age Distribution (Fig. 613). These malignant bone neoplasms can appear at any age, but mostly in the 5th to 7th decades of life. Our youngest patient was 11 years old and our oldest 94. The average age is about 50, making it significantly higher than that of patients with an osteosarcoma.

The tumor usually presents with slowly increasing local swelling and pain. In many cases these symptoms may be present from a few months to as much as 3 years before the lesion is discovered. The laboratory findings are unremarkable (normal alkaline phosphatase). It is true, however, that a large number of local pathological fractures have been reported in the region of the tumor. Apart from those in association with a bone infarct and (rarely) with a prosthesis (e.g. a total hip replacement), the foci of a malignant fibrous histiocytoma have been found in osteosarcomas and undifferentiated chondrosarcomas, or in the presence of Paget's osteitis deformans.

The **radiograph** of a malignant fibrous histiocytoma is characterized by an indistinctly bordered osteolytic zone lying eccentrically in the marrow cavity of the bone, where it has brought about endosteal erosion of the cortex. The lesion usually develops in a metaphysis and can spread into the epiphysis. Lesions of the shaft also appear, and the bone may be slightly elevated. The bone-building periosteal reaction is minimal, even when the cortex has been penetrated. In **Fig. 614** one can see a malignant fibrous histiocytoma in the proximal part of the right femur. This tumor has caused a pathological fracture of the femoral neck, which was at first stabilized osteosynthetically. One can still clearly recognize the position of the angle plate by the surrounding bone reaction *(1)*. The tumor arose in the region of the trochanter and has broken through the cortex over a wide front *(2)*. Both in the marrow cavity and in the cortex there are confluent osteolytic foci, providing evidence of aggressive tumor growth. The irregular increase in density of the structures *(3)* may well be due to the earlier fracture, since no calcification or reactive bone deposition occurs in histiocytomas. The tumor has extended far into the femoral shaft *(4)*.

In **Fig. 615** there is extensive destruction of the bony structures in the whole of the proximal part of the tibia. A large zone of densification is plainly visible *(1)* with roundish sclerotic foci at the periphery. Here it as a matter of an old bone infarct. On the other hand, the entire tibial head is set through with single and confluent osteolytic foci *(2)*, which are also to be seen in the cortex *(3)*. No periosteal reaction can be discerned. The bone is only slightly elevated. In this case a malignant fibrous histiocytoma has developed at the site of a bone infarct. The radiograph shows all the criteria of malignancy. The components of this infarct are only indistinctly detectable radiologically, and they are overlaid by the moth-eaten appearance of the bone destruction caused by the malignant histiocytoma. Since a malignant histiocytoma presents no pathognomonic radiological appearance, the final diagnosis must depend upon a biopsy.

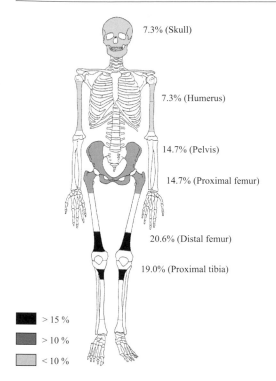

7.3% (Skull)

7.3% (Humerus)

14.7% (Pelvis)

14.7% (Proximal femur)

20.6% (Distal femur)

19.0% (Proximal tibia)

> 15 %

> 10 %

< 10 %

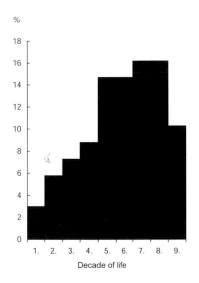

Fig. 612. Localization of the malignant fibrous histiocytomas (93 cases); others: 16.4%

Fig. 613. Age distribution of the malignant fibrous histiocytomas (93 cases)

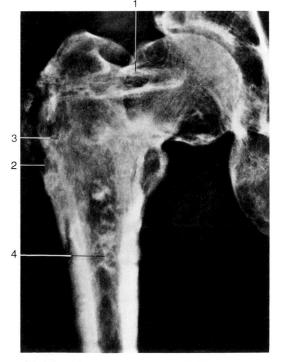

Fig. 614. Malignant fibrous histiocytoma (proximal femur)

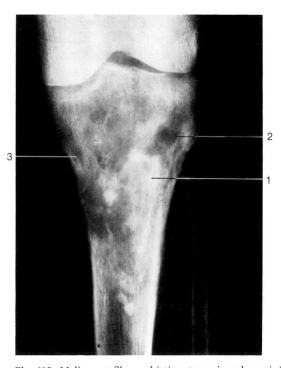

Fig. 615. Malignant fibrous histiocytoma in a bone infarct (proximal tibia)

A malignant fibrous histiocytoma can also appear in the middle of the shaft of a long bone. In the **radiograph** of **Fig. 616** there is a destructive focus of this sort in the middle of the shaft of the humerus (1). One can see here patchy osteolysis that has spread out into the spongiosa and has also destroyed the cortex on one side (2). So far no periosteal reaction can be seen; the bone in this region has a smooth border and is not elevated. The destructive focus is not surrounded by any marginal sclerosis and its border is quite indistinct. A bone lesion like this appearing on a radiograph suggests a malignant bone tumor, and it is imperative that it should be identified by means of histological examination of a bone biopsy. With some malignant fibrous histiocytomas there is marginal sclerosis, and this suggests a more slowly growing tumor, but this does not imply a better prognosis. Even with sclerotically demarcated malignant fibrous histiocytomas, lung metastases have been found within 2 years. In about 15% of patients with a malignant fibrous histiocytoma a pathological fracture occurs. In some malignant fibrous histiocytomas, patchy calcifications and zonal ossifications appeared on the radiograph as conspicuous shadows.

This is a proliferating and destructively growing tumor that stimulates the autochthonous bone tissue to a massive acceleration in reactive new bone building. As a result of this, it is not surprising to find a strong stepping up of activity in the **bone scintigram** of the tissue surrounding a malignant fibrous histiocytoma. In **Fig. 617** one can see in the region of a malignant tumor in the shaft of the right humerus a strong increase in activity (1) that extends far beyond the radiologically perceptible tumor (**Fig. 616**). This is because the radionucleotide is, as a result of the remodeling, taken up by the autochthonous bone tissue adjacent to the tumor and recorded photographically. In this way the borderline region for an en bloc resection through healthy tissue is very well marked. An impressive increase in activity is also visible in the proximal part of the humerus and in the shoulder joint (2), and this must be investigated by further radiological examination. However, there is not necessarily any causal relationship between the malignant tumor in the shaft of the humerus (1) and the increased activity in the shoulder joint. Bone remodeling processes there may be due to some other cause.

Histologically a malignant fibrous histiocytoma consists of highly cellular tumorous tissue in which no deposition of osteoid or bone building is present. In **Fig. 618** one can see the densely packed histiocytes which lie sometimes in a longitudinal (1) and sometimes in a transverse (2) direction. This tissue pattern is very characteristic of malignant fibrous histiocytomas. The histiocytic tumor cells have unambiguously polymorphic cells of varying sizes, which sometimes possess swollen nuclei with prominent nucleoli (3). Many of the nuclei are strongly hyperchromatic (4) and reveal pathological mitoses. Multinucleated histiocytic tumor cells are also scattered about in the tissue (5). In addition to the histiocytes, there are also numerous fibroblasts (6) which are likewise polymorphic and have hyperchromatic nuclei. These are also tumor cells. They lay down varying numbers of collagen fibers which are deposited between the tumorous cells. In a few places a fiber-rich fibrosis of the tumorous tissue with a storiform pattern may be present, and zones reminiscent of a fibrosarcoma (p. 333) can occur. Other regions contain only a few discrete collagen fibers, or are completely free of them and consist exclusively of dense collections of pathological histiocytes.

Under the **higher magnification** of **Fig. 619** the histiocytic nature of the tumorous tissue becomes very clear. The histiocytes have large, variously shaped and swollen nuclei (1), in which massive nucleoli are often visible (2). Many nuclei have several nucleoli (3). The nuclei are of different sizes and clearly polymorphic. The cytoplasm is abundant, the cell membranes are indistinct and faded. In the center one can see a histiocytic giant cell (4) with a pathological mitosis. Sometimes phagocytosed particles (e.g. hemosiderin particles or erythrocytes) can be seen in the cytoplasm of the histiocytes. In one such histiocyte-rich area of the tumor there are only a few fine collagen fibers (5). It consists of a polymorphic cellular tumorous tissue with fairly numerous abnormal mitoses, thus indicating a malignant tumor.

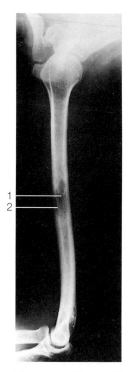

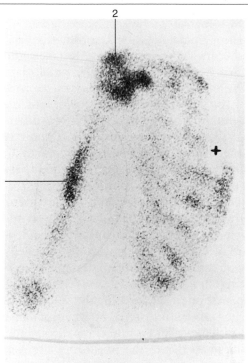

Fig. 616. Malignant fibrous histiocytoma (humeral shaft)

Fig. 617. Malignant fibrous histiocytoma (humeral shaft, scintigram)

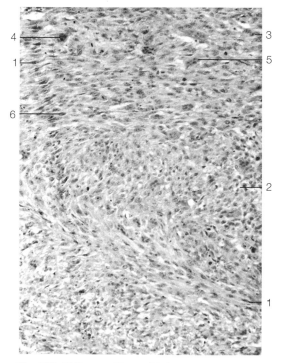

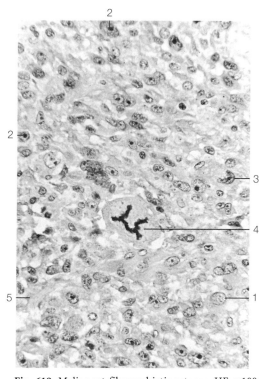

Fig. 618. Malignant fibrous histiocytoma; HE, ×51

Fig. 619. Malignant fibrous histiocytoma; HE, ×100

The **histological picture** of a malignant fibrous histiocytoma can be extraordinarily variable, and many other lesions have to taken into account when considering the differential diagnosis. The decisive histological criteria are: (a) a mixing of biphasic cells (histiocytes, fibroblasts) with fibroblastic and histiocytic differentiation, (b) a so-called "storiform" (tapestry-like) tissue pattern, (c) cells showing the cytological characteristics of malignancy. These characteristics – polymorphy and hyperchromatic nuclei, pathological mitoses – are more frequently seen in the histiocytic region of the tumor. It is important to recognize the histiocytic nature of the tumor cells with their capacity both for phagocytosis (iron, lipids) and for differentiating into fibroblasts.

In **Fig. 620** one can see a highly cellular malignant fibrous histiocytoma in which a loose network of plaited collagen fibers is discernible, and which gives rise to the storiform pattern of the tissue. Even at low power magnification the two cell populations, which are mingled together, are visible. There are spindle-shaped fibroblasts with elongated nuclei (1) which produce the collagen fibers. Histiocytes (2) with large roundish or indented nuclei and abundant cytoplasm are seen strewn about or collected together in groups. Variable numbers of multinucleated histiocytic giant cells (3) are always to be seen. The variation in size and hyperchromasia of the nuclei is striking, and this, together with pathological mitoses, confirms the malignant nature of the neoplasm.

In **Fig. 621** a fiber-rich malignant fibrous histiocytoma appears in which the storiform pattern of the tissue is clearly seen. The loosely placed collagen fibers are formed into whorls (1) and are woven together like a mat. In spite of the nuclear polymorphy the fibroblasts (2) are clearly distinguishable from the histiocytic cellular elements (3). Once again several multinucleated giants cells (4) are scattered about in the area.

Figure 622 shows, under **higher magnification**, a predominantly histiocytic histiocytoma with less fibrogenesis. Most striking is the very marked nuclear polymorphy and hyperchromasia, indicating the malignant nature of the growth. There are elongated spindle-cells with polymorphic nuclei (1), as well as large histiocytes (2), also with polymorphic nuclei and pale, patchy, foamy cytoplasm. In tumors like this, one also frequently finds complexes of foam cells. The tumor cells often look very like lipoblasts, with the result that the histological distinction between this tumor and a liposarcoma can be difficult and sometimes even impossible.

In **Fig. 623** one can see a malignant fibrous histiocytoma under **higher magnification** in which the fiber production of the fibroblasts is more strongly marked. The course of the collagen fibers (1), which run in different directions, creates the characteristic storiform pattern. In this tumor the nuclear polymorphy is only moderately apparent. In contrast to the very narrow fibroblastic nuclei (2) with their dense chromatin content, the histiocytic cellular elements have oval or roundish nuclei with loosely distributed chromatin (3). A few histiocytes have a richly eosinophilic cytoplasm (4) and recall the appearance of muscle cells. Others have a honeycomb-like or foamy cytoplasm (5).

If there is a predominance of spindle-cells with a plentiful formation of collagen fibers the **differential diagnosis** of a fibrosarcoma of bone (p. 330) must be excluded. Foci with uniform histiocytes cause one to think of a histiocytic lymphoma or a Hodgkin's lymphoma (p. 358), if the histiocytes are similar to Sternberg's giant cells. Foci of epithelioid histiocytes can look very like a carcinomatous metastasis. Numerous multinucleate giant cells in a stroma of pleomorphic spindle-cells suggest the possibility of a malignant osteoclastoma (p. 337). If the histiocytes are arranged in groups around a vessel, or the vessel is bordered by a single histiocytic cellular layer with a fibrous stroma between them, a hemangiopericytoma or a hemangioendothelioma (p. 376) must also be considered. The extracellular matrix in a histiocytoma can look very like osteoid, so that distinguishing between a malignant fibrous histiocytoma and an undifferentiated osteosarcoma can be very difficult or even impossible. This plethora of differential diagnostic possibilities do make the diagnosis, especially from a bone biopsy, very uncertain. It is entirely conceivable that a malignant fibrous histiocytoma may be diagnosed bioptically but which, on later examination of the tissue extracted at operation, turns out to be an osteosarcoma.

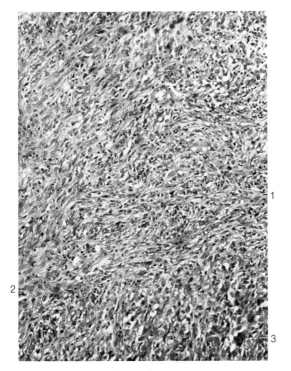

Fig. 620. Malignant fibrous histiocytoma; HE, ×25

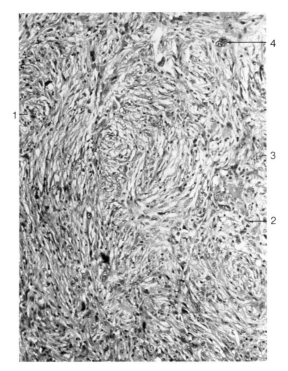

Fig. 621. Malignant fibrous histiocytoma; HE, ×40

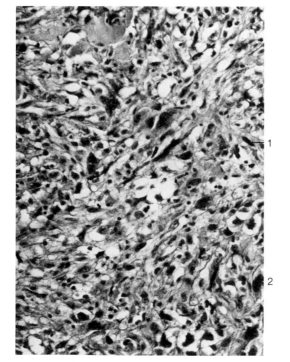

Fig. 622. Malignant fibrous histiocytoma; HE, ×64

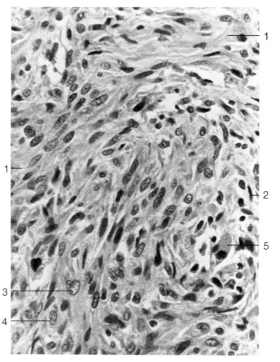

Fig. 623. Malignant fibrous histiocytoma; HE, ×100

Fibrosarcoma of Bone (ICD-O-DA-M-8810/3)

A malignant neoplasm can develop from the connective tissue of the skeleton which is structurally the same as a similar soft tissue sarcoma. *A fibrosarcoma of bone is a primary malignant neoplasm, which usually arises in the marrow cavity and consists histologically of sarcomatous connective tissue in which no tumorous bony, osteoid or cartilaginous structures have differentiated.* Among malignant bone tumors this neoplasm has a relatively good prognosis. Locally it produces severe bone destruction which looks radiologically like an osteolytic focus. Histologically the tumor can appear to be so highly differentiated that it may be difficult to distinguish it from a benign fibrous neoplasm. On the other hand, fibrosarcomatous areas can be present in other malignant tumors (e.g. in a fibroblastic osteosarcoma). With an incidence of 10% the fibrosarcoma is a relatively rare malignant bone neoplasm. About 25% of fibrosarcomas arise secondarily after irradiation of the bone. This kind of neoplasm can also develop in the cortex or in the periosteum.

Localization (Fig. 624). The usual predilection sites include the long bones, particular those of the lower limb. Here one finds 68.5% of all fibrosarcomas, of which 45.2% are located near the knee. It can, however, also attack any other bone, although most of these have been reported as single isolated occurrences. Within the long bones it is usually the metaphyses which are involved, and in this the tumor is similar to the osteosarcoma (p. 275). The tumor can, however, also arise in the region of the diaphysis. A few fibrosarcomas originate in the periosteal connective tissue. In the case of multiple osseous fibrosarcomas occurring it is necessary to ensure that these are not metastases from a sarcomatous tumor somewhere in the soft parts.

Age Distribution (Fig. 625). The usual age for this growth to appear is in the 2nd or 3rd decade of life, when 68% of osseous fibrosarcomas arise – with a peak in the 2nd decade of 43%. This type of tumor has been found in children (in the 6th year of life) as well as in old people (88 years). Its appearance even in elderly patients

is one of the things that distinguishes this growth from the osteosarcoma (p. 275).

The usually very slow-growing fibrosarcomas produce no characteristic symptoms. Mostly there is some local swelling. Intermittent pain does occur, but it is often so slight that it can persist for several months. The average length of time reported in the case history is 8 months. In 14% of cases, attention is first drawn to the existence of the tumor by a pathological fracture.

Figure 626 is a **radiograph** of a fibrosarcoma of the distal femoral metaphysis. One can see an osteolytic focus *(1)* with an indistinct border lying eccentrically in the bone. There is no marginal sclerosis. The osteolytic lesion has no internal structure. The adjacent cortex is greatly narrowed *(2)* and has been broken through in places. In this case the indentation of the bone from without *(3)* is striking, and there is a parosteal shadow of the tumor in this region. This shows that the tumor has broken through the cortex and invaded the adjacent soft parts.

In the **radiograph** of **Fig. 627** one can see a large osteolytic zone in the head of the tibia *(1)* that has involved both the epiphysis and the metaphysis. It reaches as far as the articular cartilage *(2)*, although no penetration into the knee joint cavity is discernible. The osteolytic area, which has taken up the whole diameter of the tibial head, is surrounded by a wide band of marginal sclerosis *(3)*. The cortex has certainly been narrowed, but not penetrated. No bony periosteal reaction is visible. Within the osteolytic region one can see a few sparsely distributed dense linear structures. Histological examination of the tumor material showed this to be a classical fibrosarcoma which had originated in a primary osteoclastoma (p. 337). The localization in the epiphysis with encroachment into the metaphysis confirms the nature of the primary tumor. Thus, it is a very real possibility that structures characteristic of a fibrosarcoma can appear against the background of some other primary neoplasm.

In a central osseous fibrosarcoma, periosteal bone deposition seldom causes expansion of the shaft, and both spicules and a Codman's triangle are absent. In a few cases, small bony sequestra seen radiologically within the tumor can deceive one into thinking it is a case of osteomyelitis.

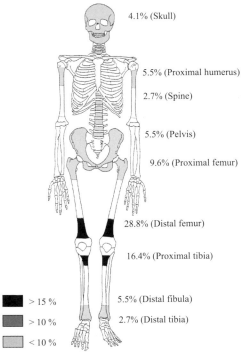

4.1% (Skull)

5.5% (Proximal humerus)

2.7% (Spine)

5.5% (Pelvis)

9.6% (Proximal femur)

28.8% (Distal femur)

16.4% (Proximal tibia)

5.5% (Distal fibula)

2.7% (Distal tibia)

> 15 %

> 10 %

< 10 %

Fig. 624. Localization of the osseous fibrosarcomas (173 cases); others: 19.2%

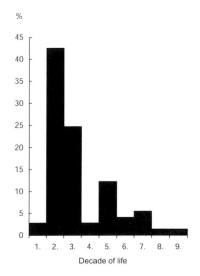

Fig. 625. Age distribution of the osseous fibrosarcomas (173 cases)

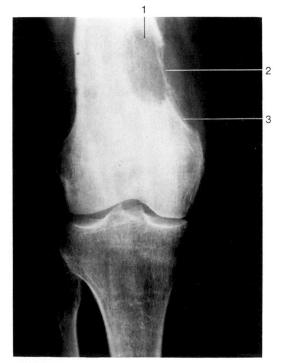

Fig. 626. Osseous fibrosarcoma (distal femoral metaphysis)

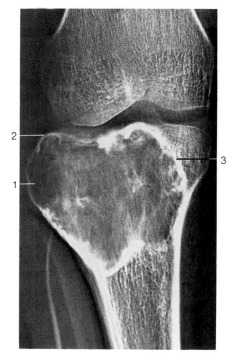

Fig. 627. Osseous fibrosarcoma (tibial head)

Figure 628 is a **macroscopic picture** of a fibrosarcoma that arose in the periosteal connective tissue of the distal part of the femur. It had developed in the popliteal fossa. This is a view of the distal femur from behind, and the articular cartilage of the femoral condyles *(1)* is clearly visible. A lumpy neoplastic outgrowth *(2)* has developed in the region of the distal femoral metaphysis and has reached far into the soft parts. It is attached to the outside of the long bone, since it had originated in the periosteal connective tissue. In advanced cases the growth of the tumor leads to erosion of the cortex, and it can also invade the marrow cavity. From the point of view of the differential diagnosis, this type of tumor must be distinguished from a juxtacortical osteosarcoma (p. 228); this can be done if different parts of it are examined histologically. The tumor is often sharply bordered from without by a connective tissue pseudocapsule, from which it can easily be shelled out. The cut surface reveals the grayish-white or grayish-red tissue of a tough elastic consistency. There is no new bone deposition. The tumorous tissue can be infiltrated and loosened by necroses, degenerative myxoid changes with the formation of cysts and hemorrhages. In the early stages the discrepancy between the palpable size of the tumor and the moderate amount of bone destruction is characteristic. Periosteal fibrosarcomas are less malignant than the intraosseous variety.

Histologically the tumorous tissue is identical with that of the soft tissue fibrosarcomas. In **Fig. 629** one can see a highly cellular, fiber-rich connective tissue arranged in streaks and whorls. Even under **lower magnification** the many clearly polymorphic spindle-shaped nuclei of varying sizes are striking. Quite a few nuclei are strongly hyperchromatic *(1)* and spindle-shaped or lumpy in appearance *(2)*. Here and there, true multinucleated giant cells *(3)* have developed. If the giant cells predominate one must consider the possibility of a fibrosarcoma which has developed on the site of a giant cell neoplasm (osteoclastoma, p. 337, see also Fig. 627). In the more mature forms of this tumor the formation of collagen fibers is prominent; but in undifferentiated fibrosarcomas they may be scarce or even absent. There is no tumorous osteoid or bone, thus distinguishing it histologically from an osteosarcoma

(p. 274). Blood capillaries *(4)* are rare in fibrosarcomas.

Under **higher magnification** the polymorphy and hyperchromasia of the cell nuclei is more clearly discernible in **Fig. 630**. In addition to the small roundish *(1)* and elongated *(2)* nuclei, one can see large, dark spindle-shaped cells *(3)*. Plentiful abnormal mitoses are also observed. The polymorphic nuclei lie in a collagenous framework that is arranged in swathes. The organization of the tumor cells into a herringbone pattern *(4)* is typical of a fibrosarcoma. Depending on the nuclear polymorphy and the differentiation of the tissue, these tumors can be subdivided into three grades of malignancy, and this is important for the prognosis. **Figure 630** shows a fibrosarcoma of grade II. No osteoid structures or tumorous bone can be identified. In places a fine-walled tumorous vessel is lying between the collagen fibers.

In **Fig. 631** a highly cellular fibrosarcoma, in which the formation of collagen fibers is poorly developed, can be seen under **higher magnification**. The narrow elongated tumor cells *(1)* are again characteristically organized into a "herring-bone" pattern of swathes and whorls. In between there are larger tumorous fibroblasts with bizarre, intensely hyperchromatic nuclei *(2)*. In the visual field shown here the nuclear polymorphy is very marked. In addition, the malignant nature of the tumorous growth is indicated by the destruction of the autochthonous bone tissue. The differential diagnosis is between a fibrosarcoma and a malignant histiocytoma (p. 324). Highly differentiated fibrosarcomas can easily be mistakenly identified as benign fibrous bone lesions (e.g. fibrous bone dysplasia, p. 318; or a non-ossifying osteofibroma, p. 308). Signs of aggressive growth on the radiograph or in the histological section must be taken into account when making a diagnosis.

After the malignant histiocytomas (p. 324) had been classified separately from the fibrosarcomas, osseous fibrosarcomas became much less common. The histological distinction is sometimes not easy, since histiocytomas can also show pronounced collagen fiber formation, and the histiocytes are often difficult to recognize. Fibrosarcomas grow relatively slowly and metastasize late. Their prognosis is therefore relatively favorable.

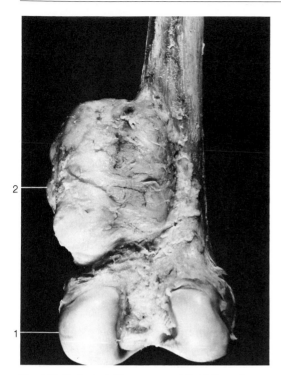

Fig. 628. Periosteal fibrosarcoma (distal femur)

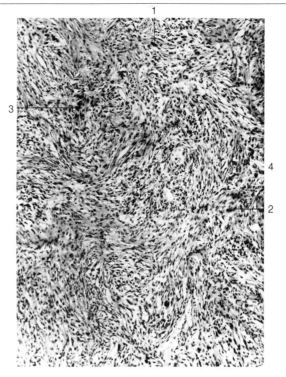

Fig. 629. Osseous fibrosarcoma; HE, ×25

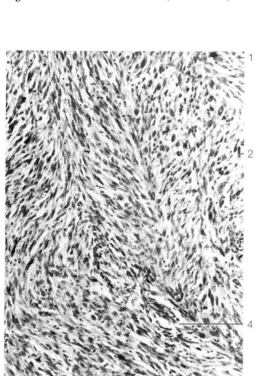

Fig. 630. Osseous fibrosarcoma; HE, ×40

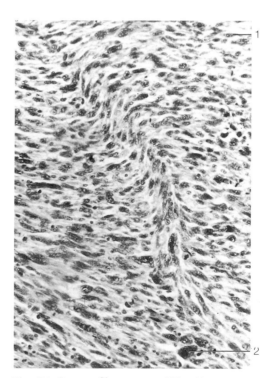

Fig. 631. Osseous fibrosarcoma; HE, ×64

The **radiograph** of an osseous fibrosarcoma is depicted in **Fig. 632**. In the proximal part of the left femur there is a large destructive osteolytic focus *(1)* below the trochanteric plane, which shows diffuse shadowing and patchy areas of translucency within. Here the original bone tissue has been completely destroyed. The tumor has also spread into the cortex *(2)*, which is also patchily loosened and thickened, and which bulges outwards. Such an expansive increase in the size of the tumor causes periosteal pain, which is mostly symptomatic of malignant growth. In the early stage the inside of the tumor is at first sharply delineated by discrete marginal sclerosis *(3)*. This is a sign of the slow early growth of the tumor, and must not be seen as a sign of its benign nature. The diffuse destruction of the cortex is a sign of malignancy.

Figure 633 shows the **radiograph** of an osseous fibrosarcoma of the tibial head. The lateral view shows this part of the bone to be is infiltrated with patchy densifications *(1)*. In between, one can see many fine osteosclerotic foci *(2)*. The lesion is not sharply demarcated within the bone, and there is no marginal sclerosis. The tumor has infiltrated the ventral cortex *(3)* and has destroyed it. This suggests a malignant tumor which must be histologically investigated by bone biopsy.

In **Fig. 634** one can see the classical **histological picture** of a fibrosarcoma as it can develop either in the soft parts or primarily within a bone. The whole tumor consists of fairly uniform connective tissue which is partly plaited, partly straggly and partly arranged in whorls. It contains many spindle-cells in unequal concentrations, which vary in size and have clearly polymorphic nuclei. Some of the nuclei are thin and spindle-shaped *(1)* and others are large and ungainly *(2)*. All the nuclei are extremely hyperchromatic. The number of pathological mitoses is variable; in highly differentiated fibrosarcomas they are few, in the undifferentiated variety, numerous. The cytoplasm of the tumor cells is scanty and indistinctly demarcated. Within the tumor one can see the "herring-bone" pattern *(3)* which is very characteristic of fibrosarcomas. The tumor is subdivided by parallel bundles of fibers running in different directions and planes, some of which have been cut longitudinally *(4)* and some transversely *(5)*. The amount of collagen varies in the individual fibrosarcomas. Usually there are only a few delicate collagen fibers between the tumor cells, sometimes broad fibers are seen which may also be hyalinized. Within the tumor there is no development of tumorous osteoid or bone, and this distinguishes the osseous fibrosarcoma from an osteosarcoma (p. 274). The original bone trabeculae are completely destroyed, so that an osteolytic focus appears on the radiograph. It is only in the marginal zones of an intraosseous fibrosarcoma that the reactive formation of new fibro-osseous trabeculae can occur. These are, however, not a product of the tumors and can be clearly distinguished histomorphologically from tumorous bone trabeculae.

Under **higher magnification** the pleomorphic nature of the tumor cells is clearly expressed in **Fig. 635**. One can observe here many small roundish cells *(1)* and also elongated spindle-cells *(2)*. Some of the cells possess large dark polymorphic nuclei *(3)* or even bizarre giant nuclei *(4)*. The so-called "herring-bone" pattern *(5)* which distinguishes the fibrosarcoma is very clearly seen in this exposure. Between the tumor cells there is a poorly developed network of collagen fibers. Tumorous osteoid and bone must be histologically excluded in the biopsy material before one can diagnose an osseous fibrosarcoma.

This tumor usually grows relatively slowly and has a relatively good prognosis. In the case of small fibrosarcomas without infiltration of the soft parts an extensive en bloc excision is sufficient; with extensive growth of the tumor, amputation is necessary. Surgical extirpation is the only effective treatment. Irradiation can only be considered as a palliative measure for inoperable cases, since the tumor is resistant to radiotherapy. The effects of chemotherapy is questionable. The prognosis depends upon the extent of the tumor, its site and the histological degree of malignancy. On average the 5-year life expectancy amounts to between 28% and 34%. About 20% of these patients survive for longer than 10 years.

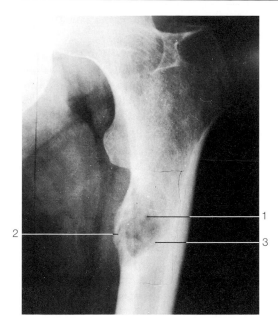

Fig. 632. Osseous fibrosarcoma (proximal femur)

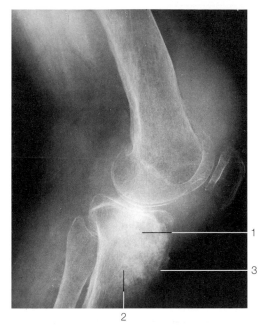

Fig. 633. Osseous fibrosarcoma (tibial head)

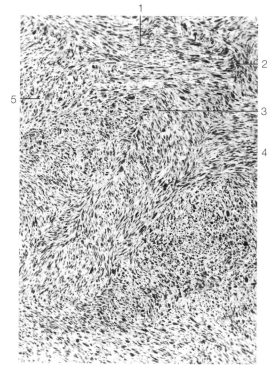

Fig. 634. Osseous fibrosarcoma; HE, ×40

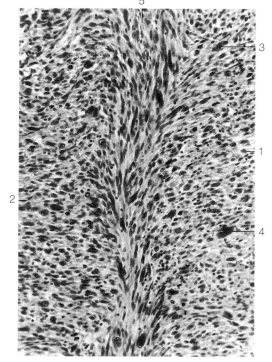

Fig. 635. Osseous fibrosarcoma; HE, ×80

Fibromatous bone tumors consists mostly of connective tissue, which is the real tissue of the neoplasm. Twelve items are assigned to this group, of which 10 are benign and only 2 are malignant. It is difficult here to distinguish "true" tumors from reactive processes or tumor-like lesions. Certainly the fibroblastic periosteal reaction of the distal femoral metaphysis (p. 314) is no bone tumor, but since it can wrongly give the radiological appearance of a tumor, it must be mentioned with the connective tissue bone tumors. Much the commonest of these is the non-ossifying bone fibroma (p. 308), although it is doubtful if it really is a tumorous growth. In most cases this harmless lesion must not be treated surgically, and it can, with increasing age of the patient, spontaneously regress without further development or become fully ossified. This is equally true of the osseous xanthofibroma (p. 312) and the fibrous cortical defect (p. 314), both of which are variants of the non-ossifying bone fibroma. Fibrous bone dysplasia (Jaffe-Lichtenstein, p. 318) and osteofibrous bone dysplasia (Campanacci, p. 316) belong both to the skeletal dysplasias (p. 56) and to the tumor-like lesions, but they are not true bone tumors. As against this, it is probable that the ossifying bone fibroma (p. 316), the osseous fibromyxoma (p. 312), the desmoplastic bone fibroma (p. 322) and the benign fibrous histiocytoma (p. 322) are indeed bone tumors. The tumorous character of the malignant fibrous neoplasms is naturally not open to question.

All these lesions have their typical **localization** within the affected bone. The fibrous bone dysplasia of Jaffe-Lichtenstein may appear either in the metaphyses or the diaphyses, while the osteofibrous bone dysplasia of Campanacci is found predominantly in the tibial diaphysis. Non-ossifying bone fibromas arise in the metaphyses, and ossifying bone fibromas are found almost exclusively in the jaw and facial skeleton.

Radiologically the benign connective tissue bone tumors appear mostly as circumscribed osteolytic areas with marginal sclerosis. They look like "bone cysts". Sometimes the lesion also presents a focus of densification (e.g. in an ossifying bone fibroma). They are fully recognizable in the radiograph as benign lesions, and quite often no treatment is necessary (e.g. for a non-ossifying bone fibroma, p. 308; or a fibrous cortical defect, p. 314). Even a fibroblastic periosteal reaction of the distal femoral metaphysis (p. 314) can be diagnosed from the radiograph alone. On the other hand, a desmoplastic bone fibroma (p. 322) and tumors showing the radiological criteria of malignancy (fibrosarcomas, malignant fibrous histiocytomas) must be histologically investigated by means of a bone biopsy.

Most of the lesions from this groups of tumors can be easily diagnosed **histologically**. The differential diagnosis between an osseous fibrosarcoma and a malignant fibrous histiocytoma can be difficult. There was a time (about 20 years ago) when the osseous fibrosarcoma (p. 330) was a familiar and not particularly rare primary malignant tumor of bone. Today we encounter the osseous malignant fibrous histiocytoma (p. 324) much more frequently. The osseous fibrosarcoma has now become exceedingly rare. Even so, the classification of the malignant fibrous histiocytoma as a separate entity among bone neoplasms is still a matter of controversy. From the point of view of diagnosis and treatment, however, this discussion is of no importance.

As regards therapy, most of the benign connective tissue tumors require no treatment at all. For the malignant neoplasms of this type, however, only surgical extirpation need be considered.

Giant Cell Tumor of Bone (Osteoclastoma) (ICD-O-DA-M-9250/1)

The giant cell neoplasms of bone present particularly serious problems with regard to diagnosis and treatment. It is especially important to distinguish them from the so-called "brown tumors" – the resorptive giant cells granulomas associated with hyperparathyroidism (p. 85). VIRCHOW classified the osteoclastomas under the myelogenous sarcomas, but stressed their largely limited malignancy as compared with the "osteoid sarcomas". At first these neoplasms were treated in the same way as osteosarcomas, but, because they were observed to run a more favorable course, they were later regarded as "benign giant cell tumors". Today we realize that the prognosis of the osteoclastomas is extremely problematic. These tumors have a strong tendency, particularly after irradiation, to undergo malignant change. Furthermore, quite apart from these secondarily malignant osteoclastomas, 10%–30% of these giant cell neoplasms are primarily malignant. They reveal a locally destructive and invasive growth and give rise to lung metastases. Generally speaking all osteoclastomas should be regarded as at least potentially malignant.

The histogenetic origin of this type of tumor is still unknown and controversial. It is assumed that the tumor cells are derived from the non-osteogenic connective tissue of the bone marrow, which accounts for their frequently quite marked fibromatous differentiation. As has been shown by the recent work of several authors, the predominating multinucleated giant cells found in this tumor are not the tumorous cells. The true proliferating tumor cells are to be found in the sarcomatous stroma of this lesion. Thus, the greater the degree of malignancy of the osteoclastoma, the more do the multinucleated osteoclastic giant cells fade into the background. They become smaller and fewer, and the sarcomatous stroma comes ever more to the fore. This implies that the name "osteoclastoma" or "giant cell neoplasm" is not really appropriate. Nevertheless, this terminology is still recognized by the WHO for this histogenetically questionable tumor.

The giant cell tumor of bone (osteoclastoma) is a primary bone tumor which undergoes locally aggressive growth, the malignancy of which may be either questionable or unambiguous. It arises osteolytically in the epiphysis of a bone, and consists histologically of a strongly vascularized spindle-cell stroma with numerous regularly distributed osteoclastic giant cells. It is always potentially malignant. This tumor constitutes about 5% of all primary bone tumors. By using histological criteria it has been possible to distinguish three degrees of differentiation:

"Benign osteoclastomas" (grade I; see Figs. 642, 643) consist of a loose and highly vascular stroma with numerous similarly shaped spindle-cells and many multinucleated giant cells which are regularly distributed throughout the tumor. The giant cells may contain more than 50 bubble-like nuclei. Mitoses are rare. Within the tumorous tissue collagenous or osseous material is scarce, and there are no cartilaginous structures. In the neighborhood of an osteoclastoma reactive bone deposition may occur. In the *"semimalignant osteoclastoma"* (grade II; see Figs. 644, 645) the spindle-cell stroma emerges further into the foreground. The spindle-cells show distinct nuclear polymorphy, and the size and chromatin content of their nuclei are variable. More mitoses are observed. The giant cells are present in smaller numbers and have fewer nuclei. The *"malignant osteoclastomas"* (grade III; see Figs. 646, 647) show marked polymorphy of cells and nuclei. The sarcomatous stroma dominates the histological picture, whereas the giant cells retreat more and more into the background.

This histological gradation is in general diagnostic use today, but the biological status of these tumors has not yet been firmly established. In our experience, however, osteoclastomas always behave at least like semimalignant tumors, since they are all locally destructive and invasive. There are, moreover, reports of osteoclastomas which in spite of their "benign" appearance have produced lung metastases, although no sarcomatous change is evident in the tumor picture. The histological level of differentiation does not therefore allow more than limited diagnostic conclusions to be drawn. The so-called "benign" osteoclastomas (grades I and II) make up about 15% of all benign bone tumors. Approximately 0.5% of all bone sarcomas are unequivocally malignant osteoclastomas.

It is absolutely essential to bear in mind the fact that large numbers of osteoclastic giant cells can be present in various tumorous and non-tumorous bone lesions, and that these must not be confused with an osteoclastoma. These include, among others: osteosarcomas (p. 274), chondroblastomas (p. 226), osteoblastomas (p. 264), aneurysmal bone cysts (p. 412) and bone granulomas (p. 195).

Localization (Fig. 636). True osteoclastomas arise in the epiphysis and spread out into the metaphysis (see Fig. 378). It is the long bones that are mostly affected. The region of the knee (distal part of the femur, proximal part of the tibia or fibula) is the most frequent site, where 42.1% of all osteoclastomas are recorded. We found this tumor most often in the leg bones. The second most common site is the femur. Of the giant cell lesions of the jaw bones, which often appear before the 15th year, the most usual is a reparative giant cell granuloma (p. 204) which must be distinguished from the true osteoclastomas. Osteoclastomas in the neighborhood of the knee are particularly prone to malignancy, although the giant cell neoplasms in the pelvis also show a high percentage of malignant cases. The recurrence rate amounts to 40%–60%. In the spinal column, including the sacrum, 6.2% of osteoclastomas have been observed, and here they must be distinguished from the more commonly encountered aneurysmal bone cyst (p. 412). Over 6% of osteoclastomas have been found in the short tubular bones of the hands and feet, where the frequently occurring giant cell reaction (p. 204) must be borne in mind. It is always necessary first of all to exclude hyperparathyroidism. A few multiple osteoclastomas have been reported.

Age Distribution (Fig. 637). It must be remembered that osteoclastomas hardly ever appear before the 10th year of life, and that after the age of 55 they are rare. They mostly arise during the 3rd decade of life, and 80% of the patients are more than 20 years old. Since primary malignant osteoclastomas can appear late in life (up to the 9th decade), every giant cell neoplasm in patients of over 40 must be suspected of malignancy. Those patients with a malignant osteoclastoma (grade III) are on average older than those with the "benign"

variety (grade I). This can partly be explained by the fact, known from experience, that sarcomatous change only takes place several years after the treatment of an earlier benign giant cell neoplasm. In this way the degree of malignity of an osteoclastoma can alter.

The predominance of women over men here is striking. A total of 58% of the patients are women, and for those of less than 20 years old this group accounts for as much as 74%. In the case of the malignant osteoclastomas, however, and among the higher age groups, men and women are equally affected.

In the **radiograph** a typical osteoclastoma appears as an osteolytic lesion with no marginal sclerosis, usually lying eccentrically in the epi-metaphyseal region where it narrows the cortex from within and expands the bone outwards. Even if the cortex remains intact there is often a bony periosteal reaction. In **Fig. 638** one can see an osteoclastoma of the distal tibial epiphysis *(1)* that has advanced far into the metaphysis *(2)* and has slightly elevated this part of the bone. In the cystic, shell-like elevation of the epi-metaphysis the normal morphology of the spongiosa has been abolished. The "bony cyst" is fuzzily demarcated from the healthy spongiosa *(3)*, and no marginal sclerosis can be seen. Irregular strips of bone reach inwards into the osteolytic area. One speaks of a so-called "soap-bubble effect" which is considered to be a pathognomonic characteristic of osteoclastomas, although this obviously only applies to slow-growing tumors. In the rapidly growing giant cell tumors (osteolytic type) no mesh of trabecular structures is visible in the radiograph. The cortex is thin and indented and in places invaded by the tumor *(4)*. No periosteal thickening *(5)* can be seen, and the tumor has not invaded the neighboring joint space *(6)*.

In **Fig. 639** one can see the **macroscopic picture** of a malignant osteoclastoma of the lumbar column. This part of the spine of a 49-year-old woman has been sawn through in the frontal plane to show the normal vertebral bodies *(1)* and the intervertebral discs *(2)*. The 2nd lumbar vertebra is completely destroyed and has broken down on one side *(3)*. On the other side there is soft, grayish-red tumorous tissue *(4)* which has destroyed the cortex. The section also shows many cysts, hemorrhages, necroses and irregular bone trabeculae.

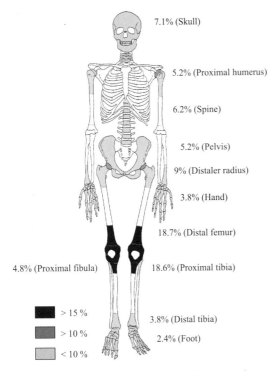

7.1% (Skull)

5.2% (Proximal humerus)

6.2% (Spine)

5.2% (Pelvis)

9% (Distaler radius)

3.8% (Hand)

18.7% (Distal femur)

4.8% (Proximal fibula)   18.6% (Proximal tibia)

> 15 %

> 10 %

< 10 %

3.8% (Distal tibia)

2.4% (Foot)

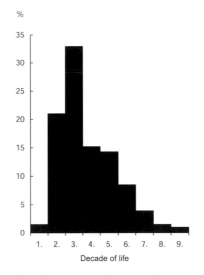

Fig. 636. Localization of the osteoclastomas (210 cases); others 15.2%

Fig. 637. Age distribution of the osteoclastomas (210 cases)

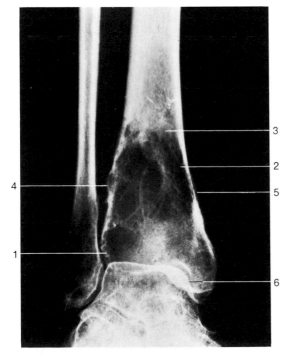

Fig. 638. Osteoclastoma (distal tibia)

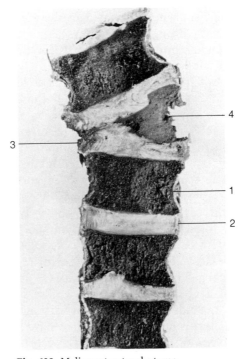

Fig. 639. Malignant osteoclastoma (body of 2nd lumbar vertebra, cut surface)

There are no sure radiological criteria for determining the degree of malignity, and even the angiographic findings provide little information on this. The tumor is heavily vascularized and there are numerous newly formed arteriolar networks and lacunae.

The **radiograph** of a truly typical osteoclastoma is shown in **Fig. 640**. One can see from the gaping epiphyseal plates *(1)* that this is a child. The tumor arose in a 14-year-old boy and is mostly lying in the distal radial metaphysis *(2)*. This part of the bone is considerably expanded as if by a cyst and there is a typical "soap bubble effect" present. One can discern the eccentric osteolysis, which is fairly sharply demarcated, although there is no marginal sclerosis. The adjacent cortex *(2)* has been severely narrowed, but is still intact. No periosteal thickening or bony periosteal reaction is visible. Within the osteolytic zone a few irregular narrow trabecular structures stand out. On one side the tumor extends right up close to the cartilaginous epiphyseal plate *(3)*, on the other side of this, however, one can recognize a clear osteolytic zone in the epiphysis itself *(4)*. This part of the bone is also elevated as if by a cyst. It is possible that the growth of this neoplasm originated in the epiphysis and grew through the epiphyseal plate into the metaphysis, where the large osteolytic tumor then developed.

In most cases a therapeutic attempt is made to shell the tumor tissue out by curettage, but one must then expect a 50%–60% recurrence rate. The most reliable treatment is therefore an en bloc resection. In **Fig. 641** one can see under a **dissecting lens** an osteoclastoma in the medial femoral condyle that had previously been curetted. The metaphysis measures 9×6 cm. It encloses a round cavity *(1)* with a diameter of 4.5 cm that is filled with a serous fluid and covered by fiber-rich connective tissue *(2)*. Between the connective tissue covering and the cortex *(3)* there are numerous neoplastic fragments *(4)* up to the size of a cherry, which reach as far as the cortex on one side and the articular cartilage on the other. These remnants of the tumor have a total surface area of 5 cm². This large section shows how difficult it is to achieve complete removal of the giant cell tumor by curettage. One must also remember that with every curettage a very large number of capillaries and sinusoids are opened and that the risk of distributing metastases hematogenously is greatly increased. With osteoclastomas that have twice undergone curettage with subsequent recurrence, it is therefore essential that block excision, resection or amputation should be carried out.

The interpretation of the **histological picture** of an osteoclastoma can be very difficult. In **Fig. 642** one can see tumorous tissue that has been assessed as a *grade I osteoclastoma*. It is richly cellular tissue with a loose, highly vascular stroma containing numerous spindle-cells *(1)*. These have uniform oval or elongated nuclei which show no hyperchromasia. Occasional mitoses may occur, but not many. In the tumorous tissue there is no osteoid, bone or cartilaginous tissue. Even so, the stroma cells have the capacity to form collagen fibers and osteoid, and small amounts of these are sometimes seen in osteoclastomas. The numerous osteoclastic giant cells *(2)* are striking. They are fairly evenly distributed throughout the tumorous tissue and lie more or less equidistant from one another. This even distribution of the giant cells is an important diagnostic observation in comparison with other giant cell bone lesions (e.g. the so-called "brown tumors", p. 85; aneurysmal bone cysts, p. 412; and giant cell reaction, p. 204).

Under **higher magnification** one can see very clearly in **Fig. 643** the highly cellular stroma with its numerous spindle-cells *(1)*. These are mononucleated cells, the cell membranes of which are often difficult to recognize and which produce cell processes. The nuclei have an evenly distributed framework of chromatin and a central nucleolus. Mitoses are rare. The osteoclastic giant cells *(2)* are very large and may have more than 50 bubble-like nuclei. These giant cells often lie in the immediate neighborhood of numerous capillaries *(3)*. Once again one can recognize the dense deposition and even distribution of the giant cells within the loose, highly cellular stroma.

The diagnosis of a **grade I osteoclastoma** is histologically only possible with adequate sections; an aspiration biopsy is not suitable here. Grade I is characterized by: (a) highly cellular densely packed giant cells which are evenly distributed, (b) giant cells with very many isomorphic nuclei, (c) a highly vascular stroma, and (d) no mitoses. One often sees giant cells in the marginal vessels, which is apparently of no significance.

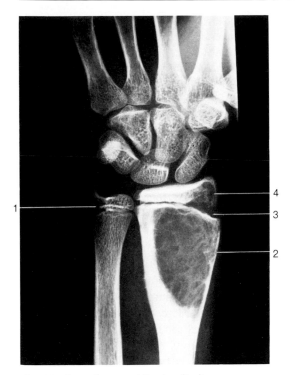

Fig. 640. Osteoclastoma (distal radius)

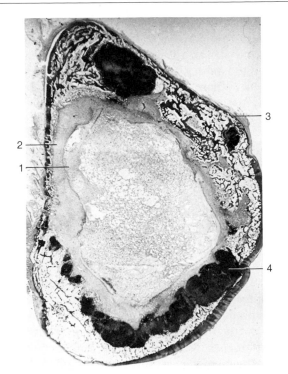

Fig. 641. Osteoclastoma after curettage; HE, ×8

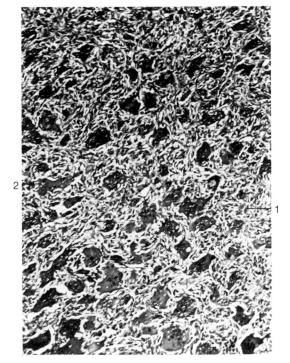

Fig. 642. Osteoclastoma Grade I; HE, ×40

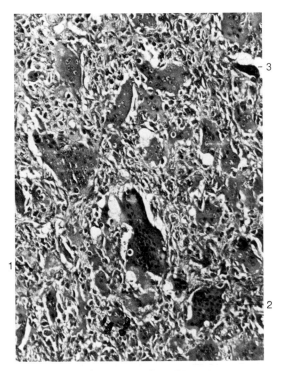

Fig. 643. Osteoclastoma Grade I; HE, ×64

With **osteoclastomas of grade II** the spindle-cell stroma comes more to the fore, while the number and size of the giant cells gets less. In **Fig 644** one can see an overall view of such a tumor. Once again there is a a highly cellular tumorous tissue in which numerous osteoclastic giant cells *(1)* are present. These giant cells are, however, lying further apart from one another and are not so evenly distributed within the tissue. In comparison with the grade I neoplasm (see Fig. 642) they are significantly smaller and have fewer nuclei, which are also smaller and no longer bubble-like. The stroma is very porous and threaded through with many capillaries *(2)*. It is often soaked in blood and fibrin, and is interspersed with inflammatory cells *(3)*: lymphocytes, plasma cells and histiocytes. One is struck be the nuclei seen in the stromal spindle-cells. These nuclei vary in size, and are partly hyperchromatic and partly also polymorphic *(4)*. More and more mitoses are present. The histological picture is, in general, significantly less restful and more polymorphic than with a grade I osteoclastoma, although there is still no unequivocally sarcomatous tissue to be seen.

Under **higher magnification** the picture in **Fig. 645** is dominated by spindle-cell stroma. It is highly cellular, very porous and threaded through with capillaries *(1)*. The stromal spindle-cells have markedly hyperchromatic nuclei, and these show a certain polymorphy. They are either elongated and oval *(2)* or roundish and lumpy *(3)*. The osteoclastic giant cells have completely retreated into the background. They are relatively small and contain few nuclei *(4)*, sometimes appearing only as shapeless clumps of chromatin where the nuclei have come together. The spindle-cell stroma, in which mitoses are usually found in large numbers, is of particular importance diagnostically. The absence of tumorous osteoid and bone is also important in making a differential diagnosis from the telangiectatic osteosarcoma (p. 283). Nevertheless, the grading of osteoclastomas depends largely on the subjective assessment of the tumorous tissue. The histological evaluation of these bone lesions requires a great deal of experience.

The appearance of *malignant osteoclastomas of grade III* is dominated by the sarcomatous stroma. As can be seen in the general view shown in **Fig. 646**, there are only a few unevenly distributed giant cells *(1)*. They are relatively small and have a few dark polymorphic nuclei. The predominant structures are those of a spindle-cell sarcoma which shows all the signs of a malignant tumor. The spindle cells *(2)* have shapeless polymorphic nuclei with a dense chromatin content. Mitoses are present in large numbers, many of which are pathological. In places *(3)* a malignant osteoclastoma can often not be distinguished from a fibrosarcoma (p. 333). If osteoid structures are observed in the neoplasms, the differential diagnosis includes the osteosarcoma (p. 279), since abnormal osteoclastic giant cells can also appear in this growth. Regions typical of an osteoclastoma must also be taken into account before the diagnosis of a malignant giant cell neoplasm can be made.

Under the **higher magnification** of **Fig. 647** the malignant character of the neoplasm is clearly and unquestionably recognizable. One can see a sarcomatous spindle-cell stroma that is more or less loosely porous. The spindle-cells have laid down a sparse framework of collagen fibers that shows up only weakly with van Gieson staining. These cells have nuclei of varying size which are sometimes elongated ovals *(1)* and sometimes roundish and lumpy *(2)*, and which have a dense chromatin content. Numerous pathological mitoses can be seen. There is considerable polymorphy and hyperchromasia of the stromal cell nuclei, indicating an unquestionably malignant growth. Osteoclastic giant cells *(3)* of varying sizes are unevenly distributed throughout the field. They possess polymorphic and hyperchromatic nuclei which often appear as shapeless irregular clumps of chromatin. Considering the obviously sarcomatous nature of the neoplasm, giant cells of this kind add confirmation to the diagnosis of a malignant osteoclastoma.

Osteoclastomas of grades I or II can sometimes change completely into a grade III osteoclastoma. The picture presented by the histological section shows the various degrees of differentiation appearing next to each other. Nevertheless, many cases are seen in which a grade I osteoclastoma, which has been accordingly classified as benign, can give rise to recurrences and even metastases. For this reason all osteoclastomas should be regarded as malignant in principle; the separating into grades then becomes of questionable significance.

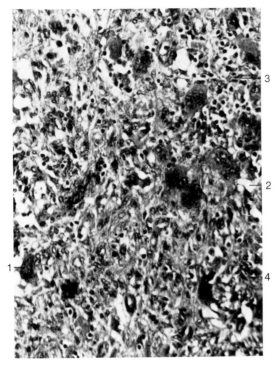

Fig. 644. Osteoclastoma Grade 2; HE, ×40

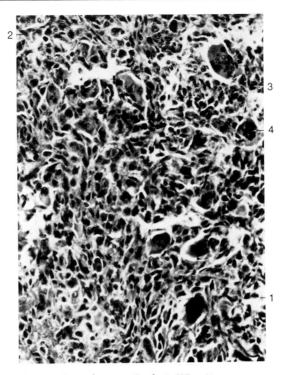

Fig. 645. Osteoclastoma Grade 2; HE, ×64

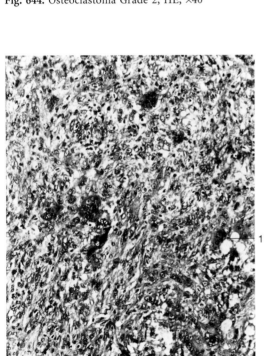

Fig. 646. Osteoclastoma Grade 3; HE, ×40

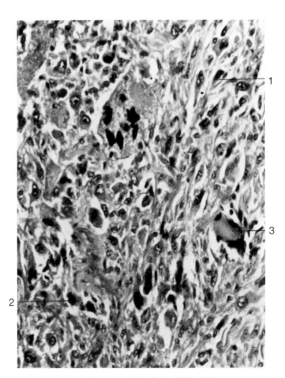

Fig. 647. Osteoclastoma Grade 3; HE, ×82

The *giant cells tumors of bone* make up a whole series of bone lesions of this type, and create a particularly difficult diagnostic and therapeutic problem. The giant cells are mostly osteoclasts, although there are some histiocytes too. Today these can be recognized by enzyme-histochemical and immunohistochemical tests. This type of giant cell appears as a macrophage both in reactive processes (e.g. a reparative giant cell granuloma of the jaw, p. 204; giant cell reaction of the short tubular bones, p. 204; foreign body reaction in the neighborhood of a prosthesis, p. 123), in hormonally controlled osteopathies (e.g. a resorptive giant cell granuloma in the presence of osteodystrophy – that is to say, the so-called "brown tumor" of hyperparathyroidism) or as Langerhans' giant cells in histiocytosis X (p. 196). In osteoclastomas they are shown by enyzmehistochemical tests (identification of tartrate-resistant acid phosphatase) to nearly always be osteoclasts.

Osteoclastomas are **localized** in the epiphyses of the long bones, which is an important diagnostic fact. Here they produce areas of osteolysis without marginal sclerosis. This radiological finding must invariably be taken into account when making a diagnosis, in order to distinguish osteoclastomas from other giant cells lesions of bone.

Radiologically these lesions appear in the epiphysis as "soap-bubble" areas of osteolysis without marginal sclerosis. This osteolysis can, however, extend radiologically right over into the adjacent metaphysis, so that it is not possible to establish whether the lesion arose in the epiphysis and extended into the metaphysis or, vice versa, whether the metaphysis was the site of origin with subsequent involvement of the epiphysis. In such cases the radiological findings offer scant information about the localization.

The **histological picture** of an osteoclastoma is determined by the numerous osteoclastic giant cells. These are, however, often present in other lesions of bone, which must be distinguished from the true osteoclastoma. This fact leads to serious problems in diagnosis which can often only be solved by taking all the clinical, radiological and histological findings together. If foci of tumorous osteoid are still found in the lesion, the exclusion of an osteosarcoma may be difficult or sometimes even impossible. In any case this is a bone tumor that is at least potentially malignant and which must therefore be treated aggressively.

Today we treat osteoclastomas – like osteosarcomas – according to the COSS protocol (p. 306). (Biopsy for diagnosis → chemotherapy → operation → postoperative chemotherapy). For osteoclastomas of low malignancy (grade I), local surgical removal of the tumor (without chemotherapy) is still necessary. An osteoclastoma should only be irradiated if it is inoperable (in the vertebral column, for instance) as a palliative measure, since it has frequently been reported that a "benign" osteoclastoma of grade I can become malignant after radiotherapy.

Osteomyelogenous Bone Tumors

Introductory Remarks

The marrow cavity plays a very important role within the skeletal system, where it is the site of origin of numerous different kinds of primary and secondary bone conditions. It is the arena for all types of inflammatory bone disease (osteomyelitis, pp. 134–141), and the target of the bone metastases (p. 396). Most of the bone granulomas (p. 195) and storage diseases (p. 183) are also found here. The marrow cavity is first and foremost the main site of activity of those diseases which originate from the hematopoietic bone marrow. Which of the tumorous osteomyelogenic diseases should really be counted as true tumors of bone is still an open and controversial question. They are all able to elicit structural bone changes that are recognizable both radiologically and – what may be useful for diagnosis – histologically. We have listed osteomyelofibrosis and osteomyelosclerosis (p. 106) among the associated bone diseases.

The main representatives of the tumorous osteomyelogenous lesions are the *leukemias.* It is true that these are strictly speaking hematological conditions. However, the functional/morphological unit comprising bone marrow and bone tissue does lead to structural changes which are apparent both in the radiograph and the histological section, thereby blurring the distinction between skeletal and hematological diseases.

Whereas chronic leukemias in adults seldom produce radiologically recognizable alterations in the skeleton, these are undoubtedly more frequent in children. Here one finds juxtaepiphyseal and, finally, a completely generalized osteoporosis, leading to patches of osteolysis, endosteal osteosclerosis and periosteal osteophytosis. The commonest juxtaepiphyseal osteoporosis appears radiologically as a translucent narrow band which takes in the whole width of the bone and is sharply set apart from the epiphyseal cartilage and the metaphyseal spongiosa. Localized osteoporoses, moth-eaten patches of osteolysis, together with endosteal and periosteal osteosclerosis, determine the radiological picture. In biopsy specimens one can see the characteristic leukemic infiltration of the marrow cavity. There are more or less well-marked signs of increased reactive bone remodeling (increased osteoblastic bone deposition and greater osteoclastic bone resorption).

Although the leukemias are malignant tumorous proliferative processes which primarily take place in the marrow cavity, these diseases are in general regarded as hematological in nature and are not classified as true afflictions of the skeleton. Nevertheless, they present diagnostic problems for the osteologist, since in quite a few bone biopsies (especially from the iliac crest) they need to be analyzed diagnostically. Because, however, they cannot be regarded as true bones diseases, the leukemias will not be dealt with in greater detail here.

Within the bone marrow cavity, however, various tissues appear from which osteomyelogenous tumors can develop, and which are certainly to be classified among primary neoplasms of bone. First and foremost here is the *medullary plasmocytoma*, which is the commonest of all primary malignant bone neoplasms. It manifests itself as an intramedullary proliferation of abnormal plasma cells, usually affecting the marrow cavities of several bones simultaneously. Other malignant osteomyelogenous tumors cannot be unambiguously associated with a particular medullary cell type, and this applies particularly to *Ewing's sarcoma.* The *primary malignant bone lymphoma* (earlier known as the "reticulum cell sarcoma") develops from the lymphatic or, less frequently, reticulohistiocytic cells of the bone marrow and constitutes an independent entity. It is a non-Hodgkin lymphoma that has arisen primarily in bone, without at first attacking the lymph nodes. Finally, a *Hodgkin's lymphoma* can manifest itself primarily in the marrow cavity, when it then counts as a primary tumor of bone.

There are other tissues apart from the bone marrow in the marrow cavity, and neoplasms may develop from these. There is the myeloid connective tissue, from which fibromas or fibrosarcomas (p. 330) may arise, and there are also the blood vessels of the marrow cavity, which can give origin to the vascular bone tumors (p. 369). Finally, the region is rich in fatty tissue, and this can also form the basis for neoplastic growth.

Osseous Lipoma (ICD-0-DA-M-8850/0)

The osseous lipoma is a benign neoplasm that arises from the fatty tissue of the bone marrow cavity and therefore develops in the marrow itself. It is a very rare primary bone neoplasm, and it is usually only diagnosed histologically in association with the radiological findings. It makes up less than 1 in 1,000 bone tumors. The lesion produces hardly any clinical symptoms and is usually only noticed because of the swelling. The cases so far reported do not enable any estimate of the average age or appearance or predilection site to be made. Radiologically it is usually seen as a translucent intraosseous focus, with that section of the bone being slightly expanded.

In **Fig. 648** the **radiograph** shows an osseous lipoma in the calcaneus (1). Here there is an oval osteolytic focus that extends on one side to the cortex (1) and on the other side is fairly sharply demarcated by discrete marginal sclerosis (2). In the center of the focus there is a very dense round shadow (3) produced by the marked central dystrophic calcification of the tumorous tissue. Lipomas may also be parosteal, where elevation of the periosteum and pressure on the nerves may produce pain.

Macroscopically there is a cystic cavity in this type of bony focus which is filled up with lobulated yellowish fatty tissue. Calcified areas may be encountered within the tumorous fatty tissue.

As can be seen in **Fig. 649**, the **histological section** also shows fatty tissue that differs only slightly from the normally occurring fat in the marrow cavity. One finds mature fat cells of different sizes (1) with small roundish isomorphic nuclei. There are no mitoses. Only very sparse narrow connective tissue septa (2) run through the growth, carrying fine blood capillaries with them. Peripherally one often finds a little sclerotic bone tissue (3), and narrow bone trabeculae may be present inside. In general this is a harmless neoplasm that can be removed by curettage.

Osseous Liposarcoma (ICD-0-DA-M-8850/3)

This fatty tissue neoplasm is also very seldom encountered as a primary bone tumor. It is a malignant tumor that arises from the fatty tissue of the marrow cavity and destroys the bone from within. Up to now only a few isolated cases have been reported in the literature, of which the exact diagnosis is sometimes doubtful. Whereas the radiograph reveals malignant tumorous growth, it is often not perfectly clear from the histological picture that the tumor has arisen from fatty tissue. There are, for instance, structural similarities with the malignant histiocytomas (p. 324). Because of the extreme rarity of this growth no information is available either about its localization or its age and sex distribution.

Figure 650 depicts the **radiograph** of a liposarcoma in the right humerus. The tumor has arisen in the proximal part of the bone (1) and then extended a long way distally (2) within the marrow cavity. One can discern the patchy osteolytic destruction of the spongiosa and erosion of the endosteal layer of the cortex (3). There are also osteolytic foci within the cortex (4) which have brought about a periosteal reaction.

The **histological picture** of this neoplasm is very similar to that of the corresponding soft tissue tumor. In **Fig. 651** one can see that the lamellar layering of the bone trabeculae (1) has been preserved. The marrow cavity is filled up with highly cellular tumorous tissue in which the variously sized complexes of large fat cells (2) with their bright cytoplasm are striking. They have small compact hyperchromatic and polymorphic nuclei. Often multinucleated giant cells with bizarre nuclei are also present. In between there are very dense collections of cells (3) with roundish polymorphic spindle-shaped nuclei.

The number of mitoses is variable. With Sudan staining, fat can be identified in all the tumor cells. In general this is a highly malignant neoplasm with a poor prognosis for which radical extirpation is the only effective treatment.

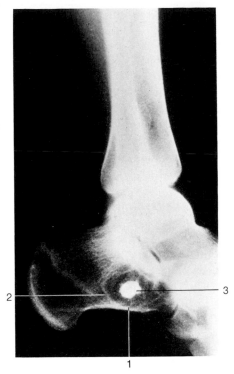

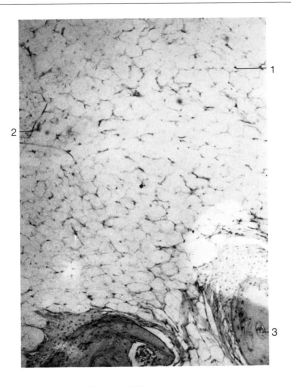

Fig. 648. Bone lipoma (calcaneus)

Fig. 649. Bone lipoma; HE, ×40

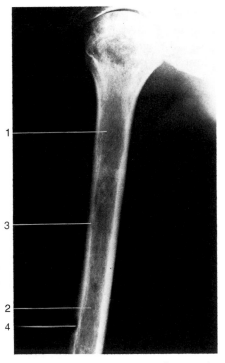

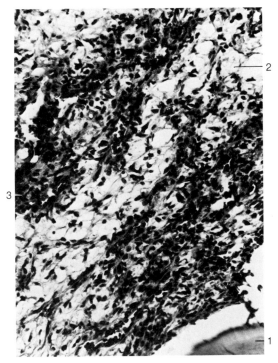

Fig. 650. Osseous liposarcoma (humerus)

Fig. 651. Osseous liposarcoma; HE, ×40

Medullary Plasmocytoma (ICD-O-DA-M-9730/3) (Multiple Myeloma)

By far the commonest malignant bone neoplasm is the medullary plasmocytoma, which makes up more than half of these tumors. It can appear as an isolated lesion in a single bone or arise in several of them simultaneously (multiple myeloma). It usually develops monotopically in one bone (e.g. femur or humerus) and them spreads with multiple foci throughout the skeleton. The tumor takes its origin from the primitive reticular cells. *There is a malignant tumorous proliferation of the plasma cells in the bone marrow which leads to local destruction of bone, and in addition to the complex syndrome known as Kahler's disease.* Clinically the predominant symptom is increasing bone pain. There may also be deformities of the affected bones with spontaneous fractures and neurological symptoms. Characteristically there is an increase in the immunoglobulins in the blood plasma (usually IgG and IgA, more rarely IgE or IgD, the so-called monoclonal immunoglobulins; partly "heavy" (H) or "light" (L) chain, or L and H antibodies), which gives rise to an increased erythrocyte sedimentation rate or altered electrophoresis (identification of paraproteins). In the kidneys pathological proteins are often excreted (Bence-Jones proteins, "light chain" protein), and this is followed by resorption and the storage of hyaline protein drops in the tubular epithelium ("plasmocytoma kidney"). In 10% of the cases a generalized amyloidosis develops. In 10%–15% of patients with a plasmocytoma a hypercalcinemia of more than 20 mg% is found, although the serum phosphates and alkaline phosphatase remain within normal limits.

Localization (Fig. 652). A medullary plasmocytoma can develop in any bone which has a marrow cavity – which is to say that almost any bone may be attacked by the tumor. Most commonly, plasmocytoma foci are found in the vertebral bodies, ribs, pelvis, skull cap, femur or sternum. The short tubular bones are only rarely affected. In about 5% of cases tumorous foci appear in the bones of the jaws, the mandible being more frequently affected than the maxilla. As far as the localization is concerned, there is no difference between the solitary and multiple myelomas. Most commonly affected is the vertebral column.

Age Distribution (Fig. 653). The higher age groups are much more often affected, more than 60% of the plasmocytomas appearing in the 6th and 7th decades of life. Before the age of 50 years plasmocytomas are extremely uncommon, and mostly single tumors. It is more frequent (73%) in men than in women.

Figure 654 shows the **radiograph** of a medullary plasmocytoma in the left humerus. Spreading of the tumor in the marrow cavity can leave the radiograph unchanged; it is only after the spongiosa has undergone considerable destruction and the compacta has been attacked from within that bone defects become visible radiologically. The left humerus depicted in **Fig. 654** shows in its proximal part an extensive expansion of the bone which reaches as far as the proximal metaphysis *(1)*. One can clearly recognize the far-reaching destruction of the spongiosa in this region, in which an osteosclerotic increase in density *(2)* is mixed up with "osteoporotic" porosity. The translucent foci are extremely patchy and are present throughout the whole marrow cavity of the bone. A few are sharply demarcated by a fine marginal sclerosis *(3)*, while others are large foci of destruction. The cortex has also become involved in the process of osteolytic destruction. In many places it has been "gnawed away" from within, as if by a rat *(4)*. Penetration of the cortex by the intramedullary tumor may cause thickening of the periosteum. A plasmocytoma can also lead to the development of a localized tumor in the affected bone which may become the site of a pathological fracture.

Thin bones (skull cap, scapula, pelvis) are very soon eaten away by the tumor. **Figure 655** shows the **radiograph** of a so-called "buck-shot skull". One can see multiple punched-out round foci of osteolysis *(1)* in the skull cap which are indeed sharply demarcated but not surrounded by marginal sclerosis. This radiograph is very characteristic of a plasmocytoma. Whereas a solitary plasmocytoma shows up on the radiograph as a punched-out defect with diffuse surrounding osteosclerosis, the multiple myeloma shows an osteoporosis-like osteolysis of the spongiosa that involves the greater part of the bone.

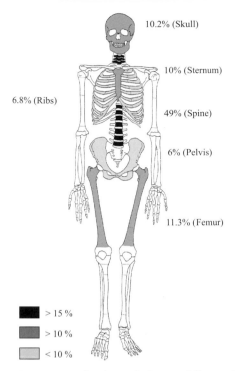

10.2% (Skull)

10% (Sternum)

6.8% (Ribs)

49% (Spine)

6% (Pelvis)

11.3% (Femur)

■ > 15 %

▨ > 10 %

▧ < 10 %

Fig. 652. Localization of the medullary plasmocytomas (1,100 cases); others: 6.7%

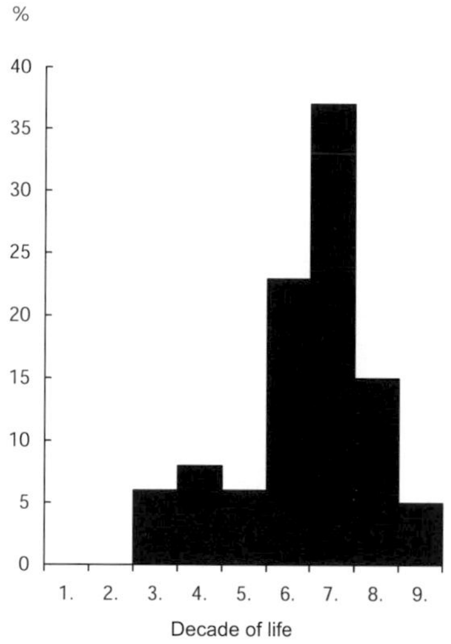

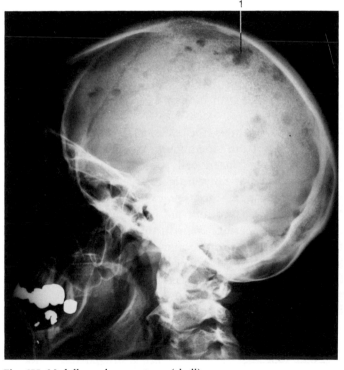

%

40

35

30

25

20

15

10

5

0

1. 2. 3. 4. 5. 6. 7. 8. 9.

Decade of life

Fig. 653. Age distribution of the medullary plasmocytomas (1,100 cases)

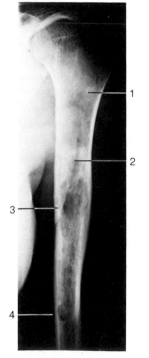

Fig. 654. Medullary plasmocytoma (left proximal humerus)

Fig. 655. Medullary plasmocytoma (skull)

The **macroscopic appearance** of a medullary plasmocytoma is represented by the sawn specimen depicted in **Fig. 656**. The cancellous bony framework work has been extensively destroyed and is only preserved in part at the cortical margin *(1)*. The entire marrow cavity has been taken over by a glassy, partly dark red *(2)*, partly grayish-white tumorous mass *(3)* of soft consistency. Parts of the bony cancellous framework may be preserved and even show a reactive increase in density, giving the radiograph a patchy, partly osteolytic, partly osteosclerotic appearance. The originally intramedullary tumor finally attacks the endosteal surface of the cortex, and we can see that its inner layer *(4)* no longer has a smooth border, but looks as though it has been irregularly gnawed. This entirely characteristic morphological picture of a plasmocytoma is often discernible in the radiograph and described as "rat-bitten". Such a type of tumorous growth can produce a reactive osteosclerotic increase in the thickness and density of the cortex *(5)* if it proceeds slowly. The tumor may, however, even penetrate the cortex and destroy it, often bringing about reactive thickening of the periosteum *(6)*. Finally, it may invade the parosteal soft parts, with a very real danger of a pathological fracture occurring. Macroscopic assessment of an intramedullary plasmocytoma is usually only possible at autopsy, and in most cases the pathologist is presented with biopsy material for diagnostic analysis.

Figure 657 depicts the classical **histological appearance** of an medullary plasmocytoma. One can see a closed cell sheet of abnormal plasma cells with very little intercellular stroma, the cells being sometimes loosely, sometimes densely packed, but not actually enclosed in any tissue coating. Even in this overall view the variously sized and polymorphic nuclei are striking. The chromatin content is variable. Some cells are weakly stained *(1)*, others are very dark *(2)*. In this tumorous tissue some large vacuoles *(3)* left over from the original fatty tissue are still visible.

Under **higher magnification** one can see in **Fig. 658** that the tumor cells are unmistakably plasma cells. They have distinct cell membranes and a richly eosinophilic cytoplasm. The nuclei are mostly round and eccentrically placed *(1)*. The chromatin within them is often minutely fragmented and concentrated in the periphery, giving rise to the so-called "wheel-spoke structure". In most cases, however, these abnormal plasma cells show a generally dense concentration of chromatin inside the nucleus. Several nucleoli are frequently present in the same nucleus. Only rarely are abnormal mitoses encountered. Multinucleated plasma cells and giant cells are also present *(2)*. Sometime one can see vacuoles and inclusions (the so-called "Russel bodies") within the cytoplasm. The most striking properties of this tumorous tissue are the differences in size of the plasma cells and their nuclei and also the distinct cellular and nuclear polymorphy. In highly differentiated plasmocytomas the plasma cells may be remarkably uniform, making it difficult to distinguish the tumor from a non-specific plasmocytosis (MGUS) or plasma cell osteomyelitis (p. 142). On the other hand, the plasma cells in an undifferentiated tumor may lose their characteristic morphological appearance, and it is then difficult to distinguish it from another malignant bone lymphoma (the reticulum cell sarcoma, p. 358). Certainly, no reticulin fibers are found in a plasmocytoma.

Figure 659 is a **cell smear** made from an intramedullary plasmocytoma, in which the morphological characteristics of the plasma cells are very clearly shown. One can again recognize the polygonal cells with their markedly eccentric nuclei. These nuclei vary in size and chromatin content, the chromatin being concentrated in such a manner as to produce the "wheel-spoke" appearance. The cytoplasm is partly eosinophilic, partly basophilic. The outline of the cell border is distinct, although no cell membrane is visible.

An **isolated plasmocytoma** is not usually accompanied by serological changes (Kahler's disease). It is a circumscribed bone tumor that calls for local surgical treatment. With a 60% survival rate of 5 years, the prognosis is relatively good, although transition into a multiple myeloma is possible. A **generalized plasmocytoma** is treated today by chemotherapy, in spite of which a 5-year survival of only just 10% can be achieved.

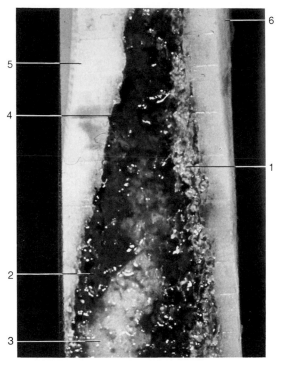

Fig. 656. Medullary plasmocytoma (femur, cut surface)

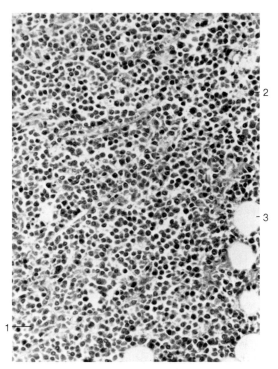

Fig. 657. Medullary plasmocytoma; HE, ×64

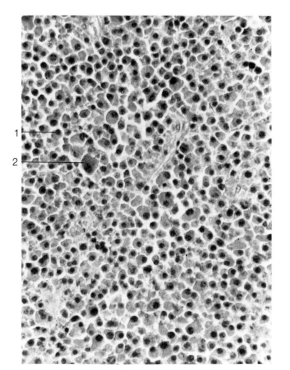

Fig. 658. Medullary plasmocytoma; HE, ×100

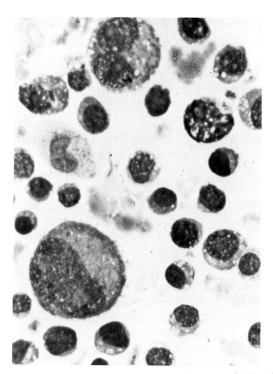

Fig. 659. Medullary plasmocytoma (cytosmear), May-Grün-wald-Giemsa, ×630

Ewing's Sarcoma (ICD-O-DA-M-9260/3)

Ewing's sarcoma accounts for up to about 8% of the malignant bone tumors. *It is a highly malignant primary bone neoplasm of children and young people. It develops in the marrow cavity, and probably arises from the immature reticular cells of the bone marrow.* Clinically the tumor, which cannot with certainty be diagnosed radiologically, imitates the signs and symptoms of osteomyelitis. Local swelling, heat, pain, fever and a raised erythrocyte sedimentation rate are the presenting symptoms of a Ewing's sarcoma. The local pain is periosteal in origin, the immediate cause being local tension, and the infiltration of the periosteum by the tumor. Pathological fractures occur in about 10% of cases.

Localization (Fig. 660). The main sites for Ewing's sarcoma are the long bones – particularly the femur, humerus and tibia – the metaphyses being more often involved than the diaphyses. It can, however, attack any bone and, in very rare cases, even the soft tissues. The pelvis is a common site, the ribs and short tubular bones are less often affected by Ewing's sarcoma. In the jaws, the mandible is more often involved than the maxilla.

Age Distribution (Fig. 661). In complete contrast to the plasmocytoma (p. 348), Ewing's sarcoma appears in children and young people, over 80% of the tumors arising in the first 2 decades, with a peak in the 2nd decade. More than 90% of these neoplasms occur before the age of thirty. It must nevertheless be emphasized that they can in fact arise at any age, although after the 30th year they are rare, and such a diagnosis should be looked at very critically.

There is no **radiological appearance** that is pathognomonic of a Ewing's sarcoma. The tumor spreads in the marrow cavity, taking in the Haversian canals and very quickly involving the whole shaft of the bone. Occasionally, however, the neoplasm remains confined to a particular region of the bone and extends itself locally. In most cases only a part of the tumor within the bone can be seen in the radiograph, and morphological examination shows that the growth has extended much further than can be seen radiologically. The most prominent feature of its growth is osteolysis. The tumor cells destroy the bone tissue and displace the osteoblasts, whereas the osteoclasts continue their full osteolytic action. In addition to the osteolysis there is also a reactive osteosclerotic process, so that small patches of translucency are seen in the tissue. This picture is described as "moth-eaten". In **Fig. 662** one can see the **radiograph** of a Ewing's sarcoma in the proximal part of the right femur. Within the marrow cavity there are irregular patches of translucency as well as patchy and diffuse densifications *(1)*. The long bone is expanded in a fusiform fashion around the tumor, and the cortex is exfoliated over some distance *(2)* and broken through *(3)*. The periosteum has been raised up by the invasion of the tumor, and marked reactive periosteal bone deposition can be seen. Several layers of bone tissue have developed below the periosteum, giving rise to a picture like an onion skin on the radiograph *(4)*. This phenomenon is present in almost all Ewing's sarcomas which lie centrally in the diaphysis of a long bone. The penetration of the cortex by the tumorous tissue can also give origin to the so-called bone spicules, where newly formed trabeculae in the periosteum are seen perpendicular to the axis of the shaft. These radial spicules are seen in 50% of Ewing's sarcomas found in the center of a long bone diaphysis.

Figure 663 depicts the **radiograph** of a Ewing's sarcoma in the head of the tibia. Immediately below the epiphyseal cartilage there is a roundish focus of destruction *(1)* which is not demarcated by any marginal sclerosis. The spongiosa in this region has been destroyed, and the bone tissue in the outer zone by osteolysis. Inside there are patchy areas of increased density. It can only be assumed that a much larger part of the marrow cavity has been invaded by the tumorous tissue. In one place *(2)* there is a small osteolytic focus in the cortex, and thickening of the periosteum *(3)* is also clearly discernible. The periosteum has been largely infiltrated by the tumor, thus leading to additional reactive new bone deposition, which can be seen in the radiograph. Invasion of the soft parts by the tumor is also possible.

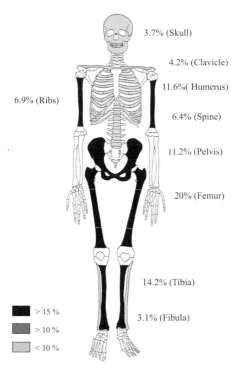

3.7% (Skull)
4.2% (Clavicle)
11.6%(Humerus)
6.9% (Ribs)
6.4% (Spine)
11.2% (Pelvis)
20% (Femur)
14.2% (Tibia)
3.1% (Fibula)
> 15 %
> 10 %
< 10 %

Fig. 660. Localization of Ewing's sarcomas (298 cases); others: 18.7%

%
50
45
40
35
30
25
20
15
10
5
0
1. 2. 3. 4. 5.
Decade of life

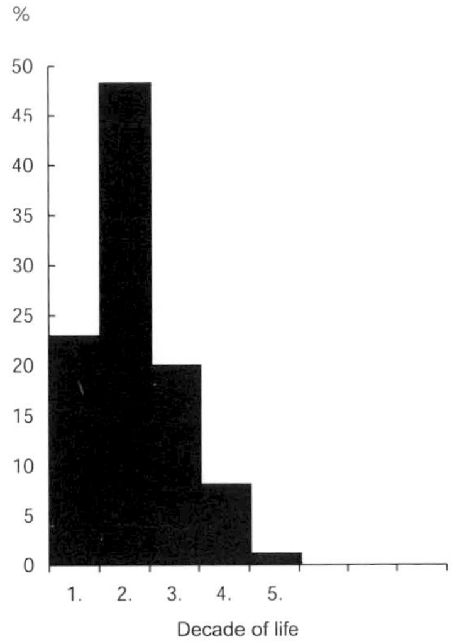

Fig. 661. Age distribution of Ewing's sarcomas (298 cases)

3
1
2
4

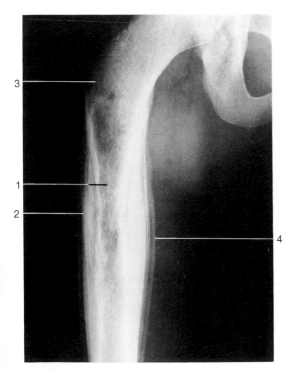

Fig. 662. Ewing's sarcoma (right proximal femur)

1
2
3

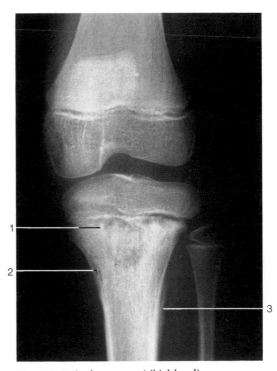

Fig. 663. Ewing's sarcoma (tibial head)

Radiologically, a Ewing's sarcoma can imitate absolutely any other bone tumor, so that a true diagnosis can only be reached by examining the histological appearance of a biopsy. **Figure 664** shows a large area of osteolysis lying centrally in the proximal part of the tibia *(1)* of a 17-year-old boy. It is sharply demarcated above by a narrow band of marginal sclerosis *(2)*, but distally the border is indistinct *(3)*. This signifies malignancy. Inside the osteolytic focus one observes only a few discrete patches of translucency. The cortex is generally intact, except at one point *(4)*, and no periosteal reaction is discernible. In this case a Ewing's sarcoma can only be diagnosed histologically.

A 24-year-old man was **examined radiologically** because of continual pain in the right foot. The lateral radiograph shown in **Fig. 665** shows only slight loosening of the cancellous structure of the calcaneus *(1)*. There are no unambiguous signs of local destruction, and the outer contours of the bone *(2)* have been fully preserved. However, the **bone scintigram** showed a high degree of activity in the calcaneus; and this, as can be seen in **Fig. 666**, does not reflect only the focus of porosity seen in the radiograph, but reveals highly concentrated activity throughout the bone *(1)*. Significantly less increased activity can be seen in the other bones, particularly in the growing regions *(2)*, but this is to be regarded as physiological. Such a radiological picture leads one at first to think of osteomyelitis; however there may be, as in this case, a Ewing's sarcoma lurking in the background.

The sawcut through the **macroscopic specimen** depicted in **Fig. 667** shows a large central focus of destruction *(1)* that is greasy and soaked with blood. It is much larger than it appears to be in the radiograph (Fig. 665). The destruction of the spongiosa reaches up in several places as far as the cortex *(2)*, which has an indistinct border and is no longer intact dorsally *(3)*. In one place *(4)* the impression is given that the tumor has already infiltrated into the soft parts. All the other bones are free from tumorous tissue.

Histologically this tumor consists of highly cellular, entirely undifferentiated tumorous tissue that is in many places necrotic and appears greasy and yellowish-red to the naked eye. It could easily be mistaken for a very active osteo-

myelitis. In order to exclude this type of inflammatory process, material should be removed for bacteriological examination at the same time as the bone biopsy – in most cases it will be found to be bacteriologically negative. In **Fig. 668** one can see densely or loosely packed "round cells" *(1)* in the marrow cavity. The very dark nuclei in some of the cell groups is striking *(2)*. No differentiated tissue structures are discernible. Peripherally *(3)* the tumorous tissue is more extensively crushed or necrotic. The spongiosa is more or less destroyed. In the center one can see a bone trabecula *(4)* that still shows the lamellar layering, although its borders are undulating and jagged. There is a broad front of new bone deposition with a few osteoblasts *(5)*. Here the original cancellous trabeculae have been extensively destroyed by the malignant tumor, giving the appearance of osteolysis on the radiograph. A few trabeculae remain and are reacting with reparative new bone deposition. This shows up as fine dense patches on the radiograph. Normally speaking, the destructive osteolytic processes in a Ewing's sarcoma exceed the reparative osteosclerotic reaction, so that a malignant tumorous osteolysis usually predominates in the radiograph.

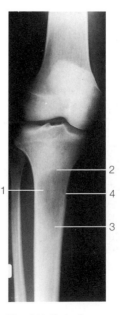

Fig. 664. Ewing's sarcoma (right proximal tibia)

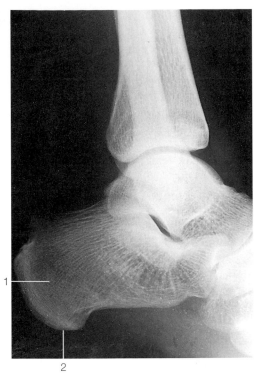

Fig. 665. Ewing's sarcoma (calcaneus)

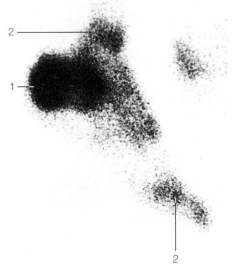

Fig. 666. Ewing's sarcoma (calcaneus, scintigram)

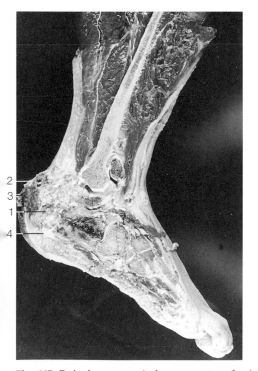

Fig. 667. Ewing's sarcoma (calcaneus, cut surface)

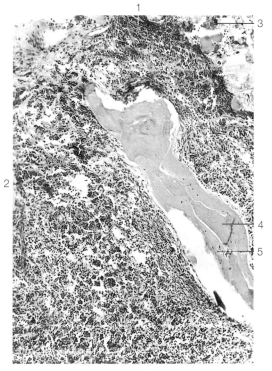

Fig. 668. Ewing's sarcoma; HE, ×64

In the **histological picture** shown in **Fig. 669** it is obvious that the tumor is composed of a highly cellular tissue in which no differentiated structures are present. The tumor cells lie together in band-shaped (1) or roundish areas (2). In between there are connective tissue septa, threaded through with dilated fine-walled blood vessels (3). The tumorous tissue is extremely vulnerable, which accounts for the large patchy or band-shaped regions of necrosis (4) in the centers of the cell groups. This tissue is best preserved around the vessels, where it presents a rosette-like appearance. Numerous pycnotic nuclei are seen at the edges of the necroses, and this highly cellular neoplastic tissue may be diffused throughout the entire bone marrow. The spongiosa is almost completely destroyed. Ewing's sarcoma is one of the most difficult of all bone tumors to recognize, because no typical structures are formed. Furthermore, there may be many crush artefacts in the biopsy, and these can render the diagnosis absolutely impossible.

Under the **higher magnification** of **Fig. 670** one can see that the whole marrow cavity is filled with tumorous tissue. It consists of dense, or sometimes loose, collections of small undifferentiated round cells (1), of which the nuclei show variable degrees of chromatin density. Very dark nuclei (2) lie next to others which are pale and distended (3). The cytoplasm of these cells is poorly developed and appears very faded at this magnification. The cell boundaries are indistinct. Sometimes stellate cells, rich in cytoplasm, are loosely but regularly distributed, reminding one of the appearance of the night sky. Within the tumorous tissue there is no intercellular material, but one can discern a narrow seam of reactive connective tissue (4) at the periphery of the tumor itself. It contains fibrocytes with elongated isomorphic nuclei, and is not a sarcomatous stroma. The remaining bone trabeculae in the spongiosa (5) are considerably deformed as a result of the reactive bone remodeling. They are in part osteosclerotically widened and have broad osteoid seams (6). Sometime one can observe deposits of osteoblasts (7). Normal areas of scar tissue may be present, which are threaded through with wide fine-walled blood vessels (8).

As can be observed in **Fig. 671**, the tumorous tissue may contain pseudoalveoli. Here there are fairly large groups of cells, bounded by narrow connective tissue septa (1). This stroma is threaded through with blood vessels (2). The tumor cells have small, very dark nuclei and sparse, scarcely recognizable cytoplasm. No silver-staining reticular fibers are formed, being present only in the neighborhood of the vessels and in the connective tissue septa. They do not belong to the tumorous tissue itself. It can be extraordinarily difficult to identify this highly cellular, undifferentiated and small-celled tumorous tissue as a Ewing's sarcoma. The differential diagnosis must also include the possibility of bone metastases, e.g. a neuroblastoma or PNET.

Figure 672 again shows a Ewing's sarcoma under **higher magnification**. At one side there is a bone trabecula with laminated layering (1) lying close to the highly cellular tumorous tissue. Some tumor cells (2) have small roundish nuclei that are fairly isomorphic. Owing to the dense condensations of chromatin they appear black. These cells have hardly any cytoplasm and are virtually naked nuclei. They are all much the same size – about two or three times as big as lymphocytes. Lying close to them, one can recognize stellate cells with abundant cytoplasm (3) which may be regularly distributed throughout the tumorous tissue, again recalling images of the night sky. These cells have fairly large spheroidal nuclei, all much the same size. They possess a loose chromatin framework, particularly at the nuclear membrane, with one or two dark nucleoli. Pathological mitoses are rare. Within the sparse cytoplasm glycogen granules can nearly always be shown up with PAS staining, although PAS-negative Ewing's sarcomas do exist. Three different types of cells can be identified cytologically: A cells = immature stem cells, B cells = dark secondary cells, C cells = differentiated reticular cells. Whether or not various other tumors, running a different course and carrying different prognoses, lie "hidden" behind the Ewing's sarcoma is still not known. Variations in the duration and course of the illness and the differing responses to the irradiation and chemotherapy usual today make one think it may be possible. Histochemical and, above all, immunohistochemical methods are being used in an attempt to analyze Ewing's sarcoma more precisely. (For further information about PNET see p. 368).

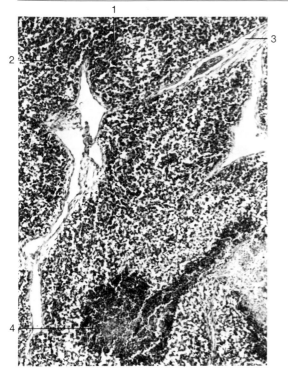

Fig. 669. Ewing's sarcoma, PAS, ×40

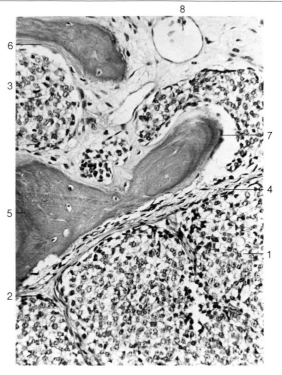

Fig. 670. Ewing's sarcoma, PAS, ×64

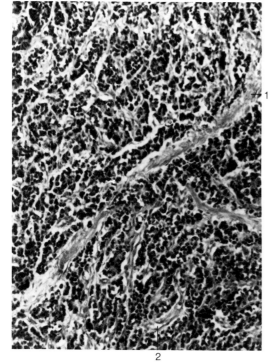

Fig. 671. Ewing's sarcoma; HE, ×64

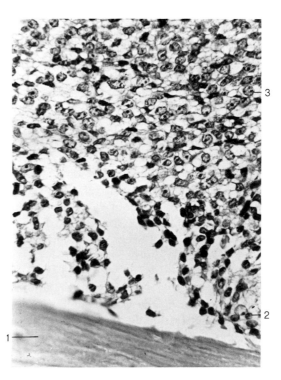

Fig. 672. Ewing's sarcoma, PAS, ×82

Malignant Lymphoma of Bone
(Non-Hodgkin Lymphoma, Reticulum Cell Sarcoma)
(ICD-O-DA-M-9640/3)

A primary bone tumor that bears great morphological similarity to Ewing's sarcoma is the bone lymphoma. *This is an isolated malignant neoplasm which is characterized by the proliferation of the lymphocytes and reticular cells of the bone marrow.* Histologically it closely resembles the malignant non-Hodgkin lymphomas of the extraskeletal lymphatic system. This tumor was formerly described as an osseous "reticulum cell sarcoma" consisting of pleomorphic cells with abundant cytoplasm, notched nuclei with prominent nucleoli and a dense fibrous network of reticulin. Since, however, it is not composed exclusively of these "histiocytic" cells, and lymphocytes and lymphoblasts are present in large numbers, this histologically inconstant neoplasm is now known as a "malignant bone lymphoma". Before the diagnosis can be confirmed, however, one must exclude the possibility that it is a bone metastasis from a malignant lymphoma from the extraskeletal lymphatic system (the lymph nodes). The malignant bone lymphoma makes up about 7% of the malignant tumors of bone. Clinically there is often a remarkable difference between the relatively good general condition of the patient and the size of the growth. It is only after a considerable time that attention is called to it by local pain and sometimes also by swelling. It is usual for 25%–50% of the affected bone to have been invaded by tumorous tissue at the time of the first examination. Nevertheless the prognosis is – particularly in comparison with Ewing's sarcoma – relatively favorable. Five-year survival is at about 30%–50%, and 10-year survival at 16%–20%. In advanced cases metastases are found in the regional lymph nodes (22%), lungs (10%) and other bones (15%).

Localization (Fig. 673). The malignant bone lymphoma can appear in any bone, but especially in the long bones (usually in the diaphysis). The principal sites are the pelvis and the neighborhood of the knee (lower end of femur, upper end of tibia), where more than half the tumors are localized. The lower end of the spinal column is often affected; 8.8% of these growths appear in the upper limb and about 4% in the jaw.

Age Distribution (Fig. 674). A malignant bone lymphoma can appear at any time, although it is more frequent in middle or old age (3rd and 6th decades). It is, however, also found in children and young people.

In **Fig. 675** one can see the **radiograph** of a malignant bone lymphoma in the proximal part of the tibia. In this region the bone tissue is extensively destroyed, although the outer shape of the bone has been preserved. Inside, there are coarse patchy osteolytic foci (1) and straggly translucencies (2). The osteolytic foci are set through with irregular zones of osteosclerosis (3). Both osteolysis and osteosclerosis are equally marked throughout the tumor, and lie close together. This results in a coarse straggly honeycomb-like structure that, from the point of view of differential diagnosis, may remind one of Paget's osteitis deformans (p. 102). The destruction of bone by the tumor had originated in the marrow cavity, but has nevertheless destroyed a large part of the cortex (4). The outline of the bony focus is undulating and uneven, and the tumor has extended proximally as far as the epiphyseal cartilage (5) and has in all probability involved the entire marrow cavity. A periosteal reaction is either absent or scarcely visible.

As can be seen in the **macroscopic picture** in **Fig. 676**, the whole of the marrow cavity has indeed been invaded by tumorous tissue and the spongiosa is almost completely destroyed. One sees large variously sized foci (1) of grayish-white soft elastic tumorous tissue. In between there are greasy foci of necrosis (2) and areas with dirty red hemorrhages. The cortex is in part narrowed and destroyed (3) and in part widened and densified by reactive osteosclerosis (4). Much infiltration of the periosteum by the tumor can be seen. Within the intramedullary tumorous tissue varying degrees of reactive bone deposition appear in many places, but there is little calcification. It is, however, the destruction of the bone which is most noticeable in this macroscopic section. In general this is not pathognomonic of a malignant bone lymphoma. In bones like these one often sees a large tumorous mass in the metaphysis extending beyond the bone itself. An extensive parosteal soft tissue tumor, which is not necessarily detectable radiographically, is also frequently met with in the macroscopic specimen. This

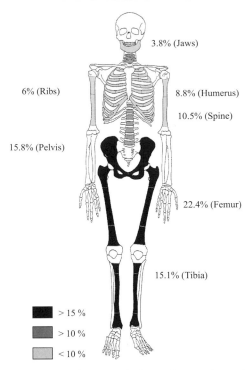

3.8% (Jaws)

8.8% (Humerus)

6% (Ribs)

10.5% (Spine)

15.8% (Pelvis)

22.4% (Femur)

15.1% (Tibia)

> 15 %

> 10 %

< 10 %

Fig. 673. Localization of the malignant bone lymphomas (315 cases); others: 17.6%

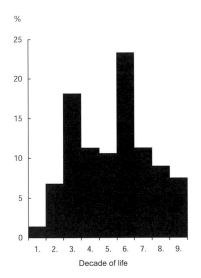

Fig. 674. Age distribution of the malignant bone lymphomas (315 cases)

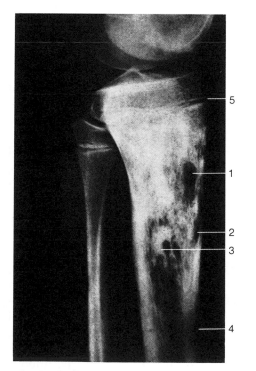

Fig. 675. Malignant bone lymphoma (proximal tibia)

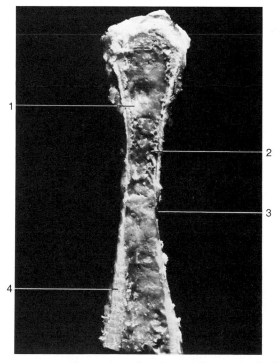

Fig. 676. Malignant bone lymphoma (tibia, cut surface)

signifies that the intramedullary tumor has already broken out of the bone.

Figure 677 shows the **a.p. radiograph** of a malignant bone lymphoma in the proximal part of the tibia of a 22-year-old man. In the sclerotically dense spongiosa *(1)* there are a few discrete regions of osteolysis *(2)*. The outer contours of the bone are intact and distinct, and no periosteal reaction is visible. The bone destruction is more clearly seen in the **lateral radiograph**. In **Fig. 678** much fine patchy osteolysis appears in the spongiosa *(1)* and the ventral cortex *(2)*. The lesion extends a long way into the tibial shaft *(3)* and is very poorly outlined. No bony periosteal reaction can be seen.

The **histological appearance** of a malignant bone lymphoma is the same as that of a malignant lymphoma that has arisen primarily in the lymph nodes. As illustrated in **Fig. 679**, the neoplastic tissue consists of a regular sheet of loosely deposited tumorous lymphocytes *(1)* which fill up the whole of the marrow cavity between the trabeculae. In contrast to Ewing's sarcoma (p. 357), there are not usually any extensive fields of necrosis. One can discern a few stout bone trabeculae *(2)* which represent an irregular front of osteosclerotic bone deposition *(3)* formed as a reaction to the growth of the tumor. There is a loose disorganized band of cells with only a very weakly developed stroma of single collagen fibers *(4)* apparent. With silver staining (Gomori, Bielschowsky or Tibor-PAP) a fine network of reticulin fibers can be seen between the tumor cells. This kind of fibrous lattice is not found in Ewing's sarcoma (p. 357). With this tissue pattern one often sees the so-called "willow catkin structures" or the formation of pseudoalveoli, when broad stretches of connective tissue subdivide the different groups of cells.

Under the **higher magnification** of **Fig. 680** one can discern densely packed collections of reticular cells between the widened bone trabeculae *(1)*, and the tumorous tissue is set through with single connective tissue septa *(2)* which sometimes carry capillaries. The neoplastic cells are polygonal and larger than those of Ewing's sarcoma (p. 357). They have large roundish nuclei which are often notched, and which sometimes contain a loose chromatin framework and prominent nucleoli *(3)*, and sometimes a very dense framework of chroma-

tin *(4)*. Some of the nuclei have several large nucleoli and are kidney-shaped. The cytoplasm varies in amount and is slightly basophilic, and the cell boundaries are not clearly distinguishable. The cells are bound together by cytoplasmic processes, but the pointed type can usually only be seen in fresh specimens. In the biopsy material the tumorous tissue is often full of crush artefacts which make the morphological analysis very difficult. There are often large necrotic fields which indicate a malignant growth. Those tumor cells which are still intact are usually rather large, but giant cells with large distended nuclei and clumps of chromatin can also be present. Mitoses are frequent. In contrast to Ewing's sarcoma, one cannot demonstrate glycogen granules in the tumor cells with PAS staining. Reactive deposition of new bone can take place within the neoplasm. In many cases numerous highly differentiated and undifferentiated lymphoblasts and lymphocytes are strewn about within a malignant bone lymphoma, and tumorous histiocytes are often encountered. If small lymphoid cells predominate in the biopsy material it may sometimes be difficult to distinguish it from a Ewing's sarcoma. Neither knotty nor follicular structures belong to the picture of an osseous lymphoma.

When diagnosing an osseous "round cell sarcoma" one must, apart from Ewing's sarcoma (p. 352) and malignant neuroblastoma (p. 388), also take the possibility of metastases from a small cell carcinoma of the bronchus into account. For this reason cytological examination of fresh tumorous tissue (e. g. an aspiration biopsy) and immunohistochemical examination (lysozyme +, S-100 protein –, cytokeratin –, vimentin +) can be helpful. Electron microscopic examination is also useful. The cells of a malignant bone lymphoma or "reticulum cell sarcoma" have nuclei of very variable size and shape, with peripheral condensation of chromatin and often prominent nucleoli. The undulating cell membranes sometimes form processes. The cytoplasm contains a fairly large number of mitochondria and ribosomes and a clearly defined Golgi apparatus. Reticulin and collagen fibrils can be demonstrated between the tumor cells. In contradistinction to Ewing's sarcoma, there are no glycogen granules in the cytoplasm.

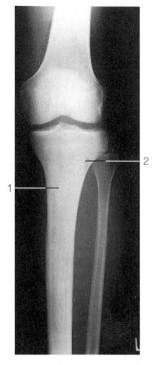

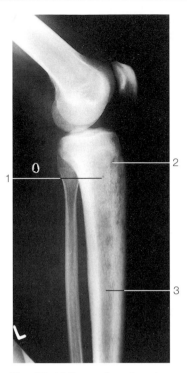

Fig. 677. Malignant bone lymphoma (proximal tibia, a.p. view)

Fig. 678. Malignant bone lymphoma (proximal tibia, lateral view)

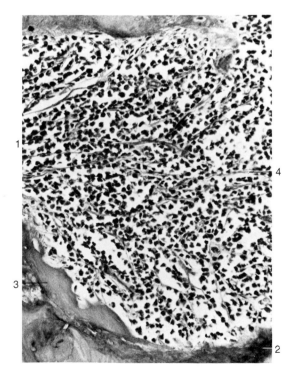

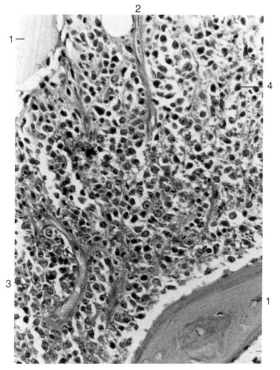

Fig. 679. Malignant bone lymphoma; HE, ×64

Fig. 680. Malignant bone lymphoma; PAS, ×82

Osseous Hodgkin Lymphoma
(Hodgkin's Disease, Malignant Lymphogranulomatosis) (ICD-O-DA-M-965/3)

About half of all lymphomas are classified under Hodgkin's lymphogranulomatosis. The lesion arises almost always in the tissue of the lymph nodes and then secondarily involves other organs, including the bones. In rare cases the disease can appear primarily within the marrow cavity, in which cases no swelling of the lymph nodes will occur. *Hodgkin's osseous lymphogranulomatosis consists of a peculiar malignant proliferation of the lymphatic tissue in the bone marrow, with the development of granulation tissue which is characterized by a mixed cytology* (reticular cells, lymphocytes, epithelioid cells, eosinophil and neutrophil granulocytes, plasma cells) *and so-called Hodgkin cells and Sternberg giant cells.* In 65% of cases it can be established that the bone marrow has been attacked, and for this reason a biopsy of the iliac crest is always indicated. Most often it is the vertebral bodies (60%), sternum (25%), femur (31%) and skull cap (3%) which are affected. With skeletal involvement, bone changes can only be detected in the radiograph in 25% of the cases.

Radiologically, osteolytic bone foci are found in about 50% of the cases, and in 10%–15% marked osteosclerosis is present. **Figure 682** depicts a so-called *ivory vertebra (1),* which should arouse suspicion of Hodgkin's disease. The entire vertebral body is sclerotically densified, without any osteolytic foci being visible. The outer contours are present and distinct, and the intervertebral spaces are unaltered *(2).* **Figure 683** shows the **radiograph** of a Hodgkin lymphoma in the shaft of the femur. One can discern several coarse or fine patches of osteolysis in the spongiosa *(1)* which are particularly concentrated at the endosteal side of the cortex. The cortex itself is unaltered *(2)* and no periosteal reaction is visible. Elsewhere, however, there is a large osteolytic focus *(3)* in the cortex which projects a central shadow, reminiscent of a sequestrum. In addition, there are small elongated osteolytic foci *(4)* in the cortex. In general the impression is given of an extensive region of bone destruction which has primarily arisen in the marrow cavity and attacked the cortex. Radiologically, a malignant tumor of the bone marrow is therefore in this case very probably the correct diagnosis.

Histologically a malignant bone lymphoma is usually easy to diagnose. It is, however, often difficult to recognize a Hodgkin lymphoma from the bone biopsy, or to distinguish between the 4 known types of Hodgkin's disease (the lymphocyte-rich, nodular sclerotic, mixed and lymphocyte-poor forms). This must be decided by examination of the lymph node. In order to diagnose an osseous Hodgkin lymphoma **(Fig. 681)** the identification of Hodgkin cells *(1)* and Sternberg giant cells *(2)* is important. Here it is a matter of large, "liquor-rich" mononucleated and multinucleated cells with extremely large nucleoli and a moderately basophilic cytoplasm. The nuclei in the Sternberg giant cells overlap one another.

In **Fig. 684** one can recognize **histologically** a typical Hodgkin lymphoma with Hodgkin cells *(1)* and Sternberg giant cells *(2).* In between there are numerous lymphocytes *(3).* Under **higher magnification** one can also see in **Fig. 685** large reticular cells *(1),* plasma cells *(2),* epithelioid cells *(3)* and eosinophils. Sprouting capillaries and a more or less pronounced scarring are also encountered. There is extensive destruction of the cancellous trabeculae in the neighborhood of the Hodgkin infiltrates. In the less common osteosclerotic form

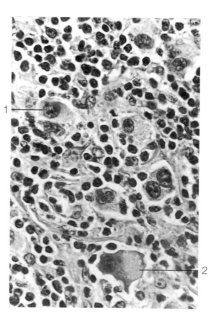

Fig. 681. Hodgkin lymphoma; HE, ×100

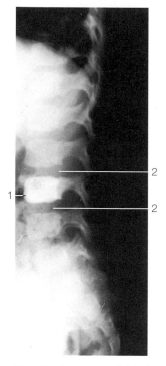

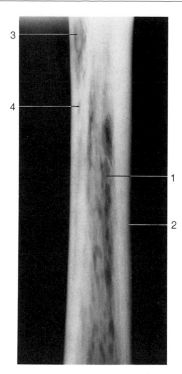

Fig. 682. Osseous Hodgkin lymphoma
(ivory vertebra, 3rd lumbar vertebra)

Fig. 683. Osseous Hodgkin lymphoma
(femoral shaft, tomogram)

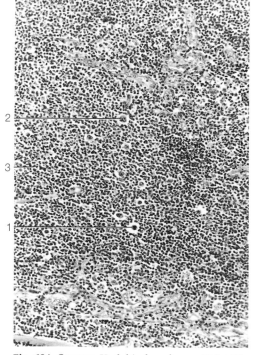

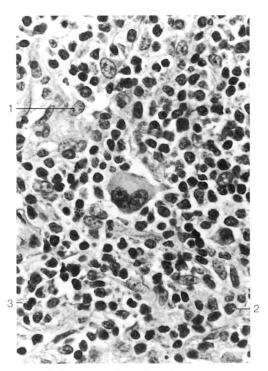

Fig. 684. Osseous Hodgkin lymphoma; PAS, ×40

Fig. 685. Osseous Hodgkin lymphoma; PAS, ×100

of Hodgkin's disease the bone is very dense, and between the sclerotically widened bone trabeculae the lymphomatous infiltrates are usually difficult to recognize.

Leukemia (ICD-O-DA-M-9800/3)

Hematological diseases can, if they include myeloid proliferation of the bone marrow, bring about structural changes in the skeleton that need to be examined osteologically in a bone biopsy. These diseases must be regarded as separate from the primary bone tumors, but they do, however, often call upon the diagnostic skills of the radiologist and the pathologist. *Leukemia is a diffuse autonomous proliferation of a strain of leukocytes in the marrow of several bones, which to a greater or lesser extent floods the peripheral bloodstream.* Radiologically demonstrable bone changes appear in about 50% of the cases of acute leukemia in childhood; in adults and in the chronic forms, skeletal involvement is less common. The most important clinical symptom is circumscribed bone pain. A hypercalcemic syndrome with metastatic calcifications in other organs can arise, so that it may be mistaken for hyperparathyroidism (p. 80).

In adult life the leukemias produce diffuse osteoporosis, osteolytic patches or the acute appearance of circumscribed osteolytic areas. In **Fig. 686** one can see numerous osteolytic patches *(1)* in the **radiograph** of the pelvis and proximal part of the femur. These are mostly in the spongiosa, but have also attacked the endosteal side of the cortex *(2)*. Between the moth-eaten areas of osteolysis there are fine and coarse sclerotic regions of increased density *(3)*. This is an *acute lymphatic leukemia* that has brought about patchy destruction of the bone.

Acute myeloid leukemia can also produce numerous osteolytic patches in the **radiograph**. In **Fig. 687** multiple fine *(1)* and coarse *(2)* bone defects are visible in the radius and ulna. These often have a punched-out appearance. In places the bone has been extensively destroyed *(3)*, and here the cortex is no longer recognizable. Endosteal sclerosis of the spongiosa *(4)* is very characteristic of leukemic infiltration and bone destruction.

In the biopsy material shown in **Fig. 688**, the **histological picture** shows that the marrow fatty tissue has disappeared and the marrow cavity is filled up with leukemic infiltrates *(1)* that originally developed in the neighborhood of the peritrabecular zone of new bone deposition. The normal hematopoietic tissue has been completely replaced. Cell morphological and histochemical criteria (the PAS reaction, peroxidase, naphthyl acetate esterase) can be used to identify the tumor cells as myeloid cells (myeloblasts, promyelocytes, monocytes, erythrocytes, megakaryocytes) which often also contain Auer's bodies. In the osteolytic foci the original cancellous trabeculae have been destroyed; peripherally they are identifiable by the osteosclerotic bone remodeling *(2)*.

Chronic lymphatic leukemia only rarely causes bone changes. In **Fig. 689** showing the **radiograph** of the humerus one can identify numerous osteolytic foci of different sizes *(1)* in the spongiosa. Some of these have become confluent. The cortex has been gnawed away from inside *(2)*. In the shaft one can observe periosteal new bone deposition *(3)*, so that here the outline of the diaphysis appears double. Between the cortex and the layer of periosteal new bone one can see a light stripe *(4)*. Such a radiographic appearance is typical of leukemic changes in the skeleton.

As can be observed in **Fig. 690**, the **histological appearance** of the marrow cavity shows it to have been filled up with relatively mature lymphocytes *(1)*. The infiltrates have spread out from the neighborhood of the larger central sinus of the marrow and replaced the residual hematopoietic tissue in the peritrabecular zone

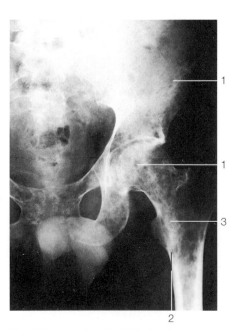

Fig. 686. Acute lymphatic leukemia (pelvis, left proximal femur)

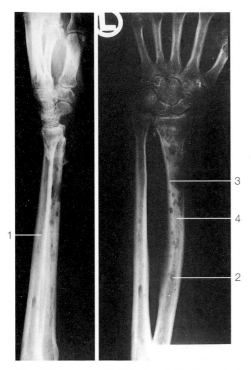

Fig. 687. Acute myeloid leukemia (radius, ulna)

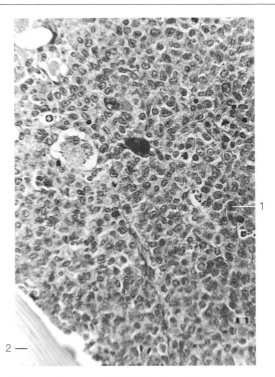

Fig. 688. Acute myeloid leukemia, PAS, ×82

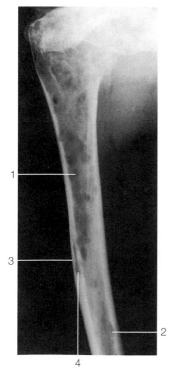

Fig. 689. Chronic lymphatic leukemia (humerus)

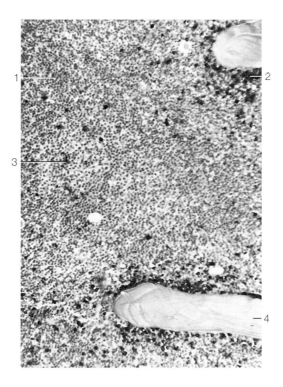

Fig. 690. Chronic lymphatic leukemia, PAS, ×40

(2). Here the granulocytes have been made conspicuously dark by their positive chloracetate esterase activity. Isolated megakaryocytes (3) are lying within the marrow infiltrate. The remaining bone trabeculae (4) are slightly thickened by sclerosis.

Malignant Mastocytosis (Mast Cell Reticulosis, Systemic Mastocytosis) (ICD-O-DA-M-9741/3)

Apart from the myeloid and lymphatic strains of bone marrow cells, other cells (plasma cells, mast cells) can also give rise to malignant tumors. In rare cases these may be formed from the mast cells of the bone marrow, and the term "mast cell reticulosis" was introduced in 1962 by LENNERT. *Malignant mastocytosis consists of a progressive neoplastic proliferation of the medullary mast cells, which frequently becomes generalized and runs a malignant course.* In this case the mast cells may flood the bloodstream (mast cell leukemia). This disease often ends up as an acute or chronic myeloid leukemia. With systemic mastocytosis the patient is in most cases also affected by infiltration of the skin (urticaria pigmentosa), the condition then being usually benign. In about 15% of cases of mastocytosis, bone changes can be detected radiologically.

In the **radiograph** malignant mastocytosis is characterized by patchy osteolysis in one region of a bone. In **Fig. 691** one can see a large poorly defined osteolytic focus in the greater trochanter *(1)*, which contains fine roundish densifications. The osteolysis has extended into the marrow cavity *(2)* where further discrete translucencies *(3)* are present. The cortex of the trochanter *(4)* has also been drawn into the lytic process, but there is no periosteal reaction.

In the **radiograph** of **Fig. 692** the lesion is also in the proximal part of the femur. The diffuse sclerotic density of the femoral neck *(1)* and proximal part of the femur is striking. In between there are fine patchy translucencies *(2)*. The lesser trochanter in particular *(3)* has a feathery outline, and the underlying cortex is osteolytically porous *(4)*. Bone changes of this sort are usually symptomless, and bone pain is rare. Pathological fractures are also uncommon with malignant mastocytosis.

Histologically one can see focally concentrated infiltrates of abnormal mast cells disseminated throughout the bone marrow. In **Fig. 693** there is in one place a bone trabecula with lamellar layering *(1)*. The marrow cavity is filled up with loose fibrous tissue *(2)*, within which collections of mast cells *(3)* can be seen. These react strongly with chloracetate esterase. The mast cells are mostly arranged in foci

around the trabeculae or arterioles. These are the same regions of the marrow for which immature granulopoiesis displays a predilection.

As can be seen in the **histological picture** of **Fig. 694**, an increasingly argyrophil myelofibrosis develops early within the zone of infiltration. Staining for reticular fibers *(1)* shows that many of these are present. In the neighborhood of a sclerotically widened bone trabecula *(2)* one sees numerous loosely distributed abnormal mast cells *(3)* which possess extremely hyperchromatic nuclei. The hematopoietic bone marrow has been displaced and the fatty marrow has been infiltrated by tumor cells. Only a few fat vacuoles remain *(4)*.

Under **higher magnification** the mast cells can be identified by their immaturity and low granulation density. At one side of **Fig. 695** one can see a sclerotically widened trabecula *(1)* with drawn-out reversal lines. In the adjacent marrow there is a porous argyrophil fibrosis *(2)*, with loosely deposited mast cells which have polymorphic nuclei *(3)*. These contain metachromatically basophilic granules *(4)* which can only be made visible by optimal fixation. Eosinophil granulocytes, lymphocytes, plasma cells and histiocytic macrophages may appear reactively around the edges of such marrow infiltrates of mast cells.

This group of primary bone tumors includes two different kinds of tissue that are found in the marrow cavity: the medullary fatty tissue and the various cells of the hematopoietic sys-

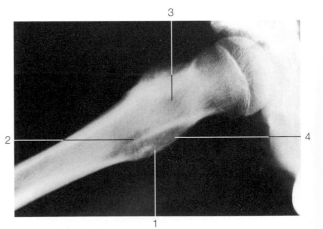

Fig. 691. Malignant mastocytosis (proximal femur, greater trochanter)

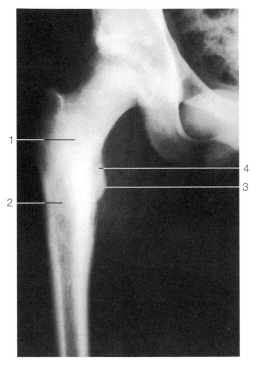

Fig. 692. Malignant mastocytosis (proximal femur)

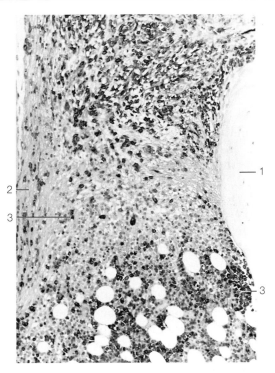

Fig. 693. Malignant mastocytosis, chloracetate esterase reaction, ×82

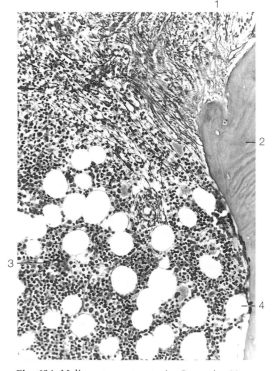

Fig. 694. Malignant mastocytosis; Gomori, ×82

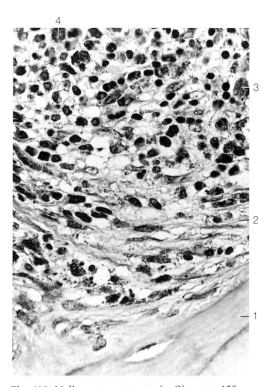

Fig. 695. Malignant mastocytosis; Giemsa, ×120

tem. Amongst the **osseous fatty tissue neoplasms** the lipoma (p. 346) is remarkable for its very high degree of differentiation, so much so that under the microscope the tumorous fatty tissue can hardly be distinguished from its normal medullary counterpart. It is certainly true that these benign tumors are sometimes overlooked and not even recorded if no clear-cut radiological signs are present. The osseous lipoma is regarded as a very rare primary bone tumor. With the osseous liposarcoma (p. 346), however, the tumorous lipoblasts may be so undifferentiated that they are hardly any longer recognizable as such. The danger exists that these equally rare neoplasms may be incorrectly classified. Radiologically they usually present themselves as osteolysis – in the case of a lipoma sometimes with central calcification.

Most **osteomyelogenic bone tumors** are "round cell sarcomas" of which the histogenesis must be established before an exact diagnosis is possible. This group includes especially the malignant lymphomas as they appear throughout the entire lymphatic system (lymph nodes, spleen etc.). Diseases of this kind are very frequent and are histologically diagnosed from an iliac crest biopsy. We distinguish histologically between Hodgkin lymphomas (p. 362) and non-Hodgkin lymphomas (p. 358). If the tumor cells are poured out into the bloodstream we call it a leukemia (p. 364). In most cases these are blood diseases. It is only when one or more bones are exclusively attacked and no extra-osseous infiltrate can be detected that a lymphoma can be regarded as a primary neoplasm of bone. Depending upon the localization of the marrow cavity, the diaphyses (or vertebral bodies, sternum and iliac wings) are infiltrated over a considerable distance. The destruction of the cancellous trabeculae may be slight, so that the tumor is not perceived radiologically. There may, however, be discrete areas of osteolysis.

The commonest osteomyelogenic bone neoplasm to be classified among the bone tumors is the medullary plasmocytoma (or myeloma, p. 348). It is also the commonest malignant bone tumor. The myeloma is usually multifocal, appearing simultaneously in different bones and producing variously sized areas of osteolysis on the radiograph. Clinically, so-called Kah-

ler's disease (p. 348) may develop, but this is not always the case. Histologically or cytologically it is possible to identify the tumor cells as plasma cells (kappa, lambda) by means of immunohistochemistry.

Much greater difficulties with the diagnosis and differential diagnosis are presented by Ewing's sarcoma, the tumorous tissue of which is completely undifferentiated and composed of various types of cells (p. 356). Clinically the patients often present with the symptoms of osteomyelitis. Even in the radiograph we find so many bone changes that, while it is indeed possible to diagnose a malignant tumor, one cannot say that it is in fact a Ewing's sarcoma. Histologically the "round cells" of a Ewing's sarcoma are characterized by the PAS-positive glycogen granules in the sparse cytoplasm. These can be confirmed immunohistochemically (see Table 5, p. 507) and the patient then treated according to the **ECESS protocol** ("cooperative Ewing's sarcoma study").

The most important of the "atypical Ewing's sarcomas" to be ruled out immunohistochemically is the **primitive neuroectodermal bone tumor (PNET)**. *This is a rare and highly malignant bone tumor, which is similar to the peripheral neuroepithelioma found in the soft parts, and to Ewing's sarcoma. It is found almost exclusively in children.* The electron microscopic findings (neurosecretory granules, intermediate filaments, neurotubule-like structures) suggest a neurogenic tumor. This kind of undifferentiated small round cell tumor is classified under PNET if, from the list of neural markers – namely, NSE, S-100 protein, GFAP (acid glial-fiber protein) and HBA71 or MIC2 – the cells can be shown immunohistochemically to express at least two. In addition it should be possible to identify Homer-Wright pseudorosettes histologically. In Ewing's sarcoma, on the other hand, no such rosettes are present and the cells express none or, at the most, one of the neural markers. In this way this special tumorous entity can be identified within the so-called "Ewing's family". It has a significantly worse prognosis than Ewing's sarcoma. This is important therefore for the prognosis and for the possible therapeutic consequences (e.g. as an indication for bone marrow transplantation).

Vascular Bone Tumors (and other Bone Tumors)

Introductory Remarks

Bones are biological organs that are composed of a number of different tissues. As in every other organ, processes of physiological remodeling and proliferation are going on which adapt themselves to the diverse functional circumstances of the organism. They also take part in the complicated metabolic activity, much of which is essential to the survival of the complete animal. Calcium metabolism is an example. Obviously such an organ must be connected to the general cardiovascular system, both to fulfil these functional commitments, and also for its own survival. For this reason the bones are supplied with blood vessels which enter them from outside, and then interlace with each other within the marrow cavity and branch out in all directions (pp. 17, 166).

As is true of the soft tissues, and in other organ systems of the body, neoplasms may develop from these blood vessels, which possess a characteristic morphology. *Hemangiomas* may develop from these vessels, and these are often regarded as local malformations – the so-called hamartomas. These are dysontogenetic neoplasms. The benign hemangiomas of bone present almost an opposing picture to that of the malignant vascular tumors: the *hemangiosarcomas*. In general, vascular neoplasms display an enormously variable radiological and histomorphological outer appearance, which can make their diagnosis extremely difficult. A proliferation of vessels and vascular buds is also found in intraosseous inflammatory granulation tissue (e.g. in osteomyelitis, p. 129). Given a limited bone biopsy, it is sometimes far from easy to distinguish between such a reactive proliferation of the blood vessels and a true vascular neoplasm. It is, however, relatively easy to recognize a *cavernous hemangioma* in which the large blood-filled spaces contain numerous erythrocytes. On the other hand, diagnostic difficulties can arise with the much rarer *osseous capillary hemangioma*. A clear distinction between a benign hemangioma of bone and an osseous hemangiosarcoma can often be exceedingly difficult, since radiologically there is bone destruction in both cases, and histologically

the nature of the bone lesion is not always apparent. Even hemangiosarcomas of bone are not always recognizable as vascular neoplasms. There are such tumors in which the malignant endothelial buds develop no lumen, so that the tumorous tissue cannot be angiographically identified as such. Histologically solid band-like endothelial sprouts are present which give the impression of metastatic tumorous tissue. It is only by using immunohistochemical methods (e.g. positive reactions against factor VIII or ulex lectin), or electron microscopic examination (characteristic structure: Palade-Weibel bodies) that the neoplastic cells can be identified as angioblasts.

The benign tumors that arise from the blood vessels of bones are histomorphologically identical with similar tumors in the soft parts. Both the *glomus tumor* and the *hemangiopericytoma* are found in bone. Finally, lymph vessels also run through the marrow cavity, and these can also be a source of neoplastic growth. From them the osseous *lymphangiomas* are derived. With the malignant variety, however, the tissue from which they are derived is no longer recognizable, so that we can only use the general term "angiosarcoma".

Whereas the benign vascular neoplasms of bone are relatively common, the corresponding angiosarcoma is a very rare primary bone neoplasm, vascular growths being essentially more often found in the soft parts and in other organs. The vascular tumors are characterized by their locally destructive growth and their sensitivity to irradiation.

In this chapter other rare bone tumors will be dealt with that are not true vascular growths. Whether the *adamantinoma of the long bones* is histogenetically of vascular origin (a "malignant angioblastoma") will be debated. The *chordoma* is an independent, non-vascular neoplasm. *Neurogenic bone tumors* which take origin from the nerve fibers of the bone are described. *Muscular bone tumors* can arise from the smooth muscle cells of the vessels. Finally, *metastatic bone neoplasms* are discussed, although here the blood vessels of the bone merely constitute a transport system for bringing the tumor cells to their destination. These various tumorous bone lesions can only be approximately identified radiologically; their clarification requires bioptical investigation.

Hemangioma of Bone (ICD-O-DA-M-9120/0)

Among the benign bone tumors, the bone hemangioma presents no great problems with regard to diagnosis and treatment. This neoplasm accounts for about 1.2% of bone tumors and is therefore relatively infrequently encountered. *The angiomas of bone are benign new growths of the blood or lymph vessels which represent a local maldevelopment (hamartoma) and are therefore described as dysontogenetic neoplasms.* Clinically they are mostly without symptoms; they may be picked up by chance or at most present with slight pain or a pathological fracture. The laboratory findings are normal. Women are twice as often affected as men.

Localization (Fig. 696). The main site is the spinal column, where almost 20% of these tumors arise, mostly in the vertebral body. Of the lesions, 16% are found in the skull, which is the second commonest site. The remainder are distributed among the other bones, the jaws being relatively often affected (9.6%). In the long bones, hemangiomas are found in the metaphyses, and the appearance of the tumorous foci in more than one bone simultaneously is not uncommon.

Age Distribution (Fig. 697). Bone hemangiomas can occur at any age. However, those arising in the soft parts (particularly the skin) are found especially in children, while bone hemangiomas appear more often in middle and late middle age. The 5th decade of life is the peak period.

When a bone hemangioma is found, it is necessary to search the skeleton for further foci. There are also a few special types. Capillary hemangiomatosis accompanied by a massive osteolysis constitutes **Gorham's syndrome**. In **Mafucci's syndrome**, multiple hemangiomas of the skeleton and soft parts appear together with an asymmetrical chondromatosis of bone. In these syndromes lymphangiomas also arise. Bone hemangiomas do not tend to undergo malignant change and their prognosis is good, lesions without symptoms requiring no treatment. Therapeutically these tumors can be removed either by local excision (with a very real danger of severe hemorrhage!) or irradiation (20–25 Gy). Superselective interventional radio-therapy by the intravascular catheter method with the administration of embolizing substances is also a possibility.

Bone hemangiomas usually have a very characteristic **radiological** appearance, so that at least a provisional diagnosis can be made. **Figure 698** depicts a bone hemangioma in the 12th thoracic vertebral body. In comparison with the other vertebral bodies *(1)*, one can discern a lattice-like honeycomb spongiosa with coarsened axial trabeculae in the affected vertebral body *(2)*. Its outer shape is preserved, and one can clearly recognize the completely intact cortex *(2)*. The intervertebral space also shows no particular alteration, thus confirming conclusively that the neoplasm is entirely concentrated in the marrow cavity and has not broken out of the bone. The full picture of a vertebral hemangioma includes a slight enlargement of the diameter of the body, together with a straggly, but still regular structure, which is predominantly organized in the vertical direction. Less commonly the bone has an alveolar structure, particularly observable in the neural arch, which is pushed up into a club-shaped protuberance. Because of the increased pressure it causes within the spinal canal, the tumorous tissue can cause the laminae to be partly resorbed, so that in the computer tomogram the neural arch appears to have been "gnawed at".

In **Fig. 699** one can see the **macroscopic picture** of a bone hemangioma of the spine. This is a case of a particularly excessive tumorous growth *(1)*. It has completely destroyed the body of the affected vertebra and also encroached upon the bodies of the adjacent vertebrae *(2)*. The cut surface of the tumor shows a sponge-like tissue drenched with hemorrhages and clots and containing hollow spaces filled to a greater or lesser extent with blood. One can clearly see it bulging into the spinal canal *(3)* with compression of the cord. The tumor is nevertheless sharply demarcated. The tissue itself soft and sponge-like and contains no hard substance. The *cystic hemangioma*, which appears between the ages of 10 and 15 years, is a particular form of the cavernous hemangioma. Here, multiple round areas of osteolysis are localized in several regions of the skeleton which may give rise to a spontaneous fracture. The lesions are benign.

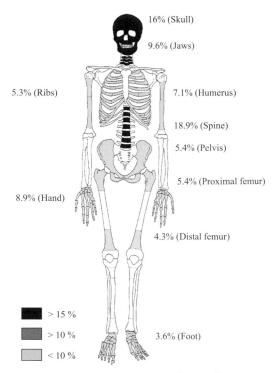

16% (Skull)

9.6% (Jaws)

5.3% (Ribs)

7.1% (Humerus)

18.9% (Spine)

5.4% (Pelvis)

5.4% (Proximal femur)

8.9% (Hand)

4.3% (Distal femur)

> 15 %

> 10 %

< 10 %

3.6% (Foot)

Fig. 696. Localization of the bone hemangiomas (118 cases); others: 15.5%

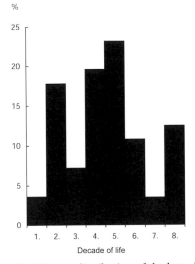

Fig. 697. Age distribution of the bone hemangiomas (118 cases)

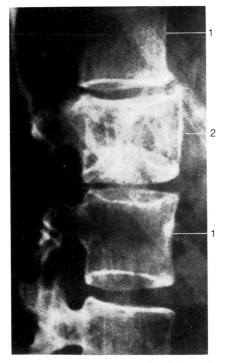

Fig. 698. Bone hemangioma (12th thoracic vertebral body)

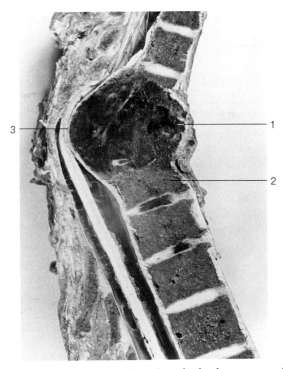

Fig. 699. Bone hemangioma (vertebral column, cut surface)

In the **radiograph** shown in **Fig. 700** one can see a hemangioma of the skull that is lying in the left occipito-parietal region *(1)*. It is a roundish focus that in places is fairly sharply demarcated, but without any marginal sclerosis. Nevertheless, it is a fairly sharply demarcated osteolytic zone, slightly elliptical in shape, within which fine patches of increased density can be seen. This gives it the internal appearance of a honeycomb. In a lateral (tangential) view one would be able to see the striped elevation of this bony focus – the stripes being due to the reactively developed bone trabeculae. This radiological phenomenon, which is known as a "sunburst", can be seen in the macroscopic photograph shown in **Fig. 702**. Thus a hemangioma of the skull presents as a sharply demarcated roundish defect of the diploe with outward bulging of the tables. In deciding the differential diagnosis of a defect in the skull cap such as this, it is essential to exclude above all an osteolytic bone metastasis or the lesions of a medullary plasmocytoma (p. 348). In this region bone hemangiomas are usually solitary.

Even so, as can be seen in the **histological picture** of such a bone hemangioma in **Fig. 701**, these lesions are very nearly always cavernous hemangiomas. **Histologically** one recognizes the broad cavernous space *(1)* which is lined by a single layer of endothelial cells *(2)*. These are completely flat and have small isomorphic nuclei. Here we have a thin-walled blood vessel, filled with blood. Only rarely are clots also present. The vessels of the tumor lie in a very loose connective tissue stroma *(3)* which contains only a few isomorphic fibrocytes. Interstitial bleeding or hemosiderin deposition is rare. In the region of the tumor the bone trabeculae are largely preserved *(4)*, although they may be osteosclerotically widened and show parallel reversal lines. Osteoclastic bone resorption and osteoblastic bone deposition are unusual in bone hemangiomas, and it is only when a pathological fracture has occurred that the fibro-osseous fracture callus may alter the appearance of the angiomatous tissue.

Figure 702 shows the **macroscopic picture** of a bone hemangioma of the skull cap. The focus has been removed with a saw and the ovaloid operation specimen carved up into slices. At the outer edges *(1)* it is clear that only healthy tissue has been cut through, leaving the tumor lying in the central region of the specimen *(2)*. It has involved the whole thickness of the skull cap and is bulging outwards *(3)*. The tumor itself is soaked through with blood. Inside the bone its margins are in places blurred or are undulating and jagged. There is no marginal sclerosis. The cut surface has the appearance of a honeycomb, showing small blood-filled cavities as well as larger "caverns". In general it resembles a soft, fragile, blood-soaked sponge, into which one can easily insert a finger. Within the bulging area one can see the radially directed, newly formed bone trabeculae (the so-called "spicules": *3*) which give the radiograph its classical "sunburst" appearance.

The rare **capillary bone hemangioma** is most frequently found in the ribs. In the long bones it arises as a cortical type at the metaphyses, projecting a single or multiple bony shell onto the radiograph, or as a central cystic type raised up like a honeycomb in which, however, the finer spongiosal structure is preserved. In **Fig. 703** one can see the **histological picture** of a capillary bone hemangioma. It consists of numerous small capillary vessels *(1)* which vary in diameter. Most of these are empty, but the larger ones contain blood. The tumorous vessels are lined with a flat single-layer endothelium. They lie in a loose connective tissue stroma, in which a few inflammatory infiltrates may be present. The trabeculae *(2)* between these vessels have been preserved, and are often even osteosclerotically widened.

While most bone tumors remain confined to the affected bone, vascular tumors may also attack the adjacent bones. This is particularly true of the *hemangiomatoses*, which may in young adults lead to the phenomenon of a so-called massive osteolysis (*Gorham's syndrome*). The clavicle is frequently affected, the process attacking the adjacent parts of the skeleton and bringing about dissolution of the bony structure. Histologically it has the morphological appearance of a cavernous hemangioma or even a lymphangioma. The cause of this condition is unknown, but it can be effectively treated by irradiation.

Among the vascular bone tumors there are a few special types which, in common with similar tumors in the soft parts, have a characteristic histological appearance but which are never-

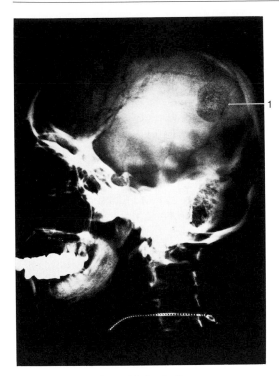

Fig. 700. Hemangioma of the skull (parieto-occipital region)

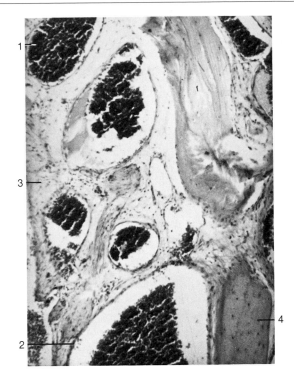

Fig. 701. Cavernous bone hemangioma; HE, ×40

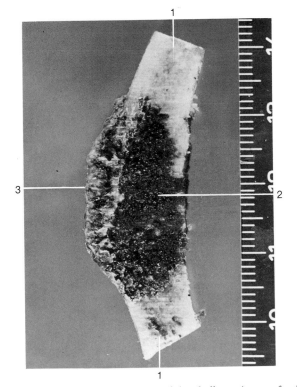

Fig. 702. Bone hemangioma of the skull cap (cut surface)

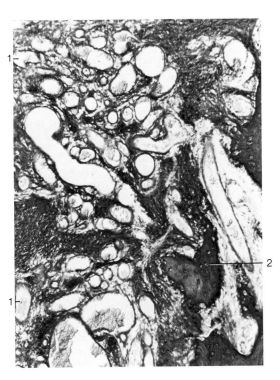

Fig. 703. Capillary bone hemangioma; van Gieson, ×25

theless comparatively rare. These include the **hemangiopericytoma** of bone. *This is an aggressively growing – on occasion even malignant – vascular bone tumor which is made up of vessels with a single-layer endothelium, but which are surrounded by proliferating cells.* The histological appearance of one of these tumors is shown in **Fig. 704.** One can observe numerous hollow vascular spaces *(1)* which are lined with a flattened endothelium. The vascular clefts are surrounded by very closely packed spindle-shaped oval cells *(2)* that can be seen in the overall view between the vascular lumens. These are relatively large spindle-shaped cells with abundant cytoplasm and dark nuclei. One can observe marked nuclear polymorphy, with dark giant nuclei *(3)* and a few multinucleated cells *(4)*. Mitoses are rare. In most cases the prognosis of these tumors cannot be assessed histologically. If the polymorphy of the cells and their nuclei is marked, if numerous abnormal mitoses are present and invasion of the cells into the lumens of the vessels can be established, then one must assume that it is a malignant tumor.

Another vascular bone tumor that is very rarely seen is the *glomus tumor.* It has a certain morphological similarity to the hemangiopericytoma, although the perivascular glomus cells are much smaller. *This is a benign osteolytic bone lesion that presents histologically with vascular structures which are surrounded by uniform roundish cells.* The end phalanges of the short tubular bones are most often affected. In **Fig. 705** one can see in the **radiograph** of a finger, a defect in the cortex of the terminal phalanx *(1)* with extensive sclerosis *(2)* in the adjacent spongiosa. A tumorous densification of the soft parts is also visible *(3)*. **Histologically** one can see in **Fig. 706** numerous drawn-out capillaries *(1)* lined with a flattened endothelium, and between them large groups of uniform cells with uniformly round nuclei *(2)* which often adhere closely to the capillaries *(3)*. These are glomus cells. Since the tumor causes severe local pain, it has to be removed surgically. Vascular bone tumors can also arise from the lymph vessels of a bone. *The bone* **lymphangioma** *is a very rare primary bone neoplasm that consists of a local aggregation of variably dilated lymph vessels and is found within the marrow cavity.* **Figure** 707 shows the **radiograph** of such a tu-

mor. There is a large cystic zone of osteolysis *(1)* that has taken up the whole width of the shaft. The lesion is fairly sharply demarcated, although there is no marginal sclerosis. The adjacent cortex *(2)* is certainly somewhat porous, but still intact. There is no thickening of the periosteum. The "bony cyst" is empty.

As is shown in the **histological photograph** of **Fig. 708**, there are large dilated lymph vessels *(1)* in the marrow cavity of the osteolytic region of the bone. Their walls are narrow and the endothelium is sparse. These vessels contain a weakly eosinophilic fluid (lymph) but no erythrocytes (blood). Between the dilated lymph vessels there is a loose fibrous stroma *(2)* in which a few inflammatory cells (plasma cells, lymphocytes, histiocytes) can be seen here and there. The cancellous trabeculae *(3)* are strongly developed, have smooth borders, and show no signs of resorptive bone destruction. In some bone lymphomas, however, there may be resorption of the local cancellous bone tissue, and this is reflected in the radiograph as a structureless osteolysis.

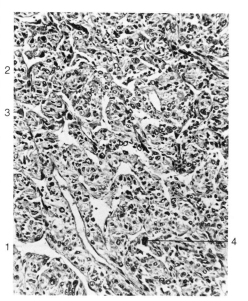

Fig. 704. Osseous hemangiopericytoma; PAS, ×40

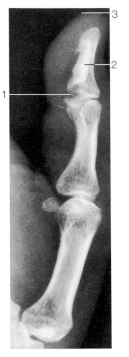

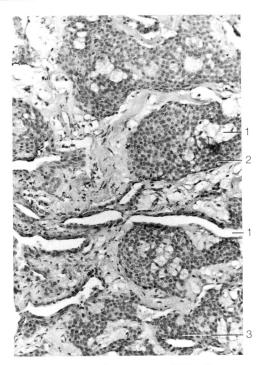

Fig. 705. Osseous glomus tumor
(terminal phalanx of a finger)

Fig. 706. Osseous glomus tumor; PAS, ×64

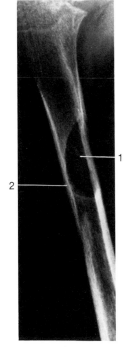

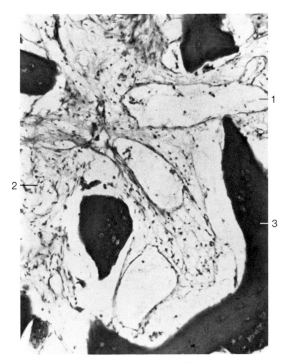

Fig. 707. Osseous lymphangioma (proximal humerus)

Fig. 708. Osseous lymphangioma; HE, ×40

Hemangiosarcoma of Bone (ICD-O-DA-M-9120/3)

Malignant vascular neoplasms very rarely appear as primary tumors of bone. So far only about 100 cases or so have been described in the literature. *The angiosarcoma is a highly malignant and destructively developing neoplasm which arises from blood vessels of a bone and consists of irregularly anastomosing vessels with an abnormal polymorphic endothelium.* Since these bizarre endothelial cells are themselves the actual tumor cells, use is often made of the synonym *"hemangioendothelioma"* to describe the tumor. In very rare cases an angiosarcoma can be identified as a *malignant hemangiopericytoma*. With such a collection of polymorphic cells as this neoplasm possesses the individual morphological variants can often not be recognized with any certainty. It may often be impossible to decide whether one is dealing with a hemangiosarcoma or a *lymphangiosarcoma*. For the purposes of diagnosis, however, the description "angiosarcoma of bone" is sufficient. The frequently multifocal appearance of this tumor (in 30% of cases) is very typical of it. It can arise in any bone at any age, although the long bones are most often attacked.

In **Fig. 709** one can see the **radiograph** of a very large soft tumorous shadow in the right humerus *(1)*, in which the original tubular bone has been completely destroyed. The shadow reaches deep into the soft parts and is very poorly demarcated. Of the humerus, one can only recognize a part of the head *(2)*, the shaft in the neighborhood of the tumor appearing as if it has been gnawed away. The entire humeral shaft is set through by an uneven finely patchy area of osteolysis *(3)*, which represents secondary bone atrophy. Osteolytic angiomatosis cannot, however, be excluded radiologically.

As shown in **Fig. 710**, the **histological section** reveals a very highly cellular, highly undifferentiated tumorous tissue. Between the tumor cells one can discern numerous spaces *(1)*, each of which represents the lumen of a blood vessel. The basal membrane *(2)* can sometimes be clearly recognized. The undifferentiated tumor cells are malignant endothelial cells. These are often lying together to form smaller or larger proliferating buds, giving the tumorous tissue a

pseudopapillary appearance. The cells vary in their size and degree of polymorphy; they have a pale cytoplasm and easily recognizable cell boundaries. A few of them possess small roundish nuclei *(3)* with light karyoplasm and a large central nucleolus. Other cells have a polymorphic, very dark giant nucleus *(4)*, and others again have several distended nuclei *(5)*. In general, the cellular and nuclear polymorphy is so marked that no doubt can exist concerning its malignancy. The number of mitoses is variable, there may be only a few present. The differential diagnosis of such a tumor can sometimes be very difficult. When epithelial-like differentiation of the tumor cells is present, one must consider a possible bone metastasis from a hypernephroid carcinoma of the kidney (renal cell carcinoma). Solid areas of endothelium can closely resemble a synovial carcinoma (p. 466). Solid fibrous regions are uncommon, but in a bone biopsy they may give the impression of an osseous fibrosarcoma (p. 330) or a malignant fibrous histiocytoma (p. 324).

The identification of tumorous vascular spaces is decisive for the diagnosis. In **Fig. 711** one can see how clearly these are shown up by silver staining. Wide cavernous *(1)* and narrow capillary vascular spaces *(2)* are mixed up with one another and bound together by anastomoses. Proliferation of the tumor cells may be seen inside or outside the reticular fibers (hemangioendothelioma/hemangiopericytoma).

In **Fig. 712** the **histological picture** of a bone angiosarcoma is depicted. Again, there is a very highly cellular tumorous tissue, harboring polymorphic cells with many ungainly hyperchromatic nuclei *(1)*. One can see many vascular cavities *(2)* against which groups of tumor cells are deposited *(3)*. One classifies such a tumor as a bone angiosarcoma of the type represented by a malignant hemangiopericytoma.

Since malignant vascular neoplasms of the same histological formation also appear in the soft parts – and more commonly there than in bone – one must always think of bone metastases when dealing with a malignant angiomatous bone tumor, especially if several foci appear at the same time. Even so, these tumors can themselves appear in several different places simultaneously.

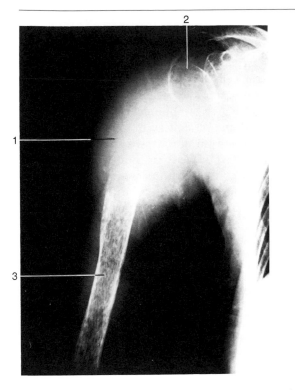

Fig. 709. Osseous hemangiosarcoma (proximal humerus)

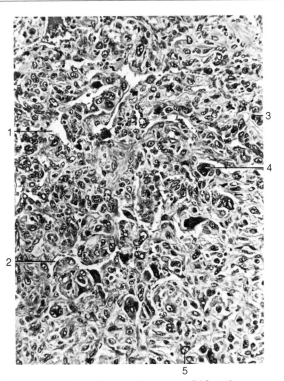

Fig. 710. Osseous hemangiosarcoma; PAS, ×40

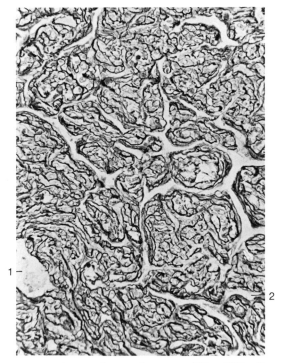

Fig. 711. Osseous hemangiosarcoma; Tibor PAP, ×40

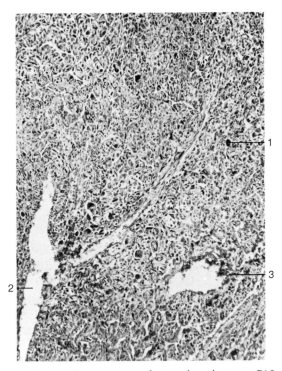

Fig. 712. Malignant osseous hemangiopericytoma; PAS, ×25

Adamantinoma of the Long Bones (ICD-O-DA-M-9261/3)

The adamantinoma of the long bones is a very rare tumor that most often appears in tibia. *It is a peculiar malignant bone neoplasm that is histologically very similar to the jaw bone adamantinoma (ameloblastoma). The histogenesis is unknown.* As a possible tissue of origin, blood vessels ("malignant angioblastoma"), the synovial membrane and scattered epithelial cells have all been suggested. The tumor usually arises in middle age and attacks men rather more often than women. It presents with swelling, which is often painful, in the middle of the leg, and is frequently traced back to an injury. The most frequent site is the shaft of the tibia, but fibula, femur, humerus, ulna or radius can also be affected. There is often a remarkable association between this tumor and a fibrous or osteofibrous bone dysplasia (pp. 316, 318).

The **radiograph** usually shows a relatively large destruction zone, which lies eccentrically in the shaft of the bone and may have a diameter of 10 cm. The cortex is often intact; the surrounding bone is sclerotic. In some cases a tumorous periosteal reaction with thickening of the cortex has been observed. In **Fig. 713** this kind of destructive lesion is lying in the tibial shaft, and one can see a polycystic osteolytic focus with a large eccentric internal zone of osteolysis *(1)* and small patchy osteolytic foci *(2)*. On one side the cortex is broken through over a wide front *(1)*. No periosteal reaction or soft tissue shadow is apparent, but there is clear marginal osteosclerosis *(3)* which has been loosened up by patches of osteolysis.

Histologically, four basic types of morphological structure can be found in long bone adamantinomas. The commonest is the *basaloid tissue pattern*, in which groups of closely packed tumor cells, surrounded by a layer of palisade cells, are found lying in a fibrous stroma (**Fig. 716**). These cell groups are enclosed by reticular fibers. In the *spindle-cell tissue pattern*, the spindle-cells are arranged in tiny whorls and resemble smooth muscle fibers or recall the patterns formed by nerve tumors. Reticular fibers enclose the individual tumor cells. With *epithelial differentiation*, there are groups of roundish or polygonal cells with an eosinophilic cytoplasm and keratohyalin granules. Reticular fibers enclose whole groups of cells. With the *tubular tissue pattern*, small flattened or cubical cells surround tissue spaces of various sizes. Blood components within the spaces suggest that they are blood vessels, and one often has the impression as of small glands lying in the middle of a fibrous stroma. Compression can cause rows of cells to infiltrate the stroma. In contrast to the situation with a synovial sarcoma (p. 466), no acid mucopolysaccharides can be demonstrated in the tumor with Alcian blue PAS staining.

Figure 714 shows the **histological appearance** of an adamantinoma with the *basaloid tissue pattern*. In the connective tissue stroma, which can show myxomatous porosity *(1)*, there are large flat or band-like complexes of tumor cells, which are bordered by palisade cells *(2)* and remind one of a basalioma. These cell nests often contain cyst-like hollow spaces *(3)*, and a squamous epithelium may also be present, prompting one to think of a bone metastasis.

Figure 715 depicts a *spindle-like adamantinoma*, in which tiny whorls and knots *(1)* can be discerned. The spindle-cells have elongated hyperchromatic nuclei of various sizes *(2)*, in which mitoses are only rarely seen. The dense, unevenly elongated cell aggregates *(3)* between the whorls are striking. They reveal no peripheral organization of the tumor cells. The narrow fissures in their centers *(4)* look like vascular clefts. Under **higher magnification** one can see in **Fig. 716** basaloid cell nests within a dense, highly fibrous stroma. The peripheral cells *(1)* are cubic or cylindrical and have roundish nuclei of uniform size. The inner cells *(2)* are more spindle-shaped or stellate, and have little cytoplasm. They are either aligned in parallel or bound together in a kind of network.

The tumor is characterized by slow, locally destructive growth, and it is only much later that metastases appear in 20% of cases. The treatment of choice is therefore an en bloc extirpation, or, with extensive tumors, amputation.

In the **a.p. radiograph** of **Fig. 718** those structures which suggest an adamantinoma of the long bones are clearly seen. There are numerous coarse patchy areas of osteolysis in the

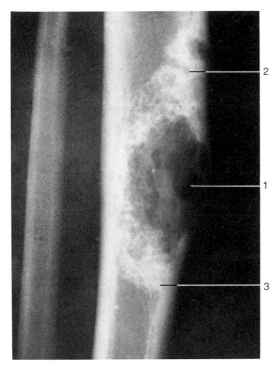

Fig. 713. Adamantinoma of the long bones (tibial shaft)

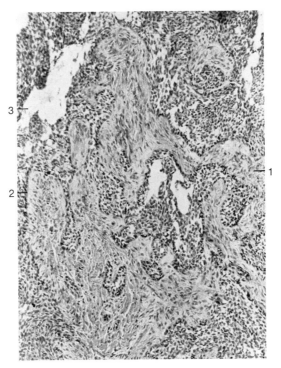

Fig. 714. Adamantinoma of the long bones; HE, ×40

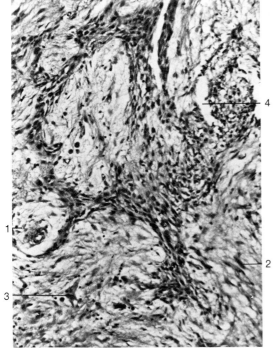

Fig. 715. Adamantinoma of the long bones; HE, ×64

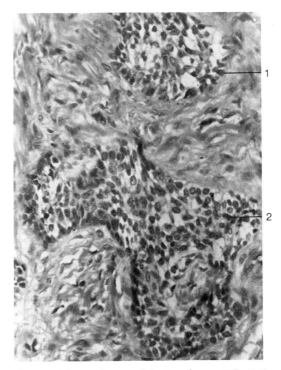

Fig. 716. Adamantinoma of the long bones; HE, ×100

tibial shaft *(1)* lying mostly within the spongiosa, which are sometimes confluent and form large regions of osteolysis *(2)*. They are fairly well demarcated by an incomplete marginal sclerosis, and often have a punched out appearance. In one place the cortex is also set through with osteolytic foci *(3)*, and here it bulges outwards. Between the patchy translucencies there are uneven sclerotic thickenings in the spongiosa. The outer contours of the long bone are sharp, and there is no periosteal reaction visible. The lesion is more clearly apparent in the **lateral view**. In **Fig. 719** one can again recognize the many coarse patches of osteolysis *(1)* in the shaft of the tibia. They give the effect as of punched out holes and are surrounded by marginal sclerosis. The cortex is much thickened ventrally *(2)* and interspersed by further similar osteolytic foci. The whole of the tibial diaphysis appears somewhat deformed. Osteolytic foci surrounded by osteosclerosis are lying also in region of the dorsal cortex *(3)*. The tumor extends over a large part of the tibial shaft. Thus an adamantinoma of the long bones can appear radiologically as a solitary circumscribed osteolytic lesion (see Fig. 713) as well as in the form of multicentric osteolytic foci.

In the **histological picture** shown in **Fig. 720** there are wide aggregations of epithelioid cells *(1)* lying in densely packed unequal groups inside the intraosseous foci. These tumor cells have nuclei which vary in size and are sometimes round, sometimes elongated and which differ in their chromatin content; those rich in chromatin *(2)* may be lying beside others which have very little. Mitoses are only rarely encountered. The cytoplasm of the tumor cells is sparsely developed and not clearly demarcated. This is the *epithelial variant* of the adamantinoma which can easily be confused in a bone biopsy with a carcinomatous bone metastasis. Between the complexes of tumor cells there is a loose connective tissue stroma *(3)* with isomorphic fibrocytes. There is no sarcomatous stroma.

Under the **higher magnification** of **Fig. 717** the connective tissue stroma dominates the picture. Here one can see isomorphic fibrocytes with greatly elongated nuclei *(1)* and a few isomorphic round cells (lymphocytes, *2*). Narrow complexes of dark cells *(3)* have been deposited which show a great similarity to the amelo-

blasts in the jaws. They have dark and only slightly polymorphic nuclei of varying size and little cytoplasm. These tumor cell complexes are poorly demarcated and show signs of infiltrating growth. This is the *spindle-cell variant* of the adamantinoma, which can again be mistaken for a bone metastasis. The diagnosis can, however, be made if the radiographic findings are also taken into account.

Figure 721 is a **histological picture** under higher magnification of the spindle-cell form of an adamantinoma. One can see many spindle-shaped tumor cells with polymorphic hyperchromatic nuclei *(1)* loosely bound together. Obviously they are not producing any collagen fibers. One trabecula *(2)* has been extensively destroyed by the tumor cells. Practically no pathological mitoses can be seen in these tumor cells. Such a tumor shows signs of malignancy. So far it has not been established whether an adamantinoma of the long bones is a vascular or an epithelial bone tumor. Even with histochemical methods (positive reaction for keratin and vimentin as well as α-SM-actin; no reaction for desmin, factor VIII or ulex I) the histogenesis cannot be decided.

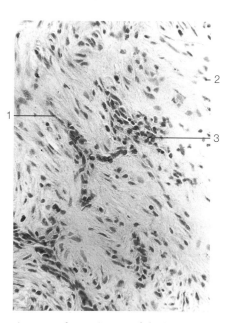

Fig. 717. Adamantinoma of the long bones; HE, ×82

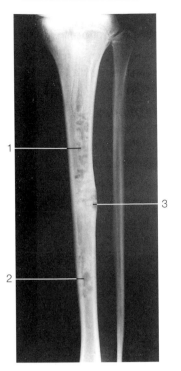

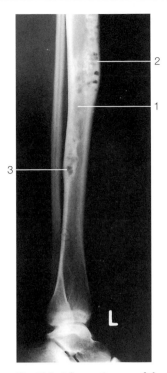

Fig. 718. Adamantinoma of the long bones (tibial shaft, a.p. view)

Fig. 719. Adamantinoma of the long bones (tibial shaft, lateral view)

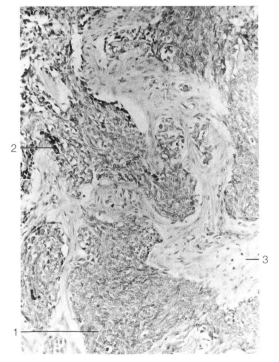

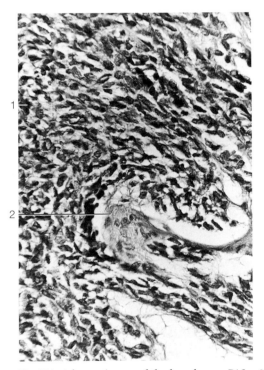

Fig. 720. Adamantinoma of the long bones; HE, ×64

Fig. 721. Adamantinoma of the long bones; PAS, ×82

Chordoma (ICD-O-DA-M-9370/3)

This neoplasm is not derived from any tissue that is present in bone, and is therefore not really a bone tumor. Nevertheless, the chordoma is classified among these tumors (p. 209) because it has a special topographical relationship to bone, appearing almost exclusively at one or other end of the spinal column. *The chordoma is a malignant tumor that develops near the axial skeleton (vertebral column) from remnants of the notochord and manifests a slow destructive growth. Metastases are unusual.* Histologically there is a certain similarity to the chondrosarcoma (p. 241). This neoplasm is quite rare (about 1% of all bone tumors) and does not usually appear before the age of 30. The principal sites are the sphenooccipital region of the skull base and the sacral component of the vertebral column, although it can arise anywhere along the course of the latter. Men are affected about twice as often as women. Clinically the tumor undergoes progressive growth with uncharacteristic pain. At the skull base its expansion can sometimes lead to fatal neurocerebral complications.

In **Fig. 772** one can see the **radiograph** of a chordoma of the sacrum *(1)*. As indicated by the arrow, the growth projects a soft roundish shadow invading the pelvis. It is not very sharply demarcated. On one side *(2)* the tumor reaches into the sacrum, where it has brought about extensive destruction. The rest of this bone is still intact. Within the tumor there are signs of lobulation, and one can see dense patchy calcifications. In general it is an osteolytically destructive growing tumor which has broken out of the bone into the pelvis, where in most cases it can be palpated.

As can be seen in the **histological picture** of **Fig. 723**, the tumorous tissue has a definitely lobular formation. One can easily discern a nodular focus *(1)* bordered by a seam of narrow connective tissue *(2)*. Such a morphological appearance is very similar to that of a chondrosarcoma (p. 241); with sphenooccipital chordomas particularly, the histological distinction can be difficult to make (the so-called ***chondroid chordoma***). Both in the center of the node and in the surrounding tumorous tissue one can recognize groups and bands of small mononuclear cells *(3)* with eosinophilic cyto-

plasm and a well marked cell boundary. In between there are abundant agglutinations of mucus *(4)*. Apart from these syncytial bands of tumor cells one can observe groups of apparently distended cells *(5)* with a very pale vacuolated cytoplasm. These are the so-called "physaliphorous" cells, which are very characteristic of a chordoma.

Under **higher magnification** these tumor cells can be more clearly perceived in **Fig. 724**. Once again one can see part of a lobule *(1)* which is bordered by a narrow connective tissue membrane *(2)*. The stroma contains much mucus *(3)* and there are groups and strings of small mononuclear cells *(4)* with a sharply demarcated strongly eosinophilic cytoplasm. Their nuclei are very compact and dark, and sometimes roundish, sometimes unevenly elongated. There is a certain amount of polymorphy. These syncytial cells occupy large areas together, between which there are physaliphorous cells *(5)* with a very pale bubble-like cytoplasm and eccentric nuclei. With mucin staining one can identify glycogen in these cells. On the other hand, the collections of mucus in the intercellular substance are not always PAS positive.

The physaliphorous cells of the chordoma can be clearly discerned under the **higher magnification** of **Fig. 725**. They have a very light glycogen-containing cytoplasm *(1)* and a small compact and very dark nucleus *(2)*. The size of the nucleus varies. Usually only a few mitoses are seen. The cell boundaries are sharp *(3)*, so that the varying size of the physaliphorous cells gives the tissue the appearance of an irregular honeycomb. This is also broken up by the deposits of mucus *(4)*.

Complete surgical removal of this slow-growing tumor is usually impossible. Palliative radiation therapy is therefore employed to delay recurrences. Metastases appear in about 10% of cases. DAHLIN has made the remarkable observation that the chondroid chordoma, which largely consists of chondrosarcomatous tumorous tissue, is associated with a survival period twice as long as that of a conventional chordoma.

In the lateral **radiograph** of the lumbar column and sacrum shown in **Fig. 726** one can see the balloon-like distension of the proximal sacral and distal lumbar components *(1)* so that

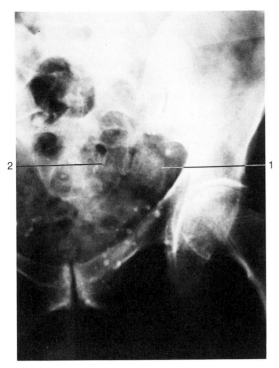

Fig. 722. Chordoma (sacrum)

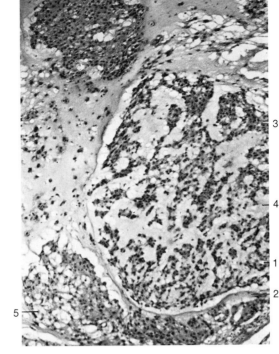

Fig. 723. Chordoma; HE, ×25

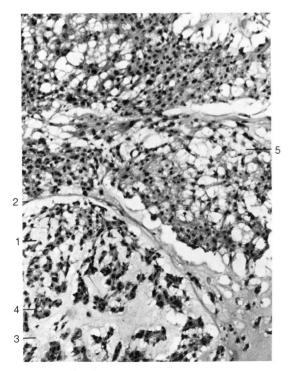

Fig. 724. Chordoma; HE, ×51

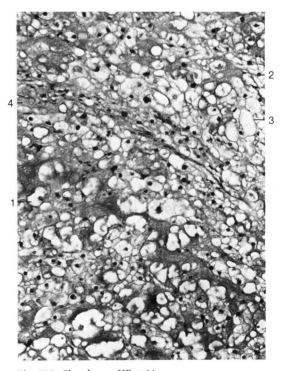

Fig. 725. Chordoma; HE, ×64

the individual vertebrae are no longer clearly distinguishable. This is due to an aggressively expanding osteolytic lesion which is very typical of the chordoma. The tumor appears as a diffuse shadow *(2)* that has expanded ventrally towards the sacrum itself. Dorsally, at the transition to the lumbar column *(3)*, one can discern a poorly demarcated zone of increased density. The two lower lumbar vertebrae (L4 and L5) have been included in the process of destruction. Parts of the tumor show fine patches of calcification *(4)*. Such a radiological appearance at the distal end of the vertebral column indicates the presence of a chordoma.

Figure 727 also shows the radiograph of a sacral chordoma. The bone structure in this region *(1)* is completely destroyed and no longer recognizable. One can only see the large diffuse shadow of the tumor reaching deep into the pelvis *(2)*. In such a case a **computer tomograph (CT)** is indicated in order to reveal the morphological details of the tumor. As shown in **Fig. 728**, this particularly emphasizes the size and extent of the growth. We can see how the tumor has destroyed the sacrum over a wide area *(1)*, and only a few parts of the bone *(2)* have remained intact. It has invaded the bones of the pelvis *(3)* and even brought about the destruction of its outer parts, and one can also see how it is bulging deep into the inside of the pelvis *(4)*. Internally the tumor consists of patchy regions of increased density, representing dystrophic calcifications. Reactive new bone deposition is not unusual in chordomas, and some lesions can be strongly osteoblastic in appearance. In a myelograph there may be, in addition to the expansive bone destruction, signs of an extradural defect or even a complete block.

The **radiograph** depicted in **Fig. 729** shows that parts of the tumorous tissue are fairly regular in form and show no signs of a lobulated or nodular structure. This is a malignant tissue in which polymorphic tumor cells are loosely bound together. One can see large polymorphic hyperchromatic nuclei *(1)* in association with small roundish *(2)* and elongated *(3)* nuclei, all of which are rich in chromatin. The cell boundaries are indistinct and the background porous and strongly mucoid. In places there are large deposits of mucus *(4)*. There are chordomas with monomorphic tumor cells and others in

which a clear nuclear polymorphy predominates. Mitoses are rare.

Chordomas of the spheno-occipital region are particularly likely to present with the **histological** morphology of a chondrosarcoma. In **Fig. 730** one can see in places a myxomatous tissue with small round cells *(1)* which corresponds to the morphological appearance of a chordoma. Adjacent to this there is a large cartilaginous area *(2)*. This is tumorous cartilage with variously sized chondrocytes which possess polymorphic hyperchromatic nuclei *(3)*. This tissue is identical with that of a chondrosarcoma (grade 2). Next to this there is a bone trabecula *(4)* which has been destroyed by the tumor and then reactively remodeled. So far, **chondroid chordomas** have only been observed in the sphenooccipital region, and in these cases the life expectation is twice as long as with a non-chondroid chordoma. These variable tissue structures can produce considerable diagnostic problems in the bone biopsy. Such an expansive and destructive tumor arising in the sacral region must be investigated bioptically. From the point of view of the differential diagnosis, giant cell tumors (p. 337), carcinomatous metastases, ependymomas or a meningocele can give rise to very similar radiological structural changes.

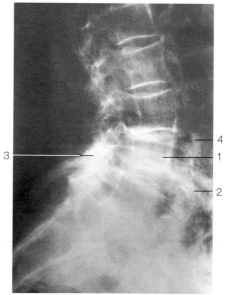

Fig. 726. Sacral chordoma

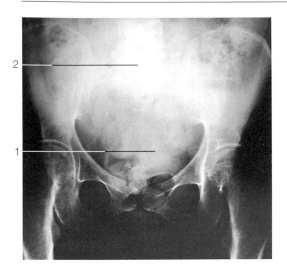

Fig. 727. Sacral chordoma

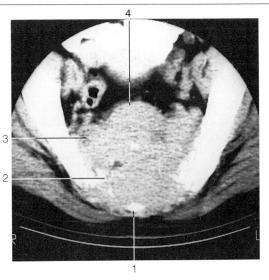

Fig. 728. Sacral chordoma (computer tomogram)

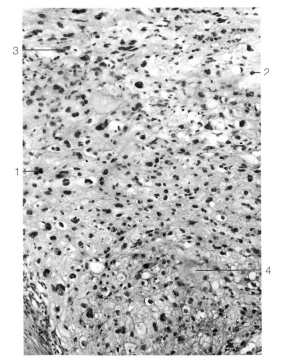

Fig. 729. Chordoma; PAS, ×82

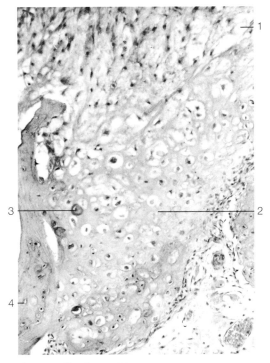

Fig. 730. Chordoma; HE, ×82

Neurogenic Bone Tumors

Osseous Neurinoma (Neurolemoma, Schwannoma) (ICD-O-DA-M-9560/0)

Primary bone tumors which arise from the nerves of the bones are extremely rare. *The osseous neurinoma is a benign tumor that is derived from the nerve sheath and has the same morphological appearance as similar tumors of the soft parts.* This neoplasm is only very rarely seen as a primary tumor of bone, and only 50 cases have appeared in the literature. The principal site is in the lower jaw, where about half of all neurinomas have been described. The predominant age of onset is in the 4th decade of life. The tumor presents with pain and swelling.

As can be seen in **Fig. 731** this slow-growing lesion appears **radiologically** as an area of circumscribed osteolysis with marginal sclerosis. There is a large zone of osteolysis *(1)* limited internally by a narrow band of marginal sclerosis *(2)* in the proximal part of the left tibia. The cortex *(3)*, which is intact but bulges slightly outwards, is also involved in the osteolytic process. In this child the focus reaches as far as, but does not encroach upon, the epiphyseal cartilage *(4)*. The tumor is situated eccentrically within the bone.

One can see **histologically** in **Fig. 732** that the components are arranged in straggly whorls *(1)* which show nuclei of varying density. The background tissue contains only a few collagen and reticular fibers. The nuclei of the neoplastic Schwann cells are characteristically arranged in regular palisade-like groups *(2)*. In between there are cell-free fibrous zones *(3)*, known as *Verocay's bodies*, which are very characteristic of the neurinoma. This is a neurinoma of Antoni type A in which fascicular structures predominate. Those defined by Antoni type B have a reticular tissue pattern with macrophages, fat and hemosiderin deposits. Thick-walled blood vessels with perivascular hyalinization *(4)* are common in the neurinoma. In benign neurinomas the cell nuclei are equally elongated and show no mitoses. Polymorphic hyperchromatic nuclei with abnormal mitoses suggest a malignant schwannoma. Histologically they reveal a morphological transition into a neurofibroma. Since osseous neurinomas are entirely benign and have a good prognosis, it is sufficient to curette the tumorous tissue, or at most remove it by en bloc excision.

Osseous Neurofibroma (ICD-O-DA-M-9540/0)

In 40% of the cases of **von Recklinghausen's neurofibromatosis**, skeletal changes occur. This is a congenital familial condition, in which complex dysplastic bone changes, which may also be generalized, appear. These consist of growth disturbances, innate deformities of the bones, dysplasia of the vertebral bodies with scoliosis, pseudoarthroses of the long bones or intraosseous and lytic eroded bone defects. *A neurofibroma is a localized benign tumor consisting of peripheral nerve cells (the Schwann cells) and loose connective tissue, rich in fibroblasts and containing mucoid material, which arises from the tissue of the perineural sheath.* Intraosseous neurofibromas are extremely rare, whereas periosteal and extraperiosteal neurofibromas are more frequently encountered. When such tumors are multiple we speak of von Recklinghausen's neurofibromatosis.

Figure 733 shows a **radiograph** of the shafts of the tibia and fibula of a 7-year-old boy with von Recklinghausen's neurofibromatosis. The tibia is obviously curved and severely sclerosed in the region of the shaft *(1)*. This sclerosis involves the cortex as well as the neighboring spongiosa. This part of the bone is covered ventrally by a greatly thickened and densified periosteum *(2)*. The adjacent soft parts *(3)* are more dense than is normal. Nevertheless, no intraosseous osteolytic foci or erosions can be observed in the case.

Figure 734 illustrates the **histological picture** of a periosteal neurofibroma. At the edge *(1)* one can see the parallel collagen fibers of the original periosteum. The adjacent tumorous tissue *(2)* is porous and strongly myxoid, with a loose background framework of collagen fibers. The Schwann cells *(3)* are loosely distributed throughout the tumor. They have small dark isomorphic nuclei which are mostly elongated or ovoid. In such neoplasms the bundles of collagen fibers and the Schwann cells may also be much more closely packed together. There is a progressive histological transition into a neurinoma. Whether neurofibrosarcomas can appear as primary neoplasms of bone is doubtful.

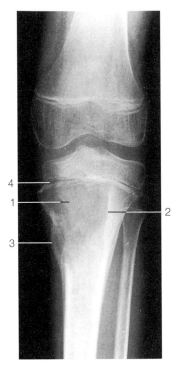

Fig. 731. Osseous neurinoma (proximal tibia)

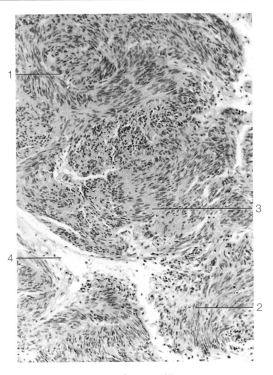

Fig. 732. Osseous neurinoma; HE, ×64

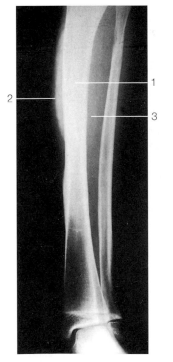

Fig. 733. Osseous neurofibroma (tibial shaft)

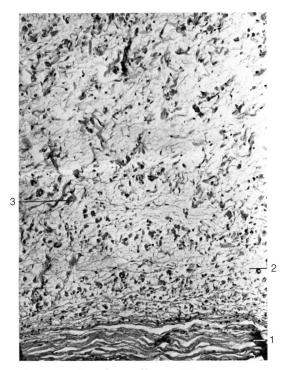

Fig. 734. Periosteal neurofibroma; HE, ×40

Neuroblastoma (Sympathicoblastoma) (ICD-O-DA-M-9490/3)

Neurogenic tumors can equally well develop in the nerves of the soft tissues as (usually less commonly) in the bones. Furthermore, malignant neurogenic tumors can produce metastases which at first give the impression of primary bone tumors and are histologically often difficult to identify. *The neuroblastoma is a highly malignant tumor that arises from undifferentiated neuroblasts (sympathicoblasts) and often produces bone metastases.* In highly differentiated neuroblastomas the ganglion cells can be identified *(ganglioneuroblastoma)*. This tumor almost only afflicts children, in 90% of cases before the age of 5, although they are seen sporadically in adults. The principal site of the primary tumor is in the retroperitoneal space, in the adrenals. In general the tumor can arise in any of the sympathetic ganglia (in the mediastinum, or the cervical or sacral regions). Metastases are found particularly in the spine, skull and long bones.

Figure 735 shows a lateral **radiograph** of the leg of a 12-year-old child, with a large area of osteolysis *(1)* in the distal part of the tibia. It is fairly sharply demarcated and has invaded the cortex. Proximal to this there are fine patches of osteolysis *(2)*. The distal epiphyseal plate *(3)* is intact and the epiphysis itself is not involved. There is a narrow band of periosteal thickening *(4)* lying on the bone at the ventral surface of the tibia.

Histologically this is an undifferentiated round cell tumor, showing destructive malignant growth, of a kind that is often difficult to classify. In **Fig. 736** one can see large groups of cells with dark nuclei *(1)* in the marrow cavity, together with many large crush artefacts *(2)*. The tumorous tissue is interspersed with wide and narrow zones of connective tissue *(3)* which contain fewer tumor cells, and which divide it up into narrow lobules. The spongiosa is extensively destroyed. There are occasional remnants of bone trabeculae *(4)* against which rows of osteoblasts have been deposited. Foci of necrosis and calcium can be present inside the tumor. The tumor cells are frequently arranged into rosettes.

Under **higher magnification** one can see in **Fig. 737** a bone trabecula *(1)* with an indistinct undulating border. Adjacent to this there is loose connective tissue *(2)* which is filling up the entire marrow cavity. Here one can see deposits of small undifferentiated tumor cells with a sparse cytoplasm *(3)*, which are striking by reason of their very dark nuclei. No rosette formation can be seen in this undifferentiated neuroblastoma. The tumorous tissue is interspersed with a few fine-walled vessels *(4)*. If isolated ganglion cells can be identified in such a tumor the diagnosis of a neuroblastoma is easily made.

The tumor cells are plain to see under the **higher magnification** in **Fig. 738**. They are about the size of lymphocytes and have only a sparse cytoplasm, which is indistinctly demarcated. The vital tumor cells have clearly hyperchromatic nuclei *(1)* which are sometimes roundish *(2)* and sometimes elongated *(3)*, thereby showing a significant degree of nuclear polymorphy. Many of the tumor cells have less dark nuclei *(4)*, indicating necrobiosis. In contrast to the malignant lymphoma, no prominent nuclei are to be seen.

In making the **differential diagnosis** of such a malignant bone lesion in children, *Ewing's sarcoma* (p. 352) will first of all come to mind. It is here that evidence of glycogen in this tumor (PAS staining) can be helpful (the neuroblastoma is often PAS negative). The neuro-specific enolase test (NSE) is positive in neuroblastomas, and neurosecretory granules and neural ramifications containing neurofibrils can be seen with the electron microscope. Clinically, vanillyl mandelic acid (VMA), homovanillyl acid (HVA) and 3-methoxy-4-hydroxyphenyl-glycol (MHPG) are found in the urine: substances which are the breakdown products of dopamine and DOPA. The *embryonic rhabdomyosarcoma*, which appears in early childhood, can on rare occasions produce skeletal metastases and must therefore also be included in the differential diagnosis.

This tumor is best identified immunohistochemically and with the electron microscope. Finally, a *malignant lymphoma* involving bone must be excluded. With young people and adults a *small cell osteosarcoma* (p. 284), a *mesenchymal chondrosarcoma* (p. 250) or a bone metastasis from a small cell bronchial carcinoma (p. 403) are differential diagnostic alternatives.

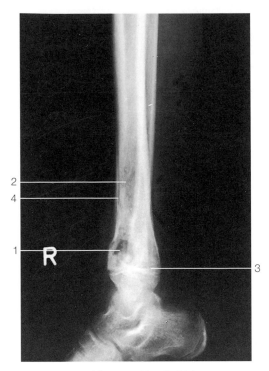

Fig. 735. Neuroblastoma (distal tibia)

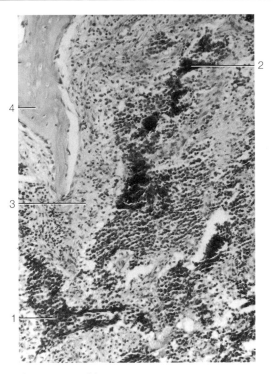

Fig. 736. Neuroblastoma; HE, ×40

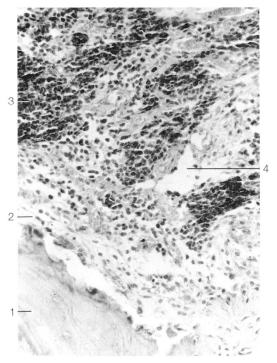

Fig. 737. Neuroblastoma; HE, ×64

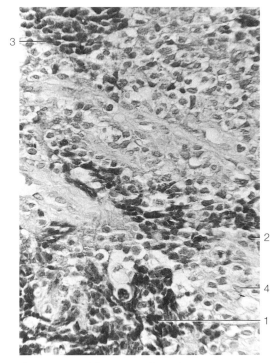

Fig. 738. Neuroblastoma; HE, ×100

Muscular Bone Tumors

Osseous Leiomyoma (ICD-O-DA-M-8890/0)

Among the spindle-celled primary bone tumors, only a few have so far been identified as neoplasms of muscle tissue. These probably arise from the smooth muscle cells of the intraosseous blood vessels. *A leiomyoma is a benign tumor consisting of smooth muscle fibers with more or less collagenous connective tissue, which must be regarded as a rarity in bone.*

The **radiograph** of one of these lesions is shown in **Fig. 740**. There is a central intraosseous focus of destruction *(1)* in the proximal part of the fibula, which in the lateral view *(2)* has the appearance of a "bony cyst". This focus is sharply demarcated and shows no internal structure. In the a.p. view *(1)*, however, the borders are indistinct and patchy. The cortex is bulging forward and also shows patches of porosity.

Histologically the tumorous tissue in **Fig. 739** consists of a loose connective tissue stroma *(1)* which is threaded through with a few vessels *(2)*, and in which lie wide smooth muscle cells *(3)* arranged almost in parallel. In one place there is a fibro-osseous trabecula *(4)*. In **Fig. 741** these smooth muscle fibers *(1)*, which determine the nature of the tumor, are more clearly seen under **higher magnification**. They have elongated isomorphic nuclei. Close to a bone trabecula *(2)* one can see loose connective tissue *(3)*.

Osseous Leiomyosarcoma (ICD-O-DA-M-8890/3)

Malignant neoplasms of muscle are also extremely seldom seen as primary bone tumors. *The leiomyosarcoma of bone arises from the smooth muscle of the intraosseous blood vessels, and is late to form metastases.* Up to the present, only isolated cases have been reported, so that it is impossible to recognize any principal sites for its appearance. Radiologically it develops as a local osteolytic zone of destruction, usually lying in the center of the bone, which can even destroy the cortex, and which in general gives the impression of a malignant bone tumor. They are more often found at the ends of the long bones than in the shaft.

In **Fig. 742** the **radiograph** shows extensive destruction of the bone structure at the distal end of the femur. The spongiosa shows "moth-eaten" osteolytic regions *(1)*, between which there are irregular zones of sclerotic thickening, so that one sees a very markedly porous tissue like a honeycomb, indicating a tumorous destruction of the bone. The cortex has also been drawn into this process *(2)*.

In the **histological picture** shown in **Fig. 743** the marrow cavity is filled with a spindle-celled tumorous tissue *(1)*, in which the fibers are often arranged in parallel. These are smooth muscle cells with clear nuclear polymorphy and hyperchromasia. One bone trabecula has remained intact *(2)* and has a broad osteoid seam *(3)*. There are abnormal mitoses in the tumorous tissue, multinucleated giant cells and many reticular fibers.

So far there has been a total of 18 intraosseous leiomyosarcomas reported in the literature. If such a histological picture is found, one must think first of all of a bone metastasis from a leiomyosarcoma of the soft parts or internal organs (uterus, stomach). It is only after

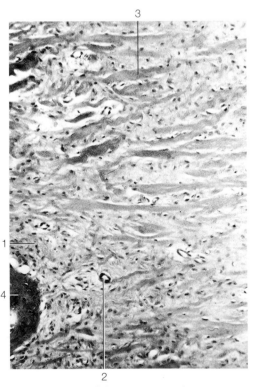

Fig. 739. Osseous leiomyoma; van Gieson, ×64

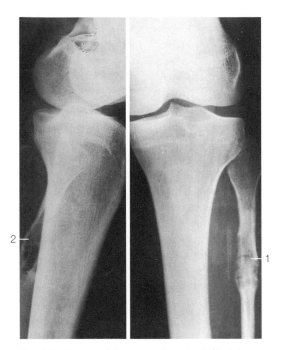

Fig. 740. Osseous leiomyoma (proximal fibula)

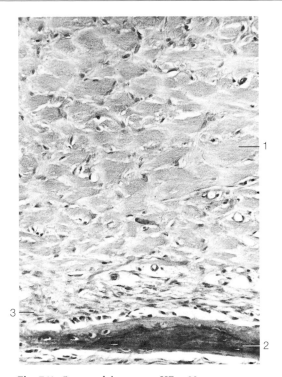

Fig. 741. Osseous leiomyoma; HE, ×82

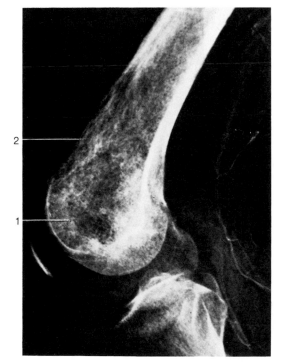

Fig. 742. Osseous leiomyosarcoma (distal femur)

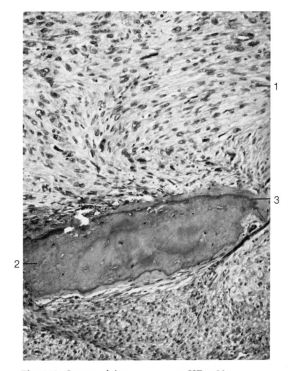

Fig. 743. Osseous leiomyosarcoma; HE, ×90

such a primary tumor has been excluded that a primary osseous leiomyosarcoma can be diagnosed. Generally speaking this tumor does not have a bad prognosis if it is completely removed surgically.

Malignant Osseous Mesenchymoma

Malignant bone tumors may occasionally appear which are seen histologically to be composed out of the differentiation of different tissues, and which cannot therefore be assigned to a particular tumor group. *The malignant mesenchymoma is characterized by the complete differentiation of several tissues, each of which represents a different kind of bone sarcoma.* In the bone this tumor usually consists of the structures of an osteosarcoma together with those of a *liposarcoma ("osteoliposarcoma")*. It is possible, however, for several other tumorous structures to be combined in such a growth. As a primary bone tumor, this neoplasm is both very rare and controversial. It was first described by SCHAJOWICZ and his coworkers in 1966, and recognized as a separate entity by the WHO.

The **radiological appearance**, which depends upon the variable differentiation of the tumor, is itself highly variable. **Figure 745** shows an example of this tumor in the distal femoral metaphysis of a 9-year-old child. One can see an eccentrically situated focus with flat patches of sclerotic thickening *(1)*. The tumor has also to an equal extent destroyed the cortex in this region *(2)*. It is indistinctly demarcated *(3)* and shows no marginal sclerosis. The epiphyseal cartilage *(4)* lies at some distance from the tumor.

Histologically it can be seen that the tumor involves at least two completely different tumorous structures. As is shown in **Fig. 746**, it consists for the greater part of closely packed cells with a strikingly pale cytoplasm *(1)* and large dark polymorphic nuclei *(2)*. Many of these cells have several nuclei *(3)*. This is a malignant lipoblast, the cytoplasm of which is seen, with appropriate staining (Sudan, oil red) to contain fat. The appearance of the tissue shows it to be identical with that of a *liposarcoma*. There is also much tumorous osteoid *(4)* and bone *(5)*, which is characteristic of an osteosarcoma (p. 274). These two tumorous tissues are mixed up together.

In many parts of the tumor there is a fine lattice work of osteoid deposits *(1)*, which is clearly seen **histologically** in **Fig. 747**. Between the thread-like strands of osteoid there are small round cells *(2)* with dark polymorphic

nuclei. A few isolated cells have hyperchromatic giant nuclei *(3)*. Some of these tumorous cells are osteoblasts and some are lipoblasts with a sudanophilic cytoplasm.

In **Fig. 748** the uneven lattice work of osteoid *(1)* is again recognizable **histologically**, and there is also differentiated tumorous bone *(2)* such as is found in osteosarcomas. Polymorphic tumor cells with hyperchromatic nuclei *(3)* are scattered among the osteosarcomatous structures. Elsewhere, the sarcomatous stroma clearly manifests itself. The proportion of liposarcomatous to osteosarcomatous tissue varies in these malignant mesenchymomas. **Figure 744** shows the **histological** appearance of round-cell tumorous tissue from a liposarcomatous area. The cells have defined polymorphic nuclei of varying sizes *(1)* and an abundant pale cytoplasm *(2)* which contains fat. This picture could pass for that of a round-cell liposarcoma such as is found in the soft parts. At the edge there is an autochthonous bone trabecula *(3)*. If in a bone biopsy only one of these structures is encountered, it is possible to arrive at a false classification of the tumor.

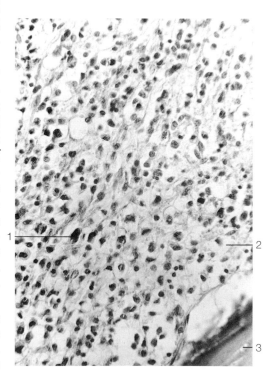

Fig. 744. Malignant osseous mesenchymoma; PAS, ×82

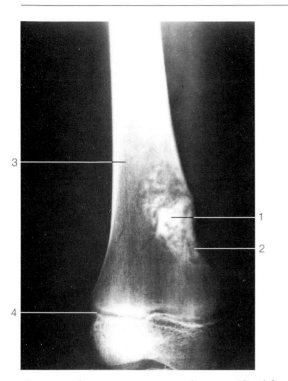

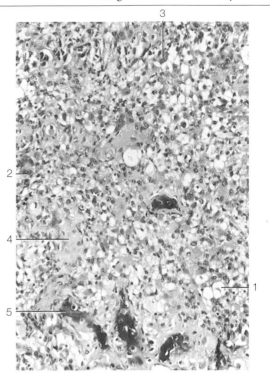

Fig. 745. Malignant osseous mesenchymoma (distal femur)

Fig. 746. Malignant osseous mesenchymoma; HE, ×40

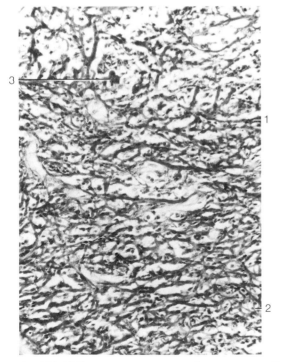

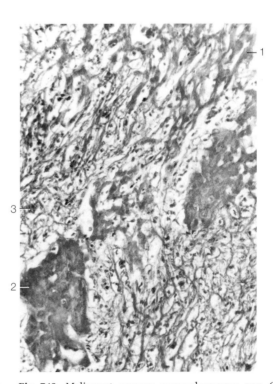

Fig. 747. Malignant osseous mesenchymoma; van Gieson, ×64

Fig. 748. Malignant osseous mesenchymoma; van Gieson, ×64

In **Fig. 751** one can see the **radiograph** of a malignant mesenchymoma in the 4th rib on the right. This region of the bone is raised up like a bubble *(1)*. The cortex is severely narrowed *(2)* and in places has been penetrated *(3)*. Within there are a few straggly densifications *(4)*.

The **histological picture** again shows a mixture of osteosarcomatous and liposarcomatous structures. In **Fig. 752** the stroma consists of round cells with polymorphic nuclei *(1)*, some of which, with their abundant light cytoplasm *(2)*, have the appearance of lipoblasts. In fact, they do contain fat. One can also see tumorous osteoid *(3)* and bone *(4)*, which are characteristic of an *osteosarcoma*. Elsewhere (**Fig. 753**) the picture reveals the morphological appearance of a *liposarcoma*. Here we can discern densely packed groups of lipoblasts with a light fat-containing cytoplasm *(1)*. The nuclei show a high degree of polymorphy and are hyperchromatic. As well as small round nuclei *(2)* there are polymorphic giant nuclei *(3)*, indicating the presence of a malignant tumor. Mitoses are rarely seen. The numerous narrow capillaries *(4)* which thread through the tumorous tissue and often present a "crowsfoot" pattern are also characteristic of this fatty neoplasm. Under **higher magnification** the marked polymorphy of the cells is seen in **Fig. 754** more clearly. Their nuclei *(1)* are variably large, dark and polymorphic. Many cells have a light cytoplasm *(2)*, are rich in fat and reveal themselves as lipoblasts. One also sees deposits of osteoid *(3)*, which does not accord with a liposarcoma and indicates a malignant mesenchymoma.

In many osseous malignant mesenchymomas other tissue structures can be detected **histologically**. Thus, in **Fig. 749** we can recognize *cartilaginous tissue* with the polymorphic hyperchromatic *(1)* nuclei of chondrocytes. The tumor has here invaded a capillary *(2)*. **Figure 750** has the **histological** appearance of an *angiomatous tissue pattern*. One sees numerous vascular clefts *(1)* and, in between, tumor cells with polymorphic nuclei *(2)* and patchy deposits of osteoid *(3)*.

A bone tumor should only be classified as a malignant mesenchymoma if unusual morphological patterns of tumorous tissue (e. g. liposarcoma + osteosarcoma) are present together.

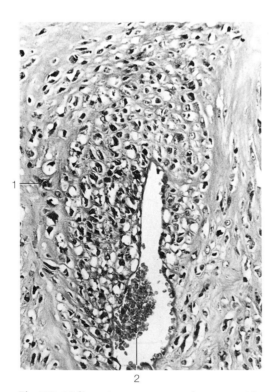

Fig. 749. Malignant osseous mesenchymoma with cartilaginous tissue; HE, ×64

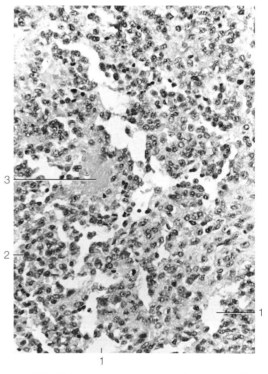

Fig. 750. Malignant osseous mesenchymoma with angiomatous structures; HE, ×64

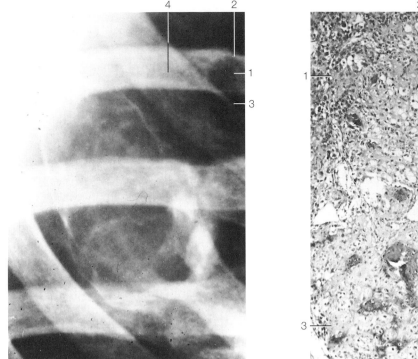

Fig. 751. Malignant osseous mesenchymoma (4th right rib)

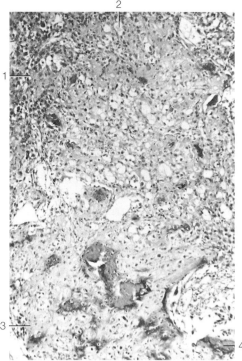

Fig. 752. Malignant osseous mesenchymoma with osteosarcomatous structures; HE, ×40

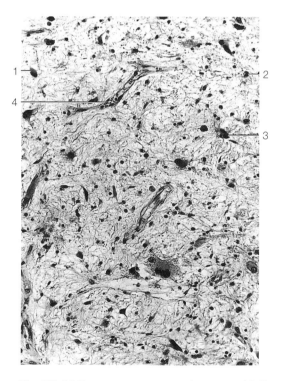

Fig. 753. Malignant osseous mesenchymoma with liposarcomatous structures; PAS, ×64

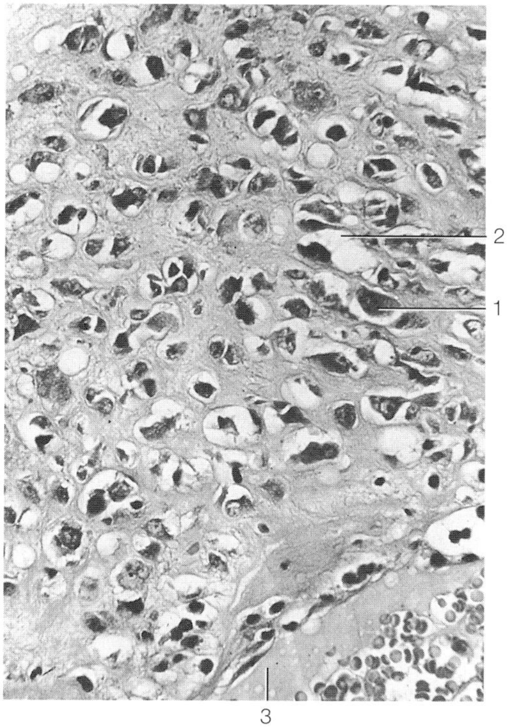

Fig. 754. Malignant osseous mesenchymoma; PAS, ×100

Osteosarcomas with various tissue structures (those of a fibrosarcoma, chondrosarcoma, histiocytoma) are not mesenchymomas and should be classified as osteosarcomas (p. 274).

Bone Metastases

With any radiologically malignant bone lesion, and particularly in older people, one must first think of a bone metastasis. These secondary bone tumors are much more frequently seen than the primary variety. About 30% of all carcinomas appear as bone metastases. Skeletal metastases are found in 70% of the patients who die of cancer, and for those tumors which tend particularly to produce secondaries in bone (carcinoma of the breast, bronchus and prostate) the figure is 85%. *One understands by the term "bone metastasis" the discontinuous spread from a primary tumor, which has developed elsewhere, of neoplastic cells into a bone, where, as a result of their proliferation, a **secondary bone tumor** has arisen.* The large majority of skeletal metastases are blood borne, the tumor cells having been carried into the marrow cavity by the nutrient arteries. One should also always expect to find lung metastases in such cases, unless there is a primary tumor in the lung (bronchial carcinoma). *Lymphogenous* metastases are theoretically possible, since both the periosteum and bone itself are connected to the lymphatics. Inside a bone, metastases my follow the *intracanalicular path,* allowing the tumor to spread discontinuously within the marrow cavity. Finally, metastases may be of the *vertebral type,* whereby tumor cells from carcinomas particularly of the prostate, lungs, breast, kidney or thyroid follow a retrograde path through the presacral and prevertebral venous plexuses to reach the vertebral column. In this case metastases do not appear beforehand in the lungs.

Figure 755 indicates the most common tumors which have a tendency to produce skeletal metastases. They make up more than 80% of all bone metastases. Naturally any malignant neoplasm can, in principle, produce metastases in bone. The main site is the vertebral column, where 62% of all metastases are found. They are more frequently seen in the lumbar than in the thoracic or cervical vertebrae. They are also frequently seen in the femur (10%), ribs (10%), skull (9%) and pelvis (5%).

A solitary bone metastasis, which is clinically observed in 25% of cases, can easily be mistaken for a primary tumor, and this must be resolved by bone biopsy. Both radiologically and histologically we see *osteolytic bone metastases,* which lead to local bone destruction, and *osteoblastic bone metastases,* where reactive osteosclerosis brings about an increase in density of the structures. Many metastases are a mixture of osteolytic and osteoblastic activity.

Figure 756 is the **radiograph** of an osteolytic bone metastasis. The bone tissue in the distal third of the left humeral shaft is completely destroyed over a wide region *(1)*. This is an osteolytic metastasis in which a patchy area of translucency is present. The osteolytic focus *(2)* is not sharply demarcated and shows no signs of marginal sclerosis. The cortex has been penetrated and on one side *(3)* even demolished. The tumorous tissue has broken out of the bone and has extended into the neighboring soft parts. In the proximal part of the humerus one can see a fracture *(4)*, which radiologically must be regarded as a pathological fracture. In this region also one finds patchy osteolytic foci in the marrow cavity. These are probably metastatic. From the radiograph alone it is, of course, impossible to identify the primary tumor.

As can be seen in the **histological picture** in **Fig. 757**, this is a metastasis from a carcinoma. One can recognize the lamellar layering of the cancellous trabeculae *(1)*, which are osteosclerotically widened and between which there is normal hematopoietic bone marrow and fatty fibrous marrow *(2)* with isomorphic elongated fibrocyte nuclei, among which a few fibro-osseous trabeculae *(3)* have differentiated. The variously sized complexes of densely packed epithelial cells *(4)* are striking. These cells also vary in size and have dark polymorphic nuclei. Here and there the cells also contain abnormal mitoses *(5)*. This is a bone metastasis from a scirrhous carcinoma of the breast. The spaces are either artefacts *(6)* or are lymph vessels *(7)* which have been filled up with tumor cells.

UEHLINGER describes particular ***patterns of distribution of skeletal metastases***: (a) In the *stem skeleton type* the metastases are symmetrically disposed in the vertebral column, pelvis, ribs, skull, and proximal parts of the humerus and femur. (b) In the *limb type* they are sporadic and mostly found asymmetrically placed and distal to the elbow or knee joint. (c) In the *periosteal type* the periosteal region of the long and short tubular bones is attacked.

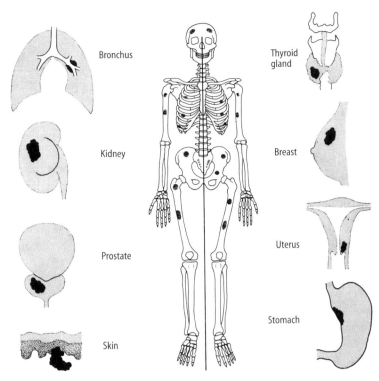

Fig. 755. Diagram showing the organs, tumors of which most frequently give rise to bone metastases

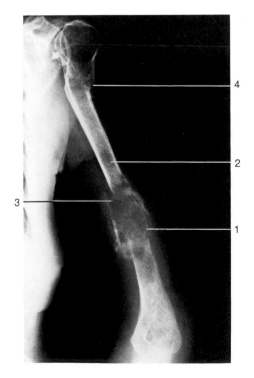

Fig. 756. Osteolytic bone metastases (humeral shaft)

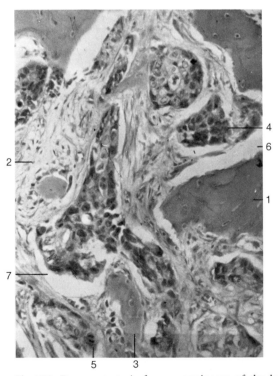

Fig. 757. Bone metastasis from a carcinoma of the breast; HE, ×82

Figure 758 shows the **histological picture** of a bone metastasis from an adenocarcinoma of the colon. Between the autochthonous cancellous trabeculae with their lamellar layers *(1)*, the marrow cavity is filled up with tumorous tissue consisting of densely packed abnormal glandular ducts *(2)*. The glands are covered with polymorphic cells. Here and there abnormal mitoses are also present. The ducts vary in size and contain abundant collections of mucus *(3)*. This kind of intraosseous tumorous tissue is readily identified as a bone metastasis from a carcinoma of the gastrointestinal tract or gallbladder.

In **Fig. 759** one can see the **radiograph** of an osteolytic bone metastasis in the proximal part of the left femur. There is a large osteolytic zone *(1)* which has occupied the greater trochanter and spread into the femoral neck. It is poorly demarcated and has no marginal sclerosis. The cortex has been eroded from within *(2)* but has not been penetrated. There is no periosteal reaction. The osteolytic area has no internal structure. Such a radiograph indicates malignant bone destruction and, in the case of an elderly patient, suggests a bone metastasis.

As can be discerned in the **histological picture** of **Fig. 760**, the cancellous bony tissue has been extensively destroyed by a malignant tumor. There are still a few peripheral autochthonous bone trabeculae *(1)* with lamellar layering and containing small osteocytes. Some osteoblasts are seen attached to the bone trabeculae *(2)*. The whole of the marrow cavity is filled up with a highly cellular tumorous tissue *(3)* containing densely packed complexes of epithelial cells with dark polymorphic nuclei and light cytoplasm. Most of the cell boundaries can be clearly seen. The tumorous tissue is threaded through by a few fine-walled capillaries *(4)*. Since there are no differentiated structures present the primary tumor cannot be established with any certainty. In this case it was a carcinoma of the breast, but other such carcinomas (bronchus, larynx, skin) can produce a similar metastatic picture.

Only a few malignant tumors produce characteristic radiological or histological bone changes from which the nature of the primary growth can be recognized. **Figure 761** shows the **radiograph** of a bone metastasis from a hypernephroid carcinoma of the kidney (renal cell carcinoma) in the proximal part of the right tibia. One can discern

several punched-out bony defects *(1)* which have no surrounding marginal sclerosis. These are found in both the marrow cavity and the cortex *(2)*. This kind of osteolytic focus is often found in such tumors. Usually there is no periosteal reaction. One intramedullary osteolytic focus *(3)* has eroded the cortex from within.

The **histological picture** of a biopsy of a bone metastasis from a hypernephroid carcinoma of the kidney (renal cell carcinoma) is often so characteristic that the primary tumor may be identified from it. In **Fig. 762** one can see on one side *(1)* a remaining trabecula from the spongiosa, which nevertheless has an undulating border. The whole of the marrow cavity has been taken up by epithelial tumorous tissue *(2)* consisting of complexes of epithelial cells with a light cytoplasm. These have small hyperchromatic and polymorphic nuclei in which almost no mitoses occur. The tumor cells are often surrounded by a sharply defined cell membrane. The tumorous tissue is interspersed with narrow connective tissue septa *(3)* in which run narrow capillaries. This reflects the endocrine formation of the primary tumor even in the metastasis.

The *distribution of skeletal metastases* can only be reliably derived from autopsy findings. However, the number of bone metastases detected radiologically is significantly in excess of those diagnosed during clinical examination.

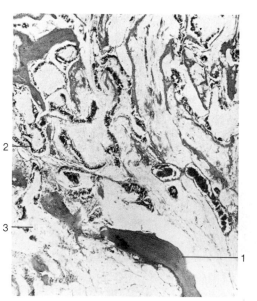

Fig. 758. Bone metastasis from an adenocarcinoma of the colon; PAS, ×51

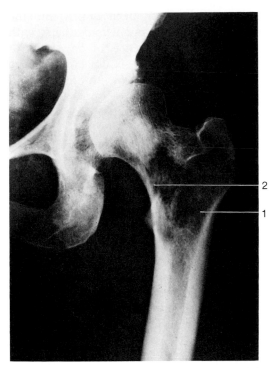

Fig. 759. Osteolytic bone metastasis (left proximal femur)

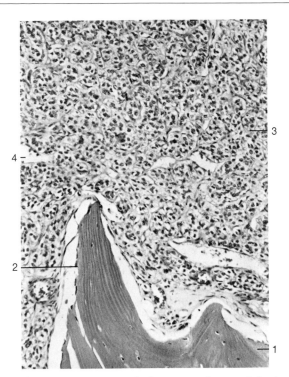

Fig. 760. Bone metastasis from a carcinoma of the breast; HE, ×40

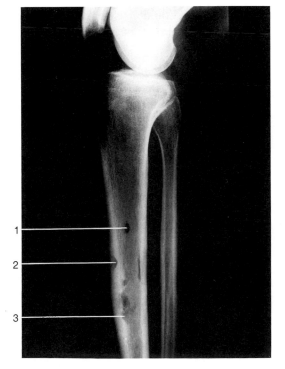

Fig. 761. Bone metastasis from a renal cell carcinoma (tibia)

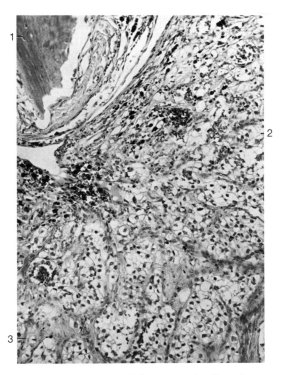

Fig. 762. Bone metastasis from a renal cell carcinoma; HE, ×25

Nevertheless, only about 50% of bone metastases are picked up radiologically. Of all bone metastases, 80% are found in the vertebral column, 40% in the femur, 25% in the ribs and 20% in the skull and pelvis. Peripheral metastases are therefore uncommon. Of all bone metastases, 90% are distributed in the stem skeleton (**Fig. 764**: the so-called *Stem skeleton type*). The number of bones affected is usually large, the distribution is symmetrical. Carcinomatous tumorous tissue is very easily laid down in well vascularized red bone marrow, and this determines the localization of the secondary deposits (vertebrae, ribs, sternum, shoulder and pelvic girdles, proximal metaphyses of humerus and femur). In only 2%–5% of all patients with carcinoma do the metastases appear in the distal parts of the limbs (**Fig. 765**: the so-called *limb type*). Here the bones on the far side of the elbow and knee joints are affected (distal tibial metaphysis, talus, calcaneus, ulna, short tubular bones of the hands and feet). Very often these are solitary metastases, particularly in the case of carcinomas of the kidney (renal cell carcinoma) or bronchus. Clinically, peripheral carcinomatous metastases present earlier than those of the stem skeleton, and often lead to spontaneous fractures. Finally, there are the *periosteal metastases,* which can be very extensive and associated with reactive periosteal new bone deposition (*coralliform type*).

Figure 763 illustrates the **histology** of a bone metastasis from a *mucoepidermoid carcinoma,* such as can arise in a salivary gland (submandibular gland). The marrow cavity is infiltrated by large groups of epithelial tumor cells *(1)*, all of which have dark polymorphic nuclei. In addition to the mucus-producing cells *(2)*, one can observe small collections of pavement epithelium *(3)*. Inside these groups of cells there are hollow cystic spaces *(4)* filled with mucus. Within the loose connective tissue stroma *(5)*, reactive fibro-osseous trabeculae *(6)* have differentiated out.

Figure 766 shows the **radiograph** of an osteolytic bone metastasis from a carcinoma of the breast in the proximal part of the left femur, which has resulted in a pathological fracture *(1)*. The ends of the fractured bone are extensively displaced. This is a fairly smooth transverse fracture running through the middle of a large, poorly demarcated osteolytic zone

(2). The cortex has also been drawn into the destructive process *(3)*, and it is feathery, with porous patches. The absence of any kind of bony or periosteal reaction is typical of such a pathological fracture (p. 126). No increase in density is observed in the region of the fracture. Such a radiological appearance urgently suggests a metastatic bone tumor.

The **macroscopic appearance** of the osseous bone metastases is extremely variable. It is determined both by the type of tumor (e.g. yellowish-red for a secondary from a renal cell carcinoma, very white from a carcinoma of the breast) and by the reaction of the bone locally (osteoblastic reactions are grayish-white, osteolytic reactions grayish-red). **Figure 767** shows a large osteolytic bone metastasis *(1)* in the proximal part of the tibia from a carcinoma of the bronchus. The tumorous tissue looks very pulpy, and its center has become necrotic *(2)*. On one side *(3)* the cortex has been destroyed and replaced by tumorous tissue. Reactive cancellous sclerosis *(4)* has developed in the neighborhood of the metastasis. If nothing has been suspected of the presence somewhere of a primary tumor, a radiograph of this kind of destructive bone lesion could itself easily be mistaken for a primary bone neoplasm. In such

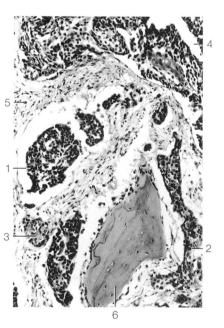

Fig. 763. Bone metastasis from a mucoepidermoid carcinoma; PAS, ×64

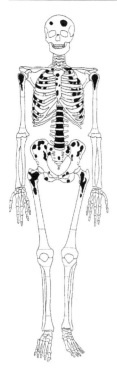

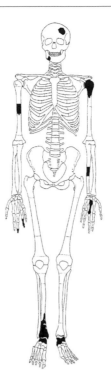

Fig. 764. Distribution pattern of bone metastases of the stem skeleton type. (After Uehlinger, from SCHINZ et al. 1981)

Fig. 765. Distribution pattern of bone metastases of the peripheral skeleton ("appendicular skeleton") type. (After Uehlinger, from SCHINZ et al. 1981)

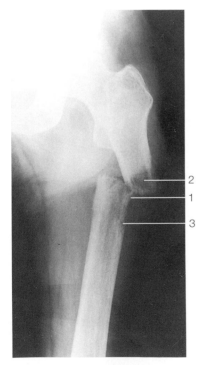

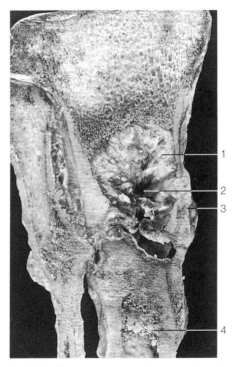

Fig. 766. Bone metastasis from a carcinoma of the breast with a pathological fracture (proximal femur)

Fig. 767. Bone metastasis from a bronchial carcinoma (proximal tibia)

cases a bone biopsy (perhaps a needle biopsy) can provide the diagnosis.

Both autoptically and on radiological examination bone metastases are most often confirmed in the vertebral column, where there is a wide spectrum of bone destruction. The fact that they are limited to the affected vertebra is characteristic of secondaries in the spine. Unlike spondylitis (p. 140) they do not usually invade the adjacent vertebrae. The intervertebral space is most often preserved, as can be confirmed radiologically. If the vertebra is sawn through the metastasis is usually easy to recognize **macroscopically. Figure 768** shows a large round focus *(1)* in the body of the 4th lumbar vertebra. It is fairly well demarcated and has a well-marked grayish-white surface, suggestive of carcinomatous tissue. The surrounding spongiosa *(2)* is filled with blood but otherwise unaltered. The adjacent intervertebral discs *(3)* are also unaltered and the outline of the vertebra is, like that of the other bodies, completely intact. In the case of purely osteoblastic spinal metastases there may be a high grade sclerotic reaction on the part of the spongiosa, with the intraosseous metastatic tumorous tissue no longer macroscopically recognizable. Radiologically one finds a so-called ivory vertebra.

In the **radiograph**, bone metastases sometimes produce a strong periosteal reaction as well as a severe local osteosclerotic lesion. In **Fig. 769** the spongiosa of the distal right femoral metaphysis is strongly sclerosed *(1)* and is continued across into the cortex. In only a few places is destructive osteolysis to be seen *(2)*. However, the massive tumorous expansion of the periosteum, both on the ventral *(3)* and (where it is more tumorous) dorsal *(4)* aspects of the femur is striking. These structural changes indicate a malignant bone lesion.

Histological examination of the biopsy material revealed the morphological appearance of a bronchial carcinoma. In **Fig. 770** there is in one place a sclerotically widened bone trabecula *(1)*. The fatty marrow has been replaced by loose connective tissue *(2)* in which shallow nodular areas of infiltrating tumorous tissue *(3)* are to be seen. This is a tumorous epithelium which is appropriate for a non-keratinizing squamous cell carcinoma. Even in this overall view the dark polymorphic nuclei of the malignant tumor cells are striking. Such osteometa-static tumorous tissue suggests a secondary from a bronchial carcinoma.

The **radiograph** of **Fig. 771** shows a pathological fracture *(1)* in the proximal part of the right femur. The fracture is gaping and the bones are badly out of line. The proximal part of the fractured bone *(2)* shows a a very cloudy increase in density of the bone structure, and this includes head, neck and intertrochanteric region. The pubic and ischial bones have also been drawn into this osteosclerotic process *(3)*. In places the pathological osteosclerosis has been rendered porous by patches of osteolysis *(4)*. A large intraosseous zone of osteolysis in the proximal part of the femoral shaft is also striking *(5)*.

This type of *osteoblastic bone metastasis* is often found in cases of prostatic carcinoma. **Histologically** we can see in **Fig. 772** newly formed osteosclerotic bone trabeculae *(1)* on which rows of active osteoblasts *(2)* have been deposited. The marrow cavity is filled with loose connective tissue *(3)*. Within there are large complexes of epithelial tumor cells *(4)*, which have a light cytoplasm and dark polymorphic nuclei. Sometimes suggestive glandular elements *(5)* can be recognized. The entire histological picture is typical of an osteoblastic secondary from a carcinoma of the prostate.

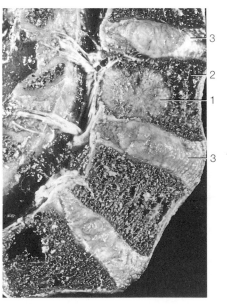

Fig. 768. Bone metastasis (4th lumbar vertebral body)

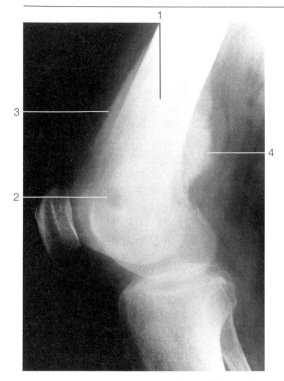

Fig. 769. Bone metastasis from a bronchial carcinoma (distal femur)

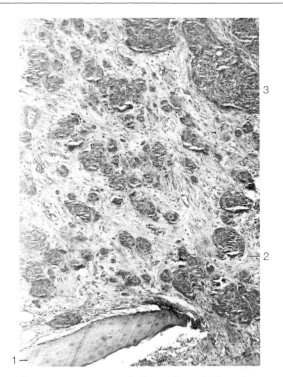

Fig. 770. Bone metastasis from a bronchial carcinoma; HE, ×40

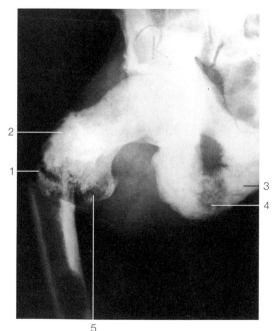

Fig. 771. Osteoblastic bone metastasis from a prostatic carcinoma with a pathological fracture (right proximal femur)

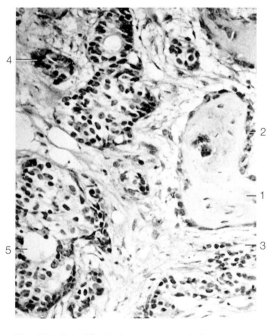

Fig. 772. Osteoblastic bone metastasis from a prostatic carcinoma; HE, ×64

Attention is often first drawn to a malignant neoplasm by a bone metastasis while the primary tumor is still unrecognized. In some cases the **histological structure** of the secondary allows conclusions to be drawn about the primary tumor. In **Fig. 773** one can see a sclerotically widened bone trabecula *(1)*, and in the marrow cavity there is an epithelial tumorous tissue of cells with abundant cytoplasm *(2)* which contain small round, slightly polymorphic nuclei. The cytoplasm is strikingly eosinophilic. These cells are arranged around hollow spaces *(3)*, making up a follicular morphological pattern which is typical of the thyroid gland. Such a histological picture of a bone metastasis suggests with fair certainty that the primary tumor is an **oncocytic thyroid carcinoma**. Highly differentiated follicular carcinomas of the thyroid often produce bone metastases, the tumorous tissue of which consists of mature follicular thyroid tissue. In other cases (e.g. various adenocarcinomas) the pathologist can, on the basis of the histological picture of the metastasis alone, indicate to the clinician which of a few possible organs might be the site of the primary tumor (e.g. the gastrointestinal tract, gallbladder, uterus etc.). Very often, when there is undifferentiated tissue in the bone metastasis, no conclusions at all can be reached concerning the nature of the primary.

The morphological appearance of skeletal metastases can take on an extraordinarily large number of different forms both radiologically and **macroscopically** and so lead to misinterpretation. Discrete bone changes can suggest benign lesions (osteomyelitis, for instance). The larger lesions do indeed indicate a malignant tumor, but it is difficult to classify it radiologically. In **Fig. 774** one can see a bone metastasis from a carcinoma of the breast in the roof of the skull. A massive spongy tumor *(1)* is clinging to the skull cap. The tumorous tissue is soaked in blood and dark red. Within, the necroses have produced numerous hollow spaces *(2)*. The skull bone has been infiltrated by the tumor and extensively destroyed *(3)*. The tu-

morous tissue has spread into the inside of the skull *(4)* and has probably infiltrated the brain. This is an osteolytic bone metastasis, which is by far the most common sort to appear, since the tumorous tissue brings about osteoclasia. Osteoblastic bone metastases, because of their inducing endosteal osteoplasia and periosteal new bone formation, are much less common. However, in the majority of bone metastases we are histologically able to recognize mixed forms of simultaneous osteolysis and osteoplasia.

Bone metastases present an enormously variable picture, with regard to the clinical symptoms, the radiological changes seen in the skeleton and the histological picture. In the case of someone suffering from cancer, it is usually impossible to detect all the bone metastases. On average, about half of the secondaries are diagnosed on clinical examination. Solitary or sporadic metastases are much more often recognized during the life of the patient. At autopsy, on the other hand, multiple bone metastases predominate, most of them in the stem skeleton. Not infrequently a carcinoma (e.g. of the stomach) is accompanied by secondaries in a very large number of bones, and we then speak of "skeletal carcinomatosis". Peripheral skeletal metastases present themselves clinically much earlier than those in the stem skeleton. In the long bones they often cause a pathological fracture to appear, but in the short or flat bones they cause periosteal irritation and early pain.

Carcinoma of the kidney particularly – less often of the bronchus – can lead to the appearance of metastases in unexpected sites. Again and again we observe local metastases in the cortex of a bone appearing as roundish-oval areas of osteolysis. They may appear one after another in the most peripheral parts of the skeleton – in the terminal phalanges of all the fingers, for instance. Cases are also always appearing in which a carcinoma of the kidney had been removed many years earlier and, after a long period of time with no symptoms, multiple secondaries suddenly appear.

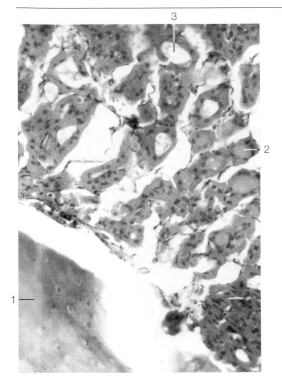

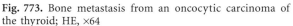

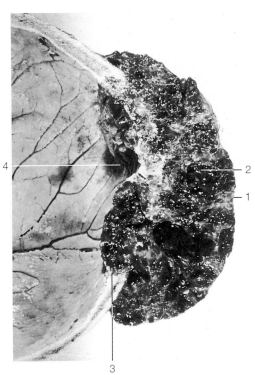

Fig. 773. Bone metastasis from an oncocytic carcinoma of the thyroid; HE, ×64

Fig. 774. Osteolytic bone metastasis from a carcinoma of the breast (skull cap)

If the metastatic tumorous tissue is carried into the bone by the bloodstream and then spreads within the marrow cavity without destroying bone tissue or stimulating new bone formation, no radiological changes are seen, and the scintigram also remains silent. The tumorous tissue itself is not visible on the radiograph, it is only after it has destroyed the bone tissue following stimulation of the osteoclasts, and is quantitatively in excess of that tissue, that the structural changes (osteolyses) become radiologically visible. However, with the modern technique of MR tomography (MRT) even the early changes can today be recognized. During these intraosseous morphological alterations the bone tissue is not directly destroyed by the tumor cells; it is apparently

much more a case of their producing an osteoclast-stimulating factor (e.g. endothelin) which brings about osteoclastic bone resorption.

In the vast majority of cases, bone metastases are derived from carcinomas which have developed in other extraosseous organs. Histologically we would expect to see associated clusters of epithelial cells in the kind of intraosseous lesion that can be identified by means of immunohistochemistry (keratin, see Table 5, p. 507). Nevertheless, mesenchymal tumors – that is to say sarcomas – can also produce bone metastases. These may be soft tissue sarcomas. If such a sarcoma first presents as a secondary in bone, it may be impossible by means of a biopsy to say whether we are dealing with a metastasis or a primary sarcoma of bone. It is known that bone sarcomas often have the identical histomorphological structure as the soft tissue variety. Even a primary malignant bone tumor can give rise to metastases in the skeleton. The medullary plasmocytoma (p. 348), for instance, usually makes a multifocal appearance in several different bones. It has been suggested that perhaps the tumor develops in one particular bone and that all the other intraosseous foci are its metastases. Another example is presented by the so-called "**skip lesions**" of the osteosarcoma (p. 276), where there is a metastasis from this mesenchymal tumor in the same bone (for example, there is an osteosarcoma in

the distal femoral metaphysis, with an intramedullary metastasis derived from it at a considerable distance from and without any relationship to the primary tumor, in the proximal part of the same femur). Multicentric osteosarcomas can also be interpreted as a particular form of metastatic spread.

To sum up, the formation of bone metastases is a particular series of events associated with the growth of malignant tumors, both carcinomas and sarcomas, which has many variants and which can give rise to many diagnostic and therapeutic problems.

Tumor-like Bone Lesions

Introductory Remarks

A tumor may be defined as a proliferation of tissue in which the growth is excessive, is not coordinated with the normal tissue, and continues even when the original stimulus is no longer active (WILLIS). Here we have, from the pathological and anatomical points of view, the principal characteristics of a true autonomously growing tumor. According to this definition a true bone tumor cannot regress by itself; at the most it can remain quiescent. There is, however, no sharp dividing line between autonomously growing neoplasms and an excessive growth of tissue, the development of which is independent of any stimulus and which can regress. In the skeleton especially we know of lesions which radiologically and biologically appear to be tumors, but which can nevertheless spontaneously regress. These local skeletal changes are collected together under the blanket term "tumor-like bone lesions".

The main characteristic of a tumor-like bone lesion is that it clinically and radiologically gives the impression of a bone neoplasm. They can appear as areas of osteosclerosis [e.g. "bone islands", p. 274; melorheostosis, p. 108; osteitis deformans (Paget), p. 102] or as osteolytic foci [e.g. eosinophilic bone granulomas, p. 196; fibrous bone dysplasia (Jaffe-Lichtenstein), pp. 56, 318; so-called "brown tumors", p. 84; reparative giant cell granulomas, p. 204; a giant cell reaction in a short tubular bone, p. 204]. Even osteomyelitis can look like a tumor radiologically. Bone lesions of this kind can bring about considerable destruction of bone, giving the impression of malignant tumorous growth (e.g. the eosinophilic granuloma). The bone can show considerable local elevation and the spongiosa be extensively obliterated, there may be erosion of the cortex, or reparative activity may bring about excessive bone remodeling. Aneurysmal cysts (p. 412) may even penetrate the cortex over a considerable area and show up as a tumor-like shadow covering the soft parts. The radiologist is not able to exclude the possibility of malignancy in such cases.

Histologically the tumor-like bone lesions can also cause the pathologist considerable difficulty. It is often a matter of a "bone cyst" which must be more precisely diagnosed. In the case of a juvenile bone cyst (p. 408) the tissue obtained by curettage is very often not pathognomonic, so that the diagnosis must be made in association with the radiograph. An aneurysmal bone cyst shows a suggestive "blow-out" appearance, with the osteolytic "neoplasm" leaving the bone and spreading into the soft parts. Histologically there is a highly cellular granulation tissue with very many multinucleated osteoclastic giant cells, so that it can be extraordinarily difficult from the curetted material to distinguish it from a true giant cell neoplasm of bone (osteoclastoma, p. 337). An aneurysmal bone cyst can also arise histomorphologically together with a true bone tumor (e.g. in a chondroblastoma, p. 226) or present the morphological appearance of a telangiectatic osteosarcoma (p. 280).

Among the tumor-like bone lesions there are many intraosseous conditions that present with giant cell granulation tissue and are difficult to distinguish from true giant cell neoplasms. A giant cell lesion in the bones of the jaw should first call to mind a reparative giant cell granuloma (p. 204); giant cell "tumors" (the so-called "brown tumors", p. 84) can also develop in cases of primary hyperparathyroidism. A "bone cyst" may be due to fibrous bone dysplasia (pp. 56, 318), an intraosseous ganglion (p. 418) or an intraosseous epidermal cyst (p. 420). Finally, there are parosseal lesions (myositis ossificans, p. 478; tumorous calcinosis, p. 484) which may give the impression of benign or malignant tumors although they are only local reactive processes.

It is necessary with all these tumor-like conditions to recognize them as reaction foci and to distinguish them from true neoplasms.

Juvenile Bone Cyst (ICD-O-DA-M-3340–4)

Osteolytic foci which are sharply demarcated and look like smooth-walled "cysts" are observed in bones with relative frequency, and it is therefore well worth classifying the various forms of bone cyst as precisely as possible. *The juvenile or solitary bone cyst is an expanding osteolytic non-tumorous condition of unknown etiology which is unicameral and surrounded by a wall of connective tissue. It is usually filled with serous fluid.* It is almost exclusively found in children and young people, 80% appearing between the ages of 3 and 14 years. Boys are more often affected than girls. Most juvenile bone cysts lie in the proximal metaphysis of the humerus or femur, where they are seen to expand. Of them 70% present with a pathological fracture. Inactive or latent cysts move ever further away from the epiphysis during skeletal growth and finally take up a position which is exclusively metaphyseal or diaphyseal. Following a fracture through the cyst, spontaneous healing can occur (15% of cases). Active cysts come to lie right up against the epiphyseal plate and lead to elevation of the bone.

In **Fig. 775** one can see the classical **radiograph** of a juvenile bone cyst in the proximal part of the right humerus. The metaphysis *(1)* is bulging outwards. Here, there is a large osteolytic cyst within the bone, which is interspersed with narrow septa *(2)*, giving it a multiloculated appearance. These are not, however, separate internal spaces. The cyst is placed centrally in the bone. The cortex has been narrowed from within *(3)*, but has not been penetrated. There is no periosteal reaction, although this may develop locally if a pathological fracture occurs. The cyst reaches as far as immediately below the epiphyseal cartilage *(4)* and is sharply separated from the diaphysis by a narrow band of marginal sclerosis *(5)*.

This type of cyst is usually curetted and the defect filled up with spongiosa. In rare cases an en bloc resection is carried out. **Figure 776** shows the **macroscopic picture** of such a resected specimen. One can see the cystically raised up part of a long bone (humerus) which has been sawn through. There is a central cyst *(1)* in the marrow cavity which has a smooth wall, and which is filled up with a gelatinous mass that is in part soaked with blood. The cortex *(2)* is intact. The cyst is incompletely subdivided into several regions by structures consisting of bone trabeculae *(3)*.

Not only is a radiograph absolutely essential for the diagnosis, but a piece of the intact wall must also be subjected to histological analysis. The **histological picture** of **Fig. 777** shows the wall of a juvenile bone cyst. It has a smooth border on all sides and no epithelial covering *(1)*. The membrane *(2)* consists of parallel layers of collagen fibers with a sparse infiltration of round cells and occasional giant cells. Sometimes there are foci of non-specific granulation tissue and a few capillaries in the cyst wall, on the outside of which many new fibro-osseous trabeculae *(3)* have been formed. Adjacent to this one can recognize the autochthonous bone tissue *(4)* which shows lamellar layering and is often osteosclerotically thickened.

Figure 778 shows the **histological picture** of a juvenile bone cyst with a very thick connective tissue wall. Towards the cavity the cyst has a smooth border *(1)*; there is no epithelial covering or lining. The wall consists of markedly fibrous connective tissue, threaded through with a few dilated blood-filled vessels *(2)*. The numerous disorganized, partly patchy, partly trabecular structures *(3)* in the cyst wall are striking, and have the appearance of cement particles. This kind of structure is often seen in juvenile bone cysts. The prognosis of such a lesion is good. In any case, juvenile bone cysts should be conservatively treated before the 10th year, since, if they are not, recurrences appear in 40% of the cases. The recurrence rate of this lesion is higher if it is at the proximal end of the humerus than when it lies in the same region of the femur or tibia. With atypical localization (e. g. in the iliac bone) and with small cysts recurrences are less common. A juvenile bone cyst can, however, occupy up to one third of a long bone, thus giving rise to severe surgical problems. In general the recurrence rate lies between 18% and 41%. Spontaneous malignant change is not to be expected.

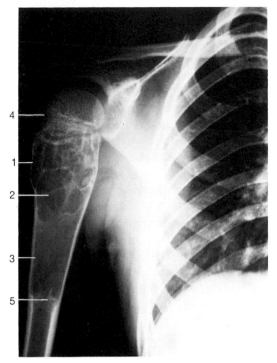

Fig. 775. Juvenile bone cyst (right proximal humerus)

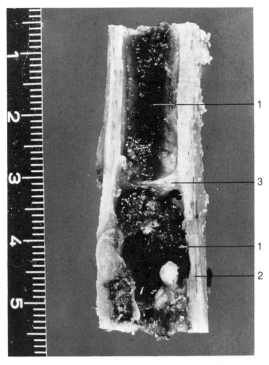

Fig. 776. Juvenile bone cyst (humerus, cut surface)

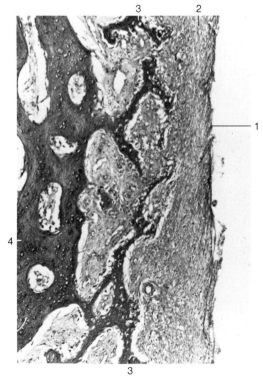

Fig. 777. Juvenile bone cyst; HE, ×25

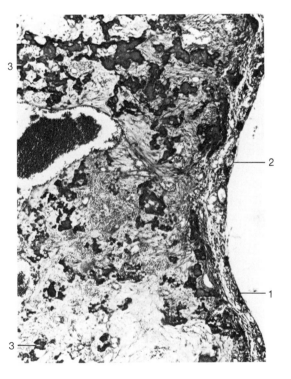

Fig. 778. Juvenile bone cyst; HE, ×25

"Cementoma" of the Long Bones
(ICD-O-DA-M-9272/0)

Generally speaking, cement, a substance having its own particular type of formation, only appears near the teeth, where it is produced by the cementoblasts. The benign cementoma can develop in the bones of the jaws. It is, however, by no means uncommon to find tumor-like lesions in the long bones (mostly in the proximal part of the femur) which consist histologically almost entirely of cement. Furthermore, we have often found deposits of cement-like material in the wall of a juvenile cyst. *A "cementoma" of the long bones is a tumor-like bone lesion, consisting of cell-free cement-like material which can be associated with a juvenile bone cyst.* Possibly this entirely benign lesion may arise in an old regressive juvenile bone cyst. Since, however, it produces a peculiarly characteristic picture on the radiograph, it is regarded as a special separate entity among the tumor-like lesions.

In **Fig. 780** the **radiograph** of such a "cementoma" can be observed. An extraordinarily radiodense round focus *(1)* is lying eccentrically placed in the trochanteric region of the femur. It is clearly demarcated, and the internal structure shows an uneven, coarsely patchy porosity *(2)*, so that it looks as if it has been broken into pieces. No cyst is to be seen. On one side the sclerosis reaches into the cortex *(3)*.

Histologically the lesion consists of broad deposits of a cement-like material *(1)*, as can be seen in **Fig. 779**. This material has a fibrillar structure, is free from cells and is interspersed by elongated, indiscriminately directed reversal lines *(2)*. Within this unevenly dense calcified material, which looks exactly like dental cement, one can observe loose connective tissue *(3)*. The "cement structures" include no deposits of active cells (cementoblasts).

In **Fig. 781** one can also see **histologically** widely distributed deposits of an almost cell-free fibrillar material *(1)* resembling cement. Close to this there are spherical corpuscles *(2)* which are unevenly calcified and which also resemble cement. Unlike osteoid seams they are bordered by fine fibrils and show no deposits of cells (such as osteoblasts, for instance). The cement-like substance lies in a fibrous stroma with isomorphic fibrocytes and a few fine-walled capillaries.

In "cementomas", which histologically show none of the structures of a juvenile bone cyst, a single roundish sclerotic focus can be seen on the **radiograph**. One can see such a focus *(1)* in **Fig. 782** in the proximal part of the femur in the intertrochanteric region. The outline is somewhat fibrous, but the focus is nevertheless fairly sharply demarcated. Inside *(2)* one can see a slight porosity, but no cystic structure. In the scintigram the lesion usually reveals no increase in activity.

Under **higher magnification** in **Fig. 783** the cement-like material *(1)* is **histologically** easily recognized. The arrangement is similar to that of fibro-osseous trabeculae, but there are no osteocytes and the material is fibrillar in formation. It does not contain any kind of cells (osteoblasts, cementoblasts) but lies within a loose connective tissue *(2)* that is threaded through by several capillaries *(3)*. A few lymphocytes have also been deposited here.

The origin and nature of the cement-like material in this kind of bone lesion are unknown. Ultramicroscopic investigations have suggested that it is a peculiar cell-free osteoid with atypical calcification that has been laid down by osteoblasts. Because of the curious radiological and histological structures it seems to be justified to classify these lesions, *"cementomas of the long bones"*, as separate entities among the tumor-like bone lesions.

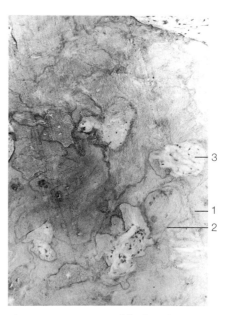

Fig. 779. Cementoma of the long bones; HE, ×64

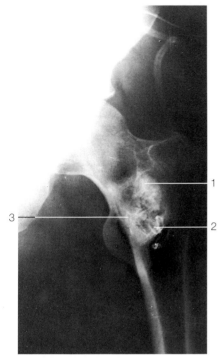

Fig. 780. Cementoma of the long bones (left proximal femur)

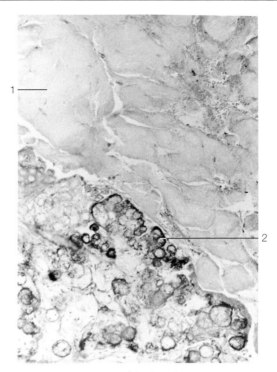

Fig. 781. Cementoma of the long bones; HE, ×64

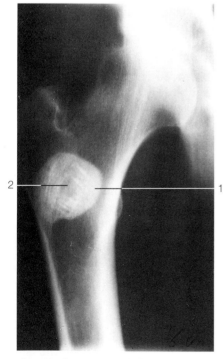

Fig. 782. Cementoma of the long bones (right proximal femur)

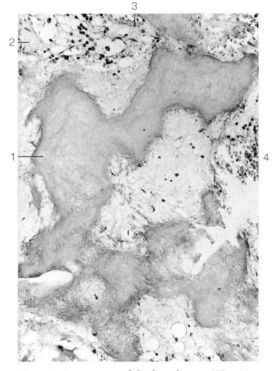

Fig. 783. Cementoma of the long bones; HE, ×82

Aneurysmal Bone Cyst (ICD-O-DA-M-3364–0)

Among the tumor-like bone lesions the aneurysmal bone cyst presents the greatest diagnostic and therapeutic problems. *This is a benign osteolytic bone lesion which consists of an intraosseous focus of destruction and an extraosseous aneurysm-like cystic portion, and which represents a particular form of local reaction on the part of the bone to previous damage.*

This means that everyone concerned in examining the lesion (radiologists, pathologists) is faced with the task of trying to discover the underlying condition, but in many cases this is unsuccessful. Behind an aneurysmal cyst may lie hidden a benign bone tumor (e.g. chondroblastoma, chondromyxoid fibroma, fibrous dysplasia) or a bone sarcoma (e.g. osteoclastoma, telangiectatic osteosarcoma). The combination of any one of these tumors or tumor-like lesions with the structures of an aneurysmal bone cyst makes the differential diagnosis extremely difficult. The lesion is quite often seen, almost always in the form of a solitary focus. Clinically it presents as a painful swelling which may remain for over a year until a rapid increase in the pain drives the patient to visit a physician. Often there has been some previous local trauma. In 4%–5% of the cases there is a pathological fracture present (e.g. a compression fracture of a vertebral body).

Localization (Fig. 784). Aneurysmal bone cysts are seen in almost all bones, including the bones of the jaws. The main sites, however, are the spinal column and the long bones. About 63% of these lesions are found in the long bones, pelvis and vertebral column. The metaphyses are most often affected, usually the distal femoral metaphysis. The epiphyseal plates have usually not been penetrated. On rare occasions the lesion can be observed in the diaphysis.

Age Distribution (Fig. 785). The aneurysmal bone cyst attacks children, young people and younger adults, about 60% of the patients being less than 20 years old. The peak period is in the 2nd decade of life, which distinguishes these lesions from osteoclastomas (p. 337). Girls and women are more often affected than men or boys.

Radiologically the aneurysmal bone cyst is characterized by an eccentric intraosseous area of osteolysis with a decidedly "blow-out" appearance, which can undergo very rapid expansion. In **Fig. 786** one can see in a lateral **radiograph** a peripheral angiogram of an aneurysmal bone cyst in the distal femoral metaphysis. Dorsally there is a hernia-like sac *(1)* attached to the bone by a broad base. One can see how on the outside of this "hernia" the lesion is restricted by the bulging periosteum. There is also a discrete area of osteolysis *(2)* within the femoral metaphysis that can be made to show up more clearly in a tomogram (CT, MRT). Destruction of the cortex is the most striking feature, and marginal sclerosis may or may not be present. The **angiogram** shows obvious hypervascularization in the neighborhood of the cyst, by which the extraosseous extension is more clearly seen. Most of the vessels within the lesion are not visible here.

In the **radiograph** of **Fig. 787** one can see an aneurysmal bone cyst in the body of the 2nd cervical vertebra. The bone of the vertebral body is strongly elevated and extensively destroyed *(1)*, and its outer contour is no longer demarcated. One can see part of the tumor expanding dorsally *(2)* where it has invaded the soft parts and expanded in the shape of a beehive over the neighboring 3rd cervical vertebra. Owing to the overlaying of the images one gets the impression that the body of this vertebra has been involved in the destruction process *(3)*. In such a case it is necessary to determine radiologically to what extent the lesion has penetrated into the spinal canal. Within this bone cyst there are numerous irregular trabeculae. Even the neighboring 1st cervical vertebra *(4)* is not clearly seen. The radiologically demonstrable extension of the process over several vertebrae is typical of the aneurysmal bone cyst, and is very seldom seen with true benign or malignant bone tumors. According to POPPE the radiograph of aneurysmal bone cysts in the vertebrae is uncharacteristic. In "blow-out" vertebrae the spongiosa of the attached transverse and articular processes is always destroyed.

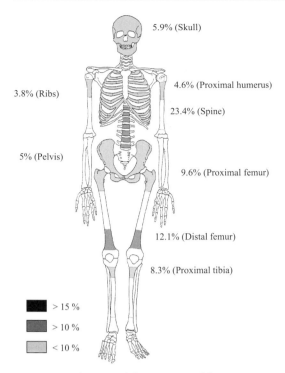

5.9% (Skull)

3.8% (Ribs)

4.6% (Proximal humerus)

23.4% (Spine)

5% (Pelvis)

9.6% (Proximal femur)

12.1% (Distal femur)

8.3% (Proximal tibia)

> 15 %

> 10 %

< 10 %

Fig. 784. Localization of the aneurysmal bone cysts (239 cases); others 27.3%

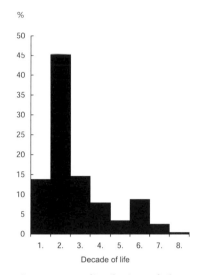

Fig. 785. Age distribution of the aneurysmal bone cysts (239 cases)

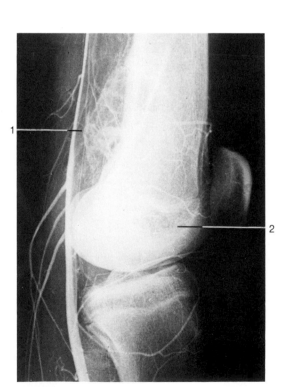

Fig. 786. Aneurysmal bone cyst (distal femoral metaphysis, angiogram)

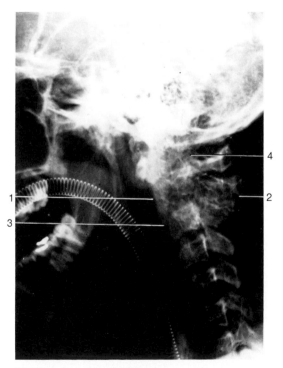

Fig. 787. Aneurysmal bone cyst (2nd cervical vertebral body)

The typical "blow-out" character of an aneurysmal bone cyst can be seen in the **radiograph** of **Fig. 788.** On the under side of the left pubis (*1*) a large cyst (*2*) is bulging downwards far into the soft tissues. It is bordered externally by a narrow shell of bone (*3*) due to new bone deposition from the elevated periosteum. Inside there are several partial trabecular thickenings. The under side of the of the pubis has been eaten away, bringing about rarefaction of the bone.

Again in **Fig. 789** one can see the **radiograph** of an extraosseous aneurysmal bone cyst. The cyst (*1*) is discernible on the right side of the body of the 1st lumbar vertebra. Again, it is also demarcated from without by a narrow shell of bone. The cyst has no internal structure. It has rarefied the bone tissue of the vertebra from the side and is sharply demarcated inside the bone by a narrow band of marginal sclerosis (*2*). A cyst of this kind often sinks downward in the shape of a beehive, and with an orthograde projection it can give the impression radiologically that two adjacent vertebrae have been destroyed by a tumor. The actual ex-

tent of the aneurysmal bone cyst can be clearly seen in a **computer tomogram.** In **Fig. 790** one can see that the cyst (*1*) has no internal structure. It is lying dorsolaterally in the vertebra and has destroyed the right transverse process and part of the neural arch. Externally, newly built bony structures (*2*) can be seen. A part of the vertebral body (*3*) has also been destroyed. This kind of extension from the lesion can easily cause the symptoms of a transverse section of the cord to develop.

The classical **radiological appearance** of an aneurysmal bone cyst is shown in **Fig. 791.** In the distal femoral metaphysis of a 9-year-old child an eccentrically placed cyst (*1*) is bulging sideways out of the bone. It has eaten away the bone tissue and shows no internal structure. In the inside of the bone it is demarcated by a band of marginal sclerosis (*2*). The outer border (*3*) can only be weakly discerned. The epiphyseal cartilage (*4*) has been preserved.

In the **overall histological section** of **Fig. 792** there are several cystic hollow spaces (*1*) within the bone, which are partly filled with blood clots (*2*). The cysts have smooth walls, and

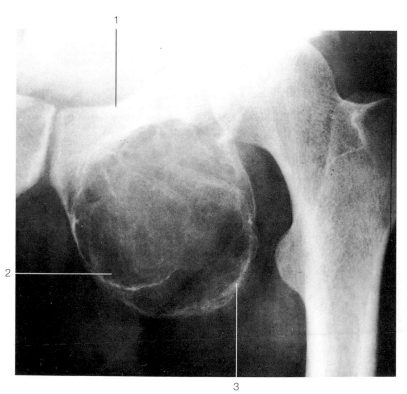

Fig. 788. Aneurysmal bone cyst (left pubic bone)

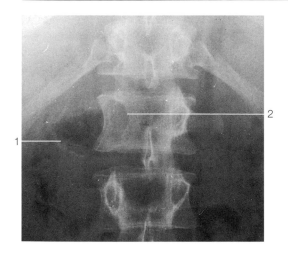

Fig. 789. Aneurysmal bone cyst (1st lumbar vertebral body)

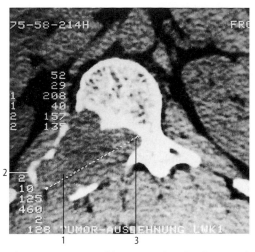

Fig. 790. Aneurysmal bone cyst (1st lumbar vertebral body, computer tomogram)

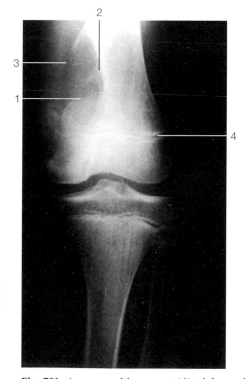

Fig. 791. Aneurysmal bone cyst (distal femoral metaphysis)

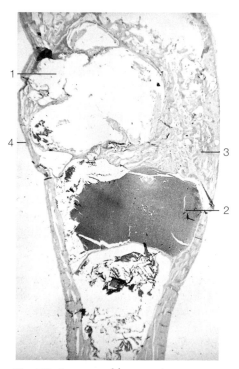

Fig. 792. Aneurysmal bone cyst (proximal tibia, hand lens: ×5)

nearby many fibro-osseous trabeculae *(3)* have differentiated out. The cyst has rarefied the cortex and is bulging outwards *(4)*.

In **Fig. 793** one can see the **macroscopic picture** of an aneurysmal bone cyst in a rib. The bone is extensively raised up over a length of about 11 cm. At one end the healthy bone of the adjacent part of the rib is still recognizable *(1)*. The extraosseous part of the lesion is significantly larger than the intraosseous. Within the flat surface there is a bone cyst with several hollow spaces of varying sizes *(2)* which are filled up with blood clots. The wall of the cyst *(3)* consists of tough connective tissue that has been fairly thickly laid down outside and which can in part be ossified. This is periosteal connective tissue that bulges out because of the expansion of the cyst, and which covers it from without. The septa which separate the spaces from one another also consist of connective tissue and often contain bone. In many aneurysmal bone cysts only a clear fluid, which may be tinged with blood, is present.

In **Fig. 794** the cystic spaces *(1)* occupy the whole **histological picture** of the aneurysmal bone cyst. These spaces are partly empty *(1)*, partly filled up with blood or blood clots *(2)*. They have smooth borders, but no epithelial lining can be recognized *(3)*. The walls of these spaces consist of loose connective and granulation tissue, within which numerous vascular clefts are present *(4)*. These distinguish the spaces themselves from dilated blood vessels such as are found in a cavernous hemangioma (p. 373). Irregular trabecular bony structures are differentiated out in the walls of the cysts *(5)*. This produces a shadow on the radiograph, showing up as a picture of trabecular internal structure. Very often such reactive new bone deposition also takes place in the surrounding periosteal mantle and provides a radiologically recognizable outer border to the aneurysmal bone cyst. Osteoid structures on which rows of osteoblasts have been deposited are also sometimes found in the cyst walls. It is difficult to distinguish such a tissue pattern from that of a telangiectatic osteosarcoma (p. 280). On occasion, differentiated cartilaginous foci can also be found in the intermediate walls, which vary in length and thickness and separate the hollow spaces from one another.

Under **higher magnification** one can discern in **Fig. 795** the hollow space in an aneurysmal bone cyst *(1)* which contains only a little blood. The cyst has a smooth border, and a lining of flattened epithelial cells *(2)* can be recognized. The wall consists of highly cellular granulation tissue in which numerous multinucleated osteoclastic giant cells are lying *(3)*. These giant cells are distributed unequally throughout the tissue and often lie together in groups. The fibrous background tissue is highly cellular and contains many fibrocytes and fibroblasts with isomorphic nuclei. However, individual mitoses can also be seen, and particularly after a previous curettage considerable mitotic activity may reveal itself. In this case the possibility of a malignant bone tumor must be included in the differential diagnosis.

In **Fig. 796** the characteristic structural formation of an aneurysmal bone cyst is clearly shown **histologically**. We can see the smoothly bordered hollow space *(1)* which has an incomplete lining of cells. The inner layer of the cyst wall *(2)* consists of loose connective tissue in which numerous isomorphic fibrocytes and fibroblasts, as well as collagen fibers, are present. Many capillaries *(3)* are also found here. In this region there may be true granulation tissue in which inflammatory infiltrates (lymphocytes, plasma cells, histiocytes and granulocytes) are also scattered about. In the outer zone *(4)* one can see granulation tissue which is still highly cellular, and in which the bandlike zone containing many multinucleated giant cells of the osteoclast type *(5)* is striking. These bring about dissolution of the autochthonous bony structures, giving the picture of an expansive osteolysis. In the curetted material, osteoclastic foci of this kind may predominate to such an extent that the differential diagnosis from an osteoclastoma (p. 337) is made much more difficult.

Although we may regard the aneurysmal bone cyst as a particular reactive process of the bone, similar to that of the reparative giant cell granuloma or giant cell reaction (p. 204), the lesions manifest a tumor-like destructive growth and, in 21% of cases, they may recur. The proliferating tissue should therefore be removed by en bloc excision or radical curettage. Radiotherapy is only indicated if the lesion is inoperable.

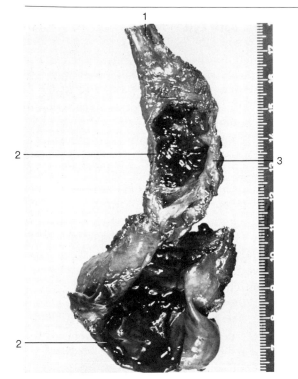

Fig. 793. Aneurysmal bone cyst (rib, cut surface)

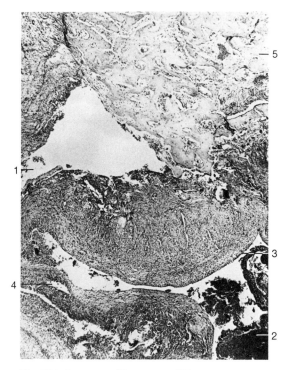

Fig. 794. Aneurysmal bone cyst; HE, ×15

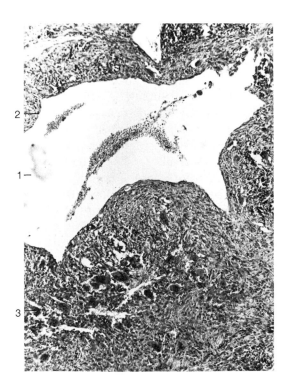

Fig. 795. Aneurysmal bone cyst; HE, ×25

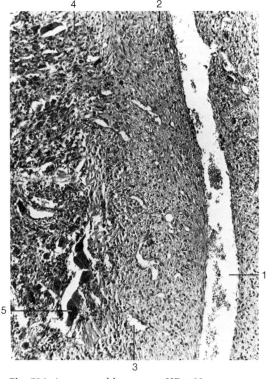

Fig. 796. Aneurysmal bone cyst; HE, ×32

Intraosseous Ganglion

When a bone cyst is found close to a joint, the possibility of an intraosseous ganglion must be considered. *This is a synovial cyst in the subchondral, juxta-articular region of a (usually degenerative) joint, which is smooth-walled and is filled with serous or mucoid fluid.* It is morphologically closely related to ganglia of the joint capsule or tendon sheath. Causally this kind of subarticular cyst can be related to earlier trauma. They are often chance findings, although they may sometimes give rise to slight pain.

In the **radiograph** of **Fig. 797** one can see an intraosseous ganglion in the distal part of the tibia *(1)*, close to the ankle joint. It is a roundish cystic osteolytic focus, lying in a highly eccentric position in the bone and completely surrounded by marginal sclerosis *(2)*. This small "bony cyst" lies close to the joint cavity *(3)* and shows no internal structure. The neighboring joint and surrounding bone show no radiological changes. However, in most cases there are more or less marked arthrotic changes in the joint.

The **histological appearance** of a typical intraosseous ganglion is depicted in **Fig. 798**. One can see a smoothly demarcated cystic hollow space *(1)* which is usually filled with serous fluid. The cyst wall – obtained by curettage – is most often submitted for a histological opinion. It consists of loose connective tissue *(2)* which here and there shows signs of myxomatous swelling *(3)*. The collagen fibers run parallel to the internal surface of the space. Many ganglia have no internal epithelial lining *(4)*, but sometimes there is a layer of synovial cells (the so-called *synovial bony cyst*). The cyst wall is threaded through with a few dilated fine-walled blood vessels *(5)*. There is a perivascular infiltrate of lymphocytes, plasma cells and histiocytes *(6)*, indicating inflammatory change. Deposits of hemosiderin may be present as a sign of earlier bleeding. There is no connection between an intraosseous ganglion and the adjacent joint. The prognosis of these cystic bone lesions is good, and after they have been shelled out and filled with bone chips they seldom recur.

Subchondral Bone Cyst

In the neighborhood of joints, particularly those of the knee and hip, solitary or multiple bone cysts may appear, the etiology of which is variable. So-called detritus cysts *(geoden)* are often encountered close to an arthrotic joint (e.g. in cases of coxarthrosis deformans, p. 424). Osteoarthritis can also lead to bone cysts arising near the joint. *A subchondral bone cyst is a solitary intraosseous cyst which appears in the neighborhood of a normal joint and shows no characteristic histological structure.* Unlike the juvenile or aneurysmal bone cysts (pp. 408, 412) it is found in the epiphysis and often extends into the metaphysis. It can be single or multichambered.

Figure 799 shows the **radiograph** of a subchondral cyst in the head of the tibia, where one can see the large cyst *(1)* lying beneath the articular cartilage *(2)*. It is sharply demarcated by marginal sclerosis, and has no internal structure. One can also see other smaller cysts in this region of the bone *(3)*. The surface of the knee joint is smooth and the joint cavity intact *(4)*. No degenerative or inflammatory changes are present.

The **histological material**, which is usually obtained by curettage, shows no particular characteristics. In **Fig. 800** one can see the smooth borders of a hollow space *(1)* surrounded by connective tissue *(2)*. The cyst has no epithelial lining *(3)*, and is most often filled with serous fluid. In the curetted material one usually finds only small scraps of connective tissue and the adjacent sclerotic bony tissue; no diagnosis can be made on this alone. Here the radiological findings are also necessary. There is no connection with the nearby joint. Clinically the subchondral bone cyst is usually symptom free, and it often turns up as a chance radiological finding. The pathogenesis is uncertain. If the radiograph is correctly interpreted, treatment is usually unnecessary. However, such a cyst may break into the joint and produce a secondary arthrosis. For this reason it should be scraped out and replaced with spongiosa if there is any pain.

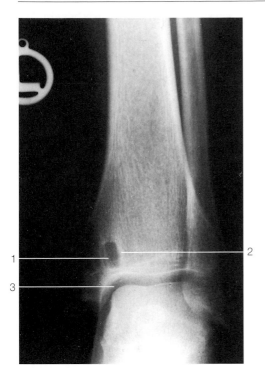

Fig. 797. Intraosseous ganglion (distal tibia)

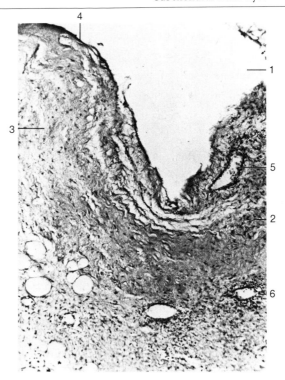

Fig. 798. Intraosseous ganglion; HE, ×25

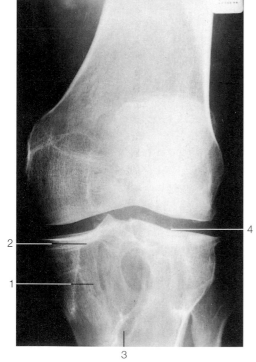

Fig. 799. Subchondral bone cyst (tibial head)

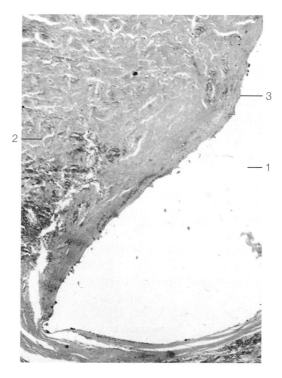

Fig. 800. Subchondral bone cyst; HE, ×40

Calcaneus Cyst

Bone cysts are frequently observed radiologically in different parts of the skeleton which are difficult to assign to any diagnostic scheme. They mostly represent chance findings. Of these, the commonest is a cystic focus appearing in the calcaneus. *A calcaneal cyst is a sharply circumscribed bone cyst in the calcaneus, which usually causes no symptoms. In rare cases a slight dragging pain may be experienced, which sends the patient to seek medical advice.* Even if such a cyst is found on the radiograph, the examination should include the search for some possible alternative cause for the pain.

In **Fig. 801** the **radiograph** of a classical calcaneal cyst can be seen *(1)*. It lies at the under side of the bone and is sharply demarcated. The adjacent cortex *(2)* is completely intact, partly sclerotically thickened and not rarefied. Proximally there are marginal sclerosis and sclerotic thickening of the bony structures *(3)*. Inside there are some discrete increases in the trabecular density. The remaining spongiosa is normally structured. The outer contour of the bone is also preserved, and no changes can be seen in the adjacent joint. These cysts usually contain a serous fluid. This type of calcaneal cyst may reach a considerable size, and can also take up a dorsal position. Nevertheless, the radiograph suggests an absolutely benign lesion, and there is usually no increased activity shown in the scintigram. Such a radiological finding is not an indication for surgical intervention. Only if there is unusual pain or a threatening fracture is curettage necessary, and then filling up the space with spongiosa.

One is usually offered broken up scraps of curetted material for **histological examination**, and this is insufficient for making the definitive diagnosis. The inclusion of a radiograph is absolutely essential. In **Fig. 802** one can see a cystic hollow space with smooth borders *(1)* which is filled up with serous fluid. The wall is composed of partly dense, partly loose connective tissue *(2)* without any epithelial lining *(3)*. This is a "simple bony cyst" of unknown etiology, although it may well be a harmless developmental disorder.

Intraosseous Epidermal Cyst

A solitary cystic bone lesion can arise because, during the development and growth of the skeleton, a group of squamous epithelial cells has been deposited in the bone, proliferating there until finally a cyst lined with this epithelium is formed. *An intraosseous epidermal cyst is a solitary benign osteolytic bone lesion which is lined by a keratinized stratified squamous epithelium and which may be filled up with horny scales.* These cysts are most often found in the skull bones or phalanges. In the latter case a traumatic origin is assumed. On occasion, cysts of this type may also be found in other bones (toes).

Whereas intraosseous epidermal cysts in the fingers usually cause a slight dragging pain, they may turn up elsewhere as chance findings. In **Fig. 803** one can see the **radiograph** of such a solitary bone cyst in the terminal phalanx of a finger *(1)*. The intraosseous cyst is in the center of the bone, which it has violently expanded almost like a bubble. The cortex is markedly narrowed from within, so that in one place it is hardly visible, but it is in no place broken through. The adjacent joint space *(2)* is fully intact. No periosteal reaction is visible. The cyst is single-chambered and has, apart from a few unspecified dense regions, no internal structure.

Histologically (**Fig. 804**) one can see a cyst that is surrounded by stratified squamous epithelium *(1)*. This appears in places as a layer of cells, but in others as a bud-like proliferation of epithelium *(2)*. The cells have small isomorphic nuclei and no mitoses can be seen. Often this is a keratinized squamous epithelium, and desquamated horny scales may be present within the cyst lumen *(3)*. Outside it is sharply demarcated *(4)*. In the curetted material from an intraosseous epidermal cyst there is often no more to be seen than a few horny scales lying between the cancellous trabeculae and some connective tissue. For a definitive diagnosis the radiological findings are always necessary. The differential diagnosis must take the radiological appearance of an enchondroma (p. 218) into account, although here the calcified patches typical of the enchondroma are absent. The prognosis of an intraosseous epidermal cyst is good, and it seldom recurs after curettage.

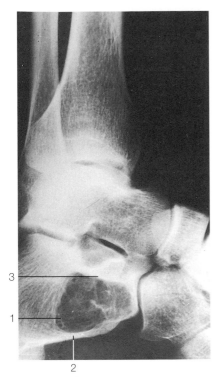

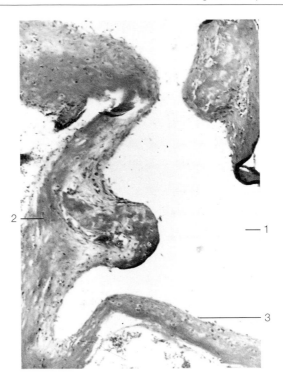

Fig. 801. Calcaneus cyst

Fig. 802. Calcaneus cyst; HE, ×25

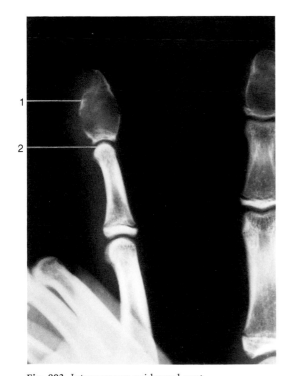

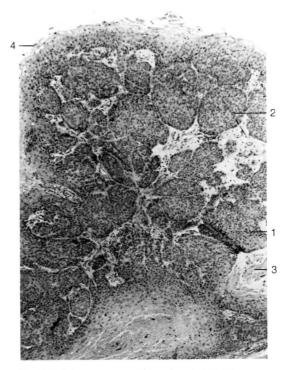

Fig. 803. Intraosseous epidermal cyst
(terminal phalanx of finger)

Fig. 804. Intraosseous epidermal cyst; HE, ×4

12 Degenerative Joint Diseases

General

Degenerative changes in the joints are so very frequently encountered that clinicians (orthopedists, surgeons, internists) as well as radiologists and pathologists are always coming across them. In the majority of cases these are the signs of wear and tear which greatly increase in old age. *Primary damage to the articular cartilage* appears in the most unlikely joints, initiating the development of **arthrosis** which leads to severe limitation of movement and causes very considerable distress to the patient. This primary impairment of function is frequently accompanied by severe pain. In spite of the very similar symptomatology, this "degenerative rheumatism" must be distinguished from "*inflammatory rheumatism*" (pp. 441 ff). Arthrosis begins as a disease of the articular cartilage when its metabolic activity is insufficient to maintain the correct functioning of the tissue. One then speaks of *primary arthrosis*. By far the most common example is encountered in the hip joint as **coxarthrosis deformans**. The patient visits the physician because of pain in the hip, coxarthrosis is diagnosed radiologically, and the femoral head (which is usually severely deformed) is in most cases removed surgically and replaced by a total endoprosthesis (TEP). The excised bone is then sent to the pathologist for macroscopic and histological examination.

This type of arthrosis can also arise as a *secondary* phenomenon. *Metabolic arthrosis* develops in the presence of general metabolic processes which cause the deposition of chondropathic metabolites. The deposition of urates in gout (p. 184), for instance, can lead to arthrosis. Similar arthrotic joint changes are found in *ochronosis* (p. 192). Arthrosis can be idiopathic, or it may be secondary to some other event. In cases of secondary arthrosis it is not always possible to discover the original disorder from a surgical specimen. In order to be able to provide an expert opinion the precise clinical findings and an exact case history are necessary.

Arthrosis can also arise as the result of long-term *unphysiological stress*. This kind of continuous unphysiological stress acting on a joint (e.g. as the result of a congenital skeletal malformation) can cause damage to the articular cartilage so that arthrosis finally develops. The radiologist, who has the whole radiological picture before him (e.g. in a case of chondrodystrophy, p. 48), can easily draw conclusions about the original stress and the development of the arthrosis. The pathologist, who has from time to time to assess a resected arthrotic joint, is dependent for information about the pathogenesis and etiology on the clinical and radiological reports available. Even pathological changes in the joint capsule or menisci can bring about arthrosis of the affected joint.

Finally, there is *arthrosis of traumatic origin,* where injury to the articular cartilage is the result of an earlier traumatic event. A long time afterwards a secondary arthrosis may develop that cannot be distinguished morphologically from the primary variety. When writing an expert report, knowledge of the case history is of decisive importance.

Localized changes in the structure of a joint are also to be counted among the degenerative joint diseases. In this way local subchondral bone necrosis with secondary degeneration of the overlying articular cartilage can lead to the clinical picture of **osteochondrosis dissicans**. If the damaged cartilage-bone complex has been pushed into the joint cavity, arthroliths (the so-called "*joint mice*") can bring about a corresponding dysfunction of the joint. The menisci can, as a result of unphysiological stress or overloading, degenerate and produce the clinical picture of **meniscopathy**. Of particular importance are degenerative changes in the spinal column, which can attack both the intervertebral discs and the vertebral joints and bodies, leading to **spondylarthrosis deformans**.

Arthrosis Deformans

Arthrosis deformans can appear in various joints and cause severe deformity of the articulating joint components, leading to a greater or lesser degree of functional impairment (shoulder joint: *omarthrosis*, proximal interphalangeal joints: *Bouchard's nodes*, distal interphalangeal joints: **Heberden's nodes**, metacarpophalangeal joint of the thumb: *rhizarthrosis*, hip joint: *coxarthrosis*, knee joint: *gonarthrosis*, vertebral column: *spondylarthrosis*). Arthrosis deformans is a common degenerative joint disease which starts off with damage to articular cartilage and is followed by secondary remodeling and deformity of the joint itself. This is not a matter of mesenchymal damage (as in the case of inflammatory rheumatism, p. 441), but a wearing out of the cartilage with consequent damage to the bone,

The first demonstrable change is a mucoid or **albuminoid granular degeneration** of the articular cartilage. In the cartilage there is a besom-twig-like arrangement of numerous yellow granules consisting of proteins and mucopolysaccharides, and microscopically visible collagen fibers (**unmasking of the fibrils**). After the collapse of the cartilage cells, the so-called **asbestos fibrosing** of the cartilage arises, accompanied by the development of cysts. These events are illustrated diagrammatically in **Fig. 805**. This destruction of the cartilaginous tissue is responsible for the reduction in the ability of the hyaline articular cartilage to resist shear forces. In this way increased pressure which can no longer be completely converted into a shearing thrust is carried over onto the bone. This results in the reactive deposition of new bone, with osteosclerosis of the subchondral spongiosa and the osteosclerotic development of peripheral osteophytes, finally resulting in partial ossification of the articular cartilage. As a consequence of this degenerative bone remodeling the head of the joint involved is severely deformed. Metabolic disturbances involving the articular cartilage lie behind a **primary arthrosis. Secondary arthrosis** may be due to various disorders of joint function (e.g. congenital displacement of the joint, fractures, inflammation, deposition of foreign material). Arthrosis deformans is frequently confined to one or more large joints. Generalized arthroses (*polyarthroses*) are most

often found in the small joints of the fingers. This is the most frequently encountered joint disease, affecting 11% of young people and 96% of those in extreme old age. Half of these people suffer from joint pains. Morphologically degenerative and reactive changes in the articular cartilage, joint capsule, subchondral bone, tendons and muscles may occur together.

In **Fig. 806** a classical **radiograph** of **coxarthrosis deformans** is depicted. The femoral head *(1)* has lost its rounded shape and is deformed. The joint cavity *(2)* is severely narrowed and scarcely recognizable, which is due to the degenerative loss of material from the articular cartilage. Within the femoral head there is a very uneven density of the bony structures *(1)* resulting from an irregular reactive spongiosal sclerosis. This starts in the subchondral zone, where it is most marked, and then in its further course takes in a large part of the head itself. In between, there are pale cystic areas *(3)* representing either gaps in the spongiosa or so-called detritus cysts (geoden) in which the mineralized tissue of the spongiosa has been destroyed. As a result of the continuous unphysiological stress acting on the socket by reason of the deformity of the femoral head, reactive osteosclerosis and new bone deposition arise here as well. On the radiograph one can see a broad band-like zone of sclerosis on the roof of the socket *(4)*. In order to preserve some degree of joint function, the socket expands, and there is a coarse osteophyte *(5)* with a drawn-out point on its lateral side.

The bizarre deformity of the structure of such a femoral head is also obvious **macroscopically**. As can be seen in the maceration specimen shown in **Fig. 807**, the surface of the cartilage *(1)* is severely roughened and furrowed, and reveals deep excoriations, in which the subchondral bone *(2)* is lying free. Coarse peripheral osteophytes *(3)* give the femoral head a mushroom-like appearance. Specimens of this kind are very familiar to the pathologist, since they are today often removed surgically (hip replacement, TEP). Such coarse deformity, with its peripheral osteophytes, and especially the severely roughened joint surface with its deep excoriations, fissures, fibrosis, defects and ulcers, can be assessed macroscopically. On the sawn surface one finds subchondral spongiosal sclerosis and detritus cysts.

Fig. 805. Diagram showing the development of arthrosis deformans. Temporal course of the joint changes: 1. normal joint. 2. early phase: asbestos fibrosing of the articular cartilage, osteochondrosis dissecans and subchondral spongiosal hypertrophy. 3. Late phase; with hyperplastic fibrosis of the joint capsule, subchondral detritus cysts and cartilaginous regeneration ("chondroblastic capsules")

Early stage

Normal

Late stage

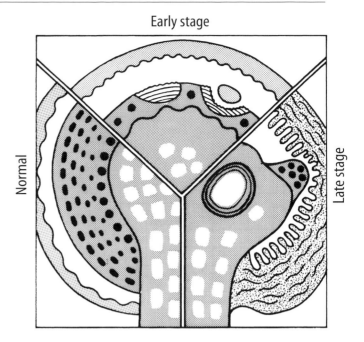

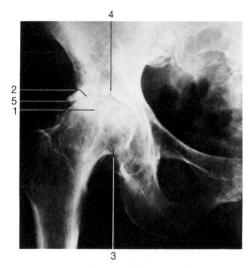

Fig. 806. Coxarthrosis deformans

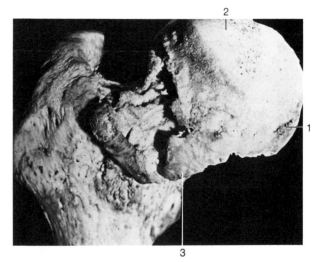

Fig. 807. Coxarthrosis deformans (femoral head, maceration specimen)

Figure 808 shows the **radiograph** of a severe *coxarthrosis deformans*, from which the condition can be diagnosed with virtually complete certainty. The contours of the joint *(1)* have been entirely eliminated by a powerful reactive osteosclerosis of both femoral head and socket. The joint cavity is practically invisible. One can see a peripheral osteophyte *(2)* at the side of the socket. At the transition between head and neck a so-called detritus cyst *(3)* can be clearly seen. The adjacent area of bone is osteoporotic *(4)*.

Figure 809 shows an **overall histological section** through an arthrotic femoral head. The head itself is no longer round, but has become deformed, and the outer contour is uneven. The layer of articular cartilage *(1)* is irregularly narrowed and, owing to the loss of chondroitin sulfate, appears rose-red with HE staining, instead of the normal dark blue. The eosinophilic reaction of the cartilaginous matrix is a sign of degeneration. The subchondral cortex *(2)* is markedly narrowed in several places, and in part osteoporotically thickened *(3)*. The spongiosa of the head *(4)* has become reticulated by osteoporosis; the cancellous trabeculae are narrowed and rarefied, but have smooth borders. In the neighborhood of the joint the marrow cavity is filled with connective tissue *(5)*, but elsewhere it contains fatty tissue *(6)* with small hematopoietic foci. At the side a peripheral bulge *(7)* can be seen.

Under the **low magnification** of **Fig. 810** one can see the very roughened surface and clefts of the cartilaginous joint surface *(1)* in which the fibers have been exposed by the loss of the matrix *(2)* and clearly lifted out of the cartilage. This roughening is particularly marked in places where the mechanical stress is greatest. The surface of the cartilage is irregularly pitted with indentations (**defects;** *3*) which have been caused by friction (traces of excoriation). These defects and a superficial *fibrillation* are the typical histological changes of arthrosis, and are signs of wear and tear. The cartilaginous matrix is eosinophilic. There is a deposition of small chondrocytes *(4)*, which may lie in more or less bubble-like chondroblastic capsules. Fibrinoid necrotic foci within which chondrocytes are no longer visible can appear in the articular cartilage *(5)*. The subchondral bone tissue is sclerotically thickened *(6)* and shows

elongated reversal lines and layers of deposited osteoblasts *(7)*. One can discern many dilated vessels *(8)* in the marrow cavity.

Under **higher magnification** the degenerative changes in the articular cartilage can be more clearly seen. In **Fig. 811** one observes greatly loosened cartilaginous tissue, in which the chondrocytes are gathered together in groups *(1)*. Many of them lie in greatly distended balloon-like chondroblastic capsules *(2)*. Large pseudocystic hollow spaces are repeatedly encountered *(3)* in which cartilage cells are no longer present. These are necrotic foci arising as a result of cartilaginous degeneration. The balloon-like chondrocytes also have small isomorphic nuclei which often appear to be pyknotic. The matrix *(4)* lying between the cartilage cells is eosinophilic and is, as a result of *demasking of the fibrils,* fibrillar.

All the structural alterations that have been described and morphologically illustrated here represent degenerative changes in the articular cartilage, and are irreversible. So far no truly effective treatment is available to bring about complete repair of this cartilage. This means that the most one can do is to minimize demands upon the joint by physiological prophylactic means, and to avoid unphysiological stress acting on the cartilage (as, for instance,

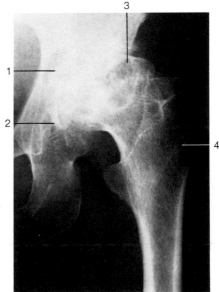

Fig. 808. Coxarthrosis deformans

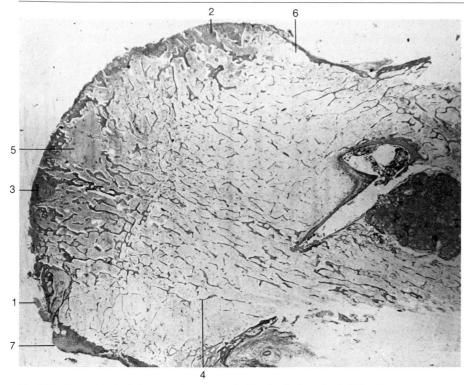

Fig. 809. Coxarthrosis deformans (macroscopic histological section); HE, ×2

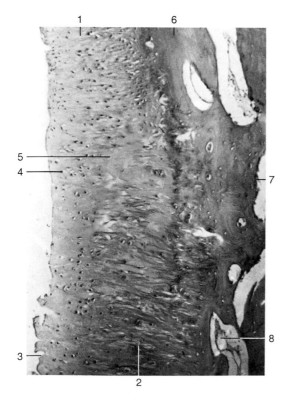

Fig. 810. Coxarthrosis deformans (articular cartilage); HE, ×25

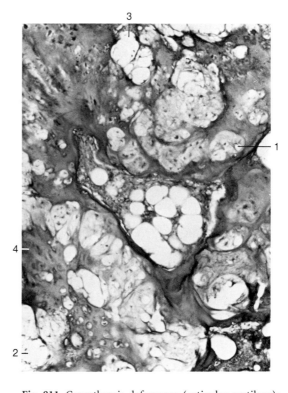

Fig. 811. Coxarthrosis deformans (articular cartilage); HE, ×40

in certain sporting activities). From the point of view of treatment, advancing arthrosis cannot be completely cured, it can only be somewhat alleviated.

In **Fig. 812** one can see the **radiograph** of a severe bilateral *coxarthrosis deformans.* It is obvious that both femoral heads are greatly deformed *(1).* The joint cavity is only in part still recognizable *(2),* being in places invisible *(3).* The spongiosa of the femoral head contains uneven areas of sclerotic thickening, and here and there translucencies representing the so-called detritus cysts *(4).* The joint socket also shows areas of sclerotic thickening, and spur-like peripheral osteophytes can be observed. In the light of a radiograph like this the diagnosis of coxarthrosis deformans can be made with certainty.

In the **overall histological view** depicted in **Fig. 813** one can see that the cartilaginous joint surface is not only narrowed *(1),* but that *spongy degeneration (with areas of bony spongiosa within the articular cartilage)* is also present *(2).* In the center there is a zone of cancellous bone tissue. Such a finding is frequent in cases of coxarthrosis.

Figure 814 shows the presence of *marginal sclerosis,* often observed particularly around a coxarthrotic femoral head. **Histologically** one can see bone trabeculae that have undergone marked sclerotic thickening *(1)* and in which elongated parallel reversal lines *(2)* reveal bone deposition. In the narrowed space between these bony structures, dilated fine-walled vessels *(3)* exemplify the condition known as *deep vascularization.*

Blood vessels sprout through the reversal lines into the degenerating articular cartilage so as to free it from fibrinoid necrotic foci. As shown in **Fig. 815,** the subchondral marrow cavity can be seen **histologically** to have undergone typical *myelofibrosis (1),* consisting of a loose or dense collagen framework with elongated fibrocyte nuclei and threaded through with dilated vessels filled with blood (capillaries; *2).* One can also see thick, osteosclerotic bone trabeculae *(3),* on which rows of osteoblasts *(4)* have been deposited.

In advanced cases, microfractures can appear within the spongiosa and form *detritus cysts* (geoden), which are detectable in the radiograph. In the **overall histological section** of **Fig. 816** one can recognize such a cyst *(1)* in the subchondral bone. The cyst is empty, but it can nevertheless be filled with connective tissue or amorphous material. The bony structure of the spongiosa surrounding it *(2)* is sclerotically thickened. Sometimes histiocytic granulation tissue may also be found here.

Unlike the situation in rheumatoid arthritis (Chapter 13) the destructive attack on the primarily degenerating articular cartilage is made exclusively from one side only; namely, from the side of the subchondral bone and myeloid tissue. At the same time the connective tissue joint capsule becomes thickened and rigid.

Fig. 812. Coxarthrosis deformans; bilateral detritus cysts

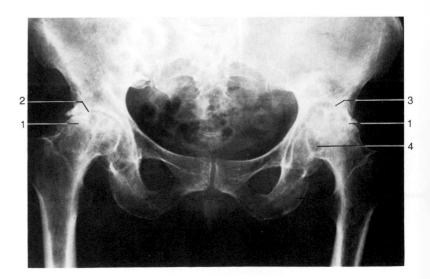

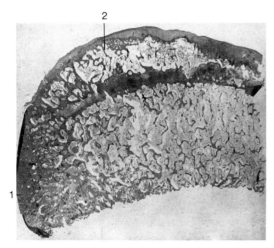

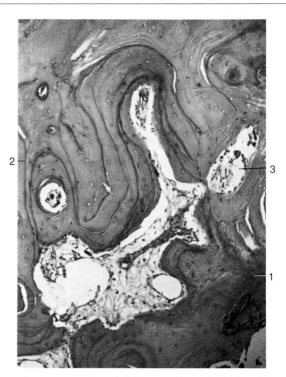

Fig. 813. Coxarthrosis deformans with spongiosal areas in the articular cartilage (overall histological section); HE, ×5

Fig. 814. Coxarthrosis deformans (marginal sclerosis); HE, ×25

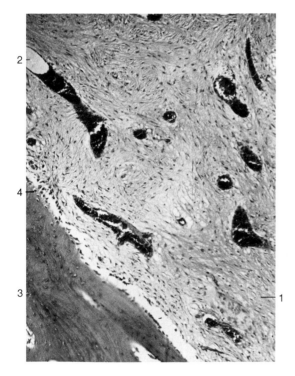

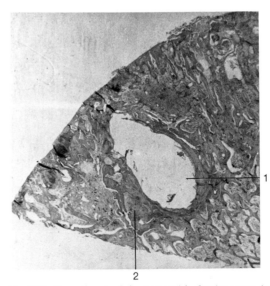

Fig. 815. Coxarthrosis deformans (myelofibrosis, deep vascularization); HE, ×25

Fig. 816. Coxarthrosis deformans with detritus cyst (overall histological section); HE, ×5

Osteochondrosis Dissecans

The development of degenerative changes in a joint can be very striking. *Osteochondrosis dissecans is a circumscribed subchondral osteonecrosis which often develops in the larger joints of adolescents and young adults, and which can lead to severe impairment of joint function.* Of these cases, 90% involve the knee joint, particularly the lateral surface of the medial condyle of the femur. Less commonly do these changes affect the elbow joint, hip joint, shoulder joint or joints of the foot. Multiple lesions may appear. Local trauma certainly plays some part in the etiology of osteochondrosis dissecans. The essential pathogenetic process may, however, be attributed to impairment of the local blood supply to the bone-cartilage region involved. The disease does after all begin at around the age of puberty, when the epiphyses are closing and the connection with the diaphyseal vascular network is still insufficiently developed. At this age the bone adjacent to the joint (particularly the knee joint) is not so well able to withstand mechanical strains. In the convex part of the joint the necrotic segment is bordered by a furrow-like indentation from the remaining bone and cartilage, as can also be seen in the radiograph. The piece of cartilage-plus-bone may be broken off under the influence of mechanical forces and come to lie within the joint cavity. This is a *free intra-articular body,* also known as a *"joint mouse".* If only a part of the degenerate and necrotic articular cartilage without any attached bone tissue becomes detached, we speak of **"Chondrosis dissecans".**

In the **lateral radiograph** of the knee joint shown in **Fig. 817** one can clearly see such a free intra-articular body *(1)*, where it lies in the joint cavity and leads to impairment of its function. There is a large corresponding defect in the joint cartilage, the so-called *"mouse bed"* *(2)*, which also impairs the function of the joint and can bring about severe arthrotic changes. Since this free lying body can inhibit the movement of the affected joint and even lock it, it must be removed surgically.

In **Fig. 818** such a "joint mouse" can be seen in the **overall histological section**. It is a piece of bone that is covered by a layer of living cartilage *(1)*. With older "joint mice", degenerative changes in the cartilage (eosinophilia of the

cartilaginous matrix, unmasking of the fibrils, mucoid degeneration, calcification) may be present. The subchondral bone, the blood supply of which has been completely cut off, is necrotic *(2)*.

Under **higher magnification** one can see in **Fig. 819** that the cartilaginous tissue of the free intra-articular body has been largely preserved, for the chondrocytes have small nuclei *(1)*. Since cartilage is nourished by the synovial fluid it is maintained in a "joint mouse" for a long time. These free intra-articular bodies are mostly surrounded by a connective tissue capsule *(2)*. At the transition to the necrotic subchondral bone tissue there are usually marked degenerative changes in the cartilage, with foci of mucoid degeneration *(3)* and necroses. Between them balloon-like chondrocytes are lying.

Figure 820 depicts the extensive necrotic bone tissue of a "joint mouse". Adjacent to the severely degenerated cartilaginous tissue *(1)* with only a few cartilage cells, there is necrotic bone tissue *(2)* in which osteocytes are no longer present; at least, the majority of the osteocyte lacunae are empty. Between these bony structures (in the marrow cavity and outside it) a richly fibrous connective tissue *(3)* has developed.

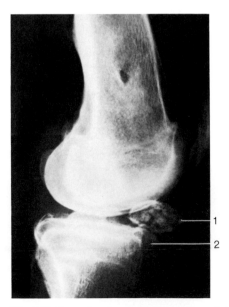

Fig. 817. Osteochondrosis dissecans (knee joint)

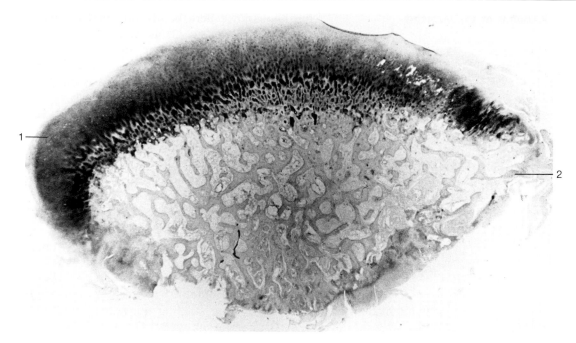

Fig. 818. Osteochondrosis dissecans ("joint mouse", macroscopic histological section); HE, ×8

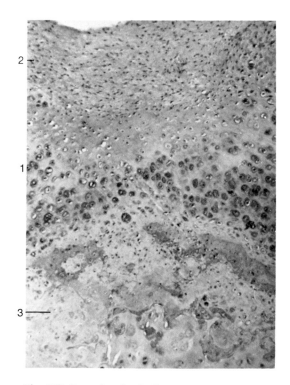

Fig. 819. Osteochondrosis dissecans; HE, ×25

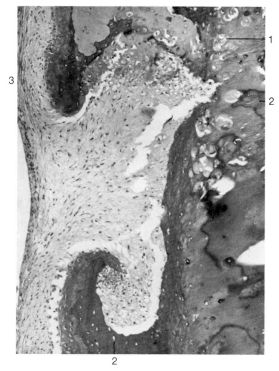

Fig. 820. Osteochondrosis dissecans; HE, ×25

Degenerative Lesions of the Meniscus

Lesions of the menisci occur very frequently, and the excised specimen is accordingly often sent to the pathologist for an assessment. Frequently an expert opinion is required, and it is at least necessary to find out whether it a matter of degenerative change or trauma (p. 434). In these cases it essential to know the time of the meniscal tear, the nature of the injury, the findings at operation and the history. *A degenerative lesion of the meniscus is brought about by excessive chronic stress acting on the knee joint, and this mostly affects the lateral meniscus.*

The medial meniscus can, however, likewise undergo degenerative changes. In this case there is usually no history of sufficient actual trauma. If the meniscus is sent for histological examination more than 5 months after the initial trauma, advanced degenerative changes are always present.

In the **radiograph** of the meniscus shown in **Fig. 821** one can see that the lateral meniscus has poorly marked contours *(1)* and a split surface, points which are very well shown up by double-contrast arthrography. On the tibial side there are additional deep lacerations *(2)*. The contrast medium often forces itself deep into the degenerative area of the meniscus *(3)*, so that this appears to have disintegrated into clumps. Also a horn of this flattened out and distorted meniscus *(4)* is softened up and heavily drenched by the contrast medium. In the **magnetic resonance tomogram** (MRT), which is today principally used with meniscal lesions, the degenerative changes in the meniscus are more clearly recognized. In **Fig. 822** one can see in a case of gonarthrosis a worn out anterior horn *(1)* and a degenerate region between the horns *(2)* with a central increase in the signal.

Figure 823 depicts the **macroscopic** picture of a meniscus removed at operation. In one place *(1)* the structure is regular. In the other parts *(2)* it is soft and porous, grayish-red and friable. At one point *(3)* a larger myxomatous focus of degeneration and a gaping tear *(4)* are clearly visible. It is this that had produced the symptoms and led to meniscectomy. At the same time a bursa *(5)* was also removed.

The **histological photograph** of the degenerative meniscal lesion depicted in **Fig. 824** shows the appearance here of necrotic fields *(1)* and cystic hollow spaces *(2)* as well as foci of mucoid degeneration *(3)* in the fiber system. With Sudan staining one can observe variably sized foci of fine fat droplets distributed throughout the meniscal tissue. These fatty changes – in contrast to traumatic meniscal lesions – are also apparent at the free edge of the meniscus. This type of degeneratively altered semilunar cartilage is less resistant and tends to tear under relatively weak mechanical stress. A tear of this kind can often appear in a primarily degeneratively altered meniscus.

Figure 825 illustrates a **histological section** of a meniscus with pronounced degenerative changes. The meniscal tissue shows marked myxomatous porosity *(1)*; the fibers are widely separated and contain only a few roundish nuclei. With Sudan staining the fatty deposits *(2)* are particularly obvious. These are arranged along the course of the fibers or appear in coarse patches *(3)*. In the intermediate regions numerous fine fat droplets *(4)* can be discerned in the meniscal tissue. In addition to the more or less pronounced myxoid porosity and splitting of the tissue, the presence of these fatty deposits within the meniscus indicates degenerative changes. These lead to the assumption that we are dealing with a primary degenerative meniscal lesion which has then brought about a secondary tear of the meniscus.

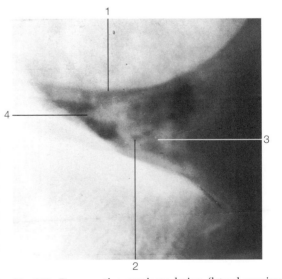

Fig. 821. Degenerative meniscus lesion (lateral meniscus – double-contrast arthrography)

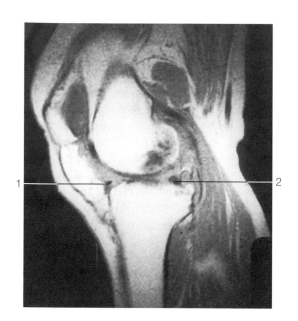

Fig. 822. Degenerative meniscus lesion (MRT)

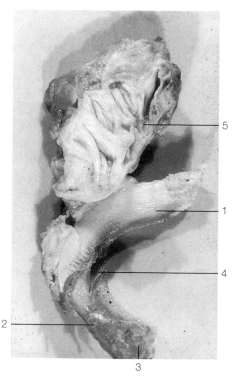

Fig. 823. Degenerative meniscus lesion (operation specimen)

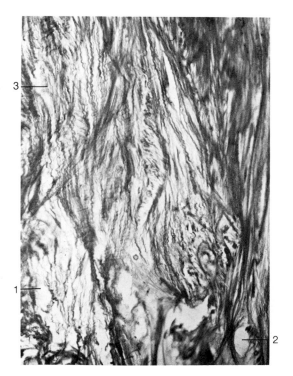

Fig. 824. Degenerative meniscus lesion; HE, ×25

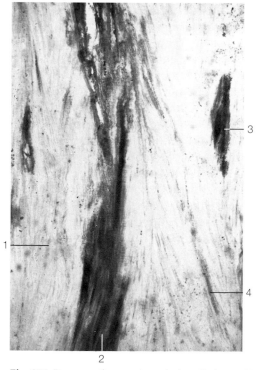

Fig. 825. Degenerative meniscus lesion, Sudan, ×64

Traumatic Lesions of the Meniscus

Particularly in cases where an expert opinion is called for, it is necessary to recognize a meniscal lesion of purely traumatic origin. The question that arises here is whether a meniscal tear has occurred because of sufficient trauma acting on a hitherto undamaged meniscus, or whether a degenerative change that was already present has finally led to a tear in response to insufficient trauma or even spontaneously. *A traumatic meniscal lesion is a mechanical tear appearing in a healthy meniscus, usually as a result of an accident during some sporting activity or at work.* With this frequent injury it is nearly always the medial meniscus which is affected (10 times more often than the lateral meniscus). One distinguishes between a complete or partial *meniscal tear* and the more frequent tear of the substance, in which case the meniscus is split. The injury results from a sudden extension with simultaneous rotation of the knee joint. The firm anchorage of the medial meniscus to the joint capsule and medial collateral ligament predisposes it to being torn.

In **Fig. 826** one can see a **radiograph** of such a traumatic meniscal lesion. In the double-contrast arthrogram the deep vertical tear *(1)* is easily recognized. There is a wide irregular air-filled gap in the smoothly contoured meniscus, the larger part of which has been torn away from its base. The outlines of the articular cartilages of the femur *(2)* and tibia *(3)* are smooth and show no signs of ulceration. Nor is there any arthrotic change in the knee joint.

Figure 827 depicts a **magnetic resonance tomogram** (MRT), and one can see a fresh arthroscopically verified tear in the region between the horns *(1)*. The tear produces a strong signal from the enclosed region within the wedge-shaped horn *(2)*.

Macroscopically a meniscus such as this reveals no damage apart from the traumatic tear. In **Fig. 828** one can see the firmly built and smoothly bordered meniscus *(1)* which here shows no signs of bleeding or foci of myxoid degeneration. At the upper end *(2)*, on the other hand, the meniscus is torn off. Here one can see split tissue that is interspersed with blood and fibrin. Even macroscopically the surgeon can see whether it is a traumatic or degenerative meniscal lesion. This must, however,

be confirmed by histological examination and documented.

Histologically one can discern in **Fig. 829** a longitudinal tear *(1)* in a meniscus (tear of the substance), the edges of which have already been smoothed out *(2)*. This points to an old injury. Within the first 3 weeks one can still observe cell damage and circumscribed necroses as well as a reactive increase in the number of cells close to the ragged edges of the tear; deposits of fibrin can also be encountered. Later these structures disappear. In the superficial layer *(3)* there is fibrous thickening which extends out into the meniscus as a narrow strip of scar tissue. Fatty deposits are a sign of secondary degeneration, traumatic meniscal lesions leaving the free margin of the meniscus clear of fat (in contrast to the degenerative lesions). Collections of fine fat droplets are very commonly observed in old traumatic meniscal lesions, particularly near the edge of the tear.

Figure 830 shows the **histological picture** of a meniscus which is essentially normal in structure. We can see orderly connective tissue with undulating collagen fibers *(1)*. Elongated and roundish isomorphic fibrocyte nuclei are strewn about *(2)*. No degenerative changes can be observed. Nevertheless one can see tears in 3 places *(3)*, the edges of which appear to be

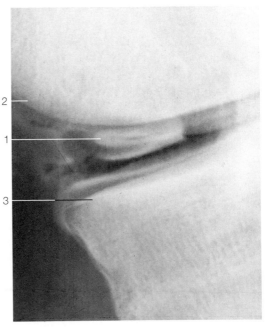

Fig. 826. Traumatic meniscus lesion (medial meniscus – double-contrast arthrography)

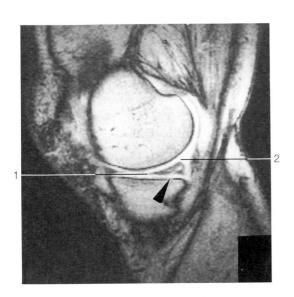

Fig. 827. Traumatic meniscus lesion (MRT)

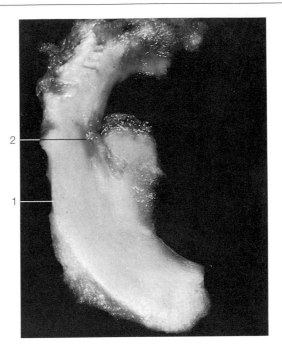

Fig. 828. Traumatic meniscus lesion (operation specimen)

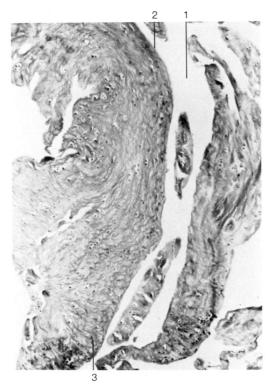

Fig. 829. Traumatic meniscus lesion; HE, ×25

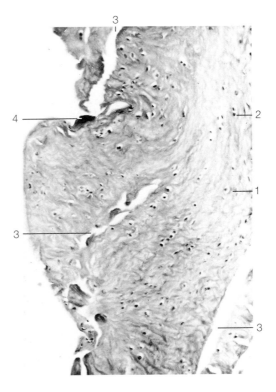

Fig. 830. Traumatic meniscus lesion; HE, ×40

frayed. Some fibrin has been deposited *(4)*, which is a reaction to the tissue damage.

By means of arthrographic transverse section pictures and MR tomograms it is possible, depending upon their nature and orientation, to distinguish between the following types of tear: 1. the vertical tear, 2. the oblique tear, 3. the horizontal tear and 4. a mixed type. With the so-called *basket-handle tear* the inner fragment is often dislocated into the joint. The radiologist can display and analyze the various types of tear very effectively with double-contrast arthrography and MR tomography, and the surgeon has the meniscus directly before him during the operation and can see the tear. Circumscribed wasting of cartilage in the neighborhood of the lesion or the arthrotic development of osteophytes are indirect indications of a meniscal injury that occurred months or years earlier (Rauber's sign).

Degenerative Changes in the Vertebral Column

Painful changes in the vertebral column are extraordinarily common and are mostly due to degenerative alterations in this complicated articular system. Depending on constitutional factors (inherited diseases) these conditions can develop as early as middle age (around 40 years) and increase in frequency as patients get older. Men are more often affected than women. The disease can begin with degeneration of the intervertebral discs *(chondrosis intervertebralis)*, whereby the influence of the altered static and functional forces acts on the adjacent bones (vertebrae) and brings about *spondylosis deformans*. These degenerative changes most often appear in the lumbar column (L 2–3, L 3–4), where the axial pressure is greatest. This leads secondarily to microfractures of the neighboring vertebral bodies followed by the repair process, which in turn leads to sclerosis of the bone next to the discs. The massive deformity of the intervertebral discs and vertebrae gives rise to severe pain ("sciatica"). Resulting from a drying-out of the anulus fibrosus and nucleus pulposus of the disc, the nucleus pulposus can be pushed medially or laterally backwards. This so-called *herniated disc* causes pressure on the spinal nerve roots and finally on the cord itself, giving rise to the vertebral

("lumbago") or root pain ("sciatica") syndromes. Whereas herniated discs are found more frequently in the lumbar column, *spondylarthrosis deformans* also frequently affects the highly motile cervical column (C4–C7). Degenerative changes in the small intervertebral joints constitute the condition termed spondylarthrosis deformans.

The diagnosis of spondylosis deformans is mostly made by means of **radiographs**. In **Fig. 831** one can see such a picture of the lumbar vertebral column in lateral view. The vertebral spongiosa *(1)* is rendered translucent by osteoporosis, and the framework of the vertebral body *(2)* is narrow and sharply demarcated. One can also recognize a marked bandlike sclerosis of the vertebral plates *(3)*. Furthermore, some of the vertebral bodies are deformed, insofar as osteophytes, rather like parrot beaks *(4)*, have developed at their upper and/or lower edges. The intervertebral discs are frequently narrowed *(5)*, thus reducing the size of the intervertebral spaces. Oblique photographs often reveal narrowing of the intervertebral foramina. This leads to compression of the spinal nerve roots ("radiculitis") and to severe back pain along the course of their distribution. If the vertebral plate is broken, the nucleus pulposus of the disc pushes like a hernia into the vertebral spongiosa, leading to the development of *Schmorl's nodes* *(6)*. Reactive cancellous sclerosis is often found in the neighborhood.

Macroscopically these degenerative changes in the vertebral column are almost exclusively found only in autopsy material. In the sagittal section through the lumbar column shown in **Fig. 832** one can see osteoporotically loosened vertebral spongiosa *(1)*, although the shape of the vertebral bodies and discs *(2)* is still well preserved. Nevertheless, marked peripheral bulges *(3)* can be seen ventrally, and these can bring about synostosis of the adjacent vertebral bodies. The anterior longitudinal ligament is thickened. This can lead to a stiffening of the vertebral column, which is often painful.

Histological pictures of such changes in the vertebral column may be found in autopsy material as well as in biopsies or operation specimens. In **Fig. 833** one can see a macroscopic section showing the development of peripheral bulges in two adjacent vertebrae *(1)* with an ir-

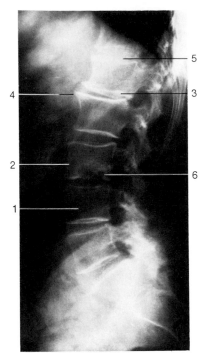

Fig. 831. Spondylarthrosis deformans (lumbar spine)

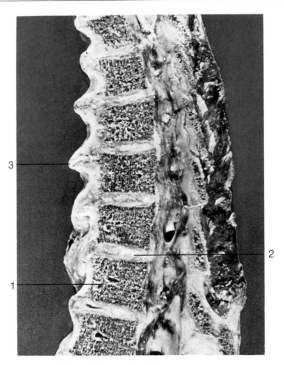

Fig. 832. Spondylarthrosis deformans (lumbar spine, surface of section)

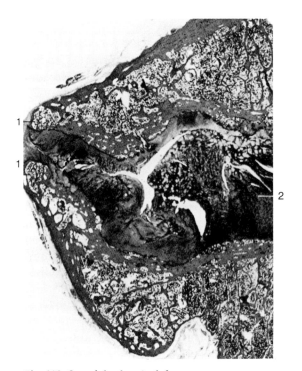

Fig. 833. Spondylarthrosis deformans
(peripheral bulges, overall histological section); HE, ×8

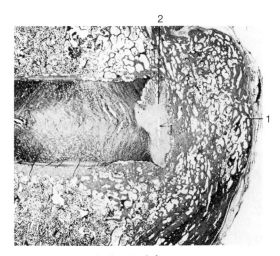

Fig. 834. Spondylarthrosis deformans
(overall histological section); HE, ×8

regular network of newly formed cancellous trabeculae. In between, the disc (2) shows marked degenerative changes. As can be seen in **Fig. 834**, the peripheral osteophytes from adjacent vertebrae are fused together (1) and the intervertebral disc is completely destroyed (2). Such changes naturally cause absolute rigidity of the part of the spine affected.

Between the covering cartilages of two adjacent vertebrae lies the **intervertebral disc**, consisting of a system of fibers enclosing the *nucleus pulposus*, which is said to represent a remnant of the notochord. The disc is bordered on the outside by the *anulus fibrosus*, which is closely bound in front and at the sides, but more loosely bound dorsally and dorsolaterally. The anterior longitudinal ligament is firmly anchored to the bodies of the vertebrae, but the posterior longitudinal ligament is only attached to the discs. In old age the anulus fibrosus dries out, shrinks, and becomes loose and easily torn. Gaps appear along the fibrils, and finally the ventral fibers are torn. The nucleus pulposus also dries out as age progresses, becomes unstable, and is pressed firmly into the gaps in the anulus fibrosus. With osteoporosis of the vertebral bodies and narrowing of their plates, the latter may be penetrated and the nucleus pulposus sink into the spongiosa.

In the lateral **radiograph** of the lumbar column shown in **Fig. 835** one can see osteoporosis of the spongiosa (1). The plates of the vertebral bodies (2) show band-like sclerotic thickening or widening and osteoporotic loosening (3). One can clearly discern the narrowing of the intervertebral space (4). There is also a dense hernia-like region of the bony structure (5) visible in the upper part of the 4th lumbar vertebra, with a *Schmorl's node*. This is a case of local penetration of the covering plate with the nucleus pulposus sinking into the vertebral body. Reactive bone deposition has produced circumscribed shadowing of the spongiosa.

This sinking of the disc tissue into the spongiosa of an adjacent vertebra can also be observed in the **macroscopic photograph** of **Fig. 836**. The central region of the disc (1) appears to have been widened – as if blown out – and has led to a more or less pronounced depression of the covering plate (2) into the underlying vertebral body. In one place (3) the nucleus pulposus of the disc has pushed like a

hernia into the spongiosa of a vertebral body, forming both macroscopically and radiologically (Figs. 831 and 835) what is known as a *Schmorl's node*. The vertebral spongiosa (4) is osteoporotically loosened, but peripheral osteophytes have not yet appeared along the edges of the vertebral body.

Degenerative changes in the spinal column can be associated with a high degree of deformity. *Kyphoscoliosis* is the curvature of a segment of the vertebral column by which on the one hand the physiological curve ("kyphosis") is increased, but on the other a lateral curvature also arises. This type of change is found in about 1% of bodies at autopsy. In 90% of the cases the cause is unknown. Sometimes it can be attributed to a congenital malformation, to adolescent kyphosis (Scheuermann's disease), to previous fully developed rickets, or to poliomyelitis, syringomyelia, Little's paralysis, neurofibromatosis or muscular dystrophy. The condition usually develops during the 2nd or 3rd year of life.

In **Fig. 837** one can see the **radiograph** of a severe kyphoscoliosis of the thoracic column. This segment of the spine is strongly curved with a convexity towards the right (1), so that the thoracic cage also appears correspondingly deformed. The density of the vertebral bodies has been increased by a reactive sclerosis and they have in places become fused together (2), and this has led to the discs being narrowed by pressure atrophy and degeneration. Kyphoscoliosis is also easily recognized **macroscopically** at autopsy. As the longitudinal section through the lumbar column in **Fig. 838** (ventral surface) shows, there is a curvature of this part of the spine which is convex towards the left (1), in which some vertebral bodies (2) show a lateral wedge-shaped narrowing.

Degenerative damage to the vertebral column practically always involves the vertebral bodies, joints and discs together, and leads to structural changes which can be seen both in macroscopic specimens and on the radiograph. In some cases a vertebral puncture is undertaken to establish the diagnosis. Often, because of a nucleotomy or laminectomy, parts of the degenerated and prolapsed disc are subjected to histological examination. Here we can observe myxoid swelling and degeneration of the tissue of the disc. Peripherally an inflammatory reac-

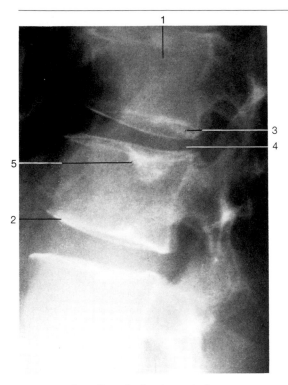

Fig. 835. Schmorl's node (lumbar spine)

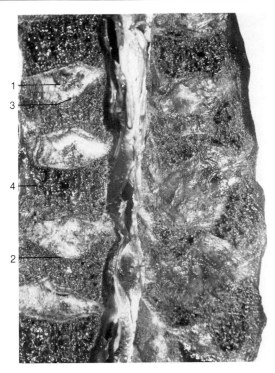

Fig. 836. Degeneratively altered lumbar spine with Schmorl's nodes (surface of section)

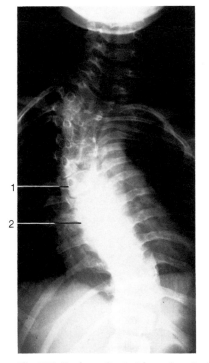

Fig. 837. Kyphoscoliosis (thoracic spine)

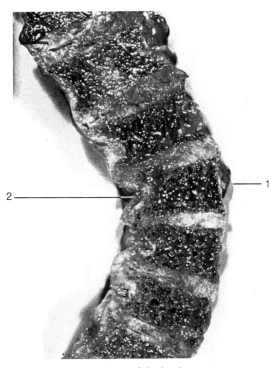

Fig. 838. Kyphoscoliosis of the lumbar spine (surface of section)

tive change is encountered. Reparative structures can be identified in association with the degenerative damage more often by a needle biopsy of the vertebra. This is a spongiosclerosis of the vertebral body with widened trabeculae, where elongated reversal lines and deposited osteoblasts are also present. The marrow cavity is filled with fibrous tissue.

In the region of the thoracic spine a particular *ankylosing hyperostosis* can appear which is associated with diabetes mellitus *(Forestier's disease)*. There is massive ossification of the anterior ligament with a clamp-like synostosis of the anterior surfaces of the vertebral bodies, which are coated as if with a layer of cake icing (p. 188).

13 Inflammatory Joint Diseases

General

As well as degenerative changes in the joint (see Chap. 12), those involving inflammation, i.e. the various forms of arthritis, present the most frequently found causes of joint damage. In this case the primary disorder is a change in the joint capsule, with the synovial membrane being the tissue in which the disease first develops. It is known that inflammation can only be built up in a tissue where blood vessels are already present, or which secondary blood vessels can invade. The joint capsule contains a double system of blood vessels, and those supplying the synovial membrane build up a dense network of anastomoses within the capillary bed. In other words, all the anatomical requirements are present for an inflammatory process to begin. If the inflammation is confined to the synovial membrane, one speaks of a *synovitis*. A non-specific synovitis is very often found histologically in a biopsy. If, however, the inflammation has involved other structures – particularly the articular cartilage – it is *arthritis*. In this case the previously intact joint cartilage is destroyed by inflammatory granulation tissue (the so-called *pannus)* which has passed into the joint cavity from the synovial membrane. This kind of damage to the articular cartilage predisposes it later to the development of secondary arthrosis (see Chap. 12). The inflammation can pass from the joint to attack the subchondral bone, or, by a reversed process, it may develop in the neighboring bone (osteomyelitis, see Chap. 7) and attack the joint secondarily. We then call it *osteoarthritis*. This results in a more or less extensive destruction of the joint, leading to a corresponding loss of function. Since there is a sensory nerve plexus in the stratum fibrosum of the joint capsule, this irritation causes joint pain, which is the principal symptom of arthritis.

As with every inflammation, a large number of damaging influences can be responsible for an attack of arthritis. Local trauma may lead to serous synovitis with hydrarthrosis (in the knee joint, for instance). Intraarticular bleeding can also cause synovial inflammation (e.g. hemarthrosis in hemophilia). Pathogenic microorganisms (bacteria, fungi, viruses) may enter a joint directly – or they may be blood borne – and cause a *purulent arthritis*. When masses of pus accumulate in the joint cavity we speak of a *joint empyema*. The most frequent organisms in young people are hemolytic staphylococci, streptococci or E. coli, and in children particularly pneumococci. Most frequently affected are the knee and hip joints. Histologically there is a *non-specific arthritis*, the morphological appearance of which gives no clue to the etiology (causative organism). The destruction of the articular cartilage and the subchondral bone, and the development of an inflammatory granulation tissue which is eventually organized, may finally bring about a fibrous ankylosis, which may ossify. In this case the joint function is completely lost. With a *specific arthritis*, conclusions may be drawn about the causative organism from the histological examination of a synovial biopsy. Such an articular inflammation may arise, for instance, during the hematogenic phase of tuberculosis *(tuberculous arthritis)*.

Immunopathological reactions may often give rise to a inflammation of the joint capsule or of the synovial membrane if immunological complexes have been built up. Lesions of this type are observed in rheumatic fever (parainfectious), in allergies, of unknown origin (idiopathic) or in cases of *progressive chronic polyarthritis* (PCP). Histologically the origin is not recognizable, which is why we speak in general terms of a *rheumatoid arthritis*. In the vertebral column this type of rheumatism is represented by *spondylitis ankylopoetica (Bechterew's disease)*. Such inflammatory joint diseases can be established and localized in the radiograph; the examination of a biopsy can provide the exact diagnosis.

Rheumatoid Arthritis

Apart from chronic non-specific synovitis, this type of joint inflammation is the most frequent to be found among specimens submitted for pathological/anatomical assessment. *It is a very slowly developing joint inflammation with no characteristic symptoms which follows an extraordinarily chronic course and, with increasing destruction of the joint, can finally bring about its complete immobility.* The etiology of the disease is so far unknown, and it has been seen in association with various infectious conditions (dysentery, tuberculosis, ulcerative colitis, scarlet fever etc.). Viruses and mycoplasms can also initiate the disease. Since no causative organism (bacteria, virus) can be detected in the affected joint in rheumatoid arthritis, one assumes that the inflammatory stimulus is an immunological reaction, an assumption for which there is some indication (identification of immunoglobulins – IgA, IgG, IgM – in the joint fluid).

Figure 839 shows the **course of rheumatoid arthritis** diagrammatically. The immunopathological reaction first initiates inflammation of the joint capsule, with exudative-proliferative synovitis. With this *exudative arthritis* the synovial membrane is, in comparison with that of a healthy joint *(1)*, thickened and soaked with edema *(2)*. There are infiltrates of granulocytes, lymphocytes and plasma cells which, together with serum, flood the joint cavity (hydrarthrosis; *3*). The synovial epithelium is activated and shows deposits of fibrin. From both the stratum synoviale *(4)* and the subarticular marrow cavity of the bone *(5)* granulation tissue *(6)*, rich in cells and vessels, grows into the articular cartilage *(7)*. With this *pannous inflammation* the articular cartilage is attacked on both sides: from the side of the joint cavity by a fibrovascular pannus *(6)*, and from the side of the marrow cavity by granulation tissue. The articular cartilage is therefore simultaneously threatened with destruction both from its surface and from the bone. This is accompanied by immunopathological reactions (IgG, IgM is the rheumatic factor, IgG-Ig-β_1C the complement), with phagocytosis of the immunocomplexes and the release of lysosomal enzymes. The organization of the pannus and its replacement by connective tissue *(8)* finally leads to *fibrous ankylosis,*

whereby the joint cavity is completely filled with fiber-rich connective tissue. The development of the pannus obliterates the joint space, as can be seen on the radiograph, whereas with simple arthrosis (Fig. 806) the cavity remains intact for a long time. Such a joint change as this produces very severe limitation of movement.

Figure 840 shows a **radiograph** of rheumatoid arthritis of the right hip joint. The femoral head is deformed and its outline no longer clearly recognizable *(1)*. Its spongiosa shows a diffuse, partly dense, partly straggly osteosclerotic thickening. Osteosclerosis can also be clearly discerned in the joint socket *(2)*. The entire region of the joint appears dense and diffusely sclerotic. The joint cavity *(3)* is greatly narrowed and, for the most part, completely abolished. The bony regions in the neighborhood of the joint *(4)* are translucent and show signs of osteoporosis. As with coxarthrosis deformans (Fig. 806) peripheral osteophytes may be present, and either condition can quickly change into the other. In most cases, rheumatoid coxarthritis can only be established histologically from the surgical specimen.

In advanced cases of rheumatoid coxarthrosis we find **macroscopically** marked deformity and destruction of the femoral head. An example of this can be seen in the maceration specimen shown in **Fig. 841**, where only part of the head is present. The surface of the joint shows deep ulcerations *(1)*; the spongiosa is in some places osteoporotic and porous *(2)*, in others sclerotic and dense *(3)*. The joint capsule has become ossified *(4)*. This unphysiological bone remodeling has spread into the shaft *(5)*.

When assessing rheumatoid arthritis macroscopically, it is the thickening of the capsule that first strikes one, in which the synovial membrane forms a grayish-red to brownish-red velvety layer. The otherwise mirror-smooth cartilaginous joint surface shows a destructive roughening, particularly at the edges of the joint space in the outer part of the joint, and is in places covered with loose granulation tissue. The articulating surfaces can be bound together by connective tissue. The framework of the subchondral spongiosa is dense; adjacently it is osteoporotic.

In an **overall histological section** through the femoral head from a case of rheumatoid arthri-

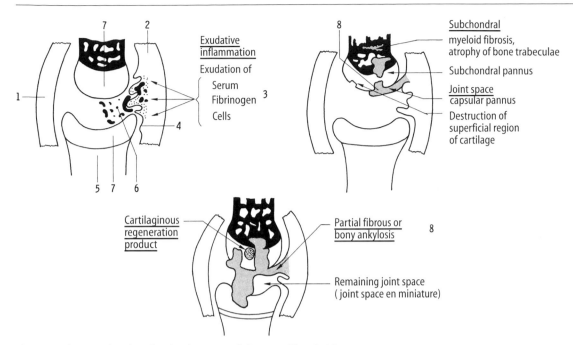

Exudative
inflammation

Exudation of

Serum
Fibrinogen   3
Cells

Subchondral
myeloid fibrosis,
atrophy of bone trabeculae

Subchondral pannus

Joint space
capsular pannus

Destruction of
superficial region
of cartilage

Cartilaginous
regeneration
product

Partial fibrous or
bony ankylosis   8

Remaining joint space
(joint space en miniature)

Fig. 839. Diagram showing the development of rheumatoid arthritis

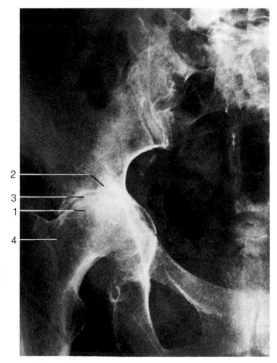

Fig. 840. Rheumatoid coxarthritis

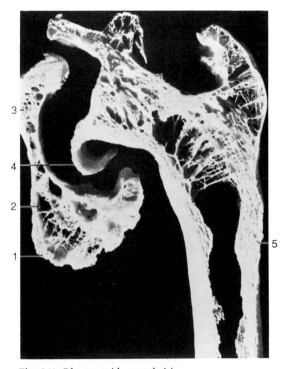

Fig. 841. Rheumatoid coxarthritis
(femoral head, maceration specimen)

tis shown in **Fig. 842**, the outline *(1)* is irregular and the normal sphericity no longer recognizable. This deformity severely impairs movement. The cartilaginous joint surface is severely narrowed and in places *(2)* no longer present. Inside the femoral head there is marked osteoporosis with rarefaction and narrowing of the cancellous trabeculae *(3)*. In some places the marrow cavity is filled with fatty tissue, and elsewhere one can see fibrous tissue and inflammatory granulation tissue *(4)* which has attacked and destroyed the articular cartilage from the direction of the bone. Invasion of the articular cartilage by a fibrovascular pannus cannot be recognized in such a specimen. To this extent it shows close similarity to coxarthrosis deformans (Fig. 809).

In **Fig. 843** one sees the classical picture of rheumatoid arthritis in **histological section**. It depicts the joint space *(1)*. Here the outside of the cartilaginous joint surface *(2)* is in part smooth, in part split *(3)*. The chondrocytes are mostly distended like balloons. Beneath the articular cartilage one can see the layer of subchondral bone *(4)*, which is in part osteosclerotically widened but which can in places be narrowed or completely absent *(5)*. The tissue of the pannus *(6)*, which has pushed itself out tongue-like from the synovial membrane into the joint cavity and lies over the cartilaginous joint surface, is characteristic of rheumatoid arthritis. It consists of inflammatory granulation tissue with numerous capillaries and capillary buds, together with infiltrates – principally of lymphocytes and plasma cells. This pannous granulation tissue burgeons out from the joint cavity into the joint cartilage and destroys it from the articular side. In addition, the joint cartilage is also under attack from the subchondral aspect. This *double-fronted attack on the articular cartilage* is pathognomonic of rheumatoid arthritis.

In the **histological picture** of **Fig. 844** one can again see a tongue-like outgrowth of inflammatory granulation tissue *(1)* which has sprouted out from the synovial membrane into the joint space. This "pannus" consists of capillaries and capillary buds, loose stromal connective tissue and infiltrates of lymphocytes, plasma cells and a few histiocytes. In other words, it is a histologically non-specific granulation tissue, the origin of which cannot be determined from the section. Furthermore, one can recognize that an entirely similar inflammatory granulation tissue *(2)* covers the cartilaginous joint surface and lies densely upon it. This granulation tissue later forces its way into the articular cartilage, destroying first the surface and later the deeper layers. Beneath this inflammatory granulation tissue ("pannus") one can still see the intact cartilaginous layer *(3)* in which the chondrocytes are often swollen, but still preserved. The layer of subchondral bone may be osteosclerotically widened, or may itself be largely destroyed by inflammatory granulation tissue (the "double-fronted attack on the articular cartilage"; *4*).

In its classic form, rheumatoid arthritis is represented by the ***progressive chronic polyarthritis (PCP)*** which is initiated by the immunopathological reactions. Here the joints are only a "battle-ground" for an immune reaction in which the heart muscle is most often attacked (rheumatic myocarditis). *In acute of rheumatism of the joints* (rheumatic fever, polyarthritis acuta serofibrinosa rheumatica) there are fleeting joint pains, particularly in the hands, feet and knee joints. *Progressive chronic polyarthritis* progresses in bursts and affects the small joints (of the fingers, toes, hands and feet) where the stiffness and deformities are found.

Rheumatoid arthritis especially attacks women between the ages of 35 and 45. The etiology is uncertain, although immune reactions and lysosomal proteases are thought to play a part. In 70%–80% of cases the rheumatic factor is positive in the serum. About 1% of the population suffer from progressive chronic polyarthritis, where there is a hereditary predisposition. A cumulative familial liability has been noted in these cases. However, the rheumatic factor is also found in healthy persons, particularly the elderly. In 60% of the patients, progressive chronic polyarthritis begins in a typical fashion with polyarticular symptoms and, above all, a symmetrical involvement of the small joints. So far the etiology of this disease remains unknown.

The *primary inflammation of the joint capsule* in progressive chronic polyarthritis leads to an exudation of blood plasma and the migration of cells (granulocytes with cytoplasmic inclusions containing the rheumatic factor, synovial cells, lymphocytes, plasma cells) into the

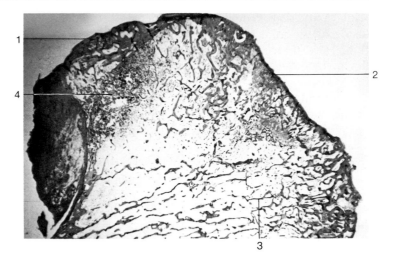

Fig. 842. Rheumatoid coxarthritis (overall histological section); HE, ×6

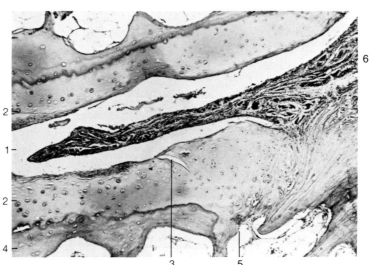

Fig. 843. Rheumatoid arthritis; HE, ×20

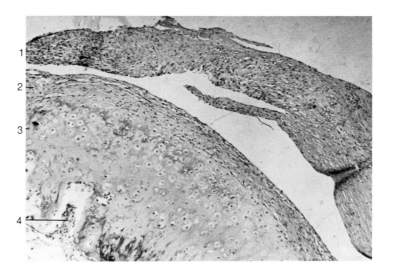

Fig. 844. Rheumatoid arthritis; HE, ×25

joint cavity. The synovial cells, which line the inside of the joint capsule, show focal destruction. Here there are homogeneous deposits of fibrin. In other places there is proliferation of the synovial membrane. As can be seen in the **histological picture** shown in **Fig. 845**, the membrane has become villous *(1)*, and these synovial villi are covered by an activated multilayered synovial epithelium *(2)*. In the connective tissue of the stratum synoviale *(3)* there are infiltrates of plasma cells and lymphocytes, which often form small lymph follicles. Here and there one can see fibrinoid necroses. These changes in the joint capsule can be early recognized morphologically by means of a capsular biopsy. Since, however, these inflammatory changes need not involve the whole of the capsule equally, a negative biopsy does not exclude progressive chronic polyarthritis. For this reason one cannot rely upon a needle biopsy for an exact diagnosis.

This is followed by the *dissolution of cartilage by granulation tissue*. The exudative stage can turn into a proliferative inflammatory process. A highly vascular granulation tissue grows out of the stratum synoviale into the joint cavity and spreads itself over the articulating joint cartilage. As can be seen in the **histological photograph** of **Fig. 846**, this inflammatory granulation tissue *(1)* is densely laid down over the articular cartilage *(2)*, from the surface of which it penetrates into the cartilage *(3)* and eventually destroys it. Furthermore, one can see that a very similar granulation tissue is entering the articular cartilage from the subchondral side *(4)* and is also destroying it. This means that the articular cartilage is being attacked from both sides, which is characteristic of rheumatoid arthritis. In other words, there is an attack from the joint cavity (by the fibrovascular pannus, *1*) and from the marrow cavity by the granulation tissue *(4)*, so that the articular cartilage is facing destruction both from its surface and from the underlying bone.

Figure 847 shows the histological picture of an advanced rheumatoid arthritis that has in places completely destroyed the articular cartilage. There is no more cartilaginous tissue present; instead, the intraarticular pannus *(1)* and

the intraosseous pannus *(2)* have joined forces. This has resulted in a moderately cellular granulation tissue with capillaries *(3)* and infiltrates of lymphocytes, plasma cells and histiocytes. The loose connective tissue stroma is in places bloated with fibrin *(4)*. The formerly subchondral bone trabeculae *(5)* are osteosclerotically widened, with elongated reversal lines and layers of deposited osteoblasts *(6)*. In places, reactive newly formed fibro-osseous trabeculae *(7)* are encountered. If the proliferating pannous tissues from the articular cartilages of both joint components finally make contact, the end result is a *fibrous ankylosis*. The joint cavity is closed by the development of the pannus, which is also apparent in the radiograph (Fig. 840).

Under **higher magnification** one can see in **Fig. 848** an exuberant proliferating formation of pannous tissue with capillaries *(1)* and dense collections of lymphocytes, plasma cells and histiocytes *(2)* that has destroyed the articular cartilage and penetrated into the subchondral bone. The still intact bone trabeculae *(3)* are osteosclerotically thickened. Bone tissue can finally differentiate within the pannus and the joint capsule, leading to a *bony ankylosis* which brings about complete immobilization of the joint. Following disuse of the diseased joint and limb, an extremely severe bone atrophy eventually develops in this part of the skeleton (immobilization osteoporosis, p. 74), which carries with it the danger of a pathological fracture. In most cases we are presented with biopsy material or a surgical specimen from a knee joint for histological examination which shows indeterminate inflammatory joint disease. From the morphological structures described we can make a diagnosis of "rheumatoid arthritis", but without being able to express an opinion about the etiology. As well as the various causative infectious diseases, a progressive chronic polyarthritis (PCP) must also be urgently considered, and this has to be clarified serologically. In 95% of these adult patients the pain first appears in the proximal interphalangeal and metacarpophalangeal joints and is intermittent in nature.

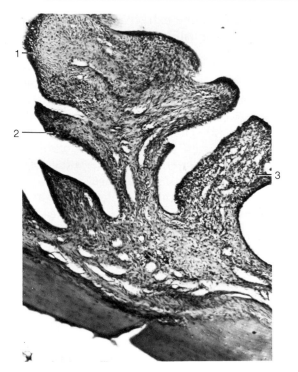

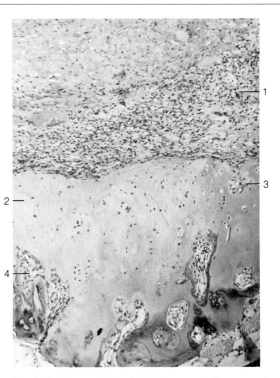

Fig. 845. Rheumatoid arthritis (proliferating synovitis villosa); HE, ×25

Fig. 846. Rheumatoid arthritis (intraarticular pannus); PAS, ×25

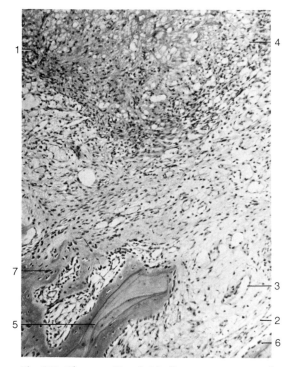

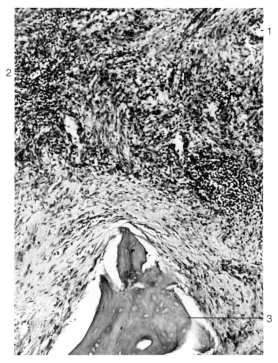

Fig. 847. Rheumatoid arthritis (intraosseous pannus); PAS, ×25

Fig. 848. Rheumatoid arthritis; HE, ×40

Non-specific Spondylitis

Inflammatory diseases of the vertebral column mostly develop in the marrow cavity of a vertebral body and lead to the clinical picture of *spondylitis*. The inflammation may involve the intervertebral discs and the neighboring vertebrae, a condition known as *spondylodiscitis*. *Spondylitis is an inflammatory bone disease of the vertebral column* (osteomyelitis) *that usually attacks one or more of the vertebral bodies, less often the neural arches or spinal processes, and frequently spreads into the neighboring joints and intervertebral discs* (spondylodiscitis) *and destroys them.* The corresponding radiological changes in structure are the result of the destructive and reparative accompaniments of the inflammatory process.

In **Fig. 849** one can see in the **a.p. radiograph** of the lumbar vertebral column, irregular sclerotic thickenings in the 4th lumbar vertebra *(1)*. The adjacent 5th lumbar vertebra also shows a similar cancellous sclerosis *(2)*. Both vertebral bodies are narrowed and deformed, and have laterally projecting peripheral osteophytes *(3)* which are joined together by bridging structures. The intervertebral space *(4)* is severely narrowed and in places absent. The plates of both vertebrae are extensively destroyed. Sclerotic increase in the spongiosal density in the 1st and 2nd lumbar vertebrae *(5)* also suggests a chronic inflammation there.

The vertebral destruction is also clearly shown in the **lateral radiograph**. In **Fig. 850** the spongiosa in the lower part of the body of the 4th *(1)* and upper part of the body of the 5th *(2)* lumbar vertebra is densely sclerosed. The large ventral spur-like osteophytes *(3)* are striking. The intervertebral space *(4)* is markedly narrowed, cloudy and dense. Severe destruction can be seen in both these adjacent vertebral bodies and also in the intervertebral discs, which is a radiological sign of spondylodiscitis. The spread of the destructive process from one vertebra to the next is very characteristic of an inflammatory process. As against this, tumorous processes (e.g. bone metastases) are usually limited to the affected vertebra, the intervertebral space remaining unaltered.

A specifically directed needle biopsy can confirm the radiological diagnosis **histologically** and at the same time extract material for bacteriological examination. **Figure 851** reveals a completely disorganized spongiosal framework in the vertebral body, with sclerotically thickened bone trabeculae *(1)* which in many cases show no lamellar layering. They contain many active osteoblasts and in places have an undulating border *(2)*. Time and again one encounters trabeculae with extensive fronts of bone deposition *(3)* and layers of osteoblasts together with a few osteoclasts in flattened resorption lacunae. The marrow cavity is filled with loose granulation tissue *(4)* which is threaded through with dilated fine-walled capillaries *(5)*. Plasma cells and lymphocytes *(6)* are loosely distributed throughout the inflammatory infiltrate. No specific inflammatory granulomas or tumor cell infiltrates can be identified. This represents the histological appearance of chronic non-specific osteomyelitis; in the vertebral column this signifies chronic spondylitis.

In **Fig. 852** the **histological findings** are similar. The marrow cavity is filled with loose inflammatory granulation tissue with scattered infiltrates of lymphocytes and plasma cells *(1)* and capillaries *(2)*. The bone trabeculae *(3)* are sclerotically thickened and edged with osteoblasts *(4)*. Intramedullary scarring with newly formed fibro-osseous trabeculae are often found with chronic spondylitis. Apart from plasma cells and lymphocytes, granulocytes are also found in the presence of recurrent chronic inflammation.

Together with degenerative changes in the vertebral column (p. 436), non-specific spondylitis is the other commonest disease of the spine found in Europe today. In adults, 50% of all cases of osteomyelitis appear in the form of a spondylitis or spondylodiscitis. Spondylitis most often attacks the lumbar and lower thoracic regions of the vertebral column. Even with an absolutely typical radiological picture, a biopsy (needle biopsy) from the affected vertebra is necessary – most of all, in order to exclude a specific type of inflammation (e.g. tuberculous spondylitis). At the same time bacteriological confirmation is often possible. With an uncharacteristic radiological picture a vertebral biopsy is necessary to exclude a possible tumor.

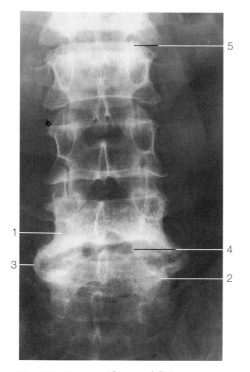

Fig. 849. Non-specific spondylitis
(4th/5th. lumbar vertebral bodies, a.p. view)

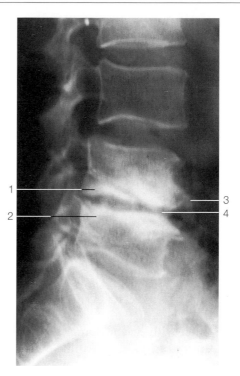

Fig. 850. Non-specific spondylitis
(4th/5th. lumbar vertebral bodies, lateral view)

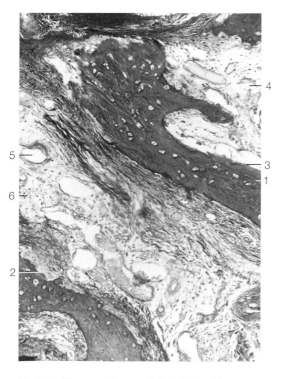

Fig. 851. Non-specific spondylitis; HE, ×64

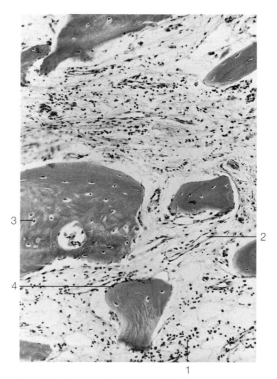

Fig. 852. Non-specific spondylitis; HE, ×64

Spondylarthritis Ankylopoetica (Bechterew's Disease)

An immunopathological inflammation due to an inherited disposition may develop particularly in the vertebral column. *Spondylarthritis ankylopoetica (Bechterew's disease) is a progressive inflammatory polyarthritis of the intervertebral joints which begins in the sacroiliac region and most often attacks the lumbar and cervical regions of the vertebral column. It eventually leads to bony ankylosis and complete rigidity of the vertebral column.* In about 20% of cases peripheral joints (shoulder, hip, knee) also develop a similar form of rheumatoid arthritis. This disease of unknown etiology starts predominantly in the 3rd decade of life and in many cases produces a progressive state of invalidism that increases after the age of 50. In 90% of cases it affects men with a leptosomal habitus. The disease slowly advances, leading to a rounded hunchback condition, immobility and pain.

This ankylosing spondylarthritis has a characteristic **radiological picture**. As shown in **Fig. 853**, one sees in a lateral radiograph of the lumbar column an ossification of the anterior longitudinal ligament *(1)* which gives the spine the appearance of a *bamboo rod*. The intervertebral joints are bridged over at the ends by ossified bars *(2)*. The intervertebral discs *(3)* may be masked by the ossification of the longitudinal ligaments. Straggly osteoporosis is seen in the vertebral bodies *(4)*.

Figure 854 shows a **maceration specimen** of such a spinal column. The joint space between the vertebral bodies has been lost and the discs are completely ossified *(1)*. This *synostosis* leads to a bony stiffening of the joints of the spine. The vertebral bodies *(2)* become fused together by the intermittent but advancing ossification, and peripheral bulges can be seen *(3)*. One also observes ossification and thickening of the anterior longitudinal ligament *(4)*. The ligamenta flava are those most frequently ossified, but this often goes unrecognized in the radiograph.

Figure 855 shows a **maceration specimen** in a **longitudinal section** through such a vertebral column, where one can discern irregular osteoporosis *(1)* in the vertebral spongiosa resulting from a relieving of the load brought about by

ossification of the longitudinal ligaments. This is augmented by pain-induced immobility and the bony stiffening of the spinal column, as well as inflammatory changes in the bone marrow with deterioration of the metabolic exchange. The intervertebral discs are in many cases still intact *(2)* so that a normal intervertebral space remains. In other places, however, bony bridges *(3)* are formed between adjacent vertebra by partial ossification of the discs, and this increases the stiffening process. In addition one can see completely ossified intertransverse joints *(4)*. In the neighborhood of the anterior longitudinal ligament, bony bars *(5)* develop and span over the intervertebral space. These structural changes in the spinal column produce a kyphosis, particularly in the mid-thoracic region, and lead to changes in shape of the vertebral body, obliterating the anterior concavity to form straight surfaces (rectangular vertebral body): a process known as "squaring".

Figure 856 depicts an **overall histological section** of an intervertebral space in a case of spondylitis ankylopoetica. One can recognize the disc *(1)*, the dorsolateral part of which has, however, been replaced by cancellous bone *(2)*. The space has been bridged over by fully mineralized bone tissue *(3)* which is the cause of the stiffening. Apart from this ossification the intervertebral foramen *(4)* is visible. The calcified cartilaginous plates of the vertebral body remain at least partly intact, so that the original shape of the space can still be seen on the radiograph.

In the living patient, Bechterew's ankylosing spondylitis can be diagnosed clinically and radiologically without the help of the pathologist. We can evaluate the extent to which this progressive disease has advanced from the macroscopic appearance of the parts of the vertebral column seen at autopsy, for which purpose maceration specimens are the most suitable (Figs. 854, 855). In many cases the disease is a chance postmortem finding, its clinical course having been free of symptoms. In just 1% of cases an exuberant course of the disease can lead to complete invalidism. In half the patients additional extravertebral joint pain appears, especially in the hip and temporomandibular joints.

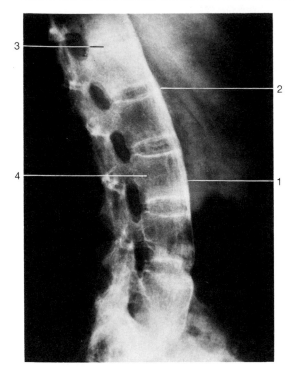

Fig. 853. Bechterew's disease (lumbar spine)

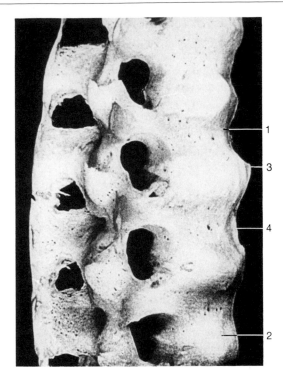

Fig. 854. Bechterew's disease
(Lumbar spine, maceration specimen)

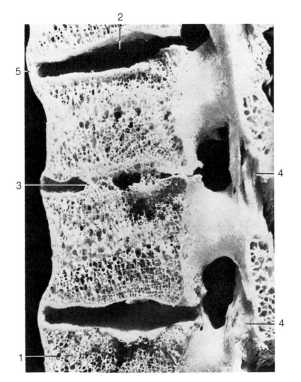

Fig. 855. Bechterew's disease
(thoracic spine, maceration specimen)

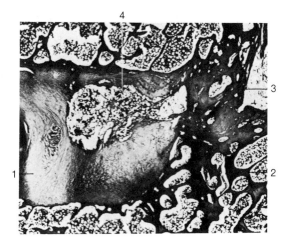

Fig. 856. Bechterew's disease (intervertebral space); HE, ×15

Non-specific and Specific Arthritis

Synovial biopsies from various joints often provide histological evidence of inflammatory changes with infiltrates of lymphocytes, plasma cells and histiocytes, without, however, allowing any conclusions to be drawn from the histological picture about their origin. In such a *non-specific synovitis* or *arthritis* the inflammatory reaction gives no hint of the underlying disease. It might be a local infection as the result of a generalized bacteremia or sepsis; such an inflammation might also result from a joint injury or the invasion of an inflammatory bone focus into a nearby joint. The most serious type of this kind of arthritis is *purulent arthritis* (pyarthrosis, joint empyema), which is most often due to hemolytic staphylococci, streptococci, E. coli or, in children, pneumococci. In most cases only a single joint is affected (knee or hip joint), and a polyarticular attack is unusual.

In the **histological picture** of **Fig. 857** one can see a chronic non-specific arthritis with a markedly villous synovial membrane in which the individual villi *(1)* are covered by a flat synovial epithelium *(2)*. The stroma of the villus has been taken over by a non-specific granulation tissue containing numerous dilated capillaries *(3)* and capillary buds, and in which, particularly around the vessels, there are collections of lymphocytes, plasma cells and histiocytes. This villous stroma may be drenched with edematous fluid containing fibrin, and also show a granulocytic infiltrate. The synovial epithelium can in places be reactively widened. Such an appearance can only mean a histologically non-specific synovitis or arthritis.

There is, however, a whole collection of inflammatory processes in joints for which the underlying disease can be established. In the case of a *specific arthritis* the histological structures found in the synovial biopsy make it possible to recognize the cause. This is particularly true of synovial inflammatory processes which contain a specific granulation tissue.

Figure 858 shows the **histological picture** of a *tuberculous arthritis*. One can discern a thickened villous synovial membrane *(1)* covered over with loose synovial epithelium *(2)*. Typical tubercles *(3)* with epithelioid cells, lymphocytes and occasional Langhans giant cells

are present in the infiltrated villous stroma. The tubercles may reveal central caseation, or they may be productive. We speak of a "tuberculoid synovitis". The identification of tubercle bacilli would lead to the diagnosis of a blood-borne tuberculous arthritis. The knee joint is most commonly affected.

Gouty arthritis (arthritis urica) is characterized by deposits of crystalline urates in the articular cartilage and subchondral bone (p. 184), which reveal the underlying disease. The main sites are the metatarsophalangeal joints, and the elbow and knee joints. In the **histological picture** shown in **Fig. 859** one can observe in the marrow cavity of the subchondral spongiosa *(1)* a roundish focus containing clusters of radially orientated birefractive crystalline sodium urate deposits *(2)*. The large brownish crystalline needles *(3)* are mostly dissolved out by formalin fixation, leaving empty spaces behind. In the neighborhood of these deposits there is a rampart of foreign body giant cells and histiocytes *(4)*. A highly cellular granulation tissue *(5)* and later a connective tissue capsule develop. This is a typical gouty tophus, which brings about a periarticular osteoclastic bone resorption and makes an exact diagnosis possible.

In cases of *systemic lupus erythematosus*, manifestations in the joints are common. As can be seen in the **histological picture** of **Fig. 860**, there is a thickened villous synovial membrane *(1)* which is covered by a multilayered synovial epithelium *(2)*. In the villous stroma there is a non-specific inflammatory granulation tissue of plasma cells and lymphocytes *(3)* as well as an influx of fibrin. Small lymph follicles may be present. Only if hematoxylin bodies can be demonstrated can this synovitis be classified as due to lupus erythematosus; otherwise it is the histological picture of a non-specific rheumatoid arthritis.

There is a whole series of other inflammatory joint diseases which show no pathognomonic histological structures. *Psoriatic arthritis* leads, about 10 years after the onset of the psoriasis, to chronic polyarthritis (fingers, toes, cervical vertebrae). Similar joint involvement is associated with Felty's syndrome.

The introduction of corticoids into a joint (particularly in the case of someone who has been injured at some sporting activity) carries with it the danger of causing damage by subse-

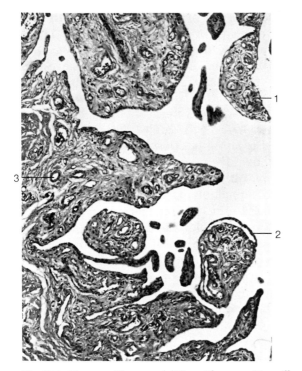

Fig. 857. Non-specific spondylitis with synovitis villosa; HE, ×25

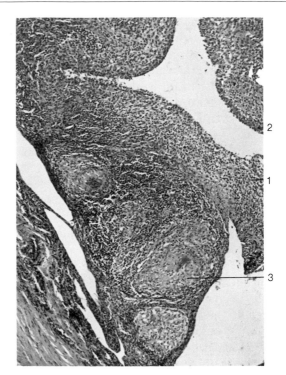

Fig. 858. Tuberculous arthritis (synovitis); HE, ×20

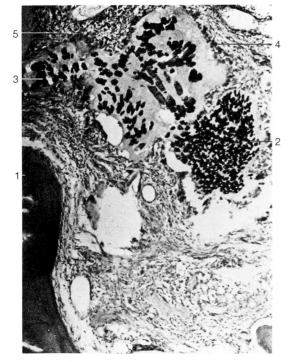

Fig. 859. Arthritis urica; HE, ×25

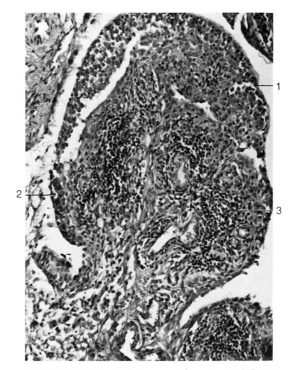

Fig. 860. Arthritis with lupus erythematosus; HE, ×40

quent non-specific arthritis. This is the so-called *cortisone arthritis.* The intraarticular administration of cortisone derivatives does indeed reduce the pain and makes it possible for the patient to continue with the physical activity, but it also leads to increased wear on the joint and, eventually, to arthrosis. The natural reparative processes are suppressed by the glucocorticoid, and progressive paraarticular osteolysis and synovitis develop, which may be followed by a bacterial arthritis. This serious complication is due to the inhibitive action of the cortisone on the resistance mechanisms.

Histologically (**Fig. 861**) one can see in biopsy material an edematously loosened synovial membrane with predominantly lymphocytic infiltrates *(1).* These are mostly concentrated beneath the synovial epithelium *(2).* They form no specific granulomas. The synovial membrane is threaded through with dilated fine-walled capillaries *(3).* Serous fluid *(4)* has collected in the joint cavity, and this leads to a painful swelling of the joint.

In the case of a bacterial infection superimposed upon an already damaged joint, a *purulent granulating synovitis* will arise. In **Fig. 862** one can see **histologically** in the synovial membrane a very highly cellular inflammatory granulation tissue with capillaries *(1)* and capillary buds and dense infiltrates of lymphocytes, plasma cells and histiocytes *(2),* and also polymorphonuclear leukocytes *(3).* In the basal layer one can again see numerous dilated blood vessels *(4).* The synovial epithelium *(5)* has mostly been detached and is no longer present. From the histological appearance there is a non-specific inflammation which gives no clue to the etiology. Only the presence of granulocytes suggests an exuberant inflammation, possibly of bacterial origin. The influence of locally applied cortisone cannot be detected, and therefore the pathologist must have the clinical information as well. If, however, such a non-specific synovitis or arthritis arises during the course of local cortisone treatment, then, professionally speaking, a causal relationship exists. The pathogenesis of these so-called "cortisone-wrecked joints" is uncertain, and such inflammatory and destructive joint changes have not been described in cases of Cushing's syndrome. It must be attributed to the direct action of cortisone on the joint structure.

Various types of **non-specific arthritis** can be triggered off by living organisms or inanimate material. Infectious arthritis is due to a living organism, and the cause can be established by bacterial analysis of the biopsy or puncture material. Usually it is a matter of gram-positive cocci, most often Staphylococcus aureus (30%–35% in adults, 40%–45% in children). Far less often (less than 1%) it is possible to identify mycobacteria, viruses, fungi or protozoa. All these organisms produce non-specific inflammation in the synovial membrane and/or the subchondral marrow cavity which provides no histological information about the exact cause. At the most a bacterial infection can be postulated (**purulent arthritis**) – particularly if collections of bacteria can be seen directly under the microscope. That applies equally to the histological identification of fungi, worms or other parasites. If a synovial biopsy reveals nothing but inflammation, we can only diagnose **synovitis**. It is only after invasion and destruction of the articular cartilage that **arthritis** can be diagnosed. In this case the biopsy material must contain tissue from the articular cartilage.

A non-specific arthritis may arise without any living agents (such as bacteria) after penetration of the synovial membrane and joint cavity, for instance by a thorn from a plant, or by spines from a sea urchin. Histologically we can find these foreign bodies in the biopsy and identify the cause. The inflammatory reaction thus triggered off, on the other hand, is completely non-specific and by itself offers no clue to the cause.

This applies equally to the microcrystalline types of arthritis due to products of the body's own metabolism. With **gouty arthritis** it is the gouty tophi which first provide the answer (pp. 184, 452). With **calcium pyrophosphate arthropathy** ("pseudogout"), deposits of crystalline calcium pyrophosphate dihydrate are found in the articular cartilage, menisci and paraarticular tissues, with the development of "chondrocalcinosis". The surrounding inflammatory reaction is non-specific. The etiology of this disease, which leads to damage to the articular cartilage, is unknown. Sometimes this type of arthritis is associated with other diseases such as hyperparathyroidism, hemochromatosis, hypothyroidosis, ochronosis, Wilson's disease, diabetes mellitus or hypophosphatasia (secondary calcium pyrophosphate arthropathy). The microcrystalline types of arthritis also include **hydroxyapatite arthropathy, oxalosis** and **cholesterol arthritis**. In every case the accompanying inflammatory reaction is histologically non-specific, and it is only after the causative metabolic product of the patient's own body has been identified in the section that the cause can be established.

The **specific types of arthritis** reveal themselves by the development of a characteristic granulation tissue in which specific granulomas are present and which histologically provides a clue to the cause. These particularly include **tuberculous arthritis, Boeck's sarcoidosis** and **syphilitic arthritis**. Other specific types of arthritis are very rare. Rheumatoid arthritis only produces a "specific" granulation tissue under certain circumstances, and can have several

causes. Arthritis appearing in the course of a systemic disease (e.g. systemic lupus erythematosus, scleroderma, panarteritis nodosa, dermatomyositis, Behçet's disease, Wegener's granulomatosis etc.) usually shows no specific granulation tissue to indicate the cause, and can only be assigned histologically to the clinically known disease.

A synovial biopsy in the case of a clinically suspected arthritis, which is very often carried out, leads in most cases only to the histological diagnosis of "non-specific exuberant" or "chronic" synovitis, which the clinician probably knew already. In particular, such a biopsy often provides identification of the causal organism, so that the histological structures already known only serve to support it. Even so, the histology can sometimes contribute decisively to establishing the final diagnosis.

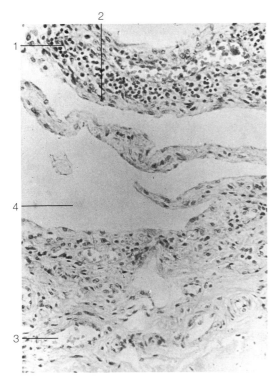

Fig. 861. Cortison arthritis (synovitis); HE, ×40

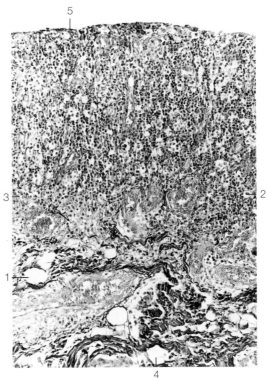

Fig. 862. Cortison arthritis (synovitis) with superimposed bacterial infection; HE, ×40

14 Tumorous Joint Diseases

General

Various kinds of primary neoplasms and tumor-like lesions can develop in the joint capsule, mostly taking origin in the synovial membrane. On the one hand these may show a certain similarity to the morphological structure of the synovial membrane, or they may show no such similarity. Some of these joint tumors are only included in this group of neoplasms because of their localization. Most of the neoplasms may be considered to be histogenetically derived from the tissues of the joint capsule. Entirely similar tumors may be observed either in the soft parts or even in the bone.

In order to understand the origin of neoplasms in the joint capsule one must call to mind the normal formation of the tissues of the capsule and the synovial membrane (p. 28). The inside of the joint cavity is lined with *synovial epithelium*. This can undergo tumorous proliferation and lead to the development of villi. Persistent and continuous movement of the affected joint results in non-specific inflammation and very often also in hemorrhage also. This leads to the picture of a so-called *pigmented villonodular synovitis*. Under these circumstances there is inflammation of the proliferating synovial villi, in which the deposition of hemosiderin pigment indicates former hemorrhages. In fact, this is a benign tumor of the joint capsule. The origin of its malignant variant – the *synovial sarcoma* – from the synovial tissue is much more difficult to recognize morphologically. In such a case there is no formation of villi, and the tumor cells grow and infiltrate and no longer resemble normal synovial epithelium.

At this point it is necessary to call attention to the fact that the tendon sheaths have a similar epithelium to the synovial membrane and that tumors similar to the primary joint neoplasms can develop from them as well. This means that a synovial sarcoma can arise close to a tendon sheath and need not necessarily be localized in the neighborhood of a joint capsule; it may thus be a completely straightforward parosteal tumor (see Chapter 15). The benign variants of the tendon sheath tumors include *de Quervain's tendovaginitis stenosans* and the *benign giant cell tumor of the tendon sheath* (localized nodular synovitis, p. 462).

Apart from the synovial epithelium the tissue of the joint capsule includes mostly connective tissue and blood vessels, lymphatics, fatty tissue and nerves. Tumors can arise from any of these, although these types of neoplasm are rare. Occasionally, however, we see *fibromas* and *fibromatosis* in a joint capsule, and sometimes even a *fibrosarcoma* may be diagnosed. Vascular tumors *(hemangiomas, lymphangiomas)* may appear which have the same histological formation in both the soft parts and in bone. Finally, *lipomas* and even *liposarcomas* have been described in the region of a joint, although it is not clear whether we are dealing with a true primary capsular neoplasm or whether the tumor has arisen in the pararticular soft parts and infiltrated into a neighboring joint capsule from outside. Tumors have been described within a joint capsule that are unambiguously soft tissue growths. These include the *epithelioid sarcoma* and the *clear-cell sarcoma* which are especially observed in the tendon sheaths. Probably these are soft tissue tumors that have invaded the tendon sheath and joint capsule.

Since both the joint capsule and the tendon sheath are derived from mesenchymal tissue, benign or malignant metaplasia can arise. Either metaplastic bone tissue or cartilaginous tissue can develop. The latter leads in the benign tumorous variants to *synovial chondromatosis*, and in the malignant form to the *synovial chondrosarcoma*. The bony neoplasms of the joint capsule include the *parosteal osteoma* and the *parosteal osteosarcoma* (p. 288). Finally, metastatic tumorous tissue can also establish itself in a joint capsule, but that is rare.

Synovial Chondromatosis (ICD-O-DA-M-7367.0)

The cartilaginous tissue in a joint capsule can differentiate metaplastically and undergo tumor-like growth. *Synovial chondromatosis (synovial osteochondromatosis) is a benign tumorous alteration of the pararticular tissue during which metaplastic nodular foci of cartilage and bone arise in the synovial membrane, which frequently lead to so-called "free joint bodies", thus impairing joint function and damaging the joint.* Changes of this sort can occasionally also occur in a tendon sheath or bursa. The cause of this new formation is unknown. Joint chondromatosis usually attacks only one joint, this being in over 50% of cases the knee. It is also often encountered in the elbow. **Macroscopically** the synovial membrane is hyperemic and thickened, and forms villi. Immediately beneath the synovial epithelium there are small grayish-white nodes of cartilaginous tissue. These changes may involve part of the joint capsule or the whole of the synovial membrane. Often the cartilaginous nodes are released into the joint cavity as "free joint bodies" (**Fig. 863**) and lead to considerable limitation of movement and damage to the joint.

In **Fig. 864** one can see a **radiograph** showing joint chondromatosis of the right elbow joint. The joint capsule is considerably thickened and interspersed with closely packed fine patchy regions of increased density *(1)* and large nodular formations which are several millimeters in diameter. The larger nodes *(2)* are themselves lobulated and nodular. Many of these formations are very radiodense, owing to calcification or even ossification. Some of these nodes are also found in the joint space *(3)*, which in places is still clearly recognizable, and they can become detached and present as so-called free joint bodies which severely impair joint function.

The **histological picture** of **Fig. 865** shows such a *"free joint body"* from a case of joint chondromatosis. Centrally one can see a roundish cartilaginous focus *(1)* which is strongly blue with HE staining. It is itself lobular in formation and has sharp borders. There are small isomorphic chondrocytes in the cartilaginous tissue, and in one place *(2)* there is characteristic calcification. The cartilaginous focus is surrounded by a thick layer of loose connective tissue *(3)* that is threaded through by a few narrow blood vessels *(4)*. The entire node has a sharp outer border with no recognizable synovial epithelial covering.

Figure 866 shows the typical **histological picture** of joint chondromatosis. The joint capsule is thickened with connective tissue and threaded through with a few fine-walled vessels *(1)*. There is no inflammatory infiltrate. In the middle of this highly fibrous connective tissue there are round nodules *(2)* of proliferating cartilaginous tissue, varying in size and surrounded by a capsule of connective tissue *(3)*. The cartilaginous nodes contain many small chondrocytes *(4)* which lie together in rounded foci. True bone tissue *(5)* has formed at the periphery of these cartilaginous nodes.

In the **histological picture** of **Fig. 867** one can again see a large cartilaginous focus *(1)* in which little groups of small chondrocytes *(2)* with roundish isomorphic nuclei are lying. Often a region of joint chondromatosis can also contain distinctly polymorphic and distended chondrocytes of various sizes with bizarre hyperchromatic nuclei. In **Fig. 867** one can also discern a synovial villus *(3)* that is covered over by narrow synovial epithelium *(4)*.

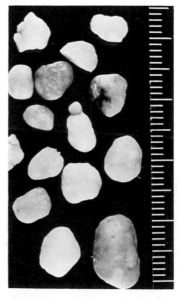

Fig. 863. Joint chondromatosis ("joint mice")

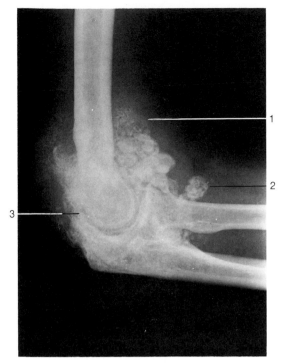

Fig. 864. Joint chondromatosis (elbow joint)

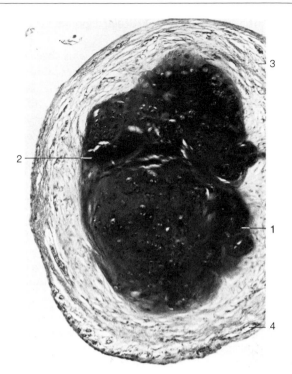

Fig. 865. Joint chondromatosis; HE, ×25

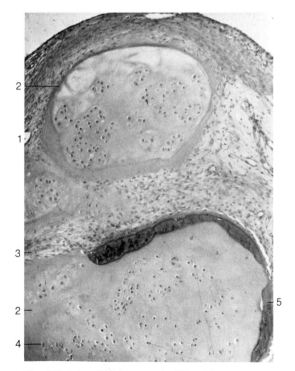

Fig. 866. Joint chondromatosis; HE, ×30

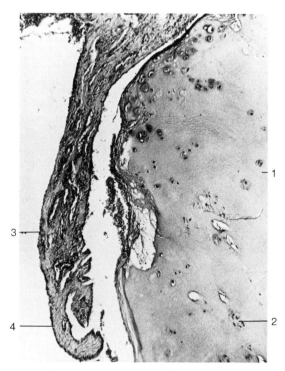

Fig. 867. Joint chondromatosis; HE, ×40

Lipoma arborescens (Diffuse Articular Lipomatosis)

Solid lipomatous tissue structures can break out at various distances from each other along the tendon sheath (endovaginal tumors), or arise like lipomas within the joint capsule. *Lipoma arborescens represents a not uncommon hyperplasia of the fatty tissue in the stroma of the synovial villi, which spreads in a papillary or polypous fashion.* Several villi are usually affected simultaneously. The lesions affects adults and is mostly sited in the knee joint, but it can appear in other joints. The main symptoms are pain and swelling of the joint, and in many cases there is also limitation of movement.

As the **radiograph** in **Fig. 868** shows, articular lipomatosis initiates no change in the bony structure. The contours of the distal parts of the femur *(1)* and the tibial head *(2)* are fully preserved and quite distinct. There are no externally caused indentations, erosions or destructive foci. The joint space *(3)* is rather wide. It is open and contains no visible deposits. The cartilaginous joint surfaces are completely smooth. The radiograph of a swollen joint such as this, with no hydrarthrosis, is virtually sufficient to exclude destructive processes such as inflammation, degeneration or a tumor.

The radiological examination can be usefully extended by computer tomography (CT) or magnetic resonance tomography (MRT). In **Fig. 869** a lipoma arborescens is more clearly shown up by **xeroradiography**. One can again see that the wrist bones *(1)*, distal parts of the ulna *(2)* and radius *(3)* are fully intact. In the joint cavity *(4)* and, seen from the side, in the capsule of the wrist joint *(5)* there are discrete, slightly villous structural thickenings corresponding to the enlarged synovial villi. These signs reveal the condition radiologically; even more so, should greater amounts of connective tissue be present in the lesions, or if there is dystrophic calcification.

Macroscopically the joint capsule is seen to be thickened and sometimes loosened by edema. Inside there are numerous deformed villi of various shapes and sizes that are distinctly yellow in color. If they have been crushed, some of these villi may become necrotic and blood-soaked.

Histologically one can see in **Fig. 870** two distinctly widened synovial villi *(1)* covered with an intact synovial epithelium *(2)*. One is struck by the large foci of mature fatty tissue *(3)* in the stroma. The fat cells are very large, have small isomorphic nuclei and themselves show no signs of polymorphy. In places the villous stroma also consists of loose connective tissue *(4)* which is largely threaded through by dilated capillaries *(5)*. Beneath the stratum synoviale there is a loose inflammatory infiltrate of lymphocytes and plasma cells *(6)*.

In **Fig. 871** one of these enlarged and ungainly synovial villi can be seen under **higher magnification**. It is clearly demarcated and covered on the outside by a single layer of synovial epithelium *(1)*. The stroma is interspersed with mature fatty tissue *(2)* of very large fat cells with small isomorphic nuclei. In between and outside there is loose connective tissue *(3)* which may be highly edematous. It contains a few capillaries *(4)*. One can also see within the villus an inflammatory infiltrate *(5)* of lymphocytes and plasma cells. There are no histological signs of a proliferative or specific inflammatory process.

Lipoma arborescens is no true neoplasm, but a tumor-like lesion that almost only appears in the larger joints. It is therefore assumed to be a reactive process that is triggered off by local trauma, a meniscal lesion (p. 434) or chronic arthritis. It is a reactive villous hyperplasia with excessive increase of the stromal fatty tissue. Not infrequently several lesions, mostly symmetrical, are observed simultaneously in several joints. An inflammatory origin is suggested by the presence of non-specific inflammatory cells in the hyperplastic villi. Since the lesion does not spontaneously regress, synoviectomy is necessary, after which recurrence is not to be expected. Lipoma arborescens must be distinguished from a true *intraarticular lipoma*. The latter is a rare benign tumor, usually found in the knee joint, that has no relationship to the synovial villi and is not covered over by synovial epithelium. *Hoffa's disease*, a traumatic inflammatory hyperplasia of the synovial fatty tissue in the neighborhood of the patellar ligament, should also not be confused with lipoma arborescens.

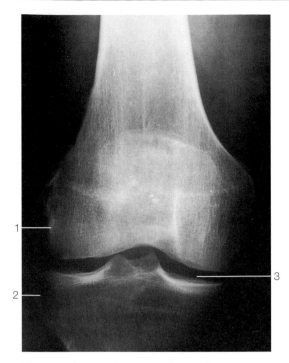

Fig. 868. Lipoma arborescens (knee joint)

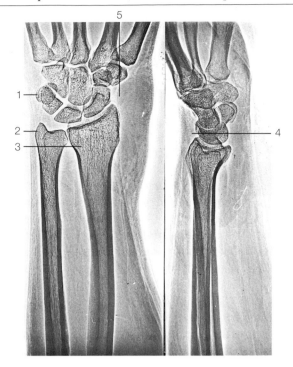

Fig. 869. Lipoma arborescens (wrist joint, xeroradiograph)

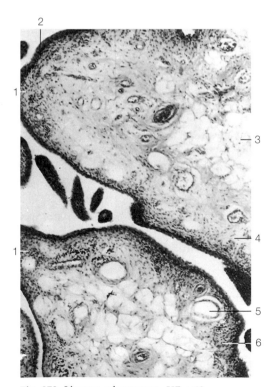

Fig. 870. Lipoma arborescens; HE, ×40

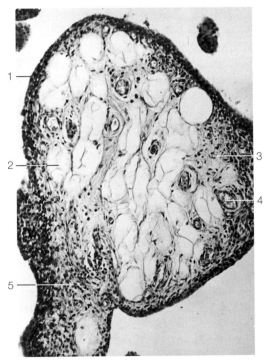

Fig. 871. Lipoma arborescens; HE, ×64

Localized Nodular Synovitis

Also to be classified among the tumorous joint changes are those lesions which can bring about an outside defect in a bone. These may develop either in the synovium of a joint capsule or in a tendon sheath. Such lesions are found relatively often in operation specimens and are described as *"benign giant cell tumors of the tendon sheath"*. *Localized nodular synovitis is a so-called "benign giant cell tumor of the tendon sheath" consisting of an augmentation of histiocytes and fibromatous cells, and it can produce sufficient pressure to cause a destructive indentation in the neighboring bone.* The principal site is in the phalanges of the hands, predominantly at the distal end of these bones. Such lesions can, however, appear in the neighborhood of the joints of the feet and hands, or in the regional joints themselves, i.e. ankle and wrist.

Figure 872 shows a classical **radiograph** of a localized nodular synovitis that has led to an osteolytic bone defect. In the region of the intermediate *(1)* and proximal *(2)* phalanges of the little toe one can discern at each site a deep concave indentation in the bone which has obviously been caused by outside pressure. In the soft parts there is a slight shadowing which indicates the presence of tumorous growth. The short tubular bones in this region are very porous, and the bone tissue has reacted to the defect with an osteosclerotic increase in density *(2)*. There are also cystic destructive foci in this bone *(3)*, but no periosteal reaction is present.

Histologically this is a highly cellular tissue that can, even within the same tumor, show very different cellular pictures. In **Fig. 873** one can see a highly cellular tumorous tissue *(1)* subdivided into nodular areas by narrow connective tissue septa *(2)*. It is in contact on one side with loosened tendinous tissue *(3)*, since the tumor has originated either from the tendon sheath or joint capsule. Even in this overall view the giant cells *(4)*, which are loosely distributed throughout the tumorous tissue, are striking. One can also observe a few bands of hyalinization. Lesions of this kind can also show dense fibrosis and extensive hyalinization, and are then much poorer in cellular content; though this provides no clues to the age of the tumor or to how much it may proliferate. The densely packed cells in this neoplasm are mostly histiocytic cells. Necrotic foci and focal deposits of hemosiderin may also be present. In a third of the cases narrow spaces *(5)* can be observed. These are lined by flat or distorted cells, presenting a certain similarity to a synovial sarcoma (p. 466). Glandular structures such as are found in a synovial sarcoma are, however, absent.

Under **higher magnification** one can see in **Fig. 874** that the lesion is predominantly histiocytic. On one side *(1)* there is a fibrillated tendon sheath and its tendon which mark off the tumor fairly sharply. The histiocytes *(2)* have elongated oval, somewhat indented nuclei with varying degrees of chromatin content and an abundant, often clear cytoplasm that may also contain hemosiderin granules. A certain amount of nuclear polymorphy and mitotic activity should not be interpreted as indicating malignancy. A few multinucleated giant cells *(3)*, variable in number and irregularly distributed, are found dispersed throughout the tumor. In some lesions, numerous giant cells and also foam cells are present.

Under **even higher magnification** a localized nodular synovitis can be seen in **Fig. 875**. The tumor contains mostly histiocytes with dark oval or roundish nuclei *(1)*. The size, shape and chromatin content of the nuclei are variable *(2)*. Nuclei which are poor in chromatin contain one or two nucleoli. Cells with abundant honeycomb-like cytoplasm (the so-called foam cells) containing sudanophilic material (fat) are strewn about. One also sees unevenly distributed multinucleated giant cells *(3)*, repeatedly interspersed by hyaline bands *(4)*. This histological picture is practically identical with that of a benign giant cell tumor of the tendon sheath (p. 476).

Depending on the localization of each, one can distinguish "localized nodular tenosynovitis" from "localized nodular joint synovitis", although the histological structures are identical. When there are extensive complexes of foam cells present, the term "fibrous xanthoma of the synovium" is often used. Clinically speaking, the lesion must be completely extirpated through healthy tissue; if excision is incomplete, a 12%–16% recurrence rate is to be expected.

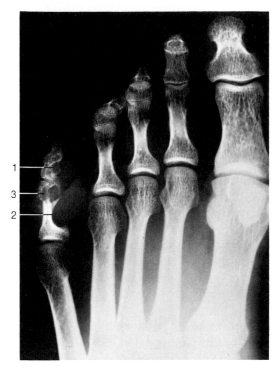

Fig. 872. Localized nodular synovitis (little toe)

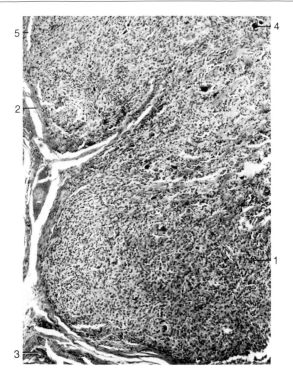

Fig. 873. Localized nodular synovitis; HE, ×20

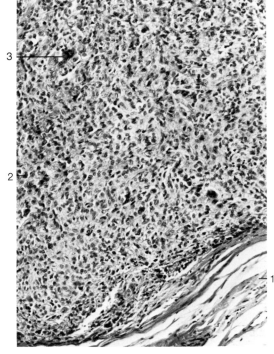

Fig. 874. Localized nodular synovitis; HE, ×40

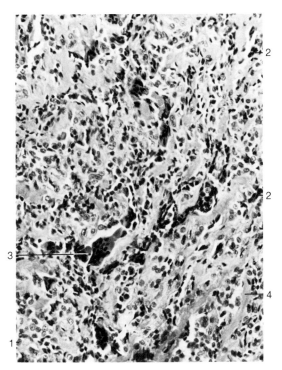

Fig. 875. Localized nodular synovitis PAS, ×64

Pigmented Villonodular Synovitis
(ICD-O-DA-M-4783.0)

Proliferation of the synovial epithelium which shows the characteristics of a benign tumor can develop in a joint capsule, tendon sheath or bursa. *Pigmented villonodular synovitis is a diffuse proliferation of the synovial epithelium and connective tissue with the formation of brown-colored villi and nodes.* This lesion is the benign counterpart of the synovial sarcoma (p. 466) and can be described as a benign tumor of the joint capsule. On the other hand the changes may be regarded as reactive and caused by inflammation, or classified under the fibrous histiocytomas. Although the proliferating tissue of the joint capsule can on occasion erode the neighboring bone, it is essentially a benign, slow-growing lesion of unknown etiology. Pigmented villonodular synovitis generally appears in middle age and leads to pain, swelling and limitation of movement of the affected joint. The fluid in the joint is increased. The knee joint is most often attacked, but it also frequently involves the hip and finger joints. Treatment consists of total synovectomy. Incomplete extirpation can lead to recurrence, in which case radiotherapy has good results.

In **Fig. 876** the **radiograph** of a left hip joint is depicted, in which the joint space *(1)* is significantly narrowed. The femoral head is deformed. There is a dense zone of osteosclerosis in the socket *(2)* and also in places in the deformed head. Most striking, however, are the periarticular erosions which have sunk osteolytic defects deeply into the head *(3)*. These destructive foci are limited by marginal sclerosis. Several of these osteolytic foci *(4)* are found in the neighborhood of the articular cartilage. Usually no osteoporosis can be seen in the surrounding regions. The soft tissues of the joint capsule are swollen and thickened. In the adjacent parariticular soft parts there is a diffuse shadowing (not recognizable in Fig. 876).

Macroscopically the tumorous tissue consists of a thickened, villous, brownish-red synovial membrane which is in places nodular. In the **histological picture** shown in Fig. 877 one can discern these densely packed synovial villi *(1)*. Some of them are narrow, some misshapen and broad. They are covered over exteriorly with flattened synovial epithelium *(2)*. The villous stroma consists of loose connective tissue which is threaded through with many fine-walled blood-filled vessels *(3)*. It is highly cellular and contains, as well as the usual inflammatory cells (lymphocytes, plasma cells), many histiocytic cells with a light cytoplasm. These are macrophages, most of which have taken up a brown hemosiderin pigment. Occasionally multinucleated giant cells are observed in the villous stroma. The mere presence of multinucleated giant cells in a synovial lesion is, however, not sufficient to justify a diagnosis of pigmented villonodular synovitis. The radiological changes, macroscopic appearance and the histological picture must together be taken into account. In the final stages of this disease, extensive hyalinization of the villous stroma is found.

In **Fig. 878** one can see a proliferating villus *(1)* from a case of pigmented villonodular synovitis. It is covered on the outside with a flattened, loose synovial epithelium *(2)*. In the highly cellular villous stroma there are abundant dark deposits of hemosiderin pigment *(3)*. Apart from this it has been infiltrated by a large number of inflammatory cells (lymphocytes, plasma cells and histiocytes). Under **higher magnification** these structures are more clearly seen. In **Fig. 879** one can discern the tip of a villus *(1)* the walls of which are raised up by nodules. It is covered over on the outside by a synovial epithelium *(2)* that is partly flattened, partly thickened. In the highly cellular stroma one can see dilated blood capillaries *(3)* and infiltrates of lymphocytes, plasma cells and histiocytes. The latter contain a brown pigment (iron pigment, *4*) that colors the entire villus. The nuclei of the histiocytes vary in size and are often hyperchromatic. Sometimes one is struck by the number of mitoses, which should nevertheless not be taken as a sign of malignant growth.

Because of its invasive and destructive growth, villonodular synovitis is classified among the semimalignant joint neoplasms. After incomplete extirpation of the diseased region of villi, 20%–25% of the cases show local recurrence. Malignant change with the development of metastases has not so far been described.

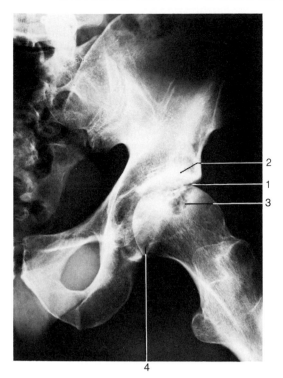

Fig. 876. Pigmented villonodular synovitis (hip joint)

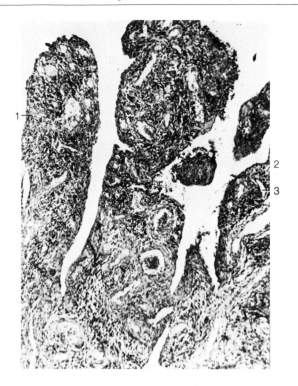

Fig. 877. Pigmented villonodular synovitis; HE, ×25

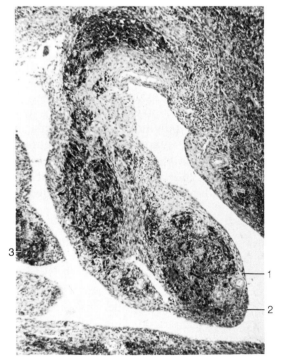

Fig. 878. Pigmented villonodular synovitis; HE, ×25

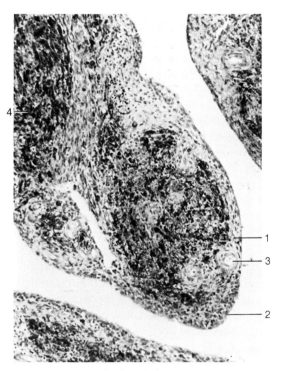

Fig. 879. Pigmented villonodular synovitis; HE, ×40

Synovial Sarcoma (ICD-O-DA-M-9040/3)

Malignant tumors which develop primarily in a joint capsule or the peritendinous soft tissues are rare. Cases of "clear cell sarcoma of the tendon sheath", "synovial chondrosarcomas" and "epithelioid sarcomas" have been described. The main representative of this group is, however, the synovial sarcoma (malignant synovioma). *This is a highly malignant mesenchymal neoplasm that usually develops in the neighborhood of the joints of the limbs, tendon sheaths or bursae and is probably derived from cells of the synovial membrane.* The tumor can, however, be found at a distance from these structures. The synovial sarcoma represents about 10% of all soft tissue sarcomas. In 70% of cases the lower limb is involved. Of the tumors, 50% are found in the region of the knee joint, 25% in the upper limbs and 5% in the trunk, head or neck. It can arise at any age, but mostly in young adult life (between 15 and 30 years of age; 50% incidence). The tumor usually presents as a painful swelling, but there may be pain alone which can last for 6 to 12 months. In 15% of the patients the symptoms have been present for 5 years, meaning that it is often a very slow growing tumor. Its marked tendency to calcification is remarkable, so that calcified masses in the soft parts should awake suspicion of a synovial sarcoma. Following surgical removal of the tumor a recurrence is found in 50%–70% of cases, indicating a deterioration in the prognosis. Early amputation should therefore be considered. Metastases appear mostly in the lungs via the blood stream, less commonly in the lymph nodes.

Figure 880 shows the **radiograph** of a synovial sarcoma of the right knee joint. A poorly demarcated tumorous mass *(1)* is clearly seen in the popliteal fossa which has invaded the joint cavity *(2)* and which is seen in the angiogram to have displaced the popliteal artery outwards *(3)*. The shadow of the neoplasm shows dense patches and marked vascularization. The adjacent bones have been eroded.

Histologically the tumorous tissue is highly cellular and consists of two different structural elements *(biphasic type)*, that is to say, cleft-shaped or acinar structures which are lined with epithelial-like cells, and areas of spindle cells. The proportional distribution of these structures is highly variable; the spindle-cell component may alone be present *(monophasic type)*, which easily leads to the diagnosis of a fibrosarcoma. In **Fig. 881** one sees highly cellular tumorous tissue consisting of densely packed spindle cells *(1)* with dark polygonal nuclei (often showing mitoses) and arranged in ridges. This type of tumorous tissue is identical with that of a fibrosarcoma (p. 333). A typical synovial sarcoma also has elongated bands of hyalinization *(2)*, and sometimes calcifications. The tumorous tissue is threaded through with dilated blood vessels *(3)*.

In **Fig. 882** one can see the epithelial-like structures **histologically**. The synovioblasts lie together in roundish groups *(1)* that are surrounded by a narrow seam of connective tissue. They have an abundant clear cytoplasm and dark polymorphic nuclei, in which atypical mitoses are repeatedly observed. These are solid epithelial-like complexes which can easily be taken in a biopsy for a carcinomatous metastasis. No cleft formation can be seen in this tumorous tissue. Collections of spindle cells *(2)* are only few in number, and are threaded through with blood capillaries *(3)*. In this tumorous tissue there are large flat necrotic areas *(4)*.

As is clear in **Fig. 883** the tumor can also have a markedly glandular appearance **histologically**. We can see large cystic cavities *(1)* which may be empty or contain blood. They are coated with large polymorphic synovioblasts *(2)*. In between, the synovioblasts are grouped around the clefts as well *(3)*. The spindle cells also represent synovioblasts, between which collagenous and reticular fibers can be identified.

The histological structures described above with their enormous variety and similarity to other malignant tumors make the diagnosis very difficult. The neoplasm takes its origin from the pararticular soft parts and rarely develops within a joint capsule. Its size and separation from the surrounding soft parts can be demonstrated by computer and magnetic resonance tomography. The tumor must be excised immediately, since with every recurrence there is a considerable deterioration in the prognosis.

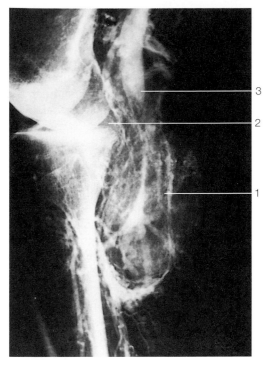

Fig. 880. Synovial sarcoma (knee joint, angiogram)

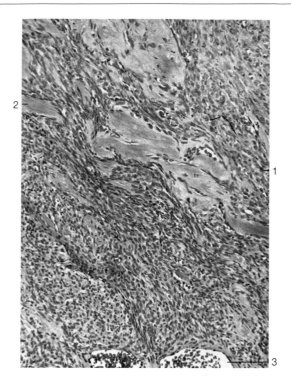

Fig. 881. Synovial sarcoma; HE, ×25

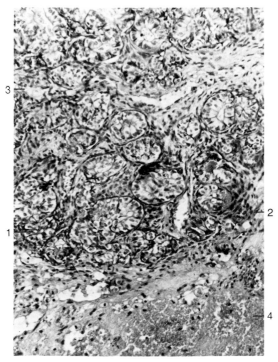

Fig. 882. Synovial sarcoma; PAS, ×40

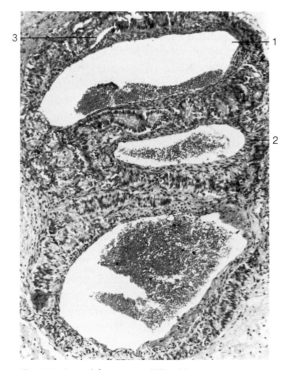

Fig. 883. Synovial sarcoma; HE, ×32

As shown in **Fig. 884** a synovial sarcoma can develop outside a joint, namely, in the neighborhood of a tendon sheath. In the lateral **radiograph** of the proximal part of the leg near the fibula one can see an oval tumorous focus in the soft parts *(1)* that is clearly shown up by its extensive calcification. The tumor is densely structured in the center and shows a fine shell-like porosity outside. The border is in places unclear *(2)* and a few discrete patches of calcification can be seen in the surrounding area also. The tumor obviously has no connection with the bone, and between it and the fibula there is a tumor-free space *(3)*. The structure of the adjacent bone is unchanged. With this sort of soft tissue focus on the radiograph one thinks at first of a calcified hematoma and then of post-traumatic myositis ossificans (p. 478). A histological examination is therefore absolutely necessary so that the whole lesion may immediately be extirpated by incising deeply into the healthy tissue.

Outside the calcified zone the highly cellular tumorous tissue has a malignant appearance **histologically**. In **Fig. 885** we can see groups of small roundish cells with little cytoplasm and hyperchromatic nuclei of various sizes *(1)*. The extensive formation of clefts *(2)* where these tumor cells are deposited is striking, so that the picture resembles that of an angioma. Closer observation, however, reveals that these clefts are not lined with endothelium and that they contain no erythrocytes. They can be contrasted with the endothelium-lined capillaries *(3)* which run through the tumorous tissue. The stroma, in which bands of hyalinization *(4)* are present, is characteristic and quite typical of a synovial sarcoma. In general it is completely undifferentiated mesenchymal tumorous tissue, which is often difficult to classify. In many tumors there are tissue structures that remind one of a hemangiopericytoma (p. 377). Staining for reticular fibers can be helpful, and equally, immunohistochemical methods may be applied. The tumor cells of a synovial sarcoma express cytokeratin and vimentin. If there are no epithelioid or glandular structures present in such a tumor it is the monophasic type of synovial sarcoma.

Another synovial sarcoma that is located away from the region of the joint can be seen in the **radiograph** of Fig. 886. Here one sees a large, poorly demarcated, soft tissue shadow *(1)* in the distal part of the leg, near the fibula. The coarse and fine calcareous deposits *(2)* near the bone are striking. This kind of patchy calcification seen in the radiograph ought to make one think of a synovial sarcoma, even when the tumor is not associated with a joint. It is obviously reaching out behind at the back of the leg, since one can see tumorous shadowing between the fibula and tibia *(3)*. The tumor can erode the bone from outside and even infiltrate into it, producing a malignant tumorous bone defect. In such cases the interpretation of the radiological findings is particularly difficult. A tumorous growth of this kind is suggested by the slightly undulating outer contours of the tibia and fibula *(4)*. In contrast to pigmented villonodular synovitis (p. 464) the bone in the neighborhood of a synovial sarcoma often shows signs of diffuse osteoporosis. In general, this type of parosseal tumor with dense or patchy calcification and possible erosion of bone should make one think of a synovial sarcoma.

In rare synovial sarcomas the epithelioid structures may predominate, so that a differential diagnosis from other tumors (e.g. a carcinomatous metastasis, malignant schwannoma, epithelioid sarcoma) must be considered. In **Fig. 887** one can see **histologically** a highly cellular, obviously malignant tumorous tissue which in this section consists entirely of epithelioid cells. The nuclei vary in size and are polymorphic. They contain one or more prominent nucleoli *(1)*. Pathological mitoses are also encountered *(2)*. A few giant nuclei are present *(3)*. The stroma is only sparsely developed. Differentiated structures (such as clefts and pseudoglands) are not present. This is a **monophasic epithelioid synovial sarcoma**. Here a malignant melanoma or a metastasis therefrom must be included in the differential diagnosis. One can see that the histological picture of the synovial sarcoma is extraordinarily variable and can often only be diagnosed by special immunohistological and electron microscopic examination (p. 507).

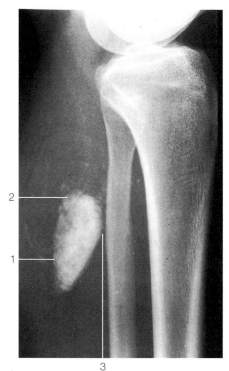

Fig. 884. Calcified synovial sarcoma (proximal part of leg)

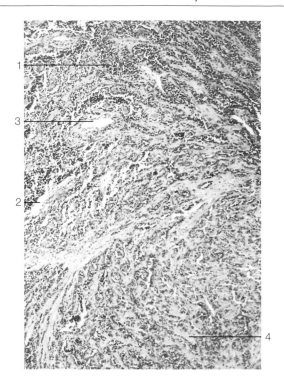

Fig. 885. Synovial sarcoma; HE, ×40

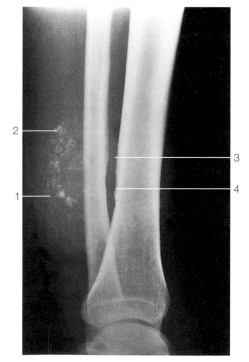

Fig. 886. Calcified synovial sarcoma (distal part of leg)

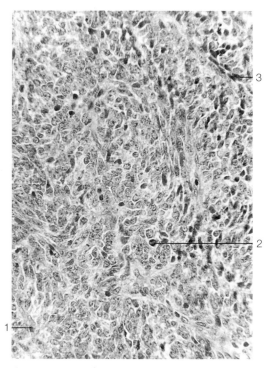

Fig. 887. Synovial sarcoma (monophasic epithelioid type); PAS, ×64

15 Parosteal and Extraskeletal Lesions

General

The individual bones of the skeleton stand in close functional relationship to the surrounding soft tissues. Even from the descriptive point of view, both are differentiated from mesenchymal tissue, so that the influence of one upon the other is mutual, and, from the structural point of view, they are very similar tissues. Topographically the bones are in close contact with the surrounding soft parts. Even with the periosteum, which is regarded as being part of the bone, the transition from bone to soft tissue has already begun. Pathological processes which develop primarily in the periosteum (for instance, periostitis ossificans, p. 160; the periosteal chondrosarcoma, p. 252; the parosteal osteosarcoma, p. 288) usually initiate a reaction both in the bone as well as in the adjacent soft tissues, where they may be identified and analyzed radiologically. The soft parts in the immediate neighborhood of the bone, which also have a close functional relationship to the skeleton, include in particular the ligaments, tendons and bursae. It is here that degenerative, inflammatory or even neoplastic conditions may develop. Such localized lesions often cause pain and other symptoms, and are therefore excised and sent to the pathologist for a histological opinion. For instance, we are often presented with a *ganglion*, which is a degenerative focus in the mesenchyme. A painful, inflammatory bursa is frequently removed from the knee or elbow joints, leading to the diagnosis by the pathologist of *bursitis*. In the same way inflammation of the tendon sheath can bring about severe pain which, because of local fibroblastic proliferation, may even awake suspicion of a tumor *(de Quervain's tendovaginitis stenosans)*. Very similar tumor-like lesions with numerous histiocytic cells and multinucleated giant cells can, as in the joint capsule (localized nodular synovitis, p. 462), also develop in a tendon sheath. This is very often a case of the so-called *benign giant cell tumor of the tendon sheath.*

A series of extraskeletal lesions are characteristically associated with the differentiation of both bone and cartilaginous tissue, so that they are morphologically similar to a bone lesion. Such changes are frequently parosseal; that is to say, they are found close to a bone. This applies particularly to *myositis ossificans* and *tumorous calcinosis.* Dystrophic foci of calcification and heterotopic bone deposition in the soft tissues can occur, of course, in practically any region (the buttock, for instance) or in any organ, and they are not restricted to the neighborhood of a bone. These degeneratively reactive lesions are not dealt with under bone diseases.

The close relationship between the skeletal system and the soft parts is shown by the fact that completely identical neoplasms can arise in either. We meet the fibrosarcoma (p. 330) or the malignant fibrous histiocytoma (p. 324) both as primary bone neoplasms and as primary soft tissue neoplasms. Even the desmoplastic osseous fibroma (p. 322) has its "brother" among the soft tissue tumors. On the other hand, tumors arise in the soft parts and sometimes even in parenchymatous organs (e.g. lung) which we otherwise find only in bone and regard as primary bone tumors. We can observe the classical *osteosarcoma* and also the *chondrosarcoma* at sites outside the skeleton. Extramedullary *plasmocytomas* have been described, and an extraskeletal *Ewing's sarcoma* postulated. Admittedly, however, such "extraskeletal bone tumors" are rare. If a neoplasm of this kind is encountered and diagnosed histologically, one should at first think of a metastasis from a primary bone tumor somewhere else, and, with this in mind, carry out an examination of the skeleton (radiograph, scintigram, CT, MRT etc.). Metastases in the soft parts or in some internal organ (in particular, in the lung) from a malignant bone tumor are much more common than "primary bone neoplasms" outside the skeleton.

Ganglion

A ganglion is very often observed in the soft parts, but intraosseous ganglia also exist (p. 418). *A ganglion is a tumor-like cystic lesion of the tendon sheath caused by mucous degeneration of collagen.* It is mostly found on the dorsal side of the wrist joint (tendon sheaths of the extensors) and less commonly on the volar side (tendon sheaths of the flexors), also on the back of the foot or at the knee joint. The etiology is unknown; probably it is a constitutional lesion. Local trauma cannot be accepted as the cause, but it can make an existing ganglion worse. Extirpation usually cures the condition.

Figure 888 depicts the **histological appearance** of a typical intraosseous ganglion. The lesion consists of a smooth-walled cyst *(1)* which is formed by a broad wall of loose connective tissue *(2)*. No epithelial lining of the cyst is discernible *(3)*, but it is filled with mucoid material *(4)*. This picture shows an **intraosseous ganglion**; at one side the bony structures are visible *(5)*. If a cyst like this is lined with synovial epithelium, one speaks of a *synovial bone cyst*. A similar lesion representing the herniation of the tendon sheath or a synovial membrane is known as a *hygroma* (e.g. of the knee joint).

The **histological picture** of a typical soft tissue ganglion is shown in **Fig. 889**. One can see here a partly dense and a partly looser highly fibrous connective tissue *(1)* threaded through by a few capillaries *(2)*. Inside this tissue a large focus of myxoid degeneration *(3)* has formed, giving the appearance of a cyst. It has no epithelial lining *(4)*. Sometimes star-shaped branching cells are seen within the mucoid ground substance, which is PAS positive. These are bound together by processes.

Chronic Bursitis

Bursae, consisting of a thin connective tissue wall lined with synovial epithelium, develop in places where there is much tissue movement (between bones, tendons, muscles or skin). An average person has about 150 of them. *Chronic non-specific bursitis is a common condition which develops without bacterial infection as a result of long-term overloading and causes painful impairment of movement at the neighboring joint.* Chronic proliferating bursitis is particularly common at the knee joint (prepatellar bursitis) and elbow joint (olecranon bursitis). Macroscopically the wall of the bursa is thickened with callous and has trabecula-like protrusions and a greasy film on the inner side. The bursa contains "rice grains" (clotted protein bodies) and frequently also blood.

In the **histological picture** of **Fig. 890** one can see the thickened wall of the inflamed bursa *(1)*, which is interspersed with granulation tissue. There are numerous capillaries *(2)* and a loose infiltrate of lymphocytes, plasma cells and histiocytes. In between there are bands of hyalinization *(3)*. On the inner side *(4)* one can see a loose synovial epithelium lining the bursa. The advancing proliferation is shown by the growth of granulation tissue, tangled vessels and connective tissue.

Under **higher magnification** one can see in **Fig. 891** the proliferating granulation tissue more clearly. There are numerous capillaries *(1)* and capillary buds, which are surrounded by an uncontrolled growth of adventitial cells, as if by a mantle. In the loose highly fibrous stroma *(2)* many fibrocytes and fibroblasts can be seen in which mitoses may be present. Exudates of protein and fibrin are deposited on the inner surface *(3)*. The lining synovial epithelium *(4)* is, for the most part, no longer present.

A particular variety of chronic bursitis is shown by the *Baker cyst* (popliteal cyst; p. 474) which lies in the popliteal fossa and is related to the knee joint. It may be very large and become inflamed as a result of pressure from the popliteus.

"**Bursitis calcarea**" is caused by the deposition of calcium in the wall of the subdeltoid bursa, and this can lead to painful humeroscapular periarthritis. In addition to these non-specific inflammatory conditions of the bursae, specific inflammation may also arise (e.g. tuberculous bursitis, rheumatoid bursitis). With direct bacterial invasion an acute purulent bursitis can develop.

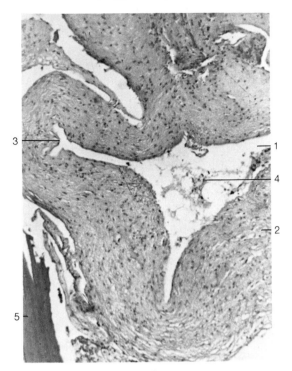

Fig. 888. Intraosseous ganglion; HE, ×25

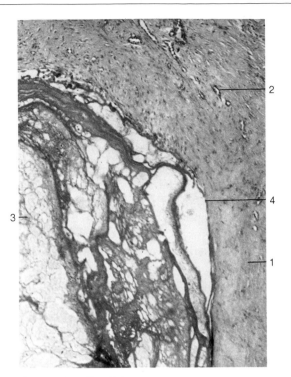

Fig. 889. Ganglion; HE, ×25

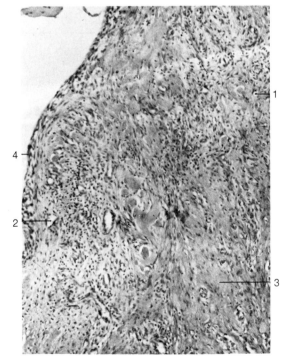

Fig. 890. Chronic bursitis; HE, ×25

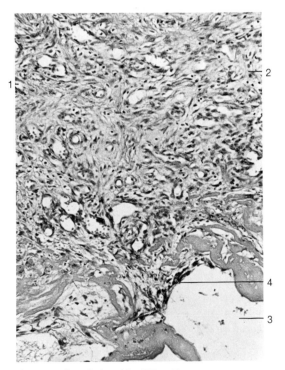

Fig. 891. Chronic bursitis; HE, ×40

Baker Cyst

Popliteal cysts and cysts in the leg in general represent bursae which serve to reduce the friction between contiguously moving components of the joint. There are up to six bursae associated with the knee joint which vary greatly in size and shape and also in the number that communicate with the joint cavity. *The Baker cyst is a hernia-like protrusion through the joint capsule at the back of the knee between the posterior surface of the tibia and the popliteus muscle (popliteal cyst) and represents a bursa specific to this muscle (subpopliteal recess).* It can become very large. Chronic compression from the popliteus can produce chronic inflammatory adhesions, leading to pressure symptoms and dragging pain.

Figure 892 illustrates the **radiograph** of a Baker cyst. In the arthrogram the cyst *(1)* is filled up with contrast medium. It is sharply marked off from the surrounding tissues. The joint cavity is also filled with contrast medium *(2)* which was able to spread from there via the two poles of the cyst *(3)* into the cyst itself. The popliteal recess *(4)*, from which the narrow neck of the cyst arises, is clearly shown. With the help of arthrography the size of the Baker cyst can be assessed, and one can see whether it has ruptured, in which case contrast medium leaks out into the surrounding region. Apertures in the wall of the cyst are a sign of hypertrophic synovitis. An uneven outer contour is indicative of inflammatory changes.

In most cases a Baker cyst is lined with synovial epithelium. In **Fig. 893** one can see the **histological picture** of such a cyst enclosing a smooth-walled hollow space *(1)*. It is lined by a single layer of very flat epithelial cells *(2)*. This is a highly atrophic synovial epithelium. It can, however, sometimes be high and stratified. The cyst has a thick wall *(3)* of collagenous connective tissue with small isomorphic fibrocytes. It therefore corresponds to the morphological formation of a bursa. The lesion is also sharply demarcated histologically. In the surrounding area there is the loosened, slightly myxoid connective tissue *(4)* of the soft parts of the knee joint. Here and in the cyst wall inflammatory infiltrates and degenerative changes are often seen.

De Quervain's Tendovaginitis Stenosans

Excessive chronic mechanical stress acting on a tendon can trigger off a chronic inflammatory reaction to the wear and tear, and this can lead to local connective tissue proliferation in the tendon sheath. *De Quervains's tendovaginitis stenosans is a local thickening of the tendon sheath caused by proliferation of the connective and scar tissue, so that the action of the tendon is impaired by narrowing of its sheath.* Most often this involves the tendons of the abductor pollicis longus and extensor pollicis brevis where they cross the radial styloid, but is can occur in other places – particularly the extensors of the wrist joint and of the forearm. Middle-aged women are especially liable to be affected. Clinically the condition presents as a palpable thickening at the site of the lesion, which is painful and causes limitation of the action of the tendon. After removal of the nodular thickening the condition is usually cured.

In **Fig. 894** one can see a broad porous tendon *(1)* with very thin elongated nuclei *(2)*. The tendon sheath *(3)* is interspersed with highly cellular granulation tissue which bulges towards the tendon. This is the active stage of the condition. In the chronic non-progressive stage there is usually no inflammatory infiltrate present. One can then see that the thickened tendon sheath consists of three layers: an inner layer of fibrocartilage with the cells arranged one behind the other, and radially orientated collagen fibers which also belong to this layer; a middle layer containing numerous blood vessels that run inwards; an outer layer of taut fibrous connective tissue.

Under **higher magnification** one can clearly see in **Fig. 895** the inflammatory granulation tissue in the locally thickened tendon sheath *(1)* with capillaries and capillary buds *(2)* and infiltrates of lymphocytes and a few plasma cells. The tendinous tissue *(3)* is here *(4)* severely narrowed. Under the continual pressure from the inflammatory proliferation on this tissue during movement, severe degenerative changes can take place in the affected part of the tendon which may even lead to its pathological rupture. In such a case the histological examination of the surgical material will verify the cause.

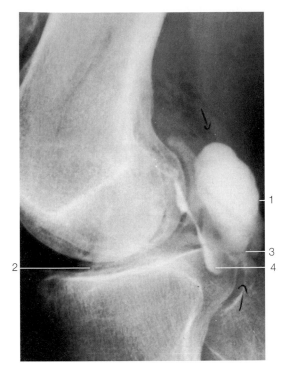

Fig. 892. Baker cyst (popliteal fossa, arthrogram)

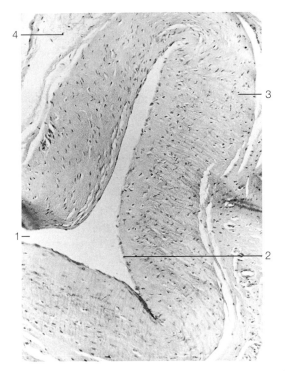

Fig. 893. Baker cyst; HE, ×20

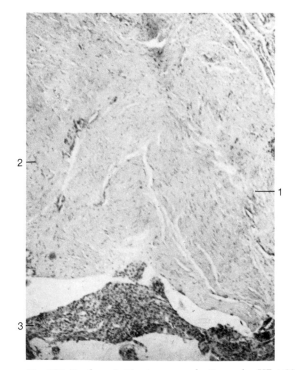

Fig. 894. Tendovaginitis stenosans de Quervain; HE, ×20

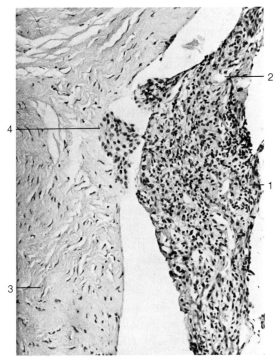

Fig. 895. Tendovaginitis stenosans de Quervain; HE, ×40

Benign Giant Cell Tumor of the Tendon Sheath

Sometimes a local proliferation in the tendon sheath cannot be attributed with certainty to a chronic inflammatory process, but has the characteristics of a neoplasm. *The benign giant cell tumor of the tendon sheath (**localized nodular synovitis**) constitutes a slow growing increase in the number of histiocytic cells and of the collagenous connective tissue, and is classified among the fibrous histiocytomas.* Of these very common lesions, 80% affect the tendon sheath, 15% the joint and 5% a bursa. It is much more frequently found in the upper limb (85%) than in the lower limb (15%), the fingers being the most usual site (70%). The knee joint is also a frequent location. It is a small nodular tumor that causes pain and limitation of movement. This tumor is not related to the giant cell neoplasms of bone (p. 337) and has no tendency to undergo malignant change. Local excision usually brings about a cure, but incomplete removal may be followed by recurrence.

Histologically one can discern in **Fig. 897** a sharply demarcated tumor *(1)* which is often surrounded by a connective tissue capsule. It lies very close to a tendon, which it often indents. The tumor itself consists of a highly cellular granulation tissue with many capillaries *(2)* and loose infiltrates, mostly of lymphocytes *(3)*. The stroma contains bands of collagenous connective tissue *(4)*. In this granulation tissue ("localized nodular synovitis") a few multinucleated giant cells *(5)* of the histiocytic type have been deposited.

Figure 898 depicts another section of this benign giant cell tumor of the tendon sheath. **Histologically** one can again see a highly cellular granulation tissue with dense infiltrates of lymphocytes *(1)*. In between there are a few plasma cells, so that one very definitely has the impression of an inflammatory process. The tissue is interspersed with uneven bands of hyalinization *(2)*. Numerous multinucleated giant cells *(3)* are irregularly distributed throughout the tissue. These are multinucleated histiocytes which do not contain acid phosphatase like osteoclasts. Nor are they tumorous giant cells. They must be regarded as part of this inflammatory process.

As shown in **Fig. 899**, the tumorous tissue can have an angiomatous appearance **histologi-**

cally. There are numerous capillary clefts *(1)*. In between there are many histiocytes and lymphocytes *(2)*. The multinucleated giant cells *(3)* are again striking. The stroma is sparsely developed *(4)* and extensively hyalinized. The *angiomatous form* of this giant cell tumor can easily be confused with a hemangioma.

Very often foam cell complexes *("xanthomatous giant cell tumor")* are encountered **histologically** in this lesion. In **Fig. 900** one can see densely packed foam cells *(1)* with clear cytoplasm and small round nuclei. In between there is a loose connective tissue stroma *(2)* that is threaded through with capillaries *(3)* and infiltrated by lymphoid inflammatory cells *(4)*. The tumor reaches right up to the border of the tendon sheath *(5)*.

Under the **higher magnification** shown in **Fig. 896** the individual cells are clearly recognizable. This is a highly cellular granulation tissue with dense infiltrates of plasma cells *(1)*, lymphocytes *(2)* and histiocytes *(3)*. In between, multinucleated histiocytic giant cells *(4)* are irregularly distributed. The wide bands of hyalinization *(5)* in this granulomatous neoplastic tissue are striking.

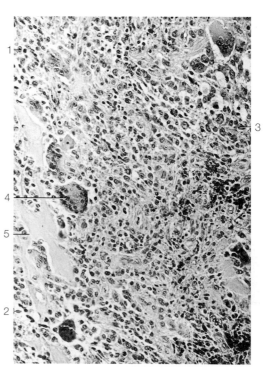

Fig. 896. Giant cell tumor of the tendon sheath; HE, ×82

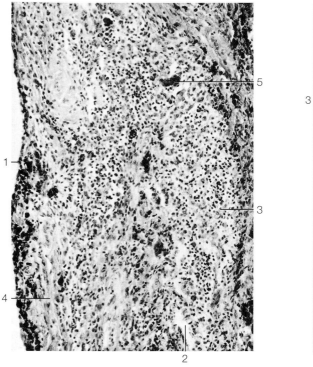

Fig. 897. Benign giant cell tumor of the tendon sheath; HE, ×64

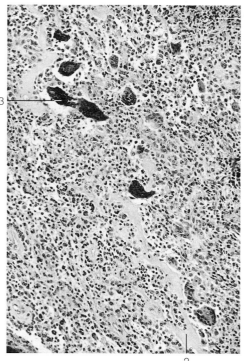

Fig. 898. Benign giant cell tumor of the tendon sheath; HE, ×64

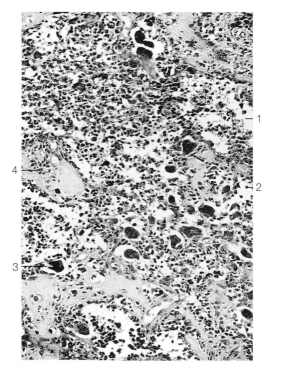

Fig. 899. Benign giant cell tumor of the tendon sheath; HE, ×64

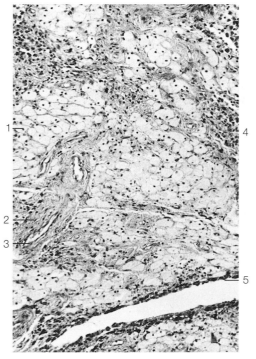

Fig. 900. Benign giant cell tumor of the tendon sheath; HE, ×64

Myositis Ossificans

Following local trauma, it is possible for a considerable amount of heterotopic bone to build up in the soft parts and give the impression of a proliferating tumor. *Localized myositis ossificans represents a benign reactive change in the parosteal soft tissues which is characterized by metaplasia and proliferation of bony and cartilaginous tissue.* The name of this lesion is not appropriate, because skeletal muscle need not be involved, an inflammatory infiltrate is often absent and, in the early stage, new bone deposition cannot yet be recognized. These changes develop within about 14 weeks after the trauma. Five months later new bone deposition takes place, and this is easily recognized on the radiograph. Of all cases, 80% are found in the arm or the thigh. It mostly affects adolescents and young adults.

Figure 902 shows the **radiograph** of a classical myositis ossificans localized near to the shaft of the femur. In this more advanced stage one can see a wide, roundish shadow, the broad base of which is adjacent to the bone *(1)*, though slightly set apart from it *(2)*. The bone itself *(3)* is unchanged. Within the lesion itself *(4)*, there is a translucent area, and outside *(5)*, increasing density.

After complete extirpation, it is possible to distinguish three different zones within this type of lesion. These are responsible for the radiological appearance, and they also characterize myositis ossificans **histologically**. As can be seen in **Fig. 903**, the center of the lesion consists of a highly cellular granulation tissue with polygonal spindle cells *(1)*, lymphocytes and numerous vessels *(2)*. Sometimes a few atypical mitoses are encountered. This is enclosed from outside by a zone, poor in cell content, where extended deposits of osteoid are found. The histological appearance of this middle zone is shown in **Fig. 904**. One can still discern areas of inflammatory granulation tissue *(1)* with lymphocytes and plasma cells as well as dilated capillaries *(2)*. In between there are extensive deposits of osteoid *(3)* containing osteoblasts. In the outermost zone, more or less mature bone has differentiated out. In **Fig. 905** one can see scarred muscle *(1)* outside the lesion and, adjacent to it, newly developed fibro-osseous trabeculae *(2)* on which rows of activated osteoblasts have been deposited. Between these bony structures there is a loose stroma which has undergone slight inflammatory change *(3)*. There is consequently an increasing maturity of the mesenchymal tissue from the center outwards until mature bone tissue is encountered at the periphery. In **Fig. 901** the characteristic triple layering of localized myositis ossificans is illustrated diagrammatically.

The triple layering that is characteristic of localized myositis ossificans comes clearly into

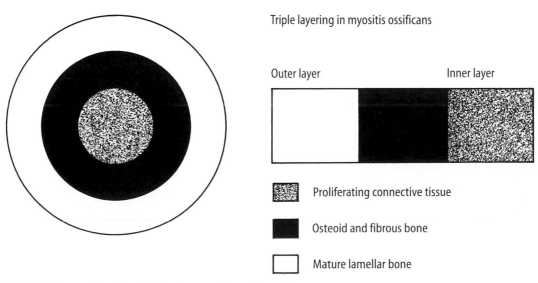

Triple layering in myositis ossificans

Outer layer   Inner layer

Proliferating connective tissue

Osteoid and fibrous bone

Mature lamellar bone

Fig. 901. Diagram showing the three layers of myositis ossificans

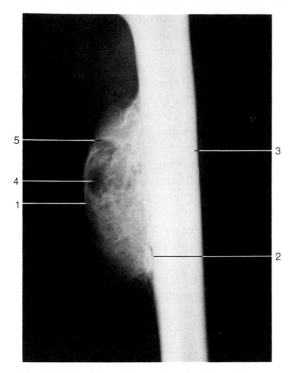

Fig. 902. Myositis ossificans (proximal femur)

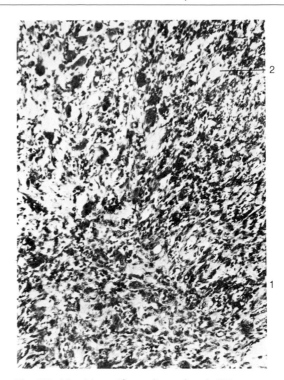

Fig. 903. Myositis ossificans (inner layer); HE, ×40

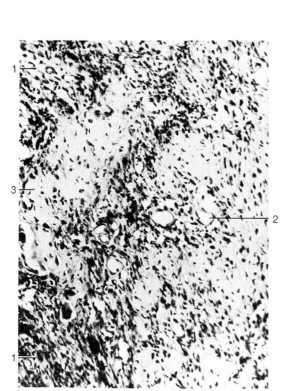

Fig. 904. Myositis ossificans (middle layer); HE, ×40

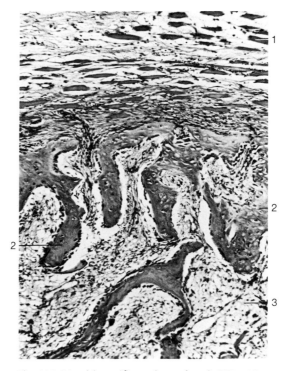

Fig. 905. Myositis ossificans (outer layer); HE, ×25

view in a **computer tomogram**. In **Fig. 906** there is on one side a transverse section through the proximal part of the right femur *(1)* which has a sharp outer contour and no sign of any defect. On the other side one can see in the soft parts at some distance from the femur a circumscribed slightly oval focus *(2)* that is bordered from without by a dense layer of bone. The center of this focal area *(3)* is translucent and has the same density as the surrounding soft tissues *(4)* – there is no increased density there. This structure is absolutely typical of a local myositis ossificans.

Figure 907 shows a **histological picture** of myositis ossificans taken from the outer zone of the lesion. One can see wide areas of fibrous bone *(1)* with large osteocytes and rows of deposited osteoblasts *(2)*. One is also struck by the metaplastic cartilaginous foci *(3)* which are not uncommonly present in this condition. In between them there is a loose connective tissue stroma *(4)* that is threaded through by fine-walled capillaries *(5)*. A larger focus with deposits of osteoid *(6)* has also settled there. The fibroblasts and fibrocytes of the stroma are completely isomorphic and show no mitoses. There is no sarcomatous stroma and no reason to suspect malignancy.

The **histological section** of **Fig. 908** is taken through the middle layer of the lesion in a case of myositis ossificans. One can see a dense network of wide osteoid trabeculae *(1)* on which layers of osteoblasts *(2)* have been deposited. There are many osteocytes *(3)*, often with dark nuclei, enclosed within the osteoid. Between these trabeculae there is a loose connective tissue stroma threaded through with many dilated capillaries *(4)*. It has also been infiltrated by a few lymphocytes.

In **Fig. 909** one can see **histologically** the innermost layer of the lesion. Here there is a loose, highly cellular granulation tissue that is threaded through with numerous dilated capillaries *(1)*. There is also a thin inflammatory infiltrate, mostly of lymphocytes *(2)*. Towards the outside, in the transition to the middle layer, one finds shapeless osteoid trabeculae *(3)* and, further out still, newly formed fibro-osseous trabeculae *(4)* with deposits of osteoblasts.

Myositis ossificans arises in various forms and can cause considerable problems in the differential diagnosis. Very rarely one comes across a *"myositis ossificans progressiva"*. This is a hereditary condition that begins in the first years of life and attacks several parts of the body simultaneously. In takes the form of advancing ossification of the skeletal muscles, ligaments, tendons and fascia, and causes immobility of the affected part of the skeleton, finally causing the death of the patient. The diagnosis is both clinical and radiological. Pathological investigation shows that the individual lesions have the same histological formation as localized myositis ossificans.

In 60%–75% of cases of **localized myositis ossificans** there has been a previous local injury (*"post-traumatic myositis ossificans"*). In 25%–40% of cases there is no history of trauma. The lesion arises in connection with a systemic disease (e.g. paraplegia, tetanus, amongst others), or else the etiology is unknown (*"idiopathic myositis ossificans"*). Localized myositis ossificans is an example of a tumor-like parosteal soft tissue lesion that is recognized by its characteristic triple-layered organization and its typical radiological and morbid anatomical appearance. The lesion is usually spherical or elliptical in shape. It must be distinguished from a calcified or ossified *soft tissue hematoma*, which also arises after local trauma. Radiologically the latter type of lesion is irregular in shape and the muscle fibers are often feathery in appearance. Ossification inside a hematoma is irregular, and there is no triple layering. The lesion can therefore be distinguished from localized myositis ossificans both radiologically and pathomorphologically. Clinically this decision is important, since myositis ossificans shows progressive growth and can recur after extirpation, whereas the calcification and ossification of a soft tissue hematoma is regressive and it does not recur after it has been removed.

Myositis ossificans undergoes *heterotopic ossification*, but can nevertheless grow and recur during the proliferative stage. It should therefore not be removed at this stage. Histologically it often shows a great similarity to an extraosseous osteosarcoma (p. 482), with which the lesion can easily be confused (it is a so-called *"pseudomalignant bone tumor of the soft tissues"*). However, with adequate knowledge of the morphology of localized myositis ossificans it is certainly possible to make the correct diagnosis.

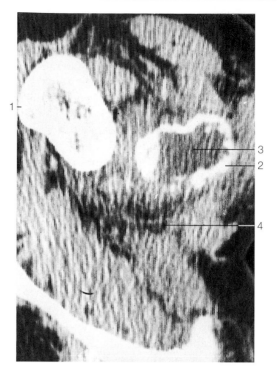

Fig. 906. Myositis ossificans (thigh, computer tomogram)

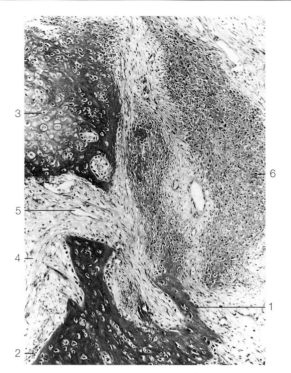

Fig. 907. Myositis ossificans (outer layer); HE, ×40

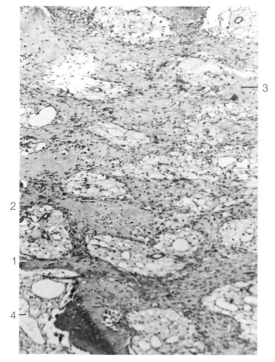

Fig. 908. Myositis ossificans (middle layer); HE, ×40

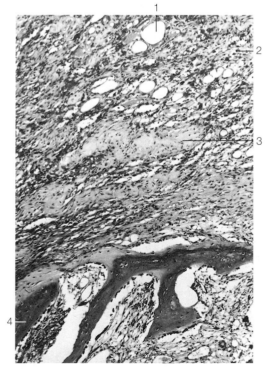

Fig. 909. Myositis ossificans (inner layer); HE, ×40

Extraosseous Osteosarcoma

This is a very rare malignant neoplasm that arises in the extraosseus soft tissues but is identical with the intraosseous osteosarcoma. The average age of the patient is usually between the 40th and 50th year, and therefore later than the age at which the intraosseous osteosarcoma appears (p. 274).

Figure 911 depicts a **radiograph** of an extraosseous osteosarcoma of the right breast. The mammogram shows an extremely densely calcified shadow in the breast *(1)* which is localized behind the mammary gland and is not in contact with the thoracic wall. The central region is so dense that no structures can be distinguished. The borders of the tumor are poorly defined. Fine processes *(2)* stream out, dense and disorganized, into the surrounding parts. The tumor reaches as far as the skin and the nipple *(3)* is drawn in.

As with myositis ossificans (p. 478) the tumor is seen **histologically** to have three layers, as is shown diagrammatically in **Fig. 910.** The arrangement is, however, the exact opposite of that in myositis ossificans, the center of the neoplasm being very densely structured whereas the periphery is seen to be more porous. This is confirmed by the histological photographs of the three layers. **Figure 912** shows the histomorphological appearance at the center of the neoplasm. One can discern the network-like arrangement of the bone structures *(1)*. These are incompletely mineralized, as is indicated by the presence of dense mesh-like patches. Within this bony area there are numerous osteocytes. In between there is only a small amount of stroma which is threaded through with wide, fine-walled blood vessels *(2)*. Thus the nucleus of the lesion consists of densely calcified tumorous bone.

Figure 913 shows loose tissue in the middle zone of the neoplasm. One can see larger areas of sarcomatous stroma *(1)* in which spindle cells with polymorphic hyperchromatic nuclei and abnormal mitoses are lying. Furthermore, there are rich deposits of osteoid *(2)* and, between them, the polymorphic nuclei of the tumorous osteoblasts *(3)*. Characteristic of this zone are the fairly numerous differentiated tumorous bone trabeculae *(4)*, which are pathognomonic of an osteosarcoma.

The histological picture of the peripheral zone is given in **Fig. 914.** This layer consists of extremely highly cellular sarcomatous stroma *(1)* with marked polymorphy and hyperchromasia of the nuclei, as well as abnormal mitoses. In between there are irregular deposits of osteoid *(2)* and abundant osteoblasts with polymorphic nuclei.

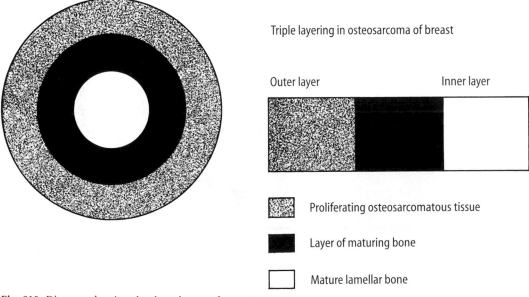

Triple layering in osteosarcoma of breast

Outer layer   Inner layer

Proliferating osteosarcomatous tissue

Layer of maturing bone

Mature lamellar bone

Fig. 910. Diagram showing the three layers of an extraosseous osteosarcoma

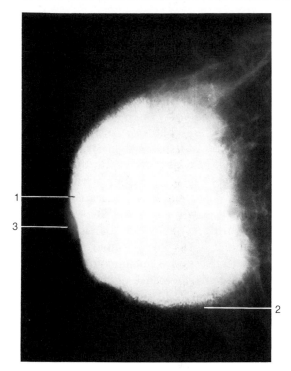

Fig. 911. Extraosseous osteosarcoma of the breast

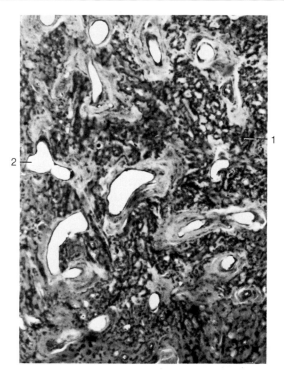

Fig. 912. Extraosseous osteosarcoma (inner layer); Azan, ×25

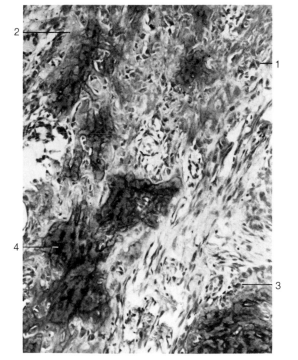

Fig. 913. Extraosseous osteosarcoma (middle layer); HE, ×40

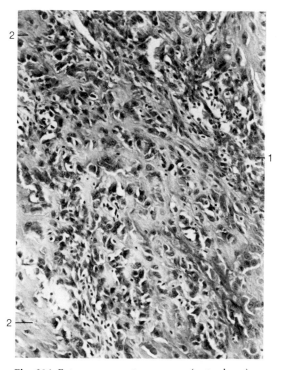

Fig. 914. Extraosseous osteosarcoma (outer layer); HE, ×40

Extraosseous Chondrosarcoma

In rare cases a true cartilaginous neoplasm can also develop in the soft tissues (or in a parenchymatous organ). *The extraosseous chondrosarcoma is a malignant cartilaginous neoplasm that arises in the soft parts and is structurally the same as an intraosseous chondrosarcoma, although it is less malignant.* This neoplasm is very rare, but several single observations have been reported (in the synovial membrane, breast, lung, heart, pharynx, larynx, orbit, beside the vertebral column and inside the cranial cavity). The commonest age for it to appear is between 40 and 50 years. Since there is no bone formation in this chondrosarcoma and only discrete focal calcifications are present, it is usually not discovered radiologically. Clinically there is an uncharacteristic tumorous mass which may cause pain. The nature of such a growth has to be elucidated histologically.

Figure 915 shows the **histological picture** of an extraosseous chondrosarcoma. Part of the tumor consists of a lobulated formation of cartilaginous tissue *(1)* in which unequally dense deposits of chondrocytes with dark polymorphic hyperchromatic nuclei *(2)* are found. Large foci of myxoid degeneration *(3)* are encountered in the tumorous cartilage, which are almost free of cells. With Alcian blue staining, large quantities of acid mucopolysaccharides can be identified. Adjoining this, there is a highly cellular mesenchymal tissue *(4)* consisting of small anaplastic cells with polymorphic hyperchromatic nuclei in which mitoses are present. Extraskeletal chondrosarcomas may therefore belong to a myxoid type or they may have the appearance of a mesenchymal chondrosarcoma (p. 250). Sometimes clefts are formed which are surrounded by tumor cells and have a resemblance to a hemangiopericytoma (see Fig. 704).

Under **higher magnification** one can see in **Fig. 916** that the tumorous cartilage has an unequal cell density. Next to clearly differentiated cartilage cells *(1)* there are small undifferentiated cells *(2)* with quite bizarre hyperchromatic nuclei.

Tumorous Calcinosis

Calcification of the parosseal soft parts can lead to severe diagnostic problems, and they can sometimes give the impression of a proliferating tumor. *Tumorous calcinosis is a condition in which nodular masses of calcium-containing material are deposited in the neighborhood of a joint.* So far, more than 50 cases have been published, in which females in the 1st and 2nd decades of life are particularly affected. There is a familial tendency and rapid growth of the lesion is often observed. The soft parts around the hip and elbow are particularly affected, although it can involve other joints, and multiple appearances are not uncommon. Local trauma is probably the cause of this tumor-like lesion, and it is likely that a metabolic disorder may also contribute. Possible hyperparathyroidism (p. 80) in particular should be investigated in these cases.

In **Fig. 917** one can see the **radiograph** of tumorous calcinosis in the region of the wrist joint. In the lateral view a shadowy focus *(1)* can be seen in the pararticular soft parts, the appearance of which suggests lobulation. Nearby there is a smaller but similarly formed focus *(2)*. Neither focus has any connection with the neighboring bones.

As can be seen in the **histological picture** of **Fig. 918**, the lesion consists of loose highly cellular granulation tissue containing only histiocytic cells *(1)*. These have bubble-like and slightly indented nuclei which are isomorphic and normochromatic. There are hardly any mitoses. In this histiocytic stroma a few non-specific inflammatory cells may be scattered about. Necrotic foci and deposits of hemosiderin are occasionally seen, and multinucleated giant cells are often present. Unequal masses of calcium salts are deposited *(2)*, which usually show a marked perifocal inflammation. After the complete surgical removal of such a lesion the condition is usually cured.

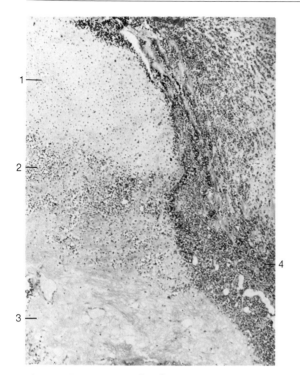

Fig. 915. Extraosseous chondrosarcoma; HE, ×20

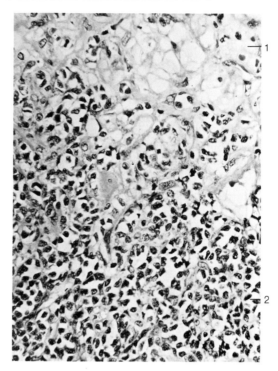

Fig. 916. Extraosseous chondrosarcoma; HE, ×100

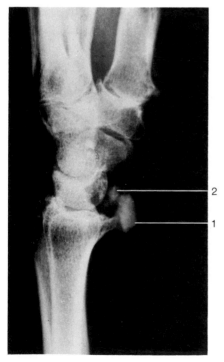

Fig. 917. Tumorous calcinosis (wrist joint)

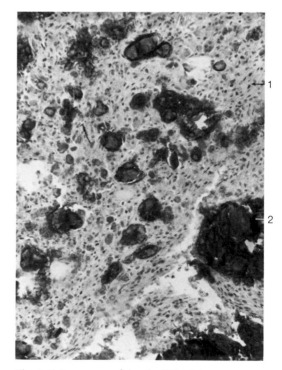

Fig. 918. Tumorous calcinosis; HE, ×40

Thibièrge-Weissenbach Syndrome

Calcification in the soft parts appearing on a radiograph should always make one think of a systemic metabolic disease. Various collagen diseases may cause calciferous foci to arise in the soft tissues. *The Thibièrge-Weissenbach syndrome consists of a multifocal parosseal deposition of calcium associated with progressive scleroderma.* *Scleroderma* is a disease of the vascular connective tissue which is probably due to an autoimmune reaction. There is an excessive increase in the number of collagen fibers in the skin and internal organs. Whereas with the benign *circumscribed form*, multiple fibrotic foci ("morpheae") develop in the skin without the serious general symptoms appearing, the *progressive diffuse form* leads to extensive subcutaneous, perivascular and submucous fibrosclerosis involving all possible internal organs (cardiac muscle, intestines, esophagus, kidneys) and finally to death. Following the arteriosclerosis, resorption processes develop particularly in the terminal phalanges of the hands and feet (*acroosteolyses*), but also in the acromion, clavicle, distal parts of the ulna and radius, and ribs. The histological background events of progressive scleroderma also take place in the joint capsules and ligaments, leading to contractures and causing progressive limitation of movement (e.g. "clawhand"). Severe non-specific *osteoporosis* often develops both in the peripheral and central parts of the skeleton.

In the **radiograph** of the left index finger of a patient with progressive scleroderma one can see in **Fig. 919** a large mulberry-like focus of calcification *(1)* in the soft tissues on the volar aspect of the terminal phalanx. This clasps the short tubular bone and projects outwards on the dorsal side *(2)*. A further large focus of calcification *(3)* can be seen in the soft tissues near the proximal end of the intermediate phalanx. In between there are other flecks of calcification *(4)*. Most of these foci are at some distance from the bone *(1)*, but they can lie so close to it that pressure defects arise *(5)*. The terminal phalanx shows signs of a slight acroosteolysis *(6)*. Such a radiological finding suggests the presence of a Thibièrge-Weissenbach syndrome and brings up the question of an existing progressive scleroderma.

Parosseal or pararticular calcification in the soft parts can, in cases of progressive scleroderma, appear in other places. In the **radiograph** of **Fig. 920** one can see such a calcification focus *(1)* on the dorsal aspect of the left wrist joint. The calcified mass is nodular and has formed a mulberry-like conglomerate of unequal density. This has no connection to the bone, and lies in the soft parts at some distance from the carpal bones. These bones *(2)* and the distal part of the radius *(3)* clearly show signs of osteoporosis.

Histologically, such a focal mass as this consists almost entirely of calcified masses without any tissue structures. In **Fig. 921** one can see coarse calcified clumps deposited *(1)* which fell to pieces during dissection. One large calcified clump *(2)* contained a great deal of calcium and stained darkly even after decalcification with acid. Unlike tumorous calcinosis (p. 484), the calcium concretions are not enclosed in a connective tissue stroma. Between them one may occasionally see a few lymphocytes *(3)*. The unequally sized calcified nodules are incompletely bordered by a broad capsule of hyalinized connective tissue *(4)*.

One can see the external capsule *(1)* under **higher magnification** in **Fig. 922**. This consists of hyalinized connective tissue, rich in collagen fibers, and containing only a few fibrocyte nuclei. Inside this, crumbling masses of calcification *(2)* are enclosed, as if in a cave. Tissue structures can no longer be discerned here. These masses are deposited in the soft parts without any signs of an inflammatory or a foreign body reaction having developed. Nevertheless, in cases of scleroderma heavy fibrotic scarring can arise in the surrounding areas. In the joint capsule, deposits of this sort can, however, produce the picture of chronic arthritis, and show arthritic changes in the soft tissues and both the collateral phenomena and the direct signs of arthritis on the radiograph. Histologically one then finds a non-specific arthritis with round cell infiltration and deposits of fibrin.

The association of a high grade osteoporosis and coarse calcification of the soft parts seen in the radiograph should make one think of scleroderma. Among the collagen diseases, dermatomyositis can also produce an interstitial calcinosis. This has a more network-like appearance radiologically.

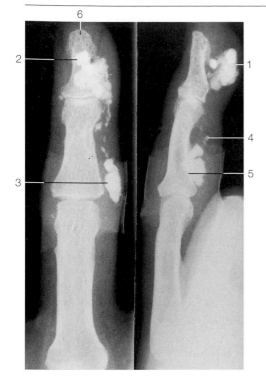

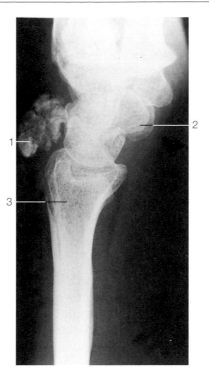

Fig. 919. Thibièrge-Weissenbach syndrome with parosseous calcium deposition (left index finger)

Fig. 920. Thibièrge-Weissenbach syndrome with parosseous calcium deposition (wrist joint)

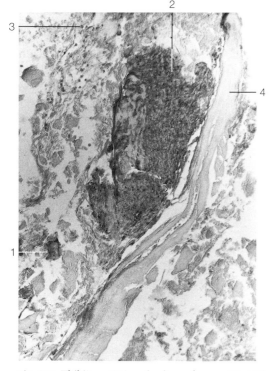

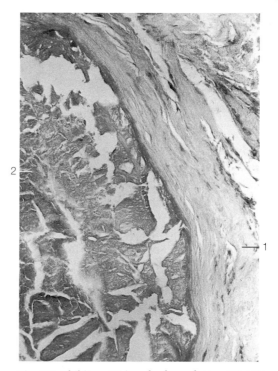

Fig. 921. Thibièrge-Weissenbach syndrome; HE, ×40

Fig. 922. Thibièrge-Weissenbach syndrome; HE, ×64

16 Examination Techniques

General

There are today an enormous number of special procedures available for examining the skeleton which can be specifically employed in difficult cases. In particular, they include techniques for carrying out radiological, pathological and anatomical investigations. In many cases of bone disease, pathologists must themselves obtain a direct impression of any radiologically observed changes in the bone, and therefore require access to the records (roentgenogram, CT, scintigram, angiogram, MRT etc.). Equally well, radiologists need to be able to recognize the macroscopic and histomorphological structural changes in bone, in order to be able to interpret and classify these with confidence as they appear on the radiograph. Interdisciplinary cooperation is often the only way of arriving at a correct diagnosis, and this must also include the clinical findings (among others, the laboratory reports).

During the last few years there has been quite a rapid development in the range of new examination techniques. In the field of radiology alone, *computer tomography* (CT) has provided an unprecedented addition to the possibilities of visualizing the various bone lesions, and providing a non-invasive method for obtaining information about the extent, biological potential and tissues of a lesion. *Magnetic resonance tomography* (MRT, NMR, MIR) has opened up unimaginable ways of obtaining insight into bone morphology without introducing the dangers of irradiation damage. These examination techniques are already in use, but they should only be employed when genuinely required. In the majority of cases one can obtain the necessary information with less expensive conventional radiological procedures. These include two *plain radiographs* (a.p. and lateral), conventional *tomography* and, when necessary, xeroradiography. In order to assess pathological remodeling in bone, one uses *scintigraphy* with radioactive nucleotides, while conventional or *digital subtraction angiography* (DSA) makes it possible to visualize the vascular structure of a bone lesion, which can provide important conclusions about the outcome.

For the pathologist the *macroscopic specimen* from the operating room is initially of major importance. The clinician provides tissue for the *histological examination,* and since this has been obtained by different methods the evaluation will vary accordingly. The preparation of the specimen (fixation, cutting) is carried out in different ways depending upon the clinical information required. When examining bone tissue, for example, it is necessary to decide whether a decalcified or undecalcified section needs to be prepared. *Histochemical methods* make it possible to visualize all kinds of histological and cytological structures. The different substances and formations, which are of such decisive significance for the precise diagnosis of many bone lesions, can be labeled by these methods. In addition to this there is *immunohistochemistry,* which has grown considerably in importance. This technique is based on the immunological reactions of cells and tissues and can lead (particularly in the case of bone tumors) to an exact identification of each type of tissue appearing in a bone lesion.

Quantitative investigations are important, particularly in dealing with the metabolic diseases, in order to assess the extent of bone resorption and thus determine the degree of bone remodeling precisely. It is here that *histomorphometry* is employed, by which the objective parameters of bone structure, remodeling and resorption can be evaluated. The quantitative and qualitative analysis of bone can also be undertaken by means of *microradiography.* These specialized radiological procedures make it possible to gain understanding of the remodeling processes and of disorders of the mineralization of bone. In the case of bone tumors, *quantitative histochemistry* is being increasingly applied to determine the content of the tumor cells. *DNA cytophotometry* of the tumor cells is particularly able to provide objective data on the degree of malignancy and therefore give information about the biological potency of the neoplasm.

In the following pages, the more important examination techniques available for the analysis of bone structures will be described.

1. Scope of Radiological Procedures for Examining the Skeleton

Radiological diagnosis is all important for the diagnosis of bone lesions. It offers the first view of the altered morphology of the bone and provides the first information about the possible nature of the lesion. The site of the lesion within the affected bone, its intraosseous and extraosseous extent, its form and structural density and many other changes which may contribute decisively to the diagnosis are here made visible. It is only after seeing the radiograph that a specifically directed biopsy can be undertaken.

The first and, as always, the most important step is the preparation of a *plain radiograph*, which should always be taken in two perpendicular planes. In **Fig. 923** one can see on the left an anteroposterior (a.p.) and on the right a lateral radiograph of the knee joint, together with the adjacent bones. In the medial part of the distal femoral metaphysis one can see a large cystic lesion *(1)*, which has pushed up the bone outwards. The lateral exposure shows that this focus has extended dorsally *(2)*. With this photographic technique the internal structure can be clearly visualized. This is a case of a *chondroblastoma* in association with an aneurysmal bone cyst (p. 412).

With some bone lesions, particularly small focal lesions, radiological sections are useful. *Tomography* allows one to visualize these within the bone, which would be impossible with a plain radiograph. **Figure 924** depicts a tomogram of the tibial shaft, in which the structures are always somewhat indistinct. One can see that the cortex on one side of the long bone *(1)* is significantly thickened in comparison with that of the other side *(2)*, and that it is also osteosclerotic. In the widest part of the cortex there is a small roundish translucency *(3)* which appears to have a central thickening. This is the nidus of an intracortical *osteoid osteoma* (p. 260). Because of the usually pronounced perifocal osteosclerosis of this tumor, it is often quite impossible to recognize the nidus, the actual pain-producing component, on an ordinary radiograph. With the help of tomography, however, it is possible to locate the tumor precisely and to remove it by specifically directed surgery.

Xeroradiography, these days a somewhat infrequently used procedure, makes it possible to visualize not only the bone structure but also the contours of a non-ossified tumor within the bone and its soft tissue components simultaneously. By increasing the contrast, the borderline between areas of differing thickness and density in the various tissues can be clearly demonstrated. The finer structures situated in the immediate vicinity of coarser ones are, on the other hand, not revealed (extinction phenomenon). By means of hardening the radiation beam, the structural elements of the bone may be visualized without loss of contrast. Whereas large areas of contrast within a bone are only imperfectly shown up, circumscribed changes in structure and soft tissue calcifications are clearly seen. In **Fig. 925** one can see a xeroradiograph of the left shoulder joint. A large tumor *(1)* has arisen within the proximal part of the humerus and grown outwards into the soft parts. Its outer border is sharply demarcated *(2)*. The tumor shows no signs of calcification. This is a *bone metastasis* from a hypernephroid carcinoma of the kidney (renal cell carcinoma). In the xeroradiograph the structure of the bone *(3)* and that of the soft tissues *(4)* are very clearly shown up.

With the assistance of nuclear medicine, additional information can be obtained on the bone metabolism. In this case, osteotropic radioactive isotopes [tracer substances: ^{18}F, ^{99m}Tc(pp)] are deposited in the bone tissue, where they cloud a photographic plate (the detector) with their own radiation. Remodeling procedures in the skeleton reveal themselves by increasing the deposition of the tracer, which is shown up by "augmented activity". **Figure 926** shows the *whole body scintigram* of a 17-year-old man, in whom the bone of the central skeleton (vertebral column *1*, pelvis *2*, thorax *3*), and the growing regions of the long bones *(4)*) are marked. The augmented activity in the right calcaneus *(5)* is striking. This is a case of *Ewing's sarcoma* which had already metastasized in the bones of the central skeleton. Whole body scintigraphy makes it possible to mark multiple foci of disease in the skeleton (e.g. metastases, systemic bone diseases). Specifically directed scintigrams of a bone lesion provide information about the local bone remodeling processes and, in the case of tumors, about the current proliferative activity.

The visualization of the vessels in a bone lesion often yields valuable information with

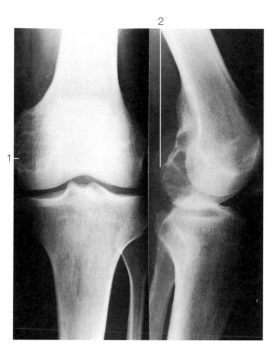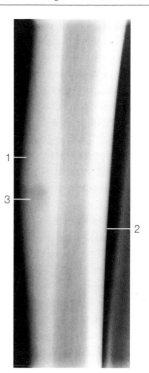

Fig. 923. Plain radiograph (chondroblastoma, distal femur)

Fig. 924. Tomogram (osteoid osteoma, tibial shaft)

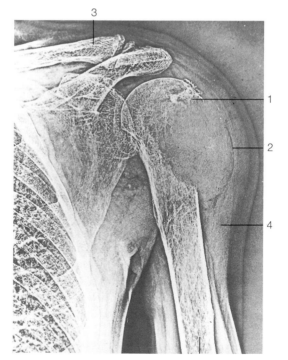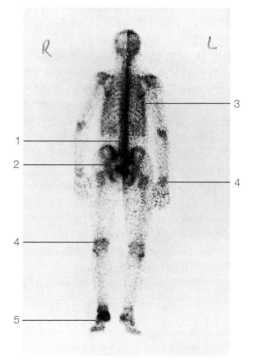

Fig. 925. Xeroradiograph
(bone metastasis, proximal humerus)

Fig. 926. Scintigram (Ewing's sarcoma, right calcaneus)

which to supplement the other radiological examinations, the most frequently employed technique being *peripheral angiography* (catheter angiography). This is a form of arteriography in which a selective iodine-containing contrast medium is injected. During the arterial phase of osteomyelitis, displaced vessels are seen in the periosteum and muscles, with a lack of vessels in the surrounding soft parts. This phase has extended into the inflammatory region, and a very early appearance of veins expresses the hyperemia of the inflamed tissue. The venous phase is characterized by increased vascularization. There is, however, no pathological vascular network present.

In contrast to this, **Fig. 927** shows a thick network of abnormal vessels in the region of an *osteosarcoma* of the left pubic bone *(1)*. These are tangled up together *(2)* and show great variation in caliber *(3)*. Particularly in the region around this malignant tumor the vessels are bundled together like the bristles of a paint brush to form a kind of cuff *(4)*. There are so-called "blood pools" and broken-down vessels. Because of the pathological anastomotic connections, the contrast medium enters the veins even during the arterial phase and spreads diffusely inside the tumor. Such an arteriogram as this indicates the presence of a malignant tumor.

With the aid of *intraosseous angiography* it has been possible to visualize the intraosseous vessels experimentally (but so far this has no clinical application!). The contrast medium is introduced through a fine hole drilled in the diaphysis and injected through a needle into these vessels. As can be seen in **Fig. 928**, the contrast medium fills the vessels *(1)* and brings the vascular network of the tumor into view. The contrast medium has spread itself out within the uneven circulation of the tumorous tissue of an *osteolytic osteosarcoma* of the head of the fibula. In the early phase, the coarse "blood pools" *(2)* fill up rapidly. At the later injection phase the medium is distributed throughout the pathological vessels of the tumorous tissue *(3)*.

Entirely new morphological aspects of various bone lesions have been revealed by axial *computer tomography* (CT). This is a radiological tomographic procedure whereby a particular three-dimensional layer of the body in the transverse plane is penetrated by a "fanbeam", while the emitting roentgen tube revolves around the patient. The CT picture consists of a matrix composed of rectangular image elements ("pixels") which represent the weakening values of three-dimensional unit volumes ("voxels"). The absorption values are stored, and a true-to-scale unlayered tomogram is reconstructed by a computer. After stepwise grading of the gray values, it is possible, by using a variable window, to visualize both the bone and the soft tissues. Tissues with low density values appear dark, those with higher values, light. **Figure 929** shows several reconstructed plane views through an *aneurysmal bone cyst* in the 1st lumbar vertebra. One can see the dense normal bone of the vertebra *(1)* and the destructive bone lesion *(2)*, which appears gray. The lesion has broken out of the bone and has spread into the adjacent soft parts *(3)*. At any desired point of the picture it is possible to obtain data (Hounsfield units) on the different degrees of radioabsorption by the various tissues (e.g. fat, bone).

With **magnetic resonance tomography** (MRT) the absorption of electromagnetic waves by atomic nuclei in an artificial magnetic field is used to produce a picture. In an external magnetic field of what is at present 0.02–2 Tesla, the summation vector of the spin ("spins") of the protons (hydrogen nuclei) is recorded; its direction can, under the resonance conditions, be influenced by high frequency impulse radiation (3 parameters: longitudinal relaxation time = **T1**, transverse relaxation time = **T2**, spin density). After cutting out the transmitter a signal is received, the intensity of which can be reproduced as a gray value in the picture. In **Fig. 930** the signal-weak bone *(1)* is shown up by negative contrast. The bone marrow, on the other hand, produces an intensive signal *(2)*. The normal soft tissue *(3)* can be distinguished from a *parosteal osteosarcoma* *(4)* by the raised signal intensity of the latter. The different gray values within the tumor *(5)* are produced by the different tissues. With MRT, not only inflammatory, degenerative, tumorous and ischemic lesions, but also traumatic soft tissue lesions can be visualized.

Using *skeletal ultrasound*, comprehensive data concerning exudates, blood vessels, menisci etc. within a *joint*, hematomas, tumors, abscesses etc. in the *soft parts* and osteolysis, exostoses, fractures etc. in *bone* can be gained.

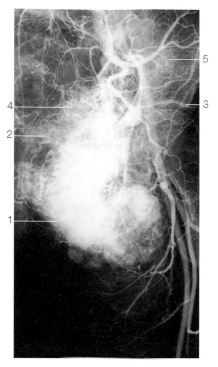

Fig. 927. Peripheral angiogram (osteosarcoma, pubic bone)

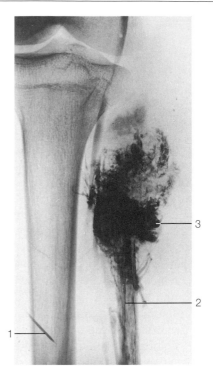

Fig. 928. Intraosseous angiogram
(osteolytic osteosarcoma, fibular head)

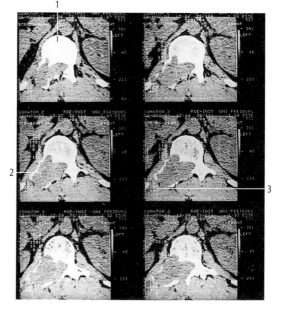

Fig. 929. Computer tomogram
(aneurysmal bone cyst, body of L 1)

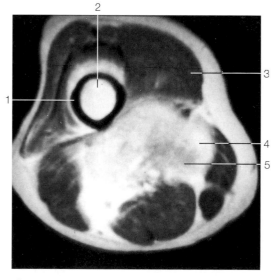

Fig. 930. MR Tomogram
(parosteal osteosarcoma, distal femur)

2. Macroscopic Specimens

With many bone lesions, larger pieces of bone and joint are removed surgically and sent to the pathologist for examination. It is essential that such a specimen should be most carefully prepared, bearing in mind that is has to provide both a comprehensive picture of the overall structural formation of the lesion as well as the basis for as precise a *macroscopic judgement* as is possible. With *inflammatory bone diseases* (osteomyelitis) the extent of the invasion of the marrow cavity by the inflammatory process should be assessed macroscopically. The amount of bone destruction and reparative remodeling (e.g. periosteal reaction, reactive osteosclerosis, involvement of the soft tissues) must be evaluated, and the color and consistency of purulent/inflammatory granulation tissue examined and recorded. Tissue should also be taken for bacteriological examination. In the case of *degenerative bone changes* (e.g. coxarthrosis deformans) changes in shape (e.g. of the femoral head) and structural changes (e.g. displacement of the articular cartilage, detritus cysts) are best observed macroscopically. The same applies to *fractures,* which can be seen in their entirety in macroscopic specimens. Particular care is needed with specimens of bone tumors. With amputation specimens the whole tumor must be laid free and completely dissected. Macroscopic analysis includes the size and extent of the tumor in all dimensions, its expansion within the bone and into the adjacent soft parts, tumorous defects or penetration of the cortex, the possible invasion of blood vessels, the appearance of the cut surface (color, hemorrhages, necroses, cysts, calcification etc.) and the consistency of the tumorous tissue. Finally, in autopsy cases, large sections of bone (e.g. from the vertebral column) may be obtained and special techniques (e.g. angiography, maceration) carried out.

Figure 931 shows a *normal macroscopic specimen* of an arm which was disarticulated because of an *osteosarcoma*. From the unfixed operation material the soft parts *(1)* were first cut into and dissected away, thus exposing the bone (humerus). One can see that only the distal part of the humerus *(2)* is present. In the proximal part there is an implanted tumor prosthesis *(3)* that was previously put into position when an osteo-

sarcoma was removed from the region by en bloc resection. The soft tissues *(4)* next to the prosthesis are hardened, mirror-smooth and gray. Tissue must be taken from this region and examined histologically in order to assess the possibility of a recurrence. There are also bloody osteolytic changes in the distal part of the humerus *(5)* which are suspiciously tumorous and must be examined histologically.

After dissection of the soft parts the bone is sawn through longitudinally. In **Fig. 932** one can see the *surface of a section* through the distal part of a femur which has been destroyed by a malignant tumor. It is a chondroblastic *osteosarcoma*. Within the marrow cavity it is in part mirror-smooth and grayish *(1)*, in part grayish-red *(2)*, and contains whitish calcifications *(3)*. The tumor occupies the entire cavity *(4)* and has broken through the cortex in several places *(5)*. It has formed a more extensive extraosseous part *(6)* that lies on the bone. Here, the soft parts have been carefully dissected away.

In order to determine the complete extent of the tumor inside and outside the bone, the excised or amputated operation specimen can be first deep-frozen and then cut into slices. This makes it possible to display both the bone and the soft parts. **Figure 933** shows such a *deep-frozen specimen* of the distal part of the femur with an *osteosarcoma*. Soft tissue *(1)* and bone *(2)* are clearly seen. Distally the spongiosa has been replaced by bone-hard tumorous tissue *(3)*. The cortex has been destroyed by the tumorous tissue *(4)* and is here soaked in blood. The tumor has grown out into the parosteal tissue *(5)*. In one place the site of a previous biopsy is clearly seen *(6)*.

One particular method of presenting systemic and local bone lesions is by *maceration*. The bone specimen is placed in a decomposing solution (hot water, enzymes) which removes all the organic material and leaves only the mineralized structures (bone) untouched. These are then bleached. The cancellous parts in particular are strikingly displayed. In **Fig. 934** one can see the *hyperplastic callus* from an infratrochanteric fracture of the femoral shaft *(1)* with displacement of the fragments *(2)* and remodeling of the spongiosa, which has been laid down along the usual tensional and pressure lines *(3)*. Ordinary fractures can also be well demonstrated as maceration specimens.

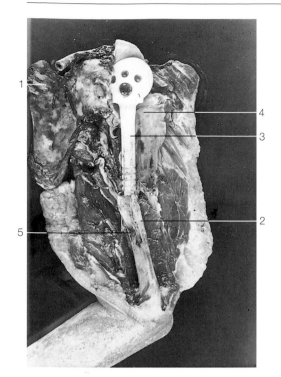

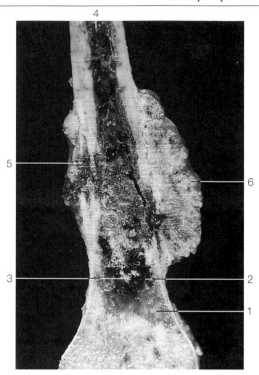

Fig. 931. Macroscopic specimen (tumor prosthesis following extirpation of osteosarcoma, proximal humerus)

Fig. 932. Macroscopic specimen – cut surface (osteosarcoma, distal femur)

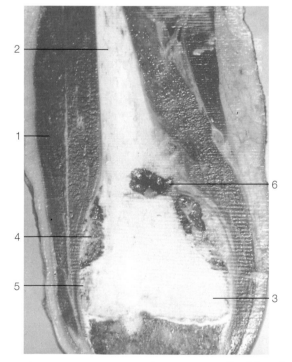

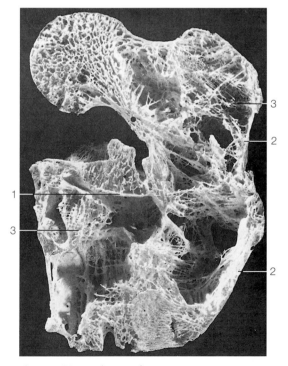

Fig. 933. Frozen specimen (osteosarcoma, distal femur)

Fig. 934. Maceration specimen (hyperplastic callus, infratrochanteric femoral fracture)

3 Bone Biopsy Techniques

The first requirement for an exact histological diagnosis is the extraction of such tissue as is specifically representative of the bone disease. This tissue can be obtained by a puncture biopsy (sample biopsy, PE), curettage, excision, resection or amputation. It is the responsibility of the clinician to provide the pathologist with representative tissue in good condition. Fragments of tissue which are too small, or tissue taken from necrotic or severely inflammatory regions, or tissue with many crush artifacts, or tissue from regions outside the actual lesion – none of these can ensure an accurate diagnosis, and may even result in an erroneous one. If the pathologist recognizes this kind of source error in a bone biopsy it must be mentioned in the report and the diagnosis recorded as conditional. Sometimes a histological section may appear under the microscope to be adequate, and the fact that it contains only perifocal tissue cannot be recognized. In this way it is easy for "osteomyelitis" (i.e. perifocal inflammation) to be diagnosed when there is in fact a malignant tumor present. This is one reason why with all diseases of bone the pathologist must always examine the relevant radiographs when making a diagnosis, in order to avoid an error. With systemic bone conditions and hematological diseases an *iliac crest biopsy* usually provides the diagnosis. This is particularly usefully in the metabolic osteopathies (see Chap. 4). It is in this connection that various biopsy techniques have been developed (Burkhardt's milling drill technique and Yamshidi's needle technique) which deliver an adequate amount of tissue. With a needle biopsy of the iliac crest or from a pathological bony focus a cylinder of tissue should be removed which is at least 2–3 cm in length and 3–4 mm wide. Such a *bone cylinder* is depicted macroscopically in **Fig. 935**.

In the case of a general bone condition (e.g. osteomyelitis) or a local bony focus (e.g. a bone tumor) representative tissue is extracted by an *open bone biopsy*, a piece of tissue being removed during the operation (excision, sample biopsy, PE). With sites that are difficult to reach (e.g. the vertebral column) a *needle puncture* is indicated, and this should be carried out under radiological control. In **Fig. 936**

one can see a lateral *radiograph* of the thoracic column. In the fused 8th thoracic vertebral body (1) a puncture needle (2) has been introduced with which to remove a representative tissue sample. Histological examination revealed only **osteoporosis** of the vertebral spongiosa.

Such a puncture cylinder is shown **histologically** under low power in **Fig. 937**. The width, shape and outer contours of the cancellous trabeculae (1) are clearly seen. The bone marrow (2) has also been completely preserved and is accessible for diagnostic examination.

With some bone lesions (amongst others, osteomyelitis of the jaws, bony cysts) the tissue is extracted by *curettage*. As is shown in **Fig. 938**, one sees numerous smaller and larger tissue fragments (1) under the microscope which should provide clues to the nature of the lesion. If one sees lobulated tumorous cartilaginous tissue there with balloon-like chondrocytes (2) the diagnosis of a **cartilaginous tumor** is easy.

The *cytological examination* of bone tumors is in practice limited to the myeloid tumors (myeloses and the plasmocytoma). Nevertheless, it allows one to draw up cytological criteria for assessing the prognosis of other skeletal tumors. In **Fig. 939** one can see a *chondroblastic osteosarcoma* with tumor cells of various sizes (1) which have slightly hyperchromatic nuclei. The nucleoli (2) are enlarged and increased in number, the cytoplasm is reduced. Tumorous giant cells (3) with increased nuclear chromatin and nucleoli are seen. This kind of cytological finding is suggestive of malignant tumor cells. Here histological examination is necessary in order to confirm the diagnosis of a malignant tumor and to allow it to be classified precisely.

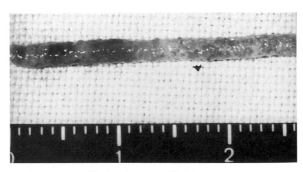

Fig. 935. Bone cylinder from needle biopsy

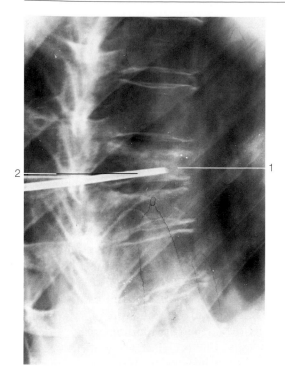

Fig. 936. Needle biopsy (compression fracture, Th 8.)

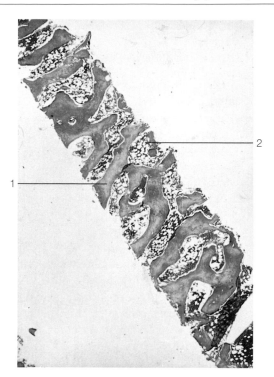

Fig. 937. Cylinder biopsy; HE, ×10

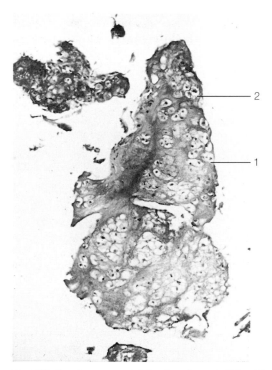

Fig. 938. Curettage material (enchondroma); HE, ×20

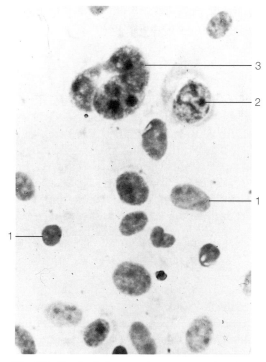

Fig. 939. Cytological smear (osteosarcoma); PAS, ×100

4 Histological Preparation

Frozen Sections (Rapid Examination)

It is sometimes desirable to be able to examine a section rapidly and obtain a diagnosis during an operation when a malignant bone tumor is suspected. In this case the softest, least calcified tissue must be taken from the suspected focus and frozen while still fresh (e.g. with carbon dioxide). The histological section is prepared in a cryostat and stained with hematoxylin and eosin (H & E). As shown in **Fig. 941**, one can see in an **osteosarcoma** highly cellular tumorous tissue with polymorphic nuclei of different sizes (1) and, in between, homogeneous tumorous osteoid (2) and bone (3). A frozen section together with the radiograph often provides evidence for a diagnosis. However, this method has only a limited application in cases of bone lesions, because with tumors that are too hard (e.g. an osteoblastic osteosarcoma) a frozen section is impossible, and important cellular details cannot be identified. A previously irradiated **osteosarcoma** certainly allows the tumorous bone (1) and osteoid (2) in **Fig. 940** to be recognized, but the sarcomatous tissue (3) shows hardly any remaining tumor cells.

Semithin Sections

A better assessment of the cytological details of bone marrow and tumor cells, particularly in iliac crest biopsies, can be gained from semithin sections of 0.2–1 μm thickness. Plastic embedding and special microtomes are required for these. A semithin section through an **adamantinoma of the long bones** is shown in **Fig. 942**. One can recognize the basaloid and epithelial tumor cells (1) within the spindle-cell tissue (2).

Fixation

Biopsy material and surgical specimens are usually fixed in *formalin* (a 30%–40% solution of formaldehyde in water). There are certain formalin mixtures available for more specific investigations (e.g. Bouin's solution, Helly's solution for the bone marrow). For iliac crest biopsies when cytological details of the bone marrow are required, fixation in *glutaraldehyde* is recom-

mended (2 ml 25% glutardialdehyde solution, 3 ml 37% formaldehyde solution, 1.58 g dehydrated calcium acetate, aqua dest. ad 100 ml. Minimum fixation time at room temperature is 8–24 h). This method is used, among other things, for semithin sections (**Fig. 942**). **Alcohol fixation** is employed when particular substances which would otherwise be dissolved out must be examined. The urate crystals in **gout**, for instance, are dissolved by formalin fixation (as seen in **Fig. 943**), leaving only circumscribed foci (1) which contain amorphous material that is not birefringent. Only the surrounding histiocytic foreign body reaction (2) makes it possible to recognize the gouty tophi histologically. With alcohol fixation (**Fig. 944**), on the other hand, the doubly refractive urate crystals (1) are preserved. One can see highly cellular inflammatory granulation tissue (2) and multinucleated foreign body giant cells (3) in the surrounding area.

The choice of special fixation methods depends upon the need to find answers to particular questions. Fixation in **acetone** is suitable for enzyme histochemistry. *Heidenhain-Susa solution* is excellent for bone sections, and for electron microscopic examination one uses *osmic acid*. The choice of the fixative depends upon each individual diagnostic requirement.

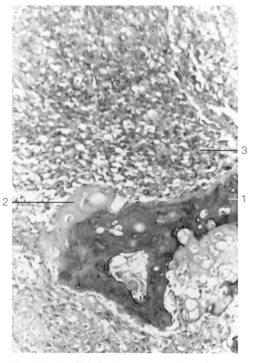

Fig. 940. Irradiated osteosarcoma; HE, ×64

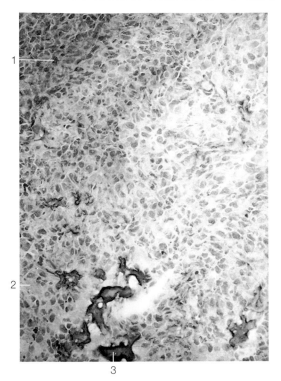

Fig. 941. Frozen section (osteosarcoma); HE, ×40

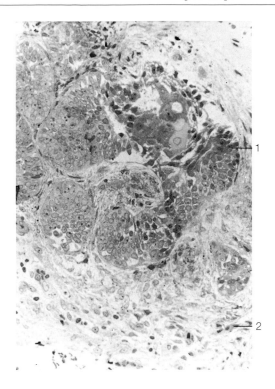

Fig. 942. Semithin section
(adamantinoma of the long bones); HE, ×40

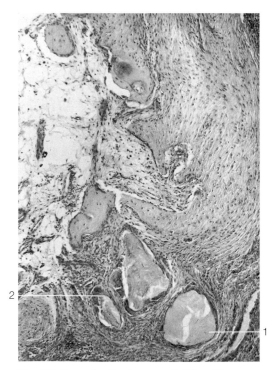

Fig. 943. Formalin fixation (gout); HE, ×40

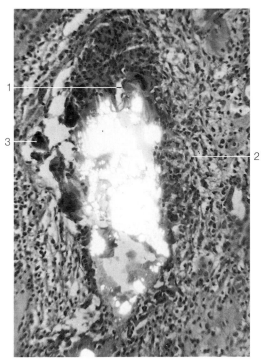

Fig. 944. Alcohol fixation (gout); HE, ×82

5 Embedding in Plastic

In order to avoid shrinkage of bone tissue and staining artifacts due to decalcification, iliac crest biopsies in particular are histologically prepared **without decalcification**. For this purpose the tissue sample must be embedded in plastic. This method for embedding bone follows short fixation in Carnoy's solution and dehydration in ascending concentrations of alcohol. The specimen is usually embedded in **methyl methacrylate** which has the same degree of hardness as bone. With special microtomes and blades it is possible to cut 5 µm sections. Thicker *ground sections* are also possible. Practically all the usual stains can be used on these sections, although the details are not always the same as in paraffin sections, because the plastic cannot be dissolved out of the tissue. Many stains and histochemical substances cannot penetrate the hydrophobic plastic embedding medium. The best results are obtained with Toluidine blue, Goldner's stain and a modification of Kossa's stain. Embedding with water-soluble *glycol methacrylate* is more suitable for water-based stains, and enzyme histochemical procedures (e.g. the identification of chloracetate esterase) are possible. What is more, the distribution of mineralized and nonmineralized bone can be assessed, and the marking of osteoid structures is particularly good, which is important for the diagnosis of osteomalacia. In **Fig. 945** one can see, embedded in plastic, an undecalcified bone section which shows the bone trabeculae in a case of *renal osteopathy*. The center is completely calcified *(1)* and appears greenish-blue with Goldner staining, whereas the varying width of the peripheral osteoid seams *(2)* is shown up in red. The bone marrow cells *(3)* are also well preserved, and the cytological details are perfectly recognizable. On the other hand, identification of the lamellar bone structure and the reversal lines is somewhat limited.

Intravital *tetracycline marking* can be used to determine the rate of mineralization within a bone, although this can only be used on undecalcified bone after embedding in plastic. Tetracycline is given by mouth with an interval of 14 days between the doses, and a biopsy from the iliac crest is then analyzed histologically. Because of its affinity for bivalent ions, this substance becomes bound to the calcium ions which are stored in the bone during deposition. As is shown in **Fig. 946**, the tetracycline becomes fluorescent under UV light. There are narrow *(1)* and wide *(2)* shining yellow bands in the osteons of the cortex which mark the mineralization fronts. Because of this double marking within a known period, the mineralization rate per unit of time can be calculated. This makes it possible to determine disorders of bone deposition and also the rate of mineralization.

6 Bone Decalcification and Paraffin Embedding

With most bone diseases the bone samples can be decalcified and embedded in paraffin. Good histological sections can be obtained after *acid decalcification* (5%–7.5% nitric acid, 5% trichloracetic acid or 5% sulphuric acid). Decalcification with chelating agents is milder *(EDTA decalcification:* 10 g disodium ethylene diamine tetra-acetic acid (Triplex III) + 3.3 g tris-(hydroxymethyl-) aminomethane (TRIS, THAM) + aqua dest. ad 100 ml; pH 7.0–7.2). The iliac crest cylinder is incubated at room temperature for about 3 days in 50 ml of the decalcifying solution. This method, developed by Schaefer (1984), can be used for all paraffin section staining and histochemical procedures. In **Fig. 947** one can see the dense, originally highly calcified bone tissue of the cortex in a section decalcified in EDTA and embedded in paraffin. The Haversian canals *(1)* and, around them, the shell-like arrangement of the reversal lines *(2)* are clearly displayed, as are the Haversian osteons *(3)* and the osteocytes *(4)*. As displayed in **Fig. 948**, the spongiosa is well preserved. The bone trabeculae *(1)* have smooth borders and show lamellar layering. In the marrow cavity the fatty tissue *(2)* and the hematopoietic cells *(3)* are clearly seen. In other words, histological examination of the majority of bone diseases can be carried out on sections decalcified in EDTA, and this will lead to a safe diagnosis. With acid decalcification, however, it is very important to ensure that the bony material is not left too long in the acid, and that it is removed precisely at the point when decalcification is complete and then embedded in paraffin.

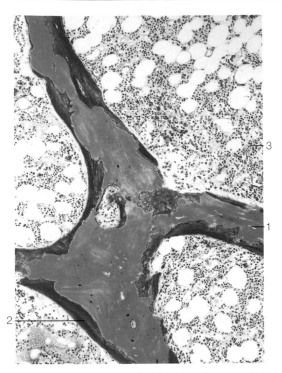

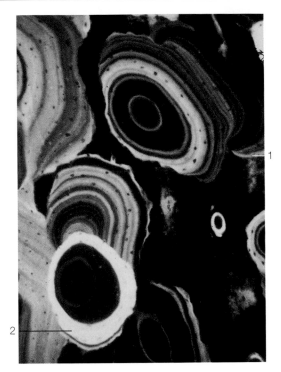

Fig. 945. Methacrylate embedding (renal osteopathy); Goldner, ×64

Fig. 946. Methacrylate embedding; tetracycline marking (ultraviolet fluorescence), ×40

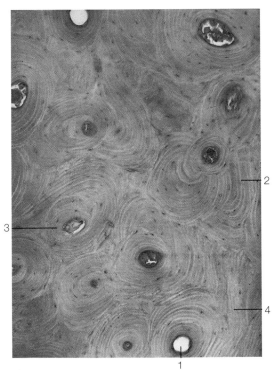

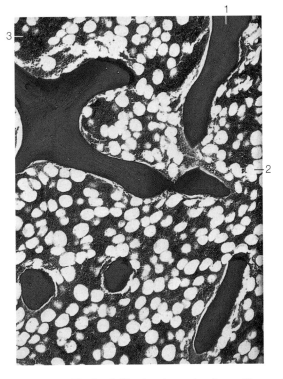

Fig. 947. EDTA decalcification (cortex); HE, ×40

Fig. 948. EDTA decalcification (spongiosa); van Gieson, ×40

7 Tissue Staining

It is not possible to recognize the individual tissue structures in unstained sections with certainty. Only deposited pigments with their own coloring (e.g. melanin, lipofuscin, hemosiderin: brown staining) can be seen. For diagnostic purposes the tissue is artificially stained, so that advantage may be taken of the particular affinity of various cellular and extracellular structures for certain stains. The discipline of histochemistry has therefore furnished us with a wealth of stains and staining methods. Many techniques for staining particular substances also require certain additional optical procedures (e.g. the identification of amyloid: Congo red together with polarized light).

The vast majority of bone diseases can be diagnosed from decalcified paraffin sections which have been stained with **hematoxylin and eosin** (HE). This standard stain shows up distinctly the contrast between the basophilic blue nucleus and the red cytoplasm. Calcium depos-its, reversal lines and cartilaginous matrix are colored blue, collagen fibers red. HE staining is basically used for all bone sections. A second routine method is *van Gieson staining* (v.G.). This is particularly suitable for the identification of collagen connective tissue, which appears red, whereas muscle and nerve fibers stain yellow. Calcified bone tissue is stained reddish-brown and osteoid red. The nuclei are black, which distinguishes them clearly from the yellow cytoplasm. This stain allows fibro-osseous trabeculae and also carcinomatous metastases to be clearly recognized, and it should be used for all bone lesions. With *van Gieson's elastic staining* the elastic fibers show up black (in the vessel wall, for instance). The trichrome stains are particularly suitable for marking connective tissue. For all bone lesions, *Masson-Goldner staining* with its excellent coloring is to be recommended. Calcified bone and connective tissue appear light green and uncalcified osteoid is colored reddish-orange. The osteoblasts and osteoclasts as well as the bone

Table 4. Histological staining

Stain	Result	Use
Hematoxylin and Eosin (HE)	**Blue:** basophilic cytoplasm, nuclei **Red:** cytoplasm, collagen fibers	All bone lesions (routine staining)
van Gieson (v.G.)	**Yellow:** cytoplasm, muscle, fibrin, amyloid **Red:** connective tissue, hyalin, osteoid	All bone lesions (routine staining)
Elastic van Gieson (EvG)	**Black:** elastic fibers **Red:** collagen fibers, osteoid	Angiomatous bone tumors, bone lymphomas, Ewing's sarcoma
Periodic Acid-Schiff Reaction (PAS)	**Purplish-red:** hydroxyl groups and amino-alcohols	Bone tumors, cartilaginous tumors, fungal osteomyelitis (routine staining)
Masson-Goldner Stain	**Reddish-orange:** connective tissue, bone marrow, uncalcified osteoid, osteoclasts, osteoblasts **Green:** calcified bone trabeculae	All bone lesions: osteopathies, osteosarcomas (routine staining)
Silver Impregnation (Gomori, Tibor-PAP, Elastic Kernecht Red)	**Black:** elastic fibers	Angiomatous bone tumors, bone lymphomas, Ewing's sarcoma
Fat Staining (Sudan-Hematoxylin, Oil Red)	**Red:** neutral fat **Blue:** cell nuclei, cytoplasm	Lipomatous bone tumors, storage diseases
Berlin Blue Staining	**Blue:** hemosiderin, Fe^{III} **Red:** cell nuclei	Tissue reaction to prostheses and metallic implants, old hemorrhages
Giemsa Staining (May-Grünwald-Giemsa)	**Blue:** cell nuclei, bacteria, basophilic substances **Red:** eosinophilic cytoplasm, granules, collagen fibers	Hematological diseases, bone lymphomas
Congo Red	**Red:** amyloid **Blue:** cell nuclei	Amyloid deposits (bone amyloidosis)
Toluidin Blue	**Blue:** basophilic cytoplasm, cell nuclei	Cartilaginous tumors, myxomas

marrow are stained red, and, owing to the iron hematoxylin, the nuclei appear black. Fibrin and erythrocytes are glowing red and muscle fibers pale red. This stain is particularly suitable for assessing osteopathies from a puncture biopsy of the iliac crest, and is also useful for identifying the tumorous osteoid in osteoid-producing growths (osteoid osteoma, osteosarcoma). Apart from HE, v.G. and *PAS staining*, all the stains shown in **Table 4** should only be used to answer particular questions.

Giemsa staining, for instance, is particularly suitable for identifying fine details (nucleus, cytoplasm) in the cells of the bone marrow, and is therefore specially to be used for all hematological diseases (e.g. leukemia) and bone lymphomas. As can be seen in **Fig. 949**, the nuclei *(1)* and cytoplasm *(2)* are stained dark blue. The cytoplasm of mature normoblasts and the granules of eosinophils are red. Mast cells are stained bluish-red. For the identification of iron deposits the *Berlin blue reaction* is used, where they appear in the cells as blue grains and indicate siderosis (at the site of an old hemorrhage is one example) or metallosis. In **Fig. 950** one

can see coarse elongated granular deposits *(1)* and even clump-like iron deposits *(2)* in a pseudocapsule near a metallic prosthesis in the hip joint, where they indicate metallosis. The nuclei of the surrounding cells appear red *(3)*, the cytoplasm is colored pink.

Included among the routine stains used for various bone lesions is *PAS staining* (the periodic acid Schiff reaction). It is effective for depicting the cellular structures in sharp relief, and should be employed whenever a tumor is suspected. The products of the tumor cells (e.g. mucus) are made visible by the red staining of the aldehyde groups with fuchsin-sulphuric acid. Basement membranes and carbohydrates show up purplish-red, whereas the cell nuclei are blue and the proteins and cytoplasm appear yellow. Fungi and parasites are recognizable in histological sections by their red coloration. A positive PAS reaction is visible in neutrophil and basophil granulocytes, glycogen fields in megakaryocytes and in the intranuclear immunoglobulin inclusions (Dutcher-Fahey bodies) in the lymphoid plasma cells of the lymphoplasmocytic immunocytoma (Waldenström's

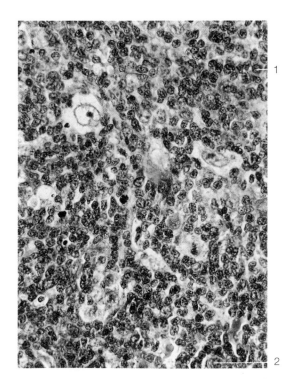

Fig. 949. Giemsa staining, ×82 (Hodgkin lymphoma)

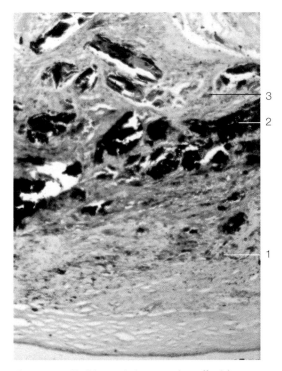

Fig. 950. Berlin blue staining, ×64 (metallosis)

disease). With many bone lesions, PAS staining is necessary for the identification of glycogen. In **Fig. 952** one can see the densely packed cells of a **Ewing's sarcoma** with roundish, variably sized nuclei *(1)* which are stained light blue. The sparse cytoplasm is shown with PAS staining to be full of red glycogen granules *(2)*. This identification of the glycogen can help to distinguish it from a round cell sarcoma of other histogenetic origin.

Silver impregnation shows up the elastic fibers in a bone lesion. The argyrophil fibers (reticular connective tissue fibers, neurofibrils) can be recognized by their black coloration, while the cellular structures recede into the background. This silver staining of the reticular fibers is therefore only of supplementary value with regard to diagnosis. The most useful silver stain is that of Gomori (others include Bielschowsky and Tibor PAP). **Figure 953** depicts a dense, narrow-mesh reticular fiber network *(1)* in an osseous **hemangiosarcoma**. Reddish tumor cells *(2)* lie between the meshes. The bone trabeculae *(3)* show up as brown. For many bone tumors (e.g. hemangiopericytoma) the presence of a reticular fiber network is of diagnostic significance; for others (e.g. Ewing's sarcoma) its absence is equally significant.

The visualization of calcium salts in bone is also based on silver staining, and completely calcified bone *(1)* appears black with *Kossa's stain* (**Fig. 951**), whereas the uncalcified osteoid shows up as impressive red seams *(2)*. The cells between the bony structures *(3)* stain pale red.

Enzymes can also be detected in paraffin sections. Neutrophil granulocytes, for instance, are very easily made recognizable by the *chloracetate esterase reaction*. In **Fig. 954** this enzyme appears in the granulocytes as fine, shining red granules *(1)*, whereas the bone marrow infiltrate of a small cell bronchial carcinoma *(2)* shows no chloracetate esterase reaction. The granulocytes are grouped together in the neighborhood of a bone trabecula *(3)*.

The *tartrate-resistant acid phosphatase reaction* (TRAP) makes it possible to identify acid phosphatase in the osteoclasts, histiocytes, phagocytic reticular cells of the bone marrow and leukemic hair cells. In particular it allows one to distinguish mononucleate osteoclasts from osteoblasts. In **Fig. 955** the osteoclasts in an **osteoblastoma** are stained red because of their

acid phosphatase content *(1)*, whereas the osteoblasts show no reaction *(2)*. Gaucher cells also show a slight positive reaction to tartrate-resistant acid phosphatase. The histochemical demonstration of particular enzymes in bone and bone marrow makes it possible to identify and quantify individual cells, this being of diagnostic importance in the case of many bone lesions. This does mean, however, that account must be taken of the various special methods of fixation, embedding and incubation, in order to be able either to elicit or to exclude enzyme identification.

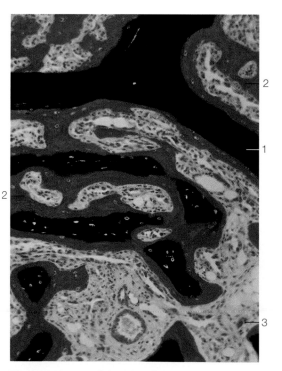

Fig. 951. Kossa staining, ×40 (bone metastasis)

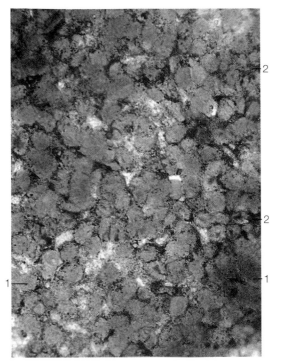

Fig. 952. PAS staining, ×160 (Ewing's sarcoma)

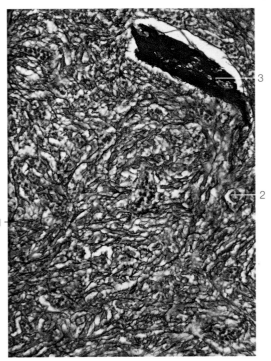

Fig. 953. Tibor PAP staining, ×40 (hemangiosarcoma)

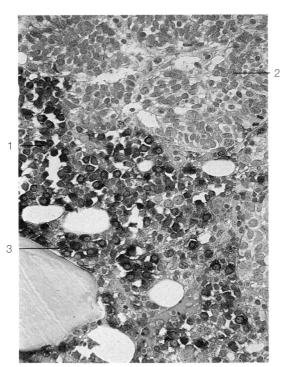

Fig. 954. Chloracetate esterase reaction, ×82 (bone metastasis from a small cell bronchial carcinoma)

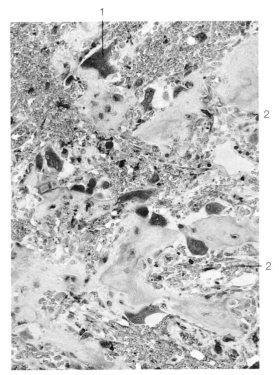

Fig. 955. Tartrate-resistant acid phosphate reaction, ×64 (osteoblastoma)

8 Diagnostic Immunohistochemistry

In recent years several substances have been tested which can identify particular tumors. Substances are produced by the tumorous tissue which can be evaluated quantitatively by various test systems. Included in these so-called **tumor markers** are plasma proteins, enzymes, hormones, proteins associated with pregnancy and oncofetal antigens. These antigenic substances can be directly identified histologically in the tissue by specific antibodies. With this type of immunohistochemical procedure, direct and indirect peroxidase techniques are employed: the peroxidase-antiperoxidase technique (PAP), the avidin-biotin-complex method (ABC) and alkaline phosphatase anti-alkaline phosphatase (APAAP). Most antigens can be identified in paraffin sections, a few require frozen sections or special methods of fixation. Histologically the action of the tumor marker serves to demonstrate the histogenetic differentiation of the tumor. With more highly differentiated bone tumors identification of the marker can identify the tissue from which they arose. In many cases this can make precise classification possible. With undifferentiated anaplastic malignant tumors, which give no specific immune reaction, the method can break down, nor can it help to distinguish between benign and malignant growths, although the identification of an epithelial or mesenchymal origin is usually possible. The ability to identify particular tumor markers is a valuable addition to conventional histological diagnosis.

In order to classify a bone tumor it is first necessary to decide whether it is of epithelial or mesenchymal origin. As is clear from **Table 5**, the identification of **cytokeratin** indicates an epithelial origin for the tumor, and therefore a bone metastasis. *Vimentin* characterizes mesenchymal tumors (sarcomas). Conventional histology must settle a questionable tumor diagnosis before the appropriate immunohistochemical reaction is brought into play. Myelomas announce themselves with *antibodies against immunoglobulins*. The monoclonal production of immunoglobulins (kappa or lambda proteins) is an indication of neoplasia. Malignant lymphomas are characterized by their surface antigens. *Antibodies against hormones* mark endocrine tumors (e. g. pancreas, thyroid). *Antibodies against oncofetal antigens* are, among other things, suitable for the identification of germ cell tumors. Cells of histiocytic origin can be recognized by *lysozyme*. Smooth muscle expresses *alpha-actin* and striped muscle *desmin*. **Myosin** can also be identified in this tissue, *myoglobin* being a specific marker for tumors of striped muscle. With *factor VIII associated antigen* (as well as *CD34*) the endothelial cells in vascular tumors (hemangioma, hemoangiosarcoma) may be visualized. Equally good results are provided by a *lectin* histochemical examination (lectin ulex europeus, peanut agglutinin: PNA). The *neuron-specific enolase* (NSE) is used with neurogenic tumors (neurinoma, neuroblastoma) and neuro-endocrine tumors, and it can be useful for identifying bone metastases from these tumors. The identification of *S-100 protein* is possible in numerous tumor cells (e. g. schwannoma, neurofibroma, melanoma, myoepithelia, Langerhans histiocytes in histiocytosis X, cartilaginous tumors, lipomatous tumors). *Osteonectin* is present in bone cells (osteoblasts, osteoclasts). *Alpha-1-antitrypsin* and *alpha-1-antichymotrypsin* are suitable for classifying a malignant histiocytoma. *Vimentin* is identifiable in large numbers of bone tumors.

In general, many immunohistochemical tests can be carried out successfully in routine laboratories, since the necessary staining sets ("kits") are available commercially. Nevertheless, it should be remembered that the use of these techniques can be extremely costly both in time and money. It must therefore be decided during the conventional histological examination which antigen is likely to occur in any particular tumor, and whether it is important for its classification. Representative tissue from the tumor and a minimum number of sections from each of the different tumorous areas must be made available. Aggressive acid decalcification is to be avoided. It therefore seems desirable to leave complicated immunohistochemical procedures, involving antibodies which are difficult to prepare, to those laboratories and institutions having the necessary experience of these particular tests and therefore able to deliver reliable and informative results. In practice, therefore, one routinely carries out a few of the available immunohistochemical reactions in one's own department, and leaves

Table 5. Diagnostic immunohistochemistry

Tumors	Cells of Origin	Antigen	Fixative
Cartilaginous Tumors Osteochondroma Enchondroma Chondroblastoma Chondromyxoid fibroma Chondrosarcoma	Cartilage cells	S-100 protein Vimentin	Formalin Alcohol
Bone Tumors Osteoma Osteoid osteoma Osteoblastoma Osteosarcoma	Bone cells (Osteoblasts, osteocytes)	Osteonectin	Formalin
Connective Tissue Tumors Bone fibromas Fibrosarcoma	Fibroblasts, fibrocytes	Vimentin	Formalin
Malignant fibroses Histiocytoma	Pluripotent mesenchyme cells	Vimentin	Formalin
Histiocytic Tumors Histiocytosis X Malignant histiocytosis	Monocytes Langerhans histiocytes	Vimentin S-100 protein Alpha-1-antitrypsin Alpha-1-antichymotrypsin Lysozyme	Formalin
Fatty Tissue Tumors Lipoma Liposarcoma	Lipoblasts	S-100 protein Vimentin	Formalin
Bone Marrow Tumors Plasmocytoma	Plasma cells	Immunoglobulins light chains (lambda, kappa) heavy chains (IgG, IgA ...) Vimentin	Formalin
Ewing's sarcoma PNET	? Neuroectodermal cells	MIC2 (HBA71), vimentin S-100 protein, GFAP, NSE, vimentin	
Vascular Tumors Hemangioma Hemangiosarcoma	Endothelial cells	Factor VIII-associated antigen Lectin (Ulex europeus) CD34, CD31	Formalin
Hemangiopericytoma	Pericytes	Vimentin	
Nerve Tumors	Nerve cells	S-100 protein Neurofilaments Neuron-specific enolase (NSE)	Formalin
Muscle Tumors Leiomyoma Leiomyosarcoma	Smooth muscle cells	Vimentin Alpha-aktin, myosin	Formalin
Rhabdomyoma Rhabdomyosarcoma	Skeletal muscle cells	Desmin, myoglobin	Formalin
Chordoma		EMA (epithelial membrane antigen), S-100 protein	Formalin
Bone Metastases Carcinoma of the kidney Carcinoma of the breast Carcinoma of the prostate Carcinoma of the thyroid gland	Tubular epithelium Ductular/lobular epithelia Glandular epithelia Thyrocytes C cells	Cytokeratin, vimentin EMA (epithelial membrane antigen), CEA, cytokeratin PSA (Prostate-specific antigen), prostatic acid phosphatase Thyroglobulin Calcitonin	Formalin

Table 5 (continued)

Tumors	Cells of Origin	Antigen	Fixative
Adenocarcinoma (Gastrointestinal tract)	Glandular epithelia	CEA, EMA, cytokeratin	
Bronchial carcinoma	Bronchial epithelium	CEA, cytokeratin	
Melanoma	Melanocytes	HMB 45, S-100 protein	
Tumors of the Joints			
Synovial sarcoma	Synovial cells	Cytokeratin, vimentin, EMA	Formalin

the rarer and more complicated procedures to laboratories which specialize in them.

S-100 protein is expressed in cartilaginous tumors, histiocytic lesions and neurogenic neoplasms. As can be seen in **Fig. 956** the cartilage cells in a **chondrosarcoma** are positively marked *(1)*. But in any case, with cartilaginous tumors the tissue is already recognizable histologically, so that immmunohistochemistry is usually superfluous. Nevertheless, the identification of S-100 protein in histiocytic lesions and neurogenic tumors can be very helpful. This marker is also effective in paraffin sections of fatty tumors that have been fixed in formalin.

Neuron-specific enolase (NSE) is a suitable marker for tumorous nerve tissue, and a *malignant neuroblastoma* thus marked is shown in **Fig. 957**. Neurogenic tumor cells have dark polymorphic nuclei *(1)*. In the cytoplasm of several cells, NSE appears in the form of fine brownish granules *(2)*. Other tumor cells contain very little or no NSE *(3)*. The immunohistochemical identification of NSE shows that we are dealing with a neurogenic tumor. For the prognosis of the tumor, on the other hand, other histological criteria are definitive.

Vimentin is a marker for mesenchymal structures, and is therefore helpful in distinguishing them from epithelial tumors. In

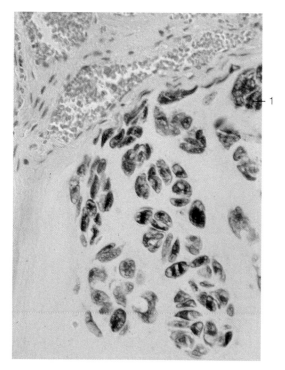

Fig. 956. S-100 protein, ×100 (chondrosarcoma)

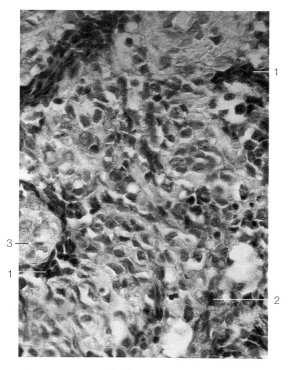

Fig. 957. NSE, ×40 (malignant neuroblastoma)

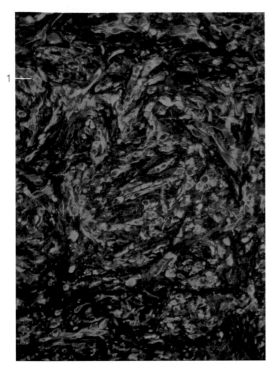

Fig. 958. Vimentin, ×40 (malignant fibrous histiocytoma) (immunofluorescence)

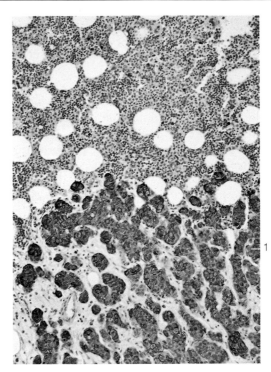

Fig. 959. Cytokeratin, ×40 (metastatic carcinoma)

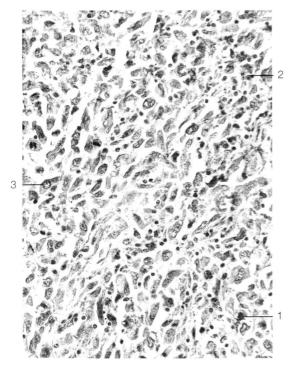

Fig. 960. Alpha-1-antichymotrypsin, ×100 (malignant fibrous histiocytoma)

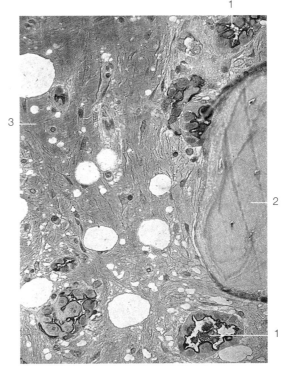

Fig. 961. PNA, ×40 (bone metastasis)

Fig. 958, the positive expression of vimentin in a **malignant fibrous histiocytoma** *(1)* can be seen. Melanomas also show a positive vimentin reaction, although in this case the identification of HMB45 is better. The same applies to **cytokeratin**, which marks epithelial tumors and is suitable for the recognition of **carcinomatous metastases** in bones. In **Fig. 959** one can see a positive cytoplasmic reaction *(1)* in the carcinomatous cells in the bone metastasis from a carcinoma of the breast. The classification of a **malignant fibrous histiocytoma** is assisted by the immunohistochemical identification of *alpha-1-antitrypsin* and *alpha-1-antichymotrypsin*. This appears in the tumor cells in **Fig. 960** as brownish – sometimes also granular – staining of the cytoplasm *(1)*. Particularly in undifferentiated tumors with roundish polymorphic *(2)* and spindle-shaped cells *(3)* this marker will reveal the histiocytic origin.

In **angiosarcomas** the tumorous endothelial cells show a positive reaction with *lectin* (peanut agglutinin, PNA). As shown in **Fig. 961**, the marker also appears in the form of reddish granules *(1)* in the glandular cells of an adenocarcinoma. This is a **bone metastasis**, in which the bone *(2)* is sclerotically widened and there is dense fibrosis *(3)* in the marrow cavity.

sured, the surface and perimeter of the cancellous bone trabecula can be calculated. **Figure 962** depicts a multiple purpose grid for the evaluation of suitably prepared structures (e.g. bone trabeculae). This allows the volume and surface densities of the trabeculae to be calculated. Measurements are carried out at a magnification of ×120–×180. Various grids have been developed which enable the parameters of different bony structures to be exactly calculated.

The individual parameters that can be obtained by bone morphometry are listed in **Table 6**. They include, amongst others, the volume and structural values of the mineralized bone and osteoid (per unit volume of total bone tissue), the width of the osteoid seams, the surface density of the osteoid and the relative osteoblast activity during *bone formation*, the structural values of *bone resorption* (interface areas of the Howship's lacunae with osteoclasts, total resorption surface area, relative osteoclast activity, osteoclast index, surface density of the total resorption area) and the *inactive spongiosal surface area*. This quantitative histomorphometry provides objective data about the structure, deposition and resorption of bone. The apposition rate of bone can be ex-

9 Histomorphometry

The purely subjective assessment of bone tissue achieved by microscopic examination can also be objectified by the collection of measurements. For this reason an increasing number of quantitative methods are being developed by which measured values can be obtained to provide objective criteria for extending and confirming the histological diagnosis. These include the morphometry of bony structures, which is particularly appropriate for osteopathies (osteoporosis, osteodystrophy, osteomalacia, renal osteopathy). Only with quantitative procedures is it possible to achieve a reliable assessment of changes in the bone structure arising in metabolic disorders or in bone reactions of exogenous origin. For *visual morphometry* a grid with 100 points and lines of semicircular undulations is introduced into the optical path of the microscope. By counting the points which lie over the structure to be mea-

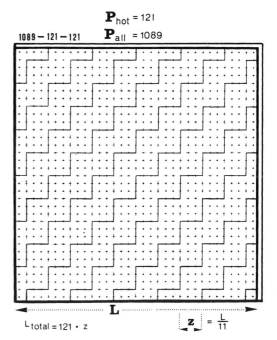

$P_{hot} = 121$

$1089 - 121 - 121$ $P_{all} = 1089$

$L_{total} = 121 \cdot z$ $z = \frac{L}{11}$

Fig. 962. Multiple purpose grid for evaluating orientated structures (bone trabeculae etc.)

Table 6. Histomorphometric parameters

Bone formation	Volume and structural values of mineralized bone and osteoid (per unit of total bone tissue)
	Width of the osteoid seam
	Surface density of the osteoid
	Relative osteoblast activity
Bone resorption	Interface areas of Howship's lacunae with osteoclasts
	Total resorption area
	Relative osteoclast activity
	Osteoclast index
	Surface density of total resorption area
	Inactive surface area of spongiosa
Tetracycline double marking	Rate of apposition of the bone

actly calculated from histomorphological analysis of *double tetracycline marking*.

As against this, bone apposition can only be derived microscopically (**Fig. 963**) from the increased and activated **osteoblasts** *(1)* which lie upon the bone *(2)*, but without gaining any information about the degree of osteoblastic activity. Even the number of **osteoclasts** (**Fig. 964**, *1*) and the depth of the resorption lacunae *(2)* can only be objectively assessed by using quantitative histomorphometry. The accuracy of this method lies between 0.5% and 3%. In any case, morphometric evaluation is only possible on suitable biopsy material, which means a spongiosal cylinder of at least 20 mm in length and with a biopsy surface of 40 mm^2.

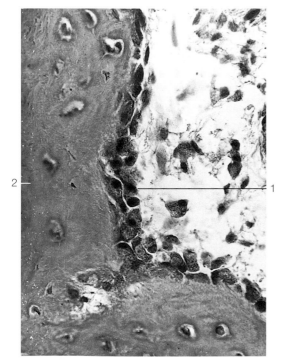

Fig. 963. Activated osteoblasts; HE, ×120

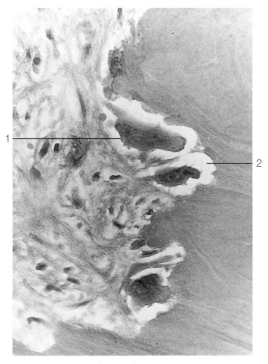

Fig. 964. Activated osteoclasts; HE, ×120

10 Microradiography

This is a special radiological method for examining bone which is particularly suitable for determining its *mineral content*. The varying mineral density in bone can also be quantitatively ascertained by measuring the absorption. The examination is carried out on ground sections about 100 µm thick which are then subjected to a previously calculated soft irradiation. The degree of absorption of the radiation is correlated with the calcium salt content (that is to say, the calcium itself). Assessment of the *bone surface* makes it possible to decide between apposition and resorption. Surfaces where bone apposition is taking place are smooth and less densely mineralized, whereas resorption surfaces are unevenly indented. After the remodeling process has come to an end, a zone with a high mineral content in the microradiograph indicates a surface where the cells are inactive. The bone cells (osteoblasts, osteocytes, osteoclasts) as well as the uncalcified osteoid are not shown up on the microradiograph. However, one can see the "empty" osteocyte lacunae in the mineralized bone very clearly, and their number and size can be used to assess pathological bone remodeling.

Figure 966 shows a microradiograph of *cortical bone tissue* from the region of the diaphysis. The narrow *(1)* and wide *(2)* Haversian canals, which have smooth borders, are striking.

The fully mineralized bone shows up as a pale area *(3)*. Darker regions in the neighborhood of the Haversian canals *(4)* indicate less mineralized bone tissue. Histological examination here also usually allows one to recognize osteoid which does not appear in the microradiograph.

In the *osteodystrophy* shown in the microradiograph of **Fig. 967**, the transformation of the bone brought about by primary hyperparathyroidism is clearly seen. One can observe the reduced mineralization *(1)* in the numerous osteons. The Haversian canals *(2)* vary in width and have in places undulating borders. An increased number of Howship's resorption lacunae *(3)* are present, indicating osteoclastic bone resorption. There is also *(4)* osteocytic osteolysis as well as periosteocytic demineralization.

It is particularly in **osteomalacia** that the marked difference in mineralization between the regions of osteoid seams and osteons can be seen. **Figure 965** shows an osteon in a stained thin section of bone. One can see the Haversian canal *(1)* and the widely deposited osteoid *(2)*. This does not show up in a microradiograph. The underlying bone tissue *(3)* and even that of the osteon *(4)* is plainly less well mineralized; this is clearly seen in the microradiograph and can be quantitatively assessed.

Figure 968 shows a microradiograph from a case of **Cushing's disease** after removal of the hormonal dysfunction. The cancellous trabeculae are partially narrowed *(1)*, without the os-

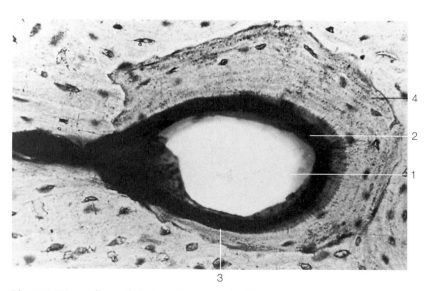

Fig. 965. Microradiograph (osteon in osteomalacia)

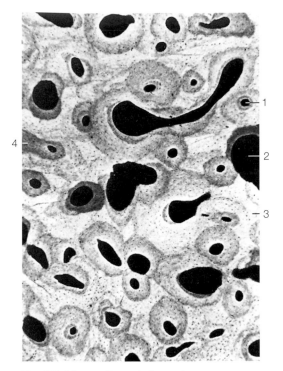

Fig. 966. Microradiograph (cortex)

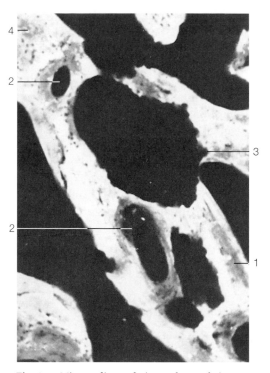

Fig. 967. Microradiograph (osteodystrophy)

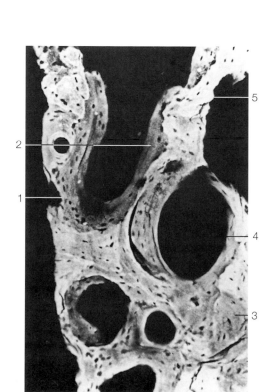

Fig. 968. Microradiograph (Cushing's disease)

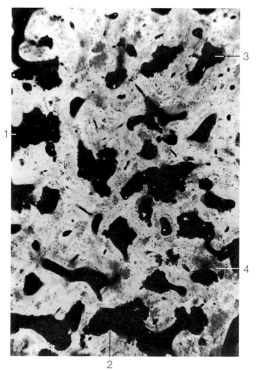

Fig. 969. Microradiograph (Paget's osteitis deformans)

teoid seams being recognizable. There are new fronts of bone deposition *(2)* which are less mineralized. Even within the old bone, mineralization defects are present *(3)*. The borders of the Haversian canals are in places smooth *(4)* and in places undulating *(5)*. The irregular porosity of the spongiosal structure is the result of bone resorption due to the disease (Cushing's osteoporosis; p. 76) and the unequal bone apposition (repair) following the removal of its cause.

In **Paget's osteitis deformans** the microradiograph displays a completely disorganized spongiosal structure. **Figure 969** shows the completely disorganized, sclerotically thickened spongiosal framework. The bone trabeculae are widened and shapeless *(1)* with partly smooth, partly undulating borders. One can see resorption lacunae which vary in depth *(2)*, indicating osteoclastic bone resorption. The mineralization of the tela ossea is uneven, with fully mineralized areas *(3)* and also numerous defects in mineralization *(4)*. Such a picture reveals very rapid bone remodeling.

11 Cytophotometry of Bone Tumors

Bone neoplasms cannot always be precisely diagnosed by radiological and histological examination. Either the exact classification of the tumor is not possible, or else a discrepancy is found between the information given by the radiograph and that of the histological section. In many cases one is not even able to assess the prognosis with sufficient certainty.

In attempting to objectify the histological and cytological pictures of a neoplastic bone lesion, we have introduced the *method of quantitative cytophotometry*. In this case the intracellular substances to be quantified are stained with a specific agent and the absorption of the transmitted light measured by means of a cytophotometer set to a specific wavelength. Taking advantage of the various possibilities offered by cytophotometry, we have carried out a quantitative evaluation of DNA in over 1,500 bone tumors. Cellular smear preparations for this were made from the tumorous tissue and subjected to Feulgen staining. The measurement of the DNA is based on the rate of reduplication of the DNA content of diploid, tetraploid and octoploid cells in normal and pathological tissue. Resting and polyploid tissues yield a frequency peak for diploid and tetraploid DNA values. Intermediate values belong either to S phase cells, or else to malignant tumor cells with aneuploid nuclei. This means that in tumor cells, and particularly in those of a malignant tumor, there is an irregular increase in the DNA which leads to a DNA stem line in the aneuploid range for highly differentiated tumors, but to no stem line at all in undifferentiated tumors. Our DNA measurements have shown that benign tumors have a diploid DNA content, whereas most malignant tumors have an aneuploid DNA distribution pattern with a stem line in the hypodiploid or hyperdiploid, in the triploid, or in the hypotetraploid or hypertetraploid ranges. Most dedifferentiated malignant tumors have no DNA stem line. With this method one can obtain information about the growth tendency and prognosis of each tumor, which can then be "graded".

The DNA distribution pattern (distribution of the ploidy stages) of tumor cells can be used, with the aid of a complex calculation (Böcking's "algorithm"), to diagnose and to grade the malignancy. Non-tumorous cell populations have a DNA content of 2c (diploid) or one of its integral powers (2c, 4c, 8c, 16c, 32c nuclei). Tumor cell nuclei usually have a raised and often aneuploid DNA content which does not correspond to any of these values. A tumor cell population can therefore be recognized from the fact that it contains aneuploid cells. The "2c deviation index" is included in the calculation, which is a measurement of the square of the deviation of the prevailing DNA value from the diploid value. With a "4.5c exceeding rate" (ER), the percentage of genuine aneuploid nuclei is shown to be above a DNA value of 4.5c, which excludes both cells in the S phase and any inaccurate measurements. Cells which are not derived from the tumor have a 4.5 ER of 0, which means that they are not aneuploid. Malignant tumor cells, on the other hand, have a 4.5 ER of more than 1 (the "aneuploidy index"). This index therefore indicates the percentage of aneuploid cells. The more malignant a tumor is, the higher is the percentage of aneuploid cells and the greater the fluctuation in the DNA values, and a DNA stem line is no longer demonstrable. Aneuploid cells have a nucleus with a DNA content between the normal stages of diploid, tetraploid, octoploid, hexadecaploid etc. The statistical evaluation of the DNA values of the cells of a bone tumor (calculated by a program available for the Hewlett Packard computer 9815 A) shows that:

1. A wider distribution of the DNA values around a peak value indicates a worse prognosis than a narrow distribution.
2. More cells in the G2 DNA synthesis phase indicate a poor prognosis.
3. A DNA stem line in the diploid and tetraploid ranges suggests a better prognosis than a stem line in the triploid or tetraploid range.
4. A high average level of ploidy indicates a worse prognosis.
5. Single very high ploidy values are signs of a deterioration of the prognosis.
6. Several DNA peaks suggest a deterioration of the prognosis.
7. With only a few diploid tumor cells the prognosis is poor.

8. In the absence of a DNA stem line and with a wider unimodal DNA distribution the prognosis is poor.

In the indisputable cases of **benign bone tumors** or tumor-like bone lesions one can nearly always expect to find cells with a diploid or euploid DNA content, corresponding to the 46 chromosomes. There is no increase in the amount of DNA present.

Jaffe-Lichtenstein fibrous bone dysplasia is an example of an absolutely benign tumor-like bone lesion. As already explained in the relevant chapters (pp. 56, 318), this is a maldevelopment of the bone-producing mesenchyme. Here the bone marrow is replaced by a fibrous marrow in which fibro-osseous trabeculae are formed directly from the connective tissue. There is a local expansion of the affected bone region, and finally the development of a curvature which can be seen in the radiograph.

In **Fig. 970a** the **radiograph** of such a bone defect can be seen in the 9th rib *(1)*. This part of the rib is expanded, the bordering cortex being completely intact but severely narrowed. In the middle of this region there is a diffuse translucency which is demarcated and shows no internal structures. In most cases such a "bony cyst" represents the monostotic form of fibrous bone dysplasia.

Histologically the lesion consists of connective tissue, rich in fibers and arranged in whorls, with isomorphic fibrocyte nuclei *(1)* in which slender arched fibro-osseous trabeculae *(2)* have differentiated out. Its typical morphological appearance is shown in **Fig. 970b**.

As can be seen in the **histogram** of **Fig. 970c**, the cytophotometric DNA measurements of the connective tissue cells and also the nuclei within the fibro-osseous trabeculae show a diploid stem line into which the hypodiploid and hyperdiploid ranges have extended somewhat. This DNA distribution diagram undoubtedly reveals a certain tendency to proliferation, but is nevertheless entirely benign.

The *juvenile bone cyst* is also an absolutely benign tumor-like bone lesion, which can nevertheless show increasingly expansive growth, but which practically never undergoes spontaneous malignant change (p. 408). In **Fig. 971a** one can see a classical **radiograph** of a juvenile bone cyst in the proximal part of the humerus *(1)*. This region of the bone has expanded to form a spindle shape, but the cortex is intact, although it is variably narrowed from within. In the center of the bone a large cystic translucency is apparent, which can show uneven patchy and straggly thickenings. This osteolytic zone stretches through the entire proximal metaphysis and reaches as far as the adjacent diaphysis. With old lesions the cyst can, with advancing growth, occupy even more of the diaphysis. Since such a region of bone is markedly less resistant mechanically, it often leads to a spontaneous (pathological) fracture which can produce considerable radiologically recognizable structural changes. The cortex is then penetrated and a reactive periostitis ossificans develops, so that increased and bizarre shadows caused by the formation of a callus can appear and a malignant bone disease cannot in the end be entirely excluded.

Histologically, parts of the cyst wall must be included in the section if a reliable diagnosis is to be made. In **Fig. 971b** one can see such a cyst wall, which consists of loose connective tissue with isomorphic fibrocytes *(1)*. Very often patchy and straggly calcifications *(2)* are deposited within. The inside of the cyst wall *(3)* is smooth and has no epithelial lining.

In **Fig. 971c** the **DNA histogram** of such a juvenile cyst is depicted. In accordance with the absolutely benign nature of this lesion the DNA measurements indicate only diploid connective tissue cells, of which the stem line (2c) has a large hypodiploid component. There are no aneuploid or polyploid cells, and the histogram reveals no tendency to proliferate.

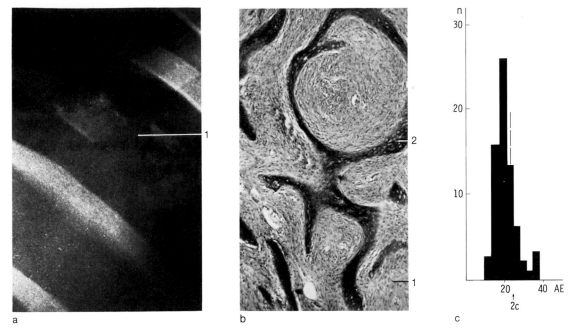

a   b   c

Fig. 970 a–c. Fibrous bone dysplasia Jaffe-Lichtenstein. **a** Radiograph: 9th rib; **b** Histology: van Gieson, ×25; **c** Histogram: DNA distribution of the connective tissue cells

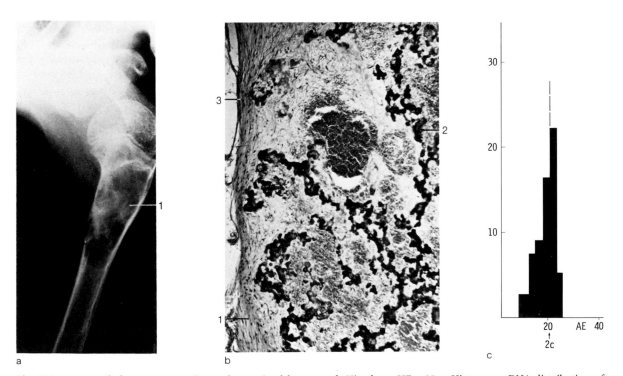

a   b   c

Fig. 971 a–c. Juvenile bone cyst **a** Radiograph: proximal humerus; **b** Histology: HE, ×25; **c** Histogram: DNA distribution of the connective tissue cells

With true **benign bone tumors** also, cyto-photometric DNA measurement of the DNA distribution in the tumor cells can reveal the benign character of the neoplasm. One relatively common benign bone tumor is the *osteoid osteoma* (p. 260). **Figure 972a** shows the **radiograph** of one of these lesions in the distal part of the tibia *(1)*. The long bone is expanded here, and an extensive area of osteosclerosis has produced a dense shadow. The "nidus", which is characteristic of the osteoid osteoma, cannot be seen in this film, having so to speak "gone underground" somewhere within the perifocal sclerosis. With a special tomographic exposure the "nidus" can usually be made visible. The outer contours of the bone in the elevated area are sharp and smooth, and no periosteal reaction can be seen.

A **histological assessment** of this lesion is only possible if the "nidus" has been included in the biopsy or excision and appears in the section. In **Fig. 972b** one can see highly cellular tumorous tissue with a loose, highly vascular stroma *(1)*. Within there are numerous irregular osteoid trabeculae *(2)* where active osteoblasts have been deposited. There are quite a number of multinucleated giant cells of the osteoclastic type. The nuclei of the fibrocytes and fibroblasts in the stroma are isomorphic, although they may often be hyperchromatic. There is no increased mitotic activity. The stroma is often interspersed with inflammatory cells.

The cytophotometric DNA measurement of the tumor cells (fibrocytes, fibroblasts, osteoblasts, osteoclasts) reveals a distribution that confirms the absolutely benign character of this tumor. In the **histogram** of **Fig. 972c** there is a single stem line in the diploid DNA range (2c). The DNA values are closely grouped around this maximum. Only a few single triploid cells are encountered, and there are no polypoid cells. There is no suggestion of a tendency to proliferate. This type of histogram is found with all benign bone tumors.

In all the **malignant bone tumors** measured by us, on the other hand, we found an aneuploid DNA distribution pattern, where sometimes a DNA stem line could no longer be discerned. The histogram differs greatly from those obtained from benign cells. Further conclusions about the degree of malignancy may be drawn from the level and distribution of the DNA values.

In the case of the *medullary plasmocytoma* (p. 348), the commonest malignant bone tumor, it is sometimes difficult to distinguish the tumorous plasma cells in the biopsy material from a reactive plasmocytosis. With the aid of DNA cytophotometry the distinction is often possible. In **Fig. 973a** one can see the **radiograph** of a medullary plasmocytoma *(1)* in the shaft of the humerus. The spongiosa has undergone extensive destruction, which is responsible for the translucency. The cortex is certainly still intact, but in places very severely narrowed. The endosteal side of the cortex has a wavy, "rat-bitten" appearance and is porous.

Histologically the marrow cavity is interspersed with densely packed, abnormal plasma cells, and the spongiosa is largely destroyed. In **Fig. 973b** there is a dense sheet of abnormal plasma cells of varying sizes and shapes. The nuclei are eccentrically located and mostly hyperchromatic and polymorphic.

The **DNA histogram** in **Fig. 973c** shows unambiguously that these are malignant tumorous plasma cells. One can recognize a shorter diploid (2c) and a very high tetraploid (4c) stem line. At 47.5% the tetraploid tumor cells predominate over the mere 12.6% of diploid plasma cells. Of the cells, 39% are aneuploid, mostly hyperdiploid, triploid or hypotetraploid. A lesser number of hypodiploid, hypertetraploid extending to octoploid cells (8c) are present. This DNA distribution pattern unambiguously indicates malignant tumorous tissue with a tendency to proliferate.

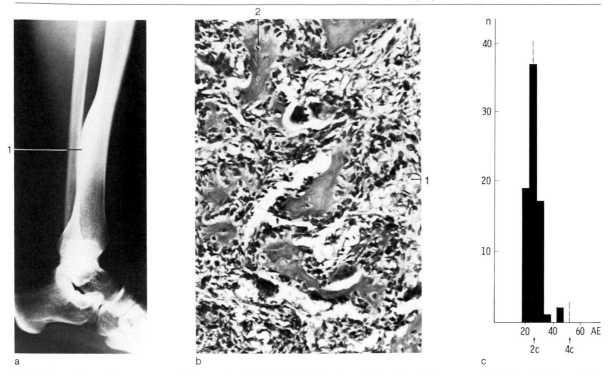

Fig. 972 a–c. Osteoid osteoma. **a** Radiograph: distal tibia; **b** Histology; HE, ×40; **c** Histogram: DNA distribution of the tumor cells

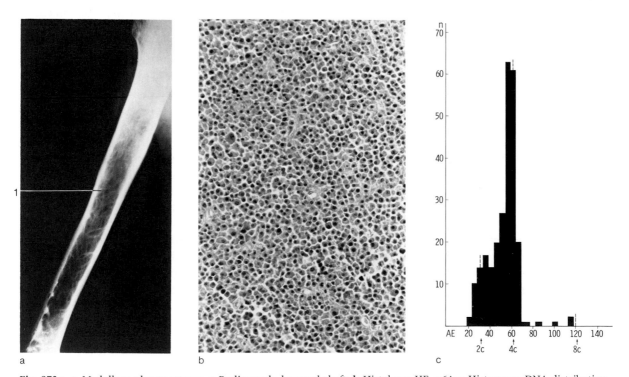

Fig. 973 a–c. Medullary plasmocytoma. **a** Radiograph: humeral shaft; **b** Histology: HE, ×64; **c** Histogram: DNA distribution of the tumor cells

The *Ewing's sarcoma* is a particularly malignant tumor that appears almost exclusively in children and young people (p. 352). It arises in the marrow cavity of a bone, where it spreads rapidly and finally involves the whole bone.

The most frequent radiological findings are destructive osteolytic foci interspersed with patchy thickenings resulting from reactive bone deposition. In **Fig. 974a** the **radiograph** shows a region of the humerus in which a Ewing's sarcoma has developed. In this film the intraosseous foci of destruction can only be guessed at. One can, however, see clear periosteal changes *(1)*, since the intramedullary tumor has penetrated the Haversian canals of the cortex and forced its way under the periosteum, which in this region is raised up. There are onion-skin thickenings in the outer layer as a result of the reactive periosteal new bone deposition. Radiologically there is a great similarity to osteomyelitis, to which most of the symptoms could apply. Such a radiological appearance must without fail be investigated by the histological examination of a representative bone biopsy.

The **microscopic interpretation** of this kind of biopsy material can present great difficulties, since there is histologically great similarity with other tumorous and non-tumorous bone lesions, and the tumorous tissue often shows extensive necroses and hemorrhages. In **Fig. 974b** one can see the typical histological picture of a Ewing's sarcoma. The tumor consists in part of loosely distributed, in part of densely packed round cells, and shows no differentiated tissue structures. The tumor cells are three times the size of lymphocytes and often lie together in nests in the middle of the loose connective tissue stroma. They have small, roundish but clearly polymorphic nuclei which are strongly hyperchromatic. Mitoses are usually only seldom encountered. The cytoplasm is sparse and not very clearly recognizable. Extended necrotic fields can make the diagnosis much more difficult.

In a Ewing's sarcoma in the humerus of a 20-year-old man the cytophotometric DNA measurement showed a DNA distribution of the tumor cells that indicated malignancy and a tendency to proliferate. In the **histogram** of **Fig. 974c** diploid cells are completely absent from the primary tumor. There is a DNA stem line in the hypertetraploid range which extends into the octoploid values (8c). Aneuploid tumor cells are also demonstrated in the triploid, hypertetraploid and hyperoctoploid ranges. In general, there is a very wide scatter of the DNA values with a clear tendency towards higher DNA values in the aneuploid range, which indicates both the malignant character of the tumor cells and a strong tendency towards proliferation. Thus the cytophotometric DNA measurements verify the presence of a tumor with a high degree of malignancy.

In this case tumorous tissue from **metastases** in the liver and spleen were also analyzed cytophotometrically. Here the **histograms** in **Figs. 974d, e** agree closely with that of the primary tumor. It is true that in the liver metastases there is a DNA stem line in the tetraploid range (4c), but this is nevertheless very wide and reaches into the hypotetraploid and hypertetraploid ranges, and there are also many aneuploid cells present. There are no diploid cells. Furthermore, hypooctoploid and hyperoctoploid cells can be observed.

The tumor cells in the spleen metastases also show a pattern of distribution that indicates a tumor with a high degree of malignancy. There are no diploid cells present, and by far the larger number of cells lie in the aneuploid range: hypotetraploid, hypertetraploid, hypooctoploid and a few hyperoctoploid cells. This histogram is practically identical with that of the primary tumor. Together, these histograms confirm the reliability of cytophotometric DNA measurements.

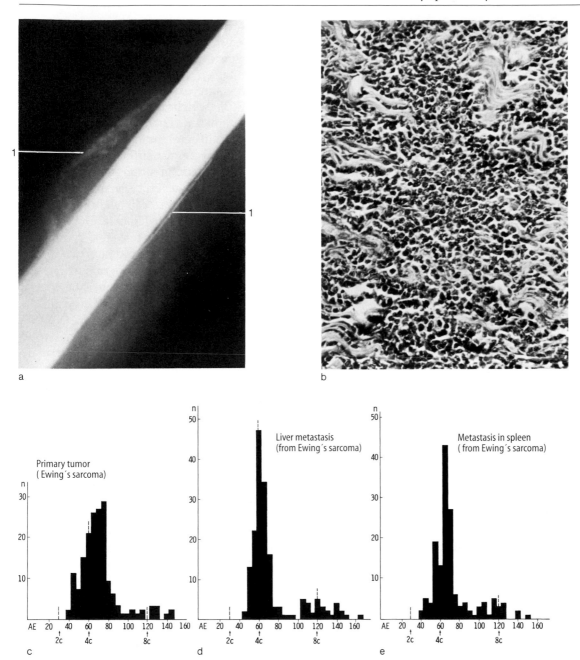

Fig. 974 a–e. Ewing's sarcoma. **a** Radiograph: Humerus; **b** Histology: HE, ×40; **c–e** Histograms of the primary tumor (**c**) and metastases in the liver (**d**) and spleen (**e**): DNA distribution of the tumor cells

Another malignant neoplasm is the *osteosarcoma*. It is regarded as highly malignant and metastasizes early. On the basis of the radiological and histological appearance, various forms of the osteosarcoma can be distinguished (p. 274), for which the prognosis also varies (osteoblastic, chondroblastic, fibroblastic, telangiectatic, parosteal osteosarcoma). It is the aim of cytophotometric DNA measurement of the tumor cells both to establish the malignant nature of the neoplasm and to assess its degree of malignancy.

As shown in the **radiograph** of **Fig. 975a**, a virtually pathognomonic radiological finding may be present. This is an osteoblastic osteosarcoma of the distal femoral metaphysis. In the distal part of the bone there is an extensive irregular sclerotic increase in density *(1)* which has taken over the entire marrow cavity and includes the cortex. The tumor has already broken out of the bone and is spreading into the covering periosteum *(2)* and into the soft parts. It reaches down as far as the cartilaginous epiphyseal plate *(3)*. Such a radiological appearance allows one to assume an osteosarcoma on the radiographic appearance alone; other cases, however, are often not so pathognomonic.

As can be seen in **Fig. 975b**, the radiological findings are confirmed **macroscopically**, and the distal femoral metaphysis is occupied by dense, bone-hard tumorous tissue *(1)*. This has spread into both the spongiosa and the cortex and is pushing out into the periosteum and the soft tissues *(2)*. It reaches down distally as far as the epiphyseal plate *(3)*.

Histologically the osteosarcoma is characterized by the presence of various tissues (sarcomatous stroma, tumorous osteoid, bone and cartilage, increased vascularity). In **Fig. 975c** the sarcomatous stroma is seen to be almost completely occupied by homogeneous eosinophilic tumorous osteoid *(1)*, in which osteoblastic tumor cells are included. These have polymorphic hyperchromatic nuclei and also show a great number of abnormal mitoses. There are in addition many osteoid and tumorous bone trabeculae *(2)*, which also contain cells with polymorphic nuclei. There are various tissue structures within the tumor, arranged somewhat like a chess board, although these are irregularly distributed. In order to obtain a representative picture, at least several tissue samples from different parts of the tumor should be examined. This is equally true for the cytological examination and for the cytophotometric DNA measurements.

Figure 975d shows the **histogram** of an osteosarcoma. As an expression of the clonal homogeneity and the strong tendency of the various tumor cells to proliferate, the DNA values are scattered over several ploidy steps up to and beyond the octoploid value (8c). There are indeed still a few diploid tumor cells (2c) measured, but most of the cells lie in the higher DNA ranges. Of the tumor cells, 98% are found in the aneuploid range, most of these being in the hyperdiploid, triploid and hypotetraploid ranges. Numerous cells lie between the tetraploid (4c) and octoploid (8c) DNA values, so that here there is no stem line. A few cells have a hyperoctoploid DNA value. Such a histogram indicates a highly malignant tumor with a strong tendency to proliferate. In spite of the inhomogeneity of the osteosarcomatous tumorous tissue, with its variable tumor cell population (osteoblastic, fibromatous, chondroblastic), the different osteosarcomas always show more or less similar histograms. From the number of aneuploid tumor cells and the extent of the displacement of the measurement values in the higher DNA ranges, conclusions may be drawn in each case about the degree of malignancy.

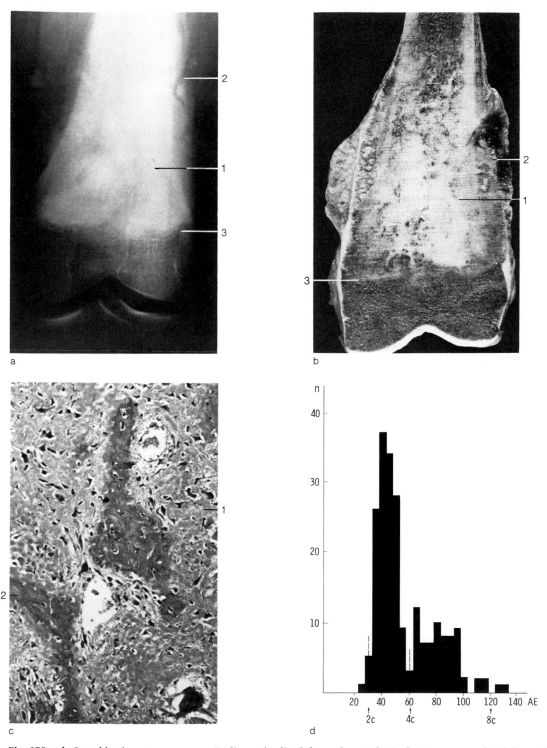

Fig. 975 a–d. Osteoblastic osteosarcoma. **a** Radiograph: distal femoral metaphysis; **b** Macroscopy: distal femoral metaphysis; **c** Histology: van Gieson, ×64; **d** Histogram: DNA distribution of the tumor cells

In those tumors where a definitive benign or malignant diagnosis has already been arrived at on the basis of radiological and histological investigations, the cytophotometric DNA measurements have shown that, in most cases, the prognosis can be read off from the histogram. DNA cytophotometry can also be of great diagnostic value when dealing with tumors where the histological structures are hard to interpret, or when it is difficult to comprehend the biological significance of the picture. This is particularly the case with *semimalignant tumors* or tumors for which the prognosis is doubtful.

One example of such a semimalignant tumor or tumor of low malignancy is the so-called *adamantinoma of the long bones* (p. 378). The **radiograph** shown in **Fig. 976a** is characterized by several large destruction foci (1) in the middle and distal parts of the tibia. Between these osteolytic areas there are irregular sclerotic thickenings. The lesion includes both the spongiosa and the cortex. The bone in this region has been forced up into a kind of hump.

As can be seen in **Fig. 976b**, the tumor consists of a loose fibrous stroma with isomorphic fibrocytes (1) with slender nuclei and deposits of elongated groups and cords of closely packed tumor cells (2) resembling nerve or muscle fibers. If there is epithelial differentiation, polygonal cells with eosinophilic cytoplasm are present here. There is often a basal tissue pattern, however, in which no marked cellular or nuclear polymorphy is present.

The adamantinoma of the long bones is one of the slow growing neoplasms with a low degree of malignancy but a high rate of recurrence. In confirmation of this the **histogram** in **Fig. 976c**, relating both to the epithelioid "ameloblasts" and also to the stromal fibroblasts, shows a DNA stem line in the tetraploid range (4c), with which are included, however, many hypotetraploid and hypertetraploid cells. The aneuploid cells which are also present indicate the semimalignant type of growth of this peculiar neoplasm. They are the expression of an ongoing increase in DNA synthesis and are also characteristic of a rising tendency to proliferate.

A rare bone tumor, which is classified as semimalignant and which can cause great diagnostic problems, is the *chondromyxoid fibroma* (p. 230). In the long bones it mostly appears in the **radiograph** as an ovoid bone cyst eccentrically situated in the metaphysis, where it is sharply demarcated by a narrow band of marginal sclerosis. In **Fig. 977a** the cytophotometrically examined chondromyxoid fibroma in the proximal part of the tibia has an extremely eccentric position (1) and is only recognizable by the widely indented erosion of the cortex.

In the **histological picture** it can be difficult to decide between a "benign" and a "malignant" lesion. As can be seen in **Fig. 977b**, the lobulated tumor is formed from a loose network of bipolar spindle-shaped and multipolar stellate cells. The highly dense accumulation of nuclei and cells in at the periphery of the lobules is characteristic. In the section, immature densely cellular areas alternate with myxomatous and chondroid regions. Its benign nature is limited, and it has a tendency to recurrence, as is observed in 25% of the cases.

As shown in the **histogram** of **Fig. 977c**, the tumor cells are polyploid with a DNA stem line in the hypotetraploid range, which corresponds with its clinically observed tendency to proliferate. The remarkably wide DNA spectrum spans both the hypodiploid and the hypertetraploid ranges, with triploid cells predominating. The rather large number of aneuploid cells indicates both the proliferative tendency and semimalignancy of the chondromyxoid fibroma. With truly malignant tumorous growth the higher aneuploid DNA values would be expected to extend beyond the octoploid range.

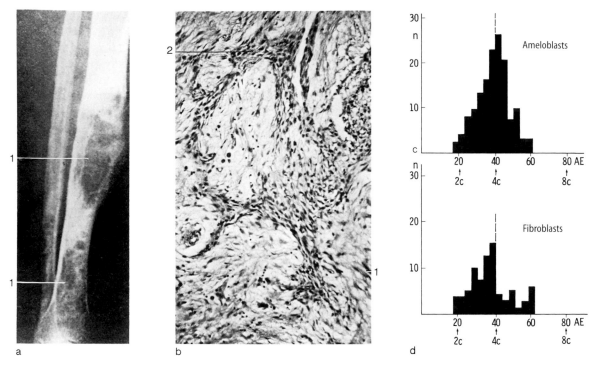

Fig. 976a–d. Adamantinoma of the long bones. a Radiograph: tibia; b Histology: HE, ×40; c–d Histogram: ameloblasts (c) and fibroblasts (d): DNA distribution of the tumor cells

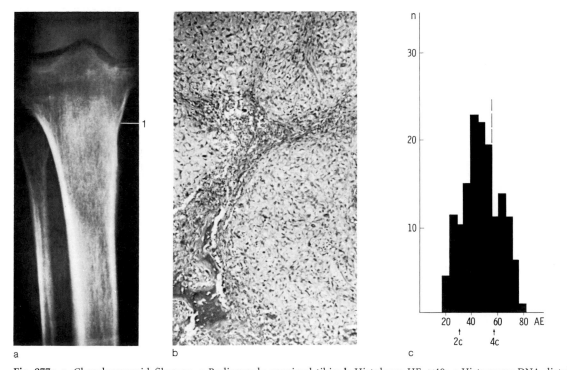

Fig. 977a–c. Chondromyxoid fibroma. a Radiograph: proximal tibia; b Histology: HE, ×40; c Histogram: DNA distribution of the tumor cells

In the case of an **osteoclastoma** (p. 337) it is known to be particularly difficult to assess the prognosis from the histological picture. Radiologically there is usually an eccentric area of osteolysis in the epiphysis which can also involve the neighboring metaphysis. Histologically we distinguish three grades of differentiation with this tumor, which can, however, be extraordinarily difficult under the microscope. Furthermore, we know that this "grading" only offers limited information about the prognosis, since metastases have even been described as arising later from a grade I osteoclastoma. However, cytophotometric DNA measurement allows one to determine the degree of differentiation objectively and to make a reliable assessment of the prognosis.

In **Fig. 978a** we can see the **histological picture** of a "benign" *osteoclastoma of grade I*. The tumor consists of a loose highly vascular stroma, in which numerous deposits of multinucleated giant cells of the osteoclastic type lie more or less equidistant from each other. The stromal spindle cells have uniform elongated elliptical nuclei with no hyperchromasia. Mitoses are rare. The giant cells are large and often have many isomorphic nuclei. In the tumorous tissue no osteoid, bone or cartilaginous tissue is encountered.

The cytophotometric DNA measurement of the cells from such a tumor confirms that it is relatively benign. The **histogram** is shown in **Fig. 978b**. We can observe a single DNA stem line in the diploid range (2c), around which the DNA values are very closely grouped. Only very few DNA values extend into the hyperdiploid range, indicating only a slight tendency to proliferate. No polyploid or aneuploid cells are present. The status of such an osteoclastoma can therefore be regarded as benign. Nevertheless, we know that even such an osteoclastoma as this may have an unpredictable prognosis, and that it can metastasize in spite of the benign histogram.

An *osteoclastoma of grade III* is quite plainly a bone sarcoma and can usually be recognized histologically as unmistakably malignant. This is confirmed by a DNA histogram which shows a malignant DNA distribution pattern.

It is particularly difficult, however, to assess the findings in a **grade II osteoclastoma**, where the histological criteria are not so distinctive. It is here that the cytophotometric DNA measurement can be very helpful. In **Fig. 979a** we can see the histological picture of a grade II osteoclastoma. In comparison with the "benign" variety the spindle-cell stroma is more in the foreground, while the number and size of the osteoclastic giant cells have been reduced, and they mostly have fewer nuclei. The distribution of the giant cells in the tumorous tissue is also less regular. The nuclei of the spindle cells are variable, being sometimes hyperchromatic and sometimes even polymorphic, and repeatedly showing mitoses. In spite, however, of a certain restlessness in the histological formation, there is no definite sarcomatous stroma present.

The tendency of the tumorous tissue to proliferate is clearly reflected in the **DNA histogram**. In **Fig. 979b** one can see that diploid tumor cells no longer occur. There is a clear DNA stem line in the tetraploid range (4c), which includes many hypotetraploid and hypertetraploid cells. Some aneuploid cells are found between the tetraploid (4c) and octoploid (8c) DNA values. A few tumor cells have a hyperoctoploid DNA content. Grade II osteoclastomas therefore show a certain polyploidy and aneuploidy of the tumor cells, which is, however, not very marked. This is an indication of a clear proliferative tendency and a propensity towards malignant change, or a potential malignancy. As yet, however, a truly malignant tumorous growth cannot be confirmed.

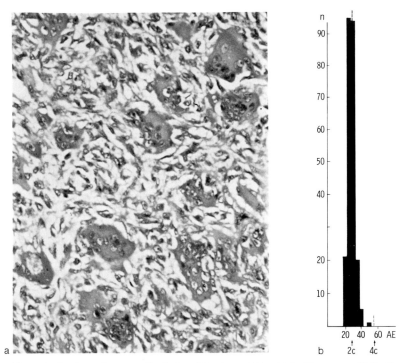

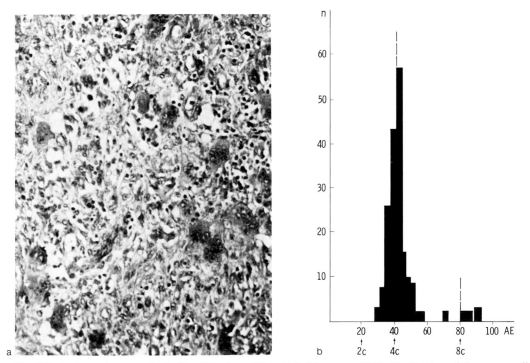

Fig. 978 a, b. Osteoclastoma Grade I. **a** Histology: HE, ×64; **b** Histogram: DNA distribution of the tumor cells

Fig. 979 a, b. Osteoclastoma Grade II. **a** Histology. HE, ×64; **b** Histogram: DNA distribution of the tumor cells

By making use of the DNA distribution pattern in individual bone tumors, one can employ a complex calculating procedure ("algorithm") to evaluate each **DNA grade of malignancy** and thus obtain information about the prognosis.

In our Department we have used cytophotometry to obtain the DNA values of tumor cells in various benign, semimalignant and malignant bone tumors. These have been brought into the calculation and the results entered in a diagrammatic survey. We also included the measurement and calculation of the values of some non-tumorous bone lesions in this procedure, in order to obtain reliable initiatory values in the purely benign range. This diagram groups together, in order of ascending malignancy, those calculated values obtained from cytophotometric measurements corresponding to the malignancy grade of each tumor. The entire peak of the rise displayed by the calculated values was divided into three parts, representing an objective classification of the malignancy grade. It was thus possible to define three grades of malignancy into which each of the measured and calculated neoplasms naturally fall.

In **Fig. 980** an overall view of these results is displayed in a **diagram**. One can see that the non-tumorous bone lesions (*synovitis* – Sy, *osteomyelitis* – OY) and benign tumors (*osteoid-osteoma* – O-O, *enchondroma* – EN) all lie on the abscissa ($y = 0$) and can therefore be characterized as benign. With the malignant bone neoplasms we distinguish **three malignancy grades**, which are shown in the diagram.

Among the *osteosarcomas* (O) the majority have a malignancy grade of 3, a few only 2 and, for one osteosarcoma, we could establish a low malignancy grade of only 1. The *medullary plasmocytoma* (P) showed with our DNA measurement malignancy grades 1 and 2. A *chondrosarcoma* (C) showed a low degree of malignancy (grade 1), although these tumors may also reach higher grades. Similarly, *osteoclastomas* (K) can show all three malignancy grades. A *hemangiosarcoma* of bone (H), a *fibrosarcoma* (F) and a *synovial sarcoma* (S) revealed themselves as neoplasms of middle malignancy (grade II). All *Ewing's sarcomas* (E) and *malignant fibrous histiocytomas* (MFH) were unmistakably of malignancy grade III.

In this diagram only a few bone sarcomas have been included according to their malignancy grades. With these neoplasms, catamnesic investigations have shown that the malignancy grade calculated by us does correlate with the recurrence rate, appearance of metastases and with the survival time. In the meantime we have carried out this examination on over 1,000 different bone neoplasms. Catamnesic examinations and survival follow-up have to a great extent confirmed the prognostic assessments arrived at by our DNA measurements. Thus the use of the latter both for distinguishing between benign and malignant tumors, and for deciding in each case the malignancy grade, has in general proved its worth. It has contributed a valuable addition to diagnostic decision-making, and should most certainly be included as a further routine investigative procedure.

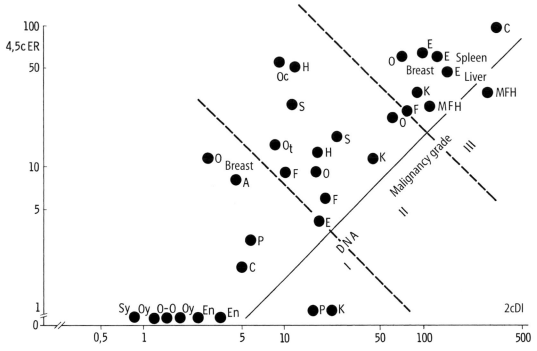

Fig. 980. Objective "grading" of bone tumors by quantitative cytophotometric DNA measurements of the tumor cells (4.5cER, 4.5c – exceeding rate; 2cDI, 2c – deviation index) (see also BÖCKING 1982). Sy = synovitis; OY = osteomyelitis; O-O = osteoid osteoma; EN = enchondroma; O = osteosarcoma; P = plasmocytoma; C = chondrosarcoma; K = osteoclastoma (giant cell tumor); H = hemangiosarcoma; F = fibrosarcoma; S = synovial sarcoma; E = Ewing's sarcoma; MFH = malignant fibrous histiocytoma

References

Chapter 1
Bones and Bone Tissue

Adler CP (1981) Störungen der Funktion des Knochens. In: Sandritter W (ed) Allgemeine Pathologie, 2nd edn. Schattauer, Stuttgart, pp 718–740

Adler CP (1992) Knochen – Gelenke. In: Sandritter W, Thomas C (eds) Histopathologie, 2n edn. Schattauer, Stuttgart, pp 290–314

Adler CP (1992) Knochen und Gelenke. In: Thomas C (ed) Grundlagen der klinischen Medizin. Schattauer, Stuttgart

Adler CP (1993) Knochen und Gelenke. In: Thomas C (ed) Makropathologie, 8th edn. Schattauer, Stuttgart, pp 147–171

Adler CP (1996) Knochen – Knorpel. In: Thomas C (ed) Spezielle Pathologie. Schattauer, Stuttgart, pp 527–593

Amstutz HC, Sissons HA (1969) The structure of the vertebral spongiosa. J Bone Joint Surg Br 51:540

Amtmann E (1971) Mechanical stress, functional adaptation and the variation structure of the human femur diaphysis. Ergebn Anat Entwickl Gesch 44:1–89

Arnott HJ, Pautard FGE (1967) Osteoblast function and fine structure. Israel J Med Sci 3:657–670

Axhausen G (1911) Über die durchbohrenden Gefäßkanäle des Knochengewebes (volkmann'sche Kanäle). Arch Klin Chir 94:296

Bargmann W (1956) Histologie und mikroskopische Anatomie des Menschen, 2nd edn. Thieme, Stuttgart

Bourne GH (1972) The biochemistry and physiology of bone. Academic Press, New York

Cohen J, Harris WH (1958) The three dimensional anatomy of Haversian systems. J Bone Joint Surg 40:419

Engfeldt B (1958) Recent observations of bone structure. J Bone Joint Surg Am 40:698

Evans FG, Riolo ML (1970) Relations between the fatigue life and histology of adult human cortical bone. J Bone Joint Surg Am 52:1579

Fischer H (1980) Mechanische Beanspruchung und biologisches Verhalten des Knochens. In: Ferner H, Staubesand J (eds) Lehrbuch der Anatomie des Menschen, vol I, 13th edn. Urban & Schwarzenberg, Munich, pp 225–242

Francillon MR (1981) Deformitäten des Skeletts. In: Schinz HR, Baensch WE, Frommhold W et al (eds) Lehrbuch der Röntgendiagnostik, vol II/part 2, 6th edn. Thieme, Stuttgart, pp 373–428

Frost HM (1960) In vivo staining of bone with tetracyclines. Stain Technol 35:135

Frost HM (1963) Bone Remodelling Dynamics. Thomas, Springfield, Ill.

Frost HM (1966) Bone dynamics in metabolic bone disease. J Bone Joint Surg 48:1192

Frost HM (1967) Bone Dynamics in Osteoporosis and Osteomalacia. Thomas, Springfield, Ill.

Garden RS (1961) The structure and function of the proximal end of the femur. J Bone Joint Surg 43:576

Gebhardt FAMW (1901) Über funktionell wichtige Anordnungsweisen der gröberen und feineren Bauelemente des Wirbelthierknochens. 1st General Part (Zweiter Beitrag zur Kenntnis des funktionellen Baues thierischer Hartgebilde). Arch Entwickl Mech Org 11:383

Gebhardt FAMW (1905–1906) Über funktionell wichtige Anordnungsweisen der gröberen und feineren Bauelementen des Wirbelthierknochens. 2nd Special Part: 1. Der Bau der Haversschen Lamellensysteme und seine funktionelle Bedeutung. Arch Enwickl Mech Org 20:187

Goldhaber P (1962) Some current concepts of bone physiology. New Engl J Med 266:924

Harris WH, Heany PR (1970) Skeletal renewal and bone disease. New Engl J Med 280:193, 253, 303

Heuck F (1970) Allgemeine Morphologie und Biodynamik des Knochens im Röntgenbild. Röntgenforsch 112:354

Jaffe HL (1972) Metabolic, degenerative, and inflammatory diseases of bones and joints. Urban & Schwarzenberg, Munich

Kopsch F (1955) Lehrbuch und Atlas der Anatomie des Menschen, vol 1, 19th edn. Thieme, Stuttgart

Kummer B (1959) Bauprinzipien des Säugerskeletts. Thieme, Stuttgart

Kummer B (1962) Funktioneller Bau und funktionelle Anpassung des Knochens. Anat Anz 111:261–293

Kummer B (1978) Mechanische Beanspruchung und funktionelle Anpassung des Knochens. Verh Anat Ges 72:21–46

Kummer B (1980) Kausale Histogenese der Gewebe des Bewegungsapparates und funktionelle Anpassung. In: Ferner H, Staubesand J (eds) Lehrbuch der Anatomie des Menschen, vol 1, 13th edn. Urban & Schwarzenberg, Munich, pp 242–256

Pauwels F (1965) Gesammelte Abhandlungen zur funktionellen Anatomie des Bewegungsapparates. Springer, Berlin Heidelberg New York

Pauwels F (1973) Atlas zur Biomechanik der gesunden und kranken Hüfte. Springer, Berlin Heidelberg New York

Peltesohn S (1933) Über die sogenannte Tibia recurvata. Z Orthop Chir 58:487–498

Schenk RK, Merz WA, Müller J (1969) A quantitative histological study on bone resorption in human cancellous bone. Acta Anat (Basel) 74:44–53

Scholten R (1975) Über die Berechnung der mechanischen Beanspruchung in Knochenstrukturen mittels für den Flugzeugbau entwickelter Rechenverfahren. Med Orthop Techn 95:130–138

Scholten R (1976) Über die Berechnung der mechanischen Beanspruchung in Knochenstrukturen. Techn Med 6:85–89

Smith JW (1960) The arrangement of collagen fibres in human secondary osteones. J Bone Joint Surg Br 42:588

Tillmann B (1969) Die Beanspruchung des menschlichen Hüftgelenks. III: Die Form der Facies lunata. Z Anat Entwickl Gesch 128:329–349

Uehlinger E (1970) Strukturwandlungen des Skelettes im Ablauf des Lebens, bei Über- und Unterbelastung und bei metabolischen Erkrankungen. Nova Acta Leopoldina 35:217–237

Vaughan JM (1975) The physiology of bone, 2nd edn. Clarendon, Oxford

Vitalli HP (1970) Knochenerkrankungen, Histologie und Klinik. Sandoz, Nürnberg

Young WR (1962) Cell proliferation and differentiation during enchondral osteogenesis in young rats. J Cell Biol 14:357

Zichner L (1970) Calcitoninwirkung auf die Osteocyten der heranwachsenden Ratte. Klin Wochenschr 48:1444

Chapter 2
Normal Anatomy and Histology

Adler CP (1981) Störungen der Funktion des Knochens. In: Sandritter W (ed) Allgemeine Pathologie, 2nd edn. Schattauer, Stuttgart, pp 717–740

Adler CP (1987) Die Bedeutung von mehrkernigen Riesenzellen in Knochentumoren und tumorähnlichen Läsionen. Verh Dtsch Ges Pathol 71:366

Adler CP (1992) Knochen – Gelenke. In: Thomas C (ed) Histopathologie, 11th edn. Schattauer, Stuttgart, pp 290–314

Adler CP (1992) Knochen und Gelenke. In: Thomas C (ed) Grundlagen der klinischen Medizin. Schattauer, Stuttgart

Adler CP (1993) Knochen und Gelenke. In: Thomas C (ed) Makropathologie, 8th edn. Schattauer, Stuttgart, pp 147–171

Adler CP (1996) Knochen – Knorpel. In: Thomas C (ed) Spezielle Pathologie. Schattauer, Stuttgart, pp 527–593

Adler CP, Klümper A (1977) Röntgenologische und pathologisch-anatomische Aspekte von Knochentumoren. Radiologe 17:355–392

Adler CP, Klümper A, Hosemann W (1983) Intraossäre Angiographie von Knochentumoren. Radiologe 23:128–136

Amato VP, Bombelli R (1959) The normal vascular supply of the vertebral colunin in the growing rabbit. J Bone Joint Surg Br 41:782–795

Amling M, Delling G (1997) Differenzierung und Funktion des Osteoklasten – Neue Ergebnisse und Modellvorstellungen. Osteologie 6:4–14

Anderson DW (1960) Studies of the lymphatic pathways of bone and bone marrow. J Bone Joint Surg Am 42:716

Anderson HC (1989) Mechanism of mineral formation in bone. Lab Invest 60:320–330

Anseroff NJ (1934) Die Arterien der langen Knochen des Menschen. Z Anat Entwickl Gesch 103:793–812

Bargmann W (1977) Histologie und mikroskopische Anatomie des Menschen, 7th edn. Thieme, Stuttgart

Brookes M (1958a) The vascular architecture of tubular bone in the rat. Anat Rec 132:25–47

Brookes M (1958b) The vascularization of long bones in the human foetus. J Anat (Lond) 92:261–267

Brookes M (1963) Cortical vascularization and growth in foetal tubular bones. J Anat (Lond) 97:597–609

Brookes M (1967) The osseous circulation. Biomed Eng 2:294–299

Brookes M (1971) The blood supply of bone. An approach to bone biology. Butterworth, London

Burkhardt R (1992) Der Osteoblast – Schlüssel zum Verständnis des Skelettorgans. Osteologie 1:139–170

Cameron DA (1963) The fine structure of bone and calcified cartilage. A critical review of the contribution of electron microscopy to the understanding of osteogenesis. Clin Orthop 26:199–228

Cohen J, Harris WH (1958) The three dimensional anatomy of Haversian systems. J Bone Joint Surg 40:419–434

Crock HV (1967) The blood supply of the lower limb bones in man. Livingstone, London

Cumming D (1962) A study of blood flow through bone marrow by a method of venous effluent collection. J Physiol (Lond) 162:13–20

Fischer H (1980) Mechanische Beanspruchung und biologisches Verhalten des Knochens. In: Staubesand J (ed) Lehrbuch der Anatomie des Menschen. Makroskopische und mikroskopische Anatomie unter funktionellen Gesichtspunkten, vol 1, 13th edn. Urban & Schwarzenberg, Munich

Frost HM (1960) In vivo staining of bone with tetracyclines. Stain Technol 35:135–138

Frost HM (1963) Bone remodelling dynamics. Thomas, Springfield, Ill.

Garden RS (1961) The structure and function of the proximal end of the femur. J Bone Joint Surg 43:576–589

Goldhaber P (1962) Some current concepts of bone physiology. N Engl J Med 266:924–931

Gurley AM, Roth SL (1992) Bone. In: Sternberg SS (ed) Histology for pathologists, chap 3. Raven, New York, pp 61–79

Hancox N (1956) The osteoclast. In: Bourne GH (ed) The biochemistry and physiology of bone. Academic Press, New York

Hert J, HladikovA J (1961) Die Gefäßversorgung des Haversschen Knochens. Acta Anat (Basel) 45:344–361

Heuck F (1979) Radiologie des gesunden Skelettes. In: Schinz HR, Baensch WE, Frommhold W et al (eds) Lehrbuch der Röntgendiagnostik, vol II/part 1, 6th edn. Thieme, Stuttgart, pp 3–143

Howe WW, Lacey T, Schwartz RP (1950) A study of the gross anatomy of the arteries supplying the proximal portion of the femur and the acetabulum. J Bone Joint Surg Am 32:856–866

Jaffe HL (1929) The vessel canals in normal and pathological bone. Am J Pathol 5:323–333

Junqueira LC, Carneiro J (1996) Histologie – Zytologie Histologie und mikroskopische Anatomie des Menschen, 4th edn. Springer, Berlin Heidelberg New York

Johnson RW (1927) A physiological study of the blood supply of the diaphysis. J Bone Joint Surg 9:153–184

Judet J, Judet R, Lagrange J, Dunoyer J (1955) A study of the arterial vascularization of the femoral neck in the adult. J Bone Joint Surg Am 37:663–680

Kelly PJ, Janes JM, Peterson LFA (1959) The effect of arteriovenous fistulae on the vascular pattern of the femora of immature dogs: a micro-angiographic study. J Bone Joint Surg Am 41:1101–1108

Klümper A (1969) Intraossäre Angiographie. Topographische und morphologische Untersuchungen zur Darstellung intraossärer Gefäße. Habilitationsschrift, Universität Freiburg

Klümper A (1976) Möglichkeiten der intraossären Angiographie zur Differentialdiagnose von Knochentumoren. Orthop Prax 10:949–953

Klümper A (1976) Grundlagen zur intraossären Angiographie am menschlichen Röhrenknochen. Fortschr Röntgenstr 125:129–136

Klümper A (1977) Differentialdiagnose aneurysmatische Knochenzyste und nicht ossifizierendes Fibrom. Fortschr Röntgenstr 127:261–264

Klümper A, Strey M, Schütz W (1968) Tierexperimentelle Untersuchungen zur intraossären Angiographie. Fortschr Röntgenstr 108:607–612

Lewis OJ (1956) The blood supply of developing long bones with special reference to the metaphysis. J Bone Joint Surg Br 38:928–933

Pauwels F (1973) Atlas zur Biomechanik der gesunden und kranken Hüfte. Prinzip, Technik und Resultate einer kausalen Therapie. Springer, Berlin Heidelberg New York

Pliess G (1974) Bewegungsapparat. In: Doerr W (ed) Organpathologie, vol III. Thieme, Stuttgart

Pommer G (1927) Über Begriff und Bedeutung der durchbohrenden Knochenkanäle. Z Mikrosk Anat Forsch 9:540–584

Pritchard JJ (1956) The osteoblast. In: Bourne GH (ed) The biochemistry and physiology of bone. Academic Press, New York

Rauber A, Kopsch F (1968) Lehrbuch und Atlas der Anatomie des Menschen, vol 1, 20th edn. Thieme, Stuttgart

Resch H, Battmarm A (1995) Die Bedeutung von Wachstumsfaktoren und Zytokinen im Knochenstoffwechsel und Remodeling. Osteologie 4:137–144

Rogers WM, Gladstone H (1950) Vascular foramina and arterial supply of the distal end of the femur. J Bone Joint Surg Am 32:867–974

Schinz HR, Baensch WE, Friedl E, Uehlinger E (1952) Lehrbuch der Röntgendiagnostik, 5th edn. Thieme, Stuttgart

Schumacher S (1935) Zur Anordming der Gefäßkanäle in der Diaphyse langer Röhrenknochen des Menschen. Z Mikrosk Anat Forsch 38:145–160

Tilling G (1958) The vascular anatomy of long bones: a radiological and histological study. Acta Radiol (Stockh) 1–107

Wilkinson LS, Pitsillides AA, Worrall JG, Edwards JCW (1992) Light microscopic characterization of the fibroblast-like synovial intimal cell (synoviocyte). Arthritis Rheum 35:1179–1184

Zheng MH, Wood DJ, Papadimitriou JM (1992) What's new in the role of cytokines on osteoblast proliferation and differentiation? Pathol Res Pract 188:1104–1121

Chapter 3
Disorders of Skeletal Development

Adler CP (1976) Knochenentzündungen. In: Thomas C, Sandritter W (eds) Spezielle Pathologie. Textbuch zu einem audiovisuellen Kurs. Schattauer, Stuttgart

Adler CP (1979) Differential diagnosis of cartilage tumors. Pathol Res Pract 166:45–58

Adler CP (1981) Störungen der Funktion des Knochens. In: Sandritter W (ed) Allgemeine Pathologie, 2nd edn, Schattauer, Stuttgart, pp 718–740

Adler CP (1992) Knochen und Gelenke. In: Thomas C (ed) Histopathologie, 11th edn. Schattauer, Stuttgart, S 290–314

Adler CP, Bollmann R (1973) Osteogenesis imperfecta congenita (Vrolik). Med Welt 24:2007–2012

Adler CP, Wenz W (1981) Intraossäre Osteolyseherde. Diagnostik, Differentialdiagnostik und Therapie. Radiologe 21:470–479

Adler CP, Klümper A, Wenz W (1979) Enchondrome aus radiologischer und pathologisch-anatomischer Sicht. Radiologe 19:341–349

Adler CP, Brendlein F, Limberg J, Böhm N (1979) Vitamin D-Mangel-Rachitis. Med Welt 30:141–146

Aegerter E, Kirkpatrick JA Jr (1968) Orthopedic diseases, 3rd edn. Saunders, Philadelphia

Agarwal RP, Sharma DK, Upadhyay VK, Goel SP, Gupta P, Singh R (1991) Hypophosphatasia. Indian Pediatrics 28:1518–1520

Albers-Schönberg H (1904) Röntgenbilder einer seltenen Knochenerkrankung. MMW 51:365

Albers-Schönberg H (1907) Eine bisher nicht beschriebene Allgemeinerkrankung des Skelettes im Röntgenbild. Fortschr Röntgenstr 11:261–263

Althoff H (1968) Marmorknochenkrankheit (Morbus Albers-Schönberg). In: Handbuch der medizinischen Radiologie, vol V/3, Springer, Berlin Heidelberg New York, pp 104

Andersen PE, Bollerslev J (1987) Heterogencity of autosomal dominant osteopetrosis. Radiology 164:223–225

Arnstein AR, Frame B, Frost HM (1967) Recent progress in osteomalacia and rickets. Ann Intern Med 67:1296–1330

Balsan S, Garabedian M (1991) Rickets, osteomalacia, and osteopetrosis. Curr Opin Rheumatol 3:496–502

Belani KG, Krivit W, Carpenter BL et al (1993) Children with mucopolysaccharidosis: perioperative care, morbidity, mortality, and new findings. J Pediatr Surg 28:403–408

Benedict PH (1962) Endocrine features in Albright's syndrome (fibrous dysplasia of bone). Metabolism 11:30–45

Bessler W, Fanconi A (1972) Die Röntgensymptome der Hypophosphatasie. Beobachtungen an 2 Brüdern mit maligner neonataler Verlaufsform. Fortschr Röntgenstr 117:58–65

Böhm N (1984) Kinderpathologie. Schattauer, Stuttgart

Bollerslev J, Nielsen HK, Larsen HF (1988) Biochemical evidence of disturbed bone metabolism and calcium homeostasis in two types of autosomal dominant osteopetrosis. Acta Med Scand 224:479–483

Bollerslev J, Mosekilde L (1993) Autosomal dominant osteopetrosis. Clin Orthop 294:45–51

Brenton DP, Krywawych S (1986) Hypophosphatasia. Clin Rheum Dis 12:771–789

Byers PH, Steiner RD (1992) Osteogenesis imperfecta. Ann Rev Med 43:269–282

Carey MC, Fitzgerald O, McKiernan E (1968) Osteogenesis imperfecta with twenty-three members of a kindred with heritable features contributed by a nonspecific skeletal-disorder. QJM (NS) 37:437–449

Czitober H (1971) Die Marmorknochenkrankheit der Erwachsenen (M. Albers-Schönberg, Osteopetrose). I. Histochemische, polarisationsoptische und mikroradiographische Untersuchungen nach intravitalen Biopsien. Wien Z Inn Med 52:245–256

Czitober H, Moser K, Gründig E (1967) Die Marmorknochenkrankheit des Erwachsenen (M. Albers-Schönberg, Osteopetrose). II. Biochemische Untersuchungen. Klin Wochenschr 45:73–77

Coley BL, Higinbotham NL (1949) The significance of cartilage in abnormal locations. Cancer (Phila) 2:777–788

Collard M (1962) Contribution l'étude de l'ostéogenèse imparfaite létale et de l'ostéopsathyrose. J Belge Radiol 45:541–580

Currarino G, Neuhauser EBD, Reyersbach GC, Sobel EH (1957) Hypophosphatasia. Am J Roentgenol 78:392–419

Eggli KD, Dorst JP (1986) The mucopolysaccharidoses and related conditions. Semin Roentgenol 21:275–294

El-Tawil T, Stoker DJ (1993) Benign osteopetrosis: a review of 42 cases showing two different patterns. Skeletal Radiol 22:587–593

Fanconi A, Prader A (1972) Hereditäre Rachitisformen. Schweiz Med Wochenschr 102:1073–1078

Faser D (1957) Hypophosphatasie. Am J Med 22:730–746

Felix R, Hofstetter W, Cecchini MG (1996) Recent developments in the understanding of the pathophysiology of osteopetrosis. Eur J Endocrinol 134:143–156

Fensom AH, Benson PF (1994) Recent advances in the prenatal diagnosis of the mucopolysaccharidoses. (Review). Prenat Diagn 14:1–12

Follis RH Jr (1953) Maldevelopment of the corium in osteogenesis imperfecta syndrome. Bull Johns Hopk Hosp 93:225–233

Franzen J, Haas JP (1961) Bevorzugt halbseitige Knochenchondromatose, eine sogenannte Ollier'sche Erkrankung. Radiol Clin (Basel) 30:28–45

Frost HM (1987) Osteogenesis imperfecta. The set point proposal (a possible causative mechanism). Clin Orthop Rel Res 216:280–297

Gerstel G (1938) Über die infantile Form der Marmorknochenkrankheit auf Grund vollständiger Untersuchung des Knochengerüstes. Frankfurt Z Pathol 51:23–42

Gilbert-Barness E (ed) (1997) Potters's pathology of the fetus and infant. Mosby, St. Louis

Godin V (1938) Über einen Fall von Marmorknochenkrankheit. Zentralbl Allg Pathol Pathol Anat 70:357–358

Grodurn E, Gram J, Brixen K (1995) Autosomal dominant osteopetrosis: bone mineral measurement of the entire skeleton of adults in two different subtypes. Bone 16:431–434

Gupta SK, Sharma OP, Malhotra S, Gupta S (1992) Cleidocranial dysostosis – skeletal abnormalities. Australas Radiol 36:238–242

Hall JG (1988) The natural history of achondroplasia. Basic Life Sci 48:3–9

Hasenhuttl K (1962) Osteopetrosis. Review of the literature and comparative studies on a case with a twenty-four year follow-up. J Bone Joint Surg Am 44:359–370

Heidger P (1936) Ein Fall von Marmorkrankheit beim Erwachsenen. Beitr Pathol Anat 97:509–525

Heys FM, Blattner RJ, Robinson HBG (1960) Osteogenesis imperfecta. and odontogenesis imperfecta: Clinic and genetic apsects in eighteen families. J Pediatr 56:234–245

Hinkel CL, DD Beiler: Osteopetrosis in adults. Am J Roentgenol 74:46–64 (1955)

Hopf M (1949) Zur Kenntnis der polyostotischen fibrösen Dysplasie (Jaffe-Lichtenstein). Radiol Clin (Basel) 18:129–158

Jaffe HL (1943) Hereditary multiple exostosis. Arch Pathol 36:335–357

Jaffe HL (1958) Solitary and multiple osteocartilaginous exostosis. In: Tumors and tumorous conditions of the bones and joints. Lea & Febiger, Philadelphia, pp 143–168

Jaffe HL (1958) Solitary enchondroma and multiple enchondromatosis. In.: Tumors and tumorous conditions of the bones and joints. Lea & Febiger, Philadelphia, pp 169–195

Jaffe HL (1972) Metabolic, degenerative, and inflammatory diseases of bones and joints. Urban & Schwarzenberg, Munich

Jervis GA, Schein H (1951) Polyostotic fibrous dysplasia (Albright's disease). Report of a case showing central nervous system changes. Arch Pathol 51:640–450

Jesserer H (1969) Zur Frage der malignen Entartung einer fibrösen Knochendysplasie. Fortschr Röntgenstr 3:251–256

Jesserer H (1971) Knochenkrankheiten. Urban & Schwarzenberg, Munich

Johnston CC Jr, Lavy N, Lord T, Vellios F, Merritt AD, Deiss WP Jr (1968) Osteopetrosis. A clinical, genetic, metabolic, and morphologic study of the dominantly inherited benign form. Medicine (Balt) 47:149–167

Keith A (1919–20) Studies on the anatomical changes which accompany certain growth-disorders of the human body. 1. The nature of the structural alterations in the disorder known as multiple exostoses. J Anat 54:101–115

Klemm GF, Kleine FD, Witkowski R, Lachrein L (1965) Familiäres Vorkommen der Osteogenesis imperfecta tarda. Beobachtungen an vier Generationen. Klin Wochenschr 43:2–27

Kovacs CS, Lambert RGW, Lavoie GJ (1995) Centrifugal osteopetrosis: appendicular sclerosis with relative sparing of the vertebrae. Skeletal Radiol 24:27–29

Kozlowski K, Sutcliff J, Barylak et al (1976) Hypophosphatasia: review of 24 cases. Pediatr Radiol 5:103–117

Kransdorf MJ, Moser RP Jr, Gilkey FW (1990) Fibrous dysplasia. Radiographics 10:519–137

Kutsumi K, Nojima T, Yamashiro K et al (1996) Hyperplastic callus formation in both femurs in osteogenesis imperfecta. Skeletal Radiol 25:384–387

Langer LO, Baumann PA, Gorlin RJ (1967) Achondroplasia. Am J Roentgenol 100:12–26

Laubmann W (1936) Über die Knochenstruktur bei Marmorknochenkrankheit. Virchows Arch Pathol Anat 296:343–357

Laurence W, Franklin EL (1953) Calcifying enchondroma of the long bones. J Bone Joint Surg Br 35:224–228

Levin LS, Wright JM, Byrd DL et al (1985) Osteogenesis imperfecta with unusual skeletal lesions: report of three families. Am J Med Genet 21:257–269

Levy WM, Aegerter EE, Kirkpatrick JA Jr (1964) The nature of cartilaginous tumors. Radiol Clin North Am 2:327–336

Lückig T, Delling G (1973) Schwere rachitische Osteopathie bei antiepileptischer Langzeitbehandlung. Dtsch Med Wochenschr 98:1036–1040

Lullmann-Rauch R, Peters A, Schleicher A (1992) Osteopenia in rats with drug-induced mucopolysaccharidosis. Arzneimittelforsch 42:559–566

Lund-Sorensen N, Gudmundsen TE, Ostensen H (1997) Autosomal dominant osteopetrosis: report of a Norwegian family with radiographic or anamnestic findings differing from the generally accepted classification. Skeletal Radiol 26:173–176

McPeak CN (1936) Osteopetrosis. Report of eight cases occuring in three generations of one family. Am J Roentgenol 36:816–829

Mankin HJ (1974) Rickets, osteomalacia and renal osteodystrophia. 1. J Bone Joint Surg Am 56:101–128

Mankin HJ (1974) Rickets, osteomalacia and renal osteodystrophia. 2. J Bone Joint Surg Am 56:352–386

Maroteaux P, Lamy M (1960) La dyschondroplasie. Semin Hp, Paris 36:182–193

Materna A (1956) Beitrag zur Kenntnis der Knochenveränderungen, hauptsächlich des Schädels bei der Marmorknochenkrankheit. Beitr Pathol Anat 116:396–421

Milgram JW, Murali J (1982) Osteopetrosis: a morphological study of twenty-one cases. J Bone Joint Surg Am 64:912–919

Montgomery RD, Standard KL (1960) Albers-Schönberg's disease: a changing concept. J Bone Joint Surg Br 42:303–312

Murdoch JL, Walker BA, Hall JG, Abbey H, Smith KK, McKusick VA (1970) Achondroplasia – a genetic and statistical survey. Ann Hum Genet 33:227–244

Murken JD (1963) Über multiple cartilaginäre Exostosen: Zur Klinik, Genetik und Mutationsrate des Krankheitsbildes. Z Menschl Vererb Konstit Lehre 36:469–505

Murray RO, Jacobson HG (1977) The radiology of skeletal disorders, 2nd edn. Churchill Livingstone, Edinburgh

Neuhauser EBD, Currarino G (1954) Hypophosphatasia. Am J Roentgenol 72:875

Nishimura G, Haga N, Ikeuchi S et al (1996) Fragile bone syndrome associated with craniognathic fibro-osseous lesions and abnormal modeling of the tubular bones: report of two cases and review of the literature. Skeletal Radiol 25:717–722

Park EA (1939) Observations of the pathology of rickets with particular reference to the changes at the cartilage shaft junctions of the growing bone. Bull N Y Acad Med 15:495–543

Pilgerstorfer W (1960) Cortison-Wirkung bei Albers-Schönbergscher Erkrankung (Marmorknochenkrankheit). Wien Z Inn Med 41:177–188

Pines B, Lederer M (1947) Osteopetrosis: Albers-Schönberg disease (marble bones). Report of a case and morphologic study. Am J Pathol 23:755–781

Pitt MJ (1991) Rickets and osteomalacia are still around. Radiol Clin North Am 29:97–118

Plenk H Jr (1974) Osteolathyrismus: Morphometrische, histochemische und mikroradiographische Untersuchungen einer experimentellen Knochenerkrankung. Verh Dtsch Ges Pathol 58:302–304

Ponseti IV (1970) Skeletal growth in achondroplasia. J Bone Joint Surg Am 52:701–716

Rathbun JC (1948) Hypophosphatasia. Am J Dis Child 75:822–831

Ritchie GMcL (1964) Hypophosphatasia: a metabolic disease with important dental manifestations. Arch Dis Child 39:584–590

Rohr HP (1963) Autoradiographische Untersuchungen über das Knorpel-/Knochen-Längenwachstum bei der experimentellen Rattenrachitis. Z Ges Exp Med 137:248–255

Rudling O, Riise R, Tornqvist K, Jonsson K (1996) Skeletal abnormalities of hands and feet in Laurence-Moon-Bardet-Biedl (LMBB) syndrome: a radiographic study. Skeletal Radiol 25:655–660

Ruprecht A, Wagner H, Engel H (1988) Osteopetrosis: report of a case and discussion of the differential diagnosis. Oral Surg Med Pathol 66:674–679

Saffran M (1995) Rickets: return of an old disease. J Am Pediatr Med Assoc 85:222–225

Salomon L (1964) Hereditary multiple exostosis. Am J Hum Genet 16:351–363

Schaefer HE (1974) Osteopetrosis Albers-Schönberg im Adoleszenten- und Erwachsenenalter. Verh Dtsch Ges Pathol 58:337–341

Schäfer EL, Sturm A Jr (1963) Zur Therapie und zum Verlauf der fibrösen Knochendysplasie. Dtsch Med Wochenschr 88:464–467

Schlesinger B, Luder J, Bodian M (1955) Rickets with alkaline phosphatase deficiency: an osteoblastic dysplasia. Arch Dis Child 30:265–276

Schmidt H, Ullrich K, Lenerke HJ von, Kleine M, Bramswig J (1987) Radiological findings in patients with mucopolysaccharidosisis I H/S (Hurler–Scheie–Syndrome). Pediatr Radiol 17:409–414

Schulz A, Delling G (1974) Zur Histopathologie und Morphometrie der Rachitis und ihrer Sonderformen. Verh Dtsch Ges Pathol 58:354–359

Scott D, Stiris G (1953) Osteogenesis imperfecta tarda. A study of three families with special references to scar formation. Acta Med Scand 145:237–257

Shapiro F (1993) Osteopetrosis: current clinical comidcrations. Clin Orthop 294:34–44

Silve C (1994) Hereditary hypophosphatasia and hyperphosphatasia. (Review). Curr Opin Rheum 6:336–339

Silvestrini G, Ferraccioli GF, Quaini F, Palummeri E, Bonucci E (1987) Adult osteopetrosis. Studies of two brothers. Appl Pathol 5:184–189

Singer FR, Chang SS (1992) Osteopetrosis (Review). Semin Nephrol 12:191–199

Smith R (1986) Osteogenesis imperfecta. Clin Rheum Dis 12:655–689

Sobel EH, Clark LC Jr, Fox RP, Robinow M (1953) Rickets, deficiency of alkaline phosphatase activity and premature loss of teeth in childhood. Pediatrics 11:309–322

Spjut HJ, Dorfman HD, Fechner RE, Ackerman IV (1971) Tumors of bone and cartilage. Armed Forces Institute of Pathology, Washington/DC

Spranger J, Langer LO, Wiedemann HR (1974) Bone dysplasias: an atlas of constitutional disorders of skeletal development. Fischer, Stuttgart

Takigawa K (1971) Chondroma of the bones of the hand: a review of 110 cases. J Bone Joint Surg Am 53:1591–1600

Uehlinger E (1949) Zur pathologischen Anatomie der frühinfantilen malignen Form der Marmorknochenkrankheit mit einfach recessivem Erbgang. Helv Paediatr Acta 4:60–76

Uehlinger E (1972) Osteogenesis imperfecta. In: Schinz HR, Baensch WE et al (eds) Lehrbuch der Röntgendiagnostik. Thieme, Stuttgart

Vetter U, Brenner R, Teller WM, Worsdorfer O (1989) Osteogenesis imperfecta. Neue Gesichtspunkte zu Grundlagen, Klinik und Therapie. Klin Pädiatr 201:359–368

Voegelin M (1943) Zur pathologischen Anatomie der Osteogenesis imperfecta Typus Lobstein Radiol Clin 12:397–415

Warzok R, Seidlitz G (1992) Muccopolysaccharidosen. Genetik, klinische Pathologie, Therapieansätze. Zentralbl Pathol 138:226–234

Wigglesworth JS, Singer DB (eds) (1991) Textbook of fetal and perinatal pathology. Blackwell, Boston

Weyers H (1968) Osteogenesis imperfecta. In: Springer, Berlin Heidelberg New York (Hdb. der medizinischen Radiologie, vol V/3)

Whyte MP, Teitelbaum SL, Murphy WA, Bergfeld MA, Avioli IV (1979) Adult hypophosphatasia. Medicine (Balt) 58:329

Chapter 4
Osteoporoses and Osteopathies

Adler CP (1981) Störungen der Funktion des Knochens. In: Sandritter W (ed) Allgemeine Pathologie, 2nd edn. Schattauer, Stuttgart, pp 718–740

Adler CP, Reinhold W-D (1989) Osteodensitometry of vertebral metastases after radiotherapy using quantitative computed tomography. Skeletal Radiol 18:517–521

Adler CP, Reinhold W-D (1991) Accuracy of vertebral mineral determination by dual-energy quantitative computed tomography. Skeletal Radiol 20:25–29

Albright F (1947) Effect of hormones on osteogenesis in man. Recent Prog Horm Res 7:293–353

Albright F, Reifenstein EC Jr (1948) The parathyroid glands and metabolic bone disease. Williams & Wilkins, Baltimore

Albright F, Smith PH, Richardson AM (1941) Postmenopausal osteoporosis. J Am Med Assoc 116:2465–2474

Bard R, Moser W, Burkhardt R et al (1978) Diabetische Osteomyelopathie: Histobioptische Befunde am Knochen und Knochenmark bei Diabetes mellitus. Klin Wochenschr 56:743–754

Bordier PJ, Marie PJ, Arnaud CD (1975) Evolution of renal osteodystrophy: Correlation of bone histomorphometry and serum mineral and immunoreactive parathyroid hormone values before and after treatment with calcium carbonate or 25-hydroxycholecalciferol. Kidney Int 7:102–112

Burkhardt R (1966) Technische Verbesserung und Anwendungsbereich der Histo-Biopsie von Knochenmark und Knochen. Klin Wochenschr 44:326–334

Burkhardt R (1979) Knochenveränderungen bei Erkrankungen des Knochenmarks. Verh Dtsch Ges Inn Med 85:323–341

Burkhardt R, Bartl R, Demmler K, Kettner G (1981) Zwölf histobioptische Thesen zur Pathogenese der primären und sekundären Osteoporose. Klin Wochenschr 59:5–18

Byers PD, Smith R (1971) Quantitative histology of bone in hyperparathyroidism: its relation to clinical features, X-rays and biochemistry. QJM 40:471–486

Delling G (1972) Metabolische Osteopathien. Fischer, Stuttgart

Delling G (1973) Age related bone changes. Curr Top Pathol 58:117–147

Delling G (1975) Endokrine Osteopathien. Fischer, Stuttgart (Veröffentlichungen aus der Pathologie, H. 98, pp 1–115)

Delling G (1979) Aussagemöglichkeiten der knochenhistologischen Untersuchungen bei Niereninsuffizienz. Mitt Klin Nephrol 8:22–41

Delling G, Lijhmann H (1979) Morphologie und Histomorphometrie der renalen Osteopathie. In: Hensch RD, Hehrmann R (eds) Renale Osteopathie: Diagnostik, präventive und kurative Therapie. Thieme, Stuttgart, pp 22–45

Delling G, Schulz A (1978) Histomorphometrische und ultrastrukturelle Skelettveränderungen beim primären Hyperparathyreoidismus. Therapiewoche 28:3646–3654

Delling G, Schulz A, Schulz W (1975) Morphologische Klassifikation der renalen Osteopathie. Mels Med Mitt 49:133–140

Delling G, Ziegler R, Schulz A (1976) Bone cells and structure of cancellous bone in primary hyperparathyroidism: a histomorphometric and electron microscopic study. Calcif Tissue Res Suppl 21:278–283

Delling H, Schulz A, Fuchs C et al (1979) Die Osteopenie als Spätkomplikation der renalen Osteopathie – Häufigkeit, Verlauf und Therapieansätze. Verb Dtsch Ges Inn Med 82:1549–1551

Dent CE, Friedmann M (1965) Idiopathic juvenile osteoporosis. QJM (NS) 34:177–210

Eichler J (1970) Inaktivitätsosteoporose. Klinische und experimentelle Studie zum Knochenumbau durch Inaktivität. In: Cotta H (ed) Aktuelle Orthopädie, Issue 3, pp 1–7. Thieme, Stuttgart (new edn: Enke, Stuttgart)

Ellegast H (1961) Zur Röntgensymptomatologie der Osteomalazie. Radiol Austriaca 11:85–114

Ellegast H (1966) Das Röntgenbild der Cortisonschäden. Wien Klin Wochenschr 78:747–755

Fanconi A, Illig R, Poley JR et al (1966) Idiopathische transitorische Osteoporose im Pubertätsalter. Helv Paediatr Acta 21:531–547

Freudenberg N, Adler CP, Halbfag H, Kröpelin T (1975) Renal Osteopathie. Med Welt (Stuttg.) 26:1061–1066

Frost M (1973) Bone remodelling and its relationship to metabolic bone diseases. Thomas, Springfield, Ill.

Frost HM, Villanueva AR, Ramser JR, Ilnick L (1966) Knochenbiodynamik bei 39 Osteoporose-Fällen gemessen durch Tetrazyklinmarkierungen. Internist (Berl) 7:572–578

Haas HG (1966) Knochenstoffwechsel- und Parathyreoidea-Erkrankungen. Thieme, Stuttgart

Henning HV, Delling G, Fuchs C, Scheler F (1977) Verlauf einer progressiven renalen Osteopathie mit Mineralisationsstörung und sekundärem Hyperparathyreoidismus unter Vitamin-D3-Therapie, nach Parathyreoidektomie und 38monatiger Heimdialyse-Behandlung. Nieren Hochdruckkrankh 4:148–154

Herrath D von, Kraft D, Schaefer K, Krempien B (1974) Die Behandlung der urämischen Osteopathie. MMW 116:1573–1578

Horowitz MC (1993) Cytokines and estrogen in bone: anti-osteoporotic effects. Science 260:626–627

Howland WJ, Pugh DG, Sprague RG (1958) Roentgenologic changes of the skeletal system in Cushing's syndrome. Radiology 71:69–78

Jesserer H (1963) Osteoporose. Wesen, Erkennung, Beurteilung und Behandlung. Blaschker, Berlin

Jesserer H (1971) Knochenkrankheiten. Urban & Schwarzenberg, Munich

Jesserer H, Zeitlhofer J (1967) Über Cortisonveränderungen am Stütz- und Bindegewebe. Arch Klin Med 213:328–338

Jowsey J (1974) Bone histology and hyperparathyroidism. Clin Endocrinol Metabol 3:267–303

Kienböck R (1901) Über akute Knochenatrophie bei Entzündungsprozessen an den Extremitäten und ihre Diagnose nach dem Röntgenbild. Wien Med Wochenschr 51:1345–1348; 1389–1392; 1427–1430; 1462–1466; 1508

Krempien B, Ritz E, Ditzen E, Hudelmeier G (1972) Über den Einfluß der Niereninsuffizienz auf Knochenbildung und Knochenresorption. Virchows Arch Abt A 355:354

Kruse HP (1978) Die primäre Osteoporose und ihre Pathogenese. Springer, Berlin Heidelberg New York

Kuhlencordt F (1978) Osteoporose. Verh Dtsch Ges Inn Med 85:269–276

Lange HP, Alluche HH, Arras D (1974) Die Entwicklung der renalen Osteopathie unter chronischer Hämodialysebehandlung bei bilateral nephrektomierten, skelettgesunden Patienten. Verh Dtsch Ges Pathol 58:366–370

Linke H (1959) Das Sudeck-Syndrom als intern-medizinisches Problem. MMW 101:658–662; 702–705

Münchow M, Kruse H-P (1995) Densitometrische Untersuchungen zum Verhalten von Kortikalis und Spongiosa bei primärer und sekundärer Osteoporose. Osteologie 4:21–26

Niethard FU, Pfeil J (1989) Orthopädie. Hippokrates, Stuttgart (Duale Reihe)

Olah AJ (1973) Quantitative relations between osteoblasts and osteoid in primary hyperparathyroidism, intestinal malabsorption and renal osteodystrophy. Virchows Arch Abt A 358:301–308

Ostertag H, Greiser E, Thiele J, Vykoupil KF (1974) Histomorphologische Unterschiede am Knochen bei primärer und sekundärer Form des Hyperparathyreodismus. Verh Dtsch Ges Pathol 58:347–350

Prechtel K, Kamke W, Lohan C, Osang M, Bartl R (1976) Morphometrische Untersuchungen über altersabhängige Knochenveränderungen am Beckenkamm und Wirbelkörper post mortem. Verh Dtsch Ges Pathol 60:356

Ritz E, Krempien B, Bommer J, Jesdinski HJ (1974) Kritik der morphometrischen Methode bei metabolischer Osteopathie. Verh Dtsch Ges Pathol 58:363–365

Ritz E, Prager F, Krempien B, Bommer J (1975) Röntgenologische Veränderungen des Skeletts bei Urämie. Nieren Hochdruckkrankh 4:109–113

Rosenkranz A, Zweymüller E (1963) Klinische und biochemische Probleme einer jahrelangen Glucocorticoidverabreichung. Z Kinderheilkd 88:91–106

Rüegsegger F, Rüegsegger E, Dambacher MA et al (1995) Natural bone loss and the effect of transdermal estrogen in the early postmenopause of healthy women. Osteologie 4:13–20

Schenk RK, Merz WA (1969) Histologisch-morphometrische Untersuchungen über Altersatrophie und senile Osteoporose in der Spongiosa des Beckenkammes. Dtsch Med Wochenschr 94:206–208

Schulz A (1975) Einbettung mineralisierten Knochengewebes für die Elektronenmikroskopie. Beitr Pathol Anat 156:280–288

Schulz W, Delling G, Heidler R, Schulz A (1975) Schweregrad, Verlauf und Therapie der renalen Osteopathie – vergleichende klinische und histomorphometrische Untersuchungen an Patienten mit chronischer Niereninsuf-

fizienz. In: Dittrich PV (ed) 5. Symposium Innsbruck 1973. Bindernagel, Treidenheim

Scola E, Schliack H (1991) Das posttraumatische Sudeck-Syndrom. Dtsch Ärztebl 88:1590–1592

Sudeck P (1901) Über die akute (reflektorische) Knochenatrophie nach Entzündungen und Verletzungen an den Extremitäten und ohne klinische Erscheinungen. Fortschr Röntgenstr 5:277–292

Sudeck P (1942) Die sogenannte akute Knochenatrophie als Entzündungsvorgang. Chirurg 15:449–458

Thorban W (1965) Der heutige Stand der Lehre vom Sudeck-Syndrom. Hippokrates (Stuttg) 10:384–387

Vitalli HP (1970) Knochenerkrankungen. Histologie und Klinik. Sandoz-Monographien

Vykoupil KF (1974) Metabolische Osteopathien im Kindesalter – Bioptische Befunde. Verh Dtsch Ges Pathol 58: 360–363

Wagner H (1965) Präsenile Osteoporose. Physiologie des Knochenumbaus und Messung der Spongiosadichte. Thieme, Stuttgart

Watson L (1974) Primary hyperparathyroidism. Clin Endocrinol Metabol 3:215–235

Wegmann A (1973) Die Alters- und Geschlechtsunterschiede des Knochenanbaus in Rippencorticalis und Beckenkammspongiosa. Acta Anat (Basel) 84:572–583

Wilde CD, Jaworski ZF, Villanueva AR, Frost HM (1973) Quantitative histological measurements of bone turnover in primary hyperparathyroidism. Calcif Tissue Res 12: 137–142

Chapter 5
Osteoscleroses

Adler CP (1992) Knochen – Gelenke. In: Thomas C (ed) Histopathologie, 11th edn. Schattauer, Stuttgart, pp 258–283

Aegerter E, Kirkpatrick JA Jr (1968) Orthopedic Diseases. Saunders, Philadelphia

Albers-Schönberg H (1915/16) Eine seltene, bisher unbekannte Strukturanomalie des Skelettes. Fortschr Röntgenstr 23:174–177

Armstrong R, Chettle DR, Scott MC, Somervaille LJ, Pendlington M (1992) Repeated measurements of tibia lead concentrations by in vivo X-ray fluorescence in occupational exposure. Br J Ind Med 49:14–16

Augenstein WL, Spoerke DG, Kulig KW et al (1991) Fluoride ingestion in children: a review of 87 cases. Pediatrics 88:907–912

Barr DGP, Prader A, Esper U et al (1971) Chronic hypoparathyroidism in two generations. Helv Paediatr Acta 26:507–521

Barry HC (1960) Sarcoma in Paget's disease of bones. Aust N Z J Surg 29:304–310

Barry HC (1969) Paget's disease of bone. Churchill Livingstone, Edinburgh

Barsony T, Schulhof O (1930) Der Elfenbeinwirbel. Fortschr Röntgenstr 42:597–609

Begemann H (1975) Klinische Hämatologie, 2nd edn. Thieme, Stuttgart

Bell NH, Avery S, Johnston CC (1970) Effects of calcitonin in Paget's disease and polyostotic fibrous dysplasia. J Clin Endocrinol 31:283–290

Berlin R (1967) Osteopoikylosis – a clinical and genetic study. Acta Med Scand 181:305–314

Beyer U, Paul D (1972) Frakturen bei ostitis deformans Paget. Zentralbl Chir 97:470–476

Block MH (1976) Text-atlas of hematology. Lea & Febiger, Philadelphia, p 287

Caffey J (1973) Paediatric X-ray diagnosis. 6th edn. Lloyd-Luke, London

Campbell CJ, Papademetrious T, Bonfigho M (1968) Melorheostosis: a report of the clinical, roentgenographic and pathological findings in fourteen cases. J Bone Joint Surg Am 50:1281–1304

Chapman GK (1992) The diagnosis of Paget's disease of bone. Aust N Z J Surg 62:24–32

Chaykin LS, Frame B, Sigler JW (1969) Spondylitis: a clue to hypoparathyroidism. Ann Intern Med 70:995–1000

Cocchi U (1952) Erbschäden mit Knochenveränderungen. In: Schinz HR, Baensch WE, Friedl E, Uehlinger E (eds) Lehrbuch der Röntgendiagnostik, vol I/I. Thieme, Stuttgart, pp 716–719

Collins DH (1956) Paget's disease of bone. Incidence and subclinical forms. Lancet 11:51–57

Collins DH (1966) Pathology of bone, chap 12. Butterworth, London, pp 228–248

Cooke BED (1956) Paget's disease of the jaws: 15 cases. Ann Roy Coll Surg Engl 19:223–240

Delling G (1975) Endokrine Osteopathien. Fischer, Stuttgart (Veröffentlichungen aus der Pathologie, Issue 98, pp 1–115)

Drury BJ (1962) Paget's disease of the skull and facial bones. J Bone Joint Surg Am 44:174–179

Edeiken J, Hodes PJ (1973) Roentgen diagnosis of diseases of bone, 2nd edn. Williams & Wilkins, Baltimore

Edholm OG, Howarth S, McMichael J (1945) Heart failure and blood flow in osteitis deformans. Clin Sci 5:249–260

Eisman JA, Martin TJ (1986) Osteolytic Paget's disease. Recognition and risks of biopsy. J Bone Joint Surg Am 68:112–117

Ellegast HH (1973) Das Röntgenbild der Knochenfluorose. Therapiewoche 23:3963–3964

Ellegast HH (1972) Exogene toxische Osteopathien. In: Schinz HR, Baensch WE et al (eds) Lehrbuch der Röntgendiagnostik. Thieme, Stuttgart

Enderle A, Willert H-G, Zichner L (1993) Die Fluorwirkung am Skelett. Osteologie 2:35–40

Erkkila J, Armstrong R, Riihimaki V et al (1992) In vivo measurements of lead in bone at four anatomical sites: long term occupational and consequent endogenous exposure. Br J Ind Med 49:631–644

Frommhold W, Glauner R, Uehlinger E, Wellauer J (eds) (1979) Lehrbuch der Röntgendiagnostik, 6th edn., vol II/1. Thieme, Stuttgart, pp 1052–1065

Erbsen H (1936) Die Osteopoikilie (Osteopathia condensans disseminata). Ergebn Med Strahlenforsch 7

Faccini JM (1969) Fluoride and bone. Calcif Tissue Res 3:1–16

Fanconi A (1969) Hypoparathyreoidismus im Kindesalter. Ergeb Inn Med Kinderheilkd (NF) 28:54–119

Fawcitt RA (1947) A case of osteo-poikilosis. BJR 20:360

Franke J (1968) Chronische Knochenfluorose. Beitr Orthop 15:680–684

Franke J, Drese G, Grau P (1972) Klinische gerichtsmedizinische und physikalische Untersuchungen eines Falles von schwerer Fluorose. Kriminal Forens Wiss 7:107–122

Fresen O (1961) On osteomyelosclerosis. Acta Pathol Jpn 11:87–108

Fritz H (1961) Die Knochenfluorose. In: Rajewski B (ed) IXth international congress of radiology, vol 1. Urban & Schwarzenberg, Munich/Thieme, Stuttgart, pp 258–260

Gallacher SJ (1993) Paget's disease of bone (Rev). Curr Opin Rheum 5:351–356

Gold RH, Mirra JM (1977) Melorheostose. Skeletal Radiol 2:57–58

Goldberg A, Seaton DA (1960) The diagnosis and management of myelofibrosis, myelosclerosis und chronic myeloid leukaemia. Clin Radiol 11:266–270

Graham J, Harris WH (1971) Paget's disease involving the hip joint. J Bone Joint Surg Br 53:650–659

Green A, Ellswood WH, Collins JR (1962) Melorheostosis and osteopoikilosis – with a review of the literature. Am J Roentgenol 87:1096–1111

Greenberg MS, Brightman VJ, Lynch MA, Ship 11 (1969) Idiopathic hypoparathyroidism, chronic candidiasis, and dental hypoplasia. Oral Surg 28:42–53

Greenspan A (1991) A review of Paget's disease: radiologic imaging, differential diagnosis, and treatment. Bull Hosp Joint Dis 51:22–33

Griffiths HJ (1992) Radiology of Paget's disease. Curr Opin Radiol 4:124–128

Grundmann E (1975) Blut und Knochenmark. In: Büchner F, Grundmann E (eds) Spezielle Pathologie, vol 11, 5th edn. Urban & Schwarzenberg, Munich, pp 67–68

Gupta SK, Gambhir S, Mithal A, Das BK (1993) Skeletal scintigraphic findings in endemic skeletal fluorosis. Nucl Med Commun 14:384–390

Haas HG (1968) Hypoparathyreoidismus. Springer, Berlin Heidelberg New York (14. Symposium der Deutschen Gesellschaft für Endokrinologie, pp 16–20)

Haas HG, Olah AJ, Dambacher M (1968) Hypoparathyreoidismus. Dtsch Med Wochenschr 93:1383–1389

Hadjipavlou A, Lander P, Srolovitz H, Enker IP (1992) Malignant transformation in Paget disease of bone. Cancer 70:2802–2808

Heuck F (1972) Skelett. In: Haubrich R (ed) Klinische Röntgendiagnostik innerer Krankheiten. Springer, Berlin Heidelberg New York

Hunstein W (1974) Das Myelofibrose-Syndrom. In: Schwiegk H (ed) Handbuch der inneren Medizin, vol 11/4. Springer, Berlin Heidelberg New York, pp 191–260

Jesserer H (1971) Knochenkrankheiten. Urban & Schwarzenberg, Munich

Jesserer H (1979) Hormonelle Knochenerkrankungen. In: Schinz HR, Baensch WE, Frommhold W et al (eds) Lehrbuch der Röntgendiagnostik vol 11/1, 6th edn. Thieme, Stuttgart, pp 901–945

Kelly PJ, Peterson LEA, Dahlin DC, Plum GE (1961) Osteitis deformans (Paget's disease of bone). A morphologic study utilizing microradiography and conventional technics. Radiology 77:368–375

Krane SM (1977) Paget's disease of bone. Clin Orthop 127:24–36

Mii Y, Miyauchi Y, Honoki K et al (1994) Electron microscopic evidence of a viral nature for osteoclast inclusions in Paget's disease of bone. Virchows Arch Pathol 424:99–104

Odenthal M, Wieneke HL (1959) Chronische Fluorvergiftung und Osteomyelosklerose. Dtsch Med Wochenschr 84:725–728

Oechslin RJ (1956) Osteomyelosklerose und Skelett. Acta Haematol (Basel) 16:214–234

Parfitt AM (1972) The spectrum of hypoparathyroidism. J Clin Endocrinol 34:152–158

Pease CN, Newton GG (1962) Metaphyseal dysplasia due to lead poisoning. Radiology 79:233–240

Pitcock JA, Reinhard EH, Justus BW, Mendelsohn RS (1962) A clinical and pathological study of seventy cases of myelofibrosis. Ann Intern Med 57:73–84

Pliess G (1974) Bewegungsapparat. In: Doerr W (ed) Organpathologie. Thieme, Stuttgart

Prescher A, Adler CP (1993) A special form of hyperostosis frontalis interna. Ann Anat 175:553–559

Roholm K (1939) Eine Übersicht über die Rolle des Fluors in der Pathologie und Physiologie. Ergebn Inn Med Kinderheilkd 57:822–915

Rohr K (1956) Myelofibrose und Osteomyelosklerose (Osteomyeloretikulose–Syndrom). Acta Haematol (Basel) 15:209–234

Rutishauser E (1941) Bleiosteosklerose. Schweiz Med Wochenschr 22:189

Sauk JJ, Smith T, Silbergeld EK, Fowler BA, Somerman MJ (1992) Lead inhibits secretion of osteonectin/SPARC without significantly altering collagen or Hsp47 production in osteoblast-like ROS 17/2.8 cells. Toxicol Acta Pharmacol 116:240–247

Schulz A, Delling G, Ringe JD, Ziegler R (1977) Morbus Paget des Knochens. Untersuchungen zur Ultrastruktur der Osteoclasten und ihrer Cytopathogenese. Virchows Arch Abt A 376:309–328

Singer FR, Mills BG (1977) The etiology of Paget's disease of bone. Clin Orthop 127:37–42

Sissons HA (1976) Paget's disease of bone. In: Ackerman AV, Spjut HJ, Abell MR (eds) Bones and joints. Williams & Wilkins, Baltimore (Int Acad Pathol Monogr 17, pp 146–156)

Soriano M, Manchon F (1966) Radiological aspects of a new type of bone fluorosis, periostitis deformans. Radiology 87:1089–1094

Stein G, Jüle S, Lange CE, Veltmann G (1973) Bandförmige Osteolysen in den Endphalangen des Handskeletts. Fortschr Röntgenstr 118:60–63

Steinbach HL (1961) Some roentgen features of Paget's disease. Am J Roentgenol 86:950–964

Stevenson CA, Watson RA (1957) Fluoride osteosclerosis. Am J Roentgenol 78:13–18

Szabo AD (1971) Osteopoikilosis in a twin. Clin Orthop 79:156–163

Taybi H, Keele D (1962) Hypoparathyroidism: a review of the literature and report of two cases in sisters, one with steatorrhea and intestinal pseudo-obstruction. Am J Roentgenol 88:432–442

Tell I, Somervaille LJ, Nilsson U et al (1992) Chelated lead and bone lead. Scand J Work Environ Health 18:113–119

Uehlinger E (1979) Ostitis deformans Paget. In: Schinz HR, Baensch WE, Frommhold W et al (eds) Lehrbuch der Röntgendiagnostik, vol 11/1, 6th edn. Thieme, Stuttgart, pp 983–1018

Vaughan JM (1975) The physiology of bone, 2nd edn. Clarendon, Oxford

Wang Y, Yin Y, Gilula LA, Wilson AJ (1994) Endemic fluorosis of the skeleton: radiographic features in 127 patients. Am J Roentgenol 162:93–98

Woodhouse NJY (1972) Paget's disease of bone. Clin Endocrinol Metab 1:125–141

Yumoto T, Hashimoto N (1963) A pathohistological investigation of myelofibrosis. Acta Haematol Jpn 26:347–370

Zipkin I, Schraer R, Schraer H, Lee WA (1963) The effect of fluoride on the citrate content of the bones of the growing rat. Arch Oral Biol 8:119–126

Chapter 6
Fractures

Adler CP (1989) Pathologische Knochenfrakturen. Definition und Klassifikation. Langenbecks Arch Chir 11[Suppl]:479–486

Adler CP (1991) Besonderheiten und erhöhte Verletzlichkeit beim krankhaft veränderten Knochen. Op J 3:4–10

Adler CP (1992) Knochen und Gelenke. In: Thomas C (ed) Histopathologie, 11th edn. Schattauer, Stuttgart, pp 290–314

Birzle H, Bergleiter R, Kuner EH (1975) Traumatologische Röntgendiagnostik. Lehrbuch und Atlas. Thieme, Stuttgart

Chew FS (1997) Skeletal radiology: the bare bones, 2nd edn. Williams & Wilkins, Baltimore

Compere EL, Banks SW, Compere CL (1966) Frakturenbehandlung. Ein Atlas für Praxis und Studium. Thieme, Stuttgart

Daffner RH, Pavlov H (1992) Stress fractures: current concepts. Am J Radiol 159:245–252

Hackenbroch M (1976) Die funktionelle Anpassungsfähigkeit des verletzten Skeletts. In: Matzen PF (ed) Callus. Nova Acta Leopoldina 223:13–31

Hellner H (1963) Frakturen und Luxationen. In: Hellner H, Nissen R, Vosschulte K (eds) Lehrbuch der Chirurgie. Thieme, Stuttgart, pp 1071–1082

Krompecher S, Tarsoly E (1976) Die Beeinflussung der Knochenbruchheilung. In: Matzen PF (ed) Callus. Nova Acta Leopoldina 223:37–50

Lee JK, Yao L (1988) Stress fracture: MR imaging. Radiology 169:217–220

Löhr J, Koch FG, Georgi P (1974) Tierexperimentelle Untersuchungen zum Einfluß des Prednisolon auf die Kallusbildung. Verh Dtsch Ges Pathol 58:297–302

Looser E (1920) Über pathologische Formen von Infraktionen und Callusbildungen bei Rachitis und Osteomalacie und anderen Knochenerkrankungen. Zentralbl Chir 47:1470–1474

Maatz R (1970) Vorgänge bei der Bruchheilung und Pseudarthrosenentstehung. In: Diethelm L, Heuck F, Olsson O et al (eds) Handbuch der medizinischen Radiologie, vol IV/1. Springer, Berlin Heidelberg New York

Maatz R (1979) Knochenbruch und Knochenbruchheilung. In: Schinz HR, Baensch WE, Frommhold W et al (eds) Lehrbuch der Röntgendiagnostik, 6th edn. vol 11/1. Thieme, Stuttgart, pp 309–433

Mason RW, Moore TE, Walker CW, Kathol MH (1996) Patellar fatigue fractures. Skeletal Radiol 25:329–332

Müller ME, Perren SM (1972) Callus und primäre Knochenheilung. Monatsschr Unfallheilk 75:442–454

Müller ME, Allgöwer M, Willenegger H (1963) Technik der operativen Frakturbehandlung. Springer, Berlin Göttingen Heidelberg

Mulligan ME, Shanley DJ (1996) Supramalleolar fatigue fractures of the tibia. Skeletal Radiol 25:325–328

Nicole R (1947) Metallschädigung bei Osteosynthesen. Helv Chir Acta 3[Suppl]:1–74

Niethard FU, Pfeil J (1989) Orthopädie (Duale Reihe). Hippokrates, Stuttgart

Perren SM, Allgöwer M (1976) Biomechanik der Frakturheilung nach Osteosynthese. In: Matzen PF (ed) Callus. Nova Acta Leopoldina 223:61–84

Rehn J (1968) Die posttraumatische Pseudarthrose, ihre Entstehung und Therapie. Monatsschr Unfallheilk 94:5–15

Rehn J (1974) Osteosynthesen bei posttraumatischer Osteomyelitis. Zentralbl Chir 99:1488–1496

Resnick JM, Carrasco CH, Edeiken J et al (1996) Avulsion fracture of the anterior inferior iliac spine with abundant reactive ossification in the soft tissue. Skeletal Radiol 25:580–584

Schauwecker F (1981) Osteosynthesepraxis. Ein Atlas zur Unfallchirurgie, 2nd edn. Thieme, Stuttgart

Schenk R (1978) Die Histologie der primären Knochenheilung im Lichte neuer Konzeptionen über den Knochenumbau. Monatsschr Unfallheilk 81:219–227

Schenk R, Willenegger H (1963) Zum histologischen Bild der sogenannten Primärheilung der Knochenkompakta nach experimentellen Osteotomien am Hund. Experientia (Basel) 19:593–595

Schenk R, Willenegger H (1964) Zur Histologie der primären Knochenheilung. Langenbecks Arch Chir 308:440–452

Schenk R, Willenegger H (1967) Morphological findings in primary fracture healing. Symp Biol Hung 7:75–86

Schenk R, Willenegger H (1977) Zur Histologie der primären Knochenheilung. Monatsschr Unfallheilk 80:155

Schink W (1969) Pathophysiologie der Pseudarthrosen. Monatsschr Unfallheilk 68:804–815

Schuster j (1975) Die Metallose. Prakt Chir 90. Enke, Stuttgart

Tscherne H, Schmit-Neuerburg KP, Greif E (1974) Die Einheilung verschiedener Knochentransplantate bei stabiler Osteosynthese. Verh Dtsch Ges Pathol 58:418–422

Umans HR, Kaye JJ (1996) Longitudinal stress fractures of the tibia: diagnosis by magnetic resonance imaging. Skeletal Radiol 25:319–324

Weller S (1973) Frakturen der oberen Gliedmaßen im Kindesalter (mit Ausnahme der Ellenbogenbrüche). Orthop Praxis 9:284–288

Weller S (1974) Konservative oder operative Behandlung von supracondylaren Oberarmfrakturen. Acta Traumatologie 4:79–83

Weller S (1974) Ellenbogengelenksnahe Unterarmfrakturen (Schriftenreihe Unfallmed. Tag. d. Landesverb. gewerbl. BG) Issue 17

Weller S (1975) Probleme der Versorgung offener Frakturen. Magyar Traumatologia 18:81–87

Weller S (1976) Die konservative Behandlung kindlicher Frakturen. Langenbecks Arch Chir 342:288–290

Weller S (1977) Schenkelhalsbruch. Dtsch Med Wochenschr 102:1266

Weller S (1978) Indikation und Technik zur operativen Behandlung der Acetabulumfrakturen. Unfallheilk 81:264

Weller S (1979) Pseudarthroses and their treatment. Eight Internat Symp Top Probl Orthop Surg, Lucerne (Switzerland) 1978. Thieme, Stuttgart

Weller S (1979) Konservative Behandlung der Oberschenkelfraktur (Schriftenreihe Unfallmed. Tag. d. Landesverb. gewerb. BG), Hannover. Issue 33:267–272

Weller S (1980) Fragen aus der Praxis. Osteosynthese. Dtsch Med Wochenschr 105:852

Weller S (1980) Hüftpfannenbrüche. Langenbecks Arch Chir 352:457–460

Weller S (1980) Indikation und Kontraindikation zur Marknagelung (Schriftenreihe Unfallmed. Tag. d. Landesverb. gewerb. BG) Issue 42:93–101

Weller S (1981) Frakturen, Luxationen und Erkrankungen von Sprunggelenk und Fuß. Bewährtes und Neues in Diagnostik und Therapie – Ergebnisse. Langenbecks Arch Chir 355:419–420

Weller S (1981) Biomechanische Prinzipien in der operativen Knochenbruchbehandlung. Akt Traumatologie 11:195–248

Weller S, Schmelzeisen H (1978) Diagnostik und Therapie von Hüftpfannenfrakturen. Beitr Orthop Traumatolog 25:436–446

Willenegger H, Perren SM, Schenk R (1971) Primäre und sekundäre Knochenbruchheilung. Chirurg 52:24–52

Chapter 7
Inflammatory Conditions of Bone

Adelaar RS (1983) Sarcoidosis of the upper extremity: case presentation and literature review. J Hand Surg 8:492

Adler CP (1976) Knochenentzündungen. In: Thomas C, Sandritter W (eds) Spezielle Pathologie. Textbuch zu einem audiovisuellen Kurs. Schattauer, Stuttgart

Adler CP (1979) Primäre und reaktive Periostveränderungen. Zur Pathologie des Periosts. Radiologe 19:293–306

Adler CP (1979) Hüftgelenkserkrankungen aus radiologischer und pathologisch-anatomischer Sicht. Röntgenpraxis 32:29–43

Adler CP (1980) Granulomatöse Erkrankungen im Knochen. Verh Dtsch Ges Pathol 64:359–365

Adler CP (1992) Knochen – Gelenke. In: Thomas C (ed) Histopathologie, 11th edn. Schattauer, Stuttgart, pp 290–314

Adler CP (1995) Ätiologie, Pathogenese und Morphologie der Osteomyelitis. Osteologie 4 [Suppl 1]:21

Aegerter E, Kirkpatrick JA Jr (1968) Orthopedic diseases: physiology, radiology, 3rd edn. Saunders, Philadelphia

Agarwal S, Shah A, Kadhi SK, Rooney RJ (1992) Hydatid bone disease of the pelvis. Clin Orthop 280:251–255

Amling M, Guthoff AE, Heise U, Delling G (1993) Echinokokkus Osteomyelitis – Beobachtung einer seltenen Primärmanifestation im Femur. Osteologie 2:175–180

Aufdermaur M (1975) Knochen. In: Büchner F, Grundmann E (eds) Spezielle Pathologie, vol 11. Urban & Schwarzenberg, Munich, p 339

Bähr R (1981) Die Echinokokkose des Menschen. Enke, Stuttgart

Barnes WC, Malament M (1963) Osteitis pubis. Surg Gynec Obstet 117:277–284

Bedacht R, Pöschl M (1971) Die chronische Osteomyelitis – Diagnose und Therapie. MMW 113:524–530

Birsner JW, Smart S (1956) Osseous coccidioidomycosis, a chronic form of dissemination. Am J Roentgenol 76:1052–1060

Björksten B, Boquist L (1980) Histopathological aspects of chronic recurrent multifocal osteomyelitis. J Bone Joint Surg Br 62:376–380

Black PH, Kunz LJ, Swartz MN (1960) Salmonellosis, a review of some unusual aspects. N Engl J Med 262:811–817

Blanche DW (1952) Osteomyelitis of infants. J Bone Joint Surg Am 34:71–85

Bonakdarpour A, Levy W, Aegerter E (1971) Osteosclerotic changes in sarcoidosis. Am J Roentgenol 113:646–649

Burri C (1974) Posttraumatische Osteitis. Akt Probl Chir, vol 18. Huber, Bern

Carr AJ, Cole WG, Roberton DM, Chow CW (1993) Chronic multifocal osteomyelitis. J Bone Joint Surg Br 75:582–591

Carter RA (1934) Infectious granulomas of bones and joints with special reference to coccidioidal granuloma. Radiology 23:1–16

Cochran W, Connolly JH, Thompson ID (1963) Bone involvement after vaccination against smallpox. Br Med J 11:285–287

Cockshott P, MacGregor M (1958) Osteomyelitis variolosa. QJM 51:369–387

Collins VP (1950) Bone involvement in cryptococcosis (torulosis). Am J Roentgenol 63:102–112

Contzen H (1961) Die sogenannte Osteomyelitis des Neugeborenen. Dtsch Med Wochenschr 86:1221–1234

Cushard WG Jr, Kohanim M, Lantis LR (1969) Blastomycosis of bone; treatment with intramedullary amphotericin-B. J Bone Joint Surg Am 51:704–712

Dalinka MK (1971) Roentgenographic features of osseous coccidioidomycosis and differential diagnosis. J Bone Joint Surg Am 53:1157–1164

Davidson JC, Palmer PES (1963) Osteomyelitis variolosa. J Bone Joint Surg Br 45:687–693

Dennison WM (1955) Haematogenous osteitis in the newborn. Lancet 11:474–476

Drescher E (1977) Ein Beitrag zu destruierenden Knochenprozessen im Frühkindesalter. Fortschr Röntgenstr 116:569–571

Dykes J, Segesman JK, Birsner W (1953) Coccidioidomycosis of bone in children. Am J Dis Child 85:34–42

Ebrahim GJ, Grech P (1966) Salmonella osteomyelitis in infants. J Bone Joint Surg Br 48:350–353

Elliott WD (1959) Vaccinial osteomyelitis. Lancet 11:1053

Exner GU (1965) Die Säuglingsosteomyelitis. In: Lange M (ed) Verb Dtsch Orthop Ges (51. Kongreß) Enke, Stuttgart, pp 140–145

Exner GU (1970) Die plasmazelluläre Osteomyelitis. Langenbecks Arch Chir 326:165–185

Felsberg GJ, Gore RL, Schweitzer ME, Jui V (1990) Sclerosing osteomyeltis of Garré (periostitis ossificans). Oral Surg Oral Med Oral Pathol 70:117–120

Fitzgerald P (1958) Sarcoidosis of hands. J Bone Joint Surg Br 40:256–261

Forschbach G (1955) Die Osteoarthropathie hypertrophiante pneumique (Zur Fernwirkung intrathorakaler Tumoren). Langenbecks Arch Chir 281:18–36

Freund E (1932) Über Osteomyelitis und Gelenkseiterung. Virchows Arch 283:325–353

Gall EA, Bennet GA, Bauer W (1951) Generalized hypertrophic osteoarthropathy. Am J Pathol 27:349–381

Garré C (1893) Über besondere Formen und Folgezustände der akuten infektiösen Osteomyelitis. Bruns' Beitr Klin Chir 10:241–298

Gehrt J, Herminghaus H (1959) Die Osteomyelitis im Säuglings- und Kindesalter. Dtsch Med Wochenschr 84:2225–2229

Giaccia L, Idriss H (1952) Osteomyelitis due to salmonella infection. J Pediatr 41:73–78

Gilmour WN (1962) Acute haematogenous osteomyelitis. J Bone Joint Surg Br 44:841–853

Green M, Nyhan W, Fonsek M (1956) Acute haematogenous osteomyelitis. Pediatrics 17:368–381

Green WT, Shannon JG (1936) Osteomyelitis of infants: a disease different from osteomyelitis of older children. Arch Surg 32:462–493

Griffiths HED, Jones DM (1971) Pyogenic infection of the spine: a review of twenty-eight cases. J Bone Joint Surg Br 53:383–391

Halbstein BM (1967) Bone regeneration in infantile osteomyelitis: report of a case with fourteen year follow-up. J Bone Joint Surg Am 49:149–152

Hardmeier T, Uehlinger E, Muggli A (1974) Primär chronische sklerosierende Osteomyelitis. Verh Dtsch Ges Pathol 58:474–477

Harris NH (1960) Some problems in the diagnosis and treatment of acute osteomyelitis. J Bone Joint Surg Br 42:535–541

Harris NH, Kirkaldy-Willis WH (1965) Primary subacute pyogenic osteomyelitis. J Bone Joint Surg Br 47:526–532

Hook EW (1961) Salmonellosis: certain factors influencing the interaction of salmonella and the human host. NY Acad Med Bull 37:499–512

Hook EW, Campbell CG, Weens HS, Cooper GR (1957) Salmonella osteomyelitis in patients with sickle-cell anemia. N Engl J Med 257:403–407

Jüngling O (1919) Ostitis tuberculosa multiplex cystica. Fortschr Röntgenstr 27:375–383

Keller H, Breit A (1979) Entzündliche Knochenerkrankungen. In: Schinz HR, Baensch WE, Frominhold W et al (eds) Lehrbuch der Röntgendiagnostik, vol II/I. Thieme, Stuttgart, pp 587–653

Kelly PJ, Martin WJ, Schirger A, Weed LA (1960) Brucellosis of the bones and joints. Experience with thirty-six patients. J Am Med Assoc 174:347–353

Kinninan JEG, Lee HS (1968) Chronic osteomyelitis of the mandible: clinical study of thirteen cases. Oral Surg 25:6–11

Kissling R, Tan K-G (1984) Echinococcus cysticus im Knochen. Röfo 141:470–471

Krempien B, Ritz E (1972) Osteomyelitis of both femora in a patient on maintenance hemodialysis with severe uremic osteopathy. Virchows Arch Abt B 356:119–126

Kulowski J (1936) Pyogenic osteomyelitis of the spine: an analysis and discussion of 102 cases. J Bone Joint Surg Br 18:343–364

Landi A, Brooks D, De Santis G (1983) Sarcoidosis of the hand: report of two cases. J Hand Surg 8:197

Langer M, Langer R, Rittmeyer K (1979) Echinococcus cysticus des Knochens. Röfo 131:217–218

Lauche A (1939) 1. Die unspezifischen Entzündungen der Knochen. In: Uehlinger E (ed) Handbuch der speziellen pathologischen Anatomie und Histologie, vol IX/4. Springer, Berlin Göttingen Heidelberg, pp 1–80

Lavalle LL, Hamm FC (1951) Osteitis pubis: its etiology and pathology. J Urol (Balt) 66:418–423

Lehmann R (1963) Zur Frage der Knochenveränderungen beim Morbus Boeck. Radiol Diagn (Berlin) 4:539–546

Lennert K (1965) Pathologische Anatomie der Osteomyelitis. In: Lange M (ed) Verh Dtsch Orthop Ges, 51. Kongreß. Enke, Stuttgart, pp 27–64

Leonard A, Cointy CM, Shapiro FL, Raij L (1973) Osteomyelitis in hemadialysis patients. Ann Intern Med 78:651–658

Lewis JW, Koss N, Kerstein MD (1975) A review of echinococcal disease. Arch Surg 181:390–396

Lindemann K (1965) Klinische Probleme der Osteomyelitis. In: Lange M (ed) Verh Dtsch Orthop Ges, 51. Kongreß. Enke, Stuttgart, pp 77–90

Lowbeer L (1948) Brucellotic osteomyelitis of the spinal column in man. Am J Pathol 24:723–724

Wdeke H, Schweiberer L (1970) Entzündliche Erkrankungen der Knochen und Gelenke. Chirurg 41:198–203

Martinelli B, Tagliapietra EA (1970) Actinomycosis of the arm. Bull Hosp Joint Dis (NY) 31:31–42

Martinez-Lavin M, Matucci-Cerinic M, Jajic I, Pineda C (1993) Hypertrophic osteoarthopathy: consensus on its definition, classification, assessment and diagnostic criteria. J Rheumatol 20:1386–1387

Mayer JB (1964) Die Osteomyelitis im Säuglings- und Kleinkindesalter. Mschr Kinderheilk 112:153–158

Mazet R (1955) Skeletal lesions in coccidioidomycosis. Arch Surg 70:497–507

Mendelsohn BG (1965) Actinomycosis of a metacarpal bone: report of a case. J Bone Joint Surg Br:739–742

Merkle E-M, Kramme E, Vogel J et al (1997) Bone and soft tissue manifestations of alveolar echinococcosis. Skeletal Radiol 26:289–292

Meyer E, Adam T (1989) Über ungewöhnliche Manifestationen der Echinokokkose. Radiologe 29:245–249

Miller D, Birsner JW (1949) Coccidioidal granuloma of bone. Am J Roentgenol 62:229–236

Mittelmeier H (1965) Osteomyelitis und Osteosynthese. In: Lange M (ed) Verh Dtsch Orthop Ges, 51. Kongreß. Enke, Stuttgart, pp 118–126

Nagel DA (1965) Chronische Osteomyelitis – ein hartnäckiges und Ausdauer erforderndes Problem. In: Lange M (ed) Verh Dtsch Orthop Ges, 51. Kongreß. Enke, Stuttgart, pp 93–96

Niethard FU, Pfeil J (1989) Orthopädie. Hippokrates, Stuttgart (Duale Reihe)

Nathan MH, Radman WP, Barton HL (1962) Osseous actinomycosis of the head and neck. Am J Roentgenol 87:1048–1053

Panders AK, Hadders HN (1970) Chronic sclerosing inflammations of the jaws; osteomyelitis sicca (Garré), chronic sclerosing osteomyelitis with fine-meshed trabecular structure, and very dense sclerosing osteomyelitis. Oral Surg 30:396–412

Pineda CJ, Martinez-Lavin M, Goobar JE et al (1987) Periostitis in hypertrophic osteoarthropathy: relationship to disease duration. Am J Roentgenol 148:773–778

Posner MA, Melendez E, Steiner G (1991) Solitary osseous sarcoidosis in a finger. J Hand Surg 16:827

Preuer H (1971) Die chronische plasmazelluläre Osteomyelitis. Eine Differentialdiagnose zum Plasmozytom. MMW 113:299–302

Putschar GJ (1976) Osteomyelitis including fungal. In: Akkerman LV, Spjut HJ, Abell MR (eds) Bones and joints. (Int Acad Pathol) Williams & Wilkins, Baltimore pp 39–60

Pygott F (1970) Sarcoidosis in bone. Postgrad Med J 46:505–506

Rasmussen H (1952) Peripheral vascular disease, with hypertrophic osteoarthropathy, as the first manifestation ofbronchial carcinoma. Acta Med Scand 66[Suppl 2]:855–862

Ravelli A (1955) Die Periostitis bzw. Osteomyelitis typhosa. Bruns' Beitr Klin Chir 191:351–357

Reischauer F (1955) Hämatogene Osteomyelitis und leichtes Trauma. Monatsschr Unfallheilk 5:97–112

Rieber A, Brambs HJ, Friedl P (1989) CT beim Echinokokkus der LWS und den paravertebralen Strukturen. Röfo 151:379–380

Rivera-Sanfeliz G, Resnick D, Haghighi P (1996) Sarcoidosis of hands. Skeletal Radiol 25:786–788

Saphra I, Winter JW (1957) Clinical manifestations of salmonellosis in man: an evaluation of 7779 human infections indentified at the New York Salmonella Center. N Engl J Med 256:1128–1134

Schilling F (1997) Die chronisch rekurrierende multifokale Osteomyelitis. Act Rheumatol 22 [Suppl]:1–16

Schmidt H (1928) Zur Statistik der Knochenerkrankungen bei Säuglingssyphilis. Z Kinderheilkd 46:661–675

Schnaidt U, Vykoupil KF, Thiele J et al (1980) Granulomatöse Veränderungen im Knochenmark. Verh Dtsch Ges Pathol 64:404–409

Schwarz J (1984) What's new in mycotic bone and joint diseases? Pathol Res Pract 178:617–634

Sciuk J, Erlemann R, Schober O, Peters PE (1992) Bildgebende Diagnostik der Osteomyelitis. Dtsch Arztebl 89:1337–1344

Scott TH, Scott MA (1984) Sarcoidosis with nodular lesions of the palm and sole. Arch Dermatol 120:1239

Sinner WN von (1990) Hydatid disease involving multiple bones and soft tissue. Case Report. Skeletal Radiol 19:312–316

Spencer RP (1988) Hepatic hypertrophic osteodystrophy detected on bone imaging. Clin Nucl Med 13:611–612

Sundaram M, McDonald D, Engel E et al (1996) Chronic recurrent multifocal osteomyelitis: an evolving clinical and radiological spectrum. Skeletal Radiol 25:333–336

Torricelli P, Martinelli C, Biagini R et al (1990) Radiographic and computed tomographic findings in hydatid disease of bone. Skeletal Radiol 19:435–439

Trueta J (1959) The three types of acute haematogenous osteomyelitis: a clinical and vascular study. J Bone Joint Surg Br 41:671–680

Trueta J (1963) Die drei Typen der akuten hämatogenen Osteomyelitis. Schweiz Med Wochenschr 93:306–312

Uehlinger E (1970) Die pathologische Anatomie der hämatogenen Osteomyelitis. Chirurg 41:193–198

Uehlinger E, Wurm K (1976) Skelettsarkoidose. Literaturübersicht und Fallbericht. Fortschr Röntgenstr 125:111–112

Uhl M, Leichsenring M, Krempien B (1995) Chronisch rezidivierende multifokale Osteomyelitis. Fortschr Röntgenstr 162:527–530

Waldvogel FA, Medoff G, MN Swartz (1971) Osteomyelitis: clinical features, therapeutic considerations and unusual aspects. Thomas, Springfield, Ill.

Weaver JB, Sherwood L (1935) Hematogenous osteomyelitis and pyarthrosis due to salmonella suipestifer. J Am Med Assoc 105:1188–1189

Widen AL, Cardon L (1961) Salmonella thyphimurium osteomyelitis with sickle cell hemoglobin C disease; a review and case report. Ann Intern Med 54:510–521

Winkelhoff B (1971) Plasmazelluläre Osteomyelitis. Bruns' Beitr Klin Chir 218:569–574

Winters JL, Cahen I (1960) Acute hematogenous osteomyelitis; a review of sixty-six cases. J Bone Joint Surg Am 42:691–704

Witorsch P, Utz JP (1968) North American blastomycosis; a study of 40 patients. Medicine (Balt) 47:169–200

Wray TM, Bryant RE, Killen DA (1973) Sternal osteomyelitis and costochondritis after median sternotomy. J Thorac Cardiovasc Surg 65:227–233

Wu P-C, Khin N-M, Pang S-W (1985) Salmonella osteomyelitis. An important differential diagnosis of granulomatous osteomyelitis. Am J Surg Pathol 9:531–537

Young WB (1960) Actinomycosis with involvement of the vertrebal column: case report and review of the literature. Clin Radiol 11:175–182

Zadek I (1938) Acute osteomyelitis of the long bones in adults. Arch Surg 37:531–545

Zeppa MA, Laorr A, Greenspan A, McGahan J, Steinbach LS (1996) Skeletal coccidioidomycosis: imaging findings in 19 patients. Skeletal Radiol 25:337–343

Zorn G (1956) Über die sklerosierende Osteomyelitis Garré. MMW 98:269–271

Chapter 8
Bone Necroses

Adler CP (1979) Hüftgelenkserkrankungen aus radiologischer und pathologisch-anatomischer Sicht. Röntgenpraxis 32:29–43

Alabi ZO, Durosinmi MA (1989) Legg-Calve-Perthes' disease associated with chronic myeloid leukaemia in a child: case report. East Afr Med J 66:556–560

Alnor PC (1980) Chronische Skelettveränderungen bei Tauchern. In: Gerstenbrand F, Lorenzoni E, Seemarm K (eds) Tauchmedizin. Pathologie, Physiologie, Klinik, Prävention, Therapie. Schlütersche Verlagsanstalt, Hannover, pp 179–188

Adler CP (1995) Durchblutung und Durchblutungsstörungen des Knochens. In: Kummer B, Koebke J, Bade H, Pesch H-J (eds) Osteologie aktuell IX. VISU-Verlag, Herzogenaurach, pp 143–159

Alnor PC, Herget R, Seusing J (1964) Drucklufterkrankungen. Barth, Munich

Amako T (1973) Bone and joint lesions in decompression sickness. Rheumatologie 3:637

Anseroff NJ (1934) Die Arterien der langen Röhrenknochen des Menschen. Z Anat Entwickl Gesch 103:793–812

Aufdermaur M (1973) Die Scheuermannsche Adoleszentenkyphose. Orthopädie 2:153–161

Bargmann W (1930) Über den Feinbau der Knochenmarkskapillaren. Z Zellforsch 11:1–22

Boettcher WG, Bonfiglio M, Hamilton HH et al (1970) Nontraumatic of the femoral head. 1. Relation of altered hemostasis to etiology. J Bone Joint Surg Am 52:312–321

Bradley J, Dandy DJ (1989) Osteochondritis dissecans and other lesions of the femoral condyles. J Bone Joint Surg Br 71:518–522

Branemark PJ (1961) Experimental investigation of microcirculation in bone marrow. Angiology 12:293–305

Brocher JEW (1973) Die Prognose der Wirbelsäulenleiden. Thieme, Stuttgart

Brookes M (1957) Vascular patterns in human long bones. J Anat 91:604–611

Brookes M (1971) The blood supply of bone. Butterworth, London

Buchner F, Zenger H, Adler CP (1992) Osteonekrose des proximalen Femur. Akt Rheumatol 17:109–112

Bullough PG, DiCarlo EF (1990) Subchondral avascular necrosis: a common cause of arthritis. Ann Rheum Dis 49:412–420

Burrows HJ (1941) Coxa Plana, with special reference to its pathology and kinship. Br J Surg 29:23–36

Burrows HJ (1959) Osteochondritis juvenilis. J Bone Joint Surg Br 41:455–456

Catto M (1965) A histological study of avascular necrosis of the femoral head after transcervical fracture. J Bone Joint Surg Br 47:777–791

Crock HV (1967) The blood supply of the lower limb bones in man. Livingstone, Edinburgh

Dale T (1952) Bone necrosis in divers (Caisson disease). Acta Chir Scand 104:153–156

Ferguson AB Jr, Gingrich RM (1957) The normal and the abnormal calcaneal apophysis and tarsal navicular. Clin Orthop 10:87–95

Ficat RP (1985) Idiopathic bone osteonecrosis of the femoral head: early diagnosis and treatment. J Bone Joint Surg Am 76:3–9

Fink B, Rilther W, Busch T, Schneider T (1993) Multiple aseptische Knochennekrosen bei chronischer Hämodialyse. Osteologie 2:228–232

Fischer E, Volk H (1970) Breite, Länge und Höhe der Wirbelkörper der unteren Hälfte der Brustwirbelsäule bei normalen Wirbelsäulen und beim Morbus Scheuermann von der Pubertät bis zum Senium. Z Orthop 107:627

Fliedner T, Sandkühler S, Stodtmeister R (1956) Untersuchungen über die Gefäßarchitektonik des Knochenmarkes der Ratte. Z Zellforsch 45:328–338

Fournier AM, Jullien G (1965) La Maladie Ostéoarticulaire des Caissons. Masson, Paris

Freehafer AA (1960) Osteochondritis dissecans following Legg-Calvé-Perthes disease. J Bone Joint Surg Am 42:777–782

Freund E (1930) Zur Deutung des Röntgenbildes der Perthesschen Krankheit. Fortschr Röntgenstr 42:435–464

Glimcher MJ, Kenzora JE (1979) The biology of osteonecrosis of the human femoral head and its clinical implications. 3. Discussion of etiology and genesis of the pathological sequelae: comments on treatment. Clin Orthop 140:273–312

Hammersen F, Seidemann I (1964) Ein Beitrag zur Angioarchitektonik der Knochenhaut. Arch Orthop Unfall Chir 56:617–633

Herget R (1952) Primäre Infarkte der langen Röhrenknochen durch lokale Zirkulationsstörungen. Zentralbl Chir 77:1372–1375

Hermans R, Fossion E, Ioannides C et al (1996) CT findings in osteoradionecrosis of the mandible. Skeletal Radiol 25:31–36

Herndorn JH, Aufranc OE (1972) A vascular necrosis of the femoral head in the adult: a review of its incidence in a variety of conditions. Clin Orthop 86:43–62

Hert J, Hladikov J (1961) Die Gefäßversorgung des Havers' schen Knochens. Acta Anat (Basel) 45:344–361

Horvath F (1980) Röntgenmorphologie des caissonbedingten Knocheninfarkts. In: Gerstenbrand F, Lorenzoni FE, Seemann K (eds) Tauchmedizin. Pathologie, Physiologie, Klinik, Prävention, Therapie. Schlütersche Verlagsanstalt, Hannover, pp 173–178

Horvath F, Viskelety T (1973) Experimentelle Untersuchungen der osteoartikulären Manifestation der Caisson-Krankheit. Arch Orthop Unfall Chir 75:28–72

Howe WW, Lacey TI, Schwartz RP (1950) A study of the gross anatomy of the arteries supplying the proximal portion of the femur and the acetabulum. J Bone Joint Surg Am 32:856–866

Hulth A (1961) Necrosis of the head of the femur: a roentgenological microradiographic and histological study. Acta Chir Scand 122:75–84

Hunter JC, Escobedo EM, Routt ML (1996) Osteonecrosis of the femoral condyles following traumatic dislocation of the knee. Skeletal Radiol 25:276–278

Jaffe HL (1929) The vessel canals in normal and pathological bones. Am J Pathol 5:323–332

Jaffe HL (1972) Metabolic, degenerative, and inflammatory diseases of bones and joints. Urban & Schwarzenberg, Munich

Johnson RW (1968) A physiological study of the blood supply of the diaphysis. Clin Orthop 56:5–11

Judet I, Judet R, Lagrange J, Dunoyer J (1955) A study of the arterial vascularization of the femoral neck in adult. J Bone Joint Surg Am 37:663–680

Kantor H (1987) Bone marrow pressure in osteonecrosis of the femoral condyle (Ahlback's disease). Arch Orthop Trauma Surg 106:349–352

Kawabata M, Ray D (1967) Experimental study of peripheral circulation and bone growth. Clin Orthop 55:177–189

Kelly PJ (1968) Anatomy, physiology and pathology of the blood supply of bones. J Bone Joint Surg Am 50:766–783

Kelly PJ, Peterson LEA (1963) The blood supply of bone. Heart Bull 12:96–99

Kienböck R (1910) Über traumatische Malazie des Mondbeins und ihre Folgezustände: Entartungsformen und Kompressionsfrakturen. Fortschr Röntgenstr 16:77–115

Klümper A (1969) Intraossäre Angiographie. Topographische und morphologische Untersuchungen zur Darstellung intraossärer Gefäße in vivo. Habilitationsschrift, Freiburg

Klümper A, Strey M, Schütz W (1968) Tierexperimentelle Untersuchungen zur intraossären Angiographie. Fortschr Röntgenstr 108:607–612

Konjetzny GE (1934) Zur Pathologie und pathologischen Anatomie der Perthes-Calvé'schen Krankheit. Acta Chir Scand 74:361–377

Laing PG (1953) The blood supply of the femoral shaft. An anatomical study. J Bone Joint Surg Br 35:462–466

Laing PG (1956) The arterial supply of the adult humerus. J Bone Joint Surg Am 38:1105–1116

Leone J, Vilque J-P, Pignon B et al (1996) Avascular necrosis of the femoral head as a complication of chronic myelogenous leukaemia. Skeletal Radiol 25:696–698

Lewis OJ (1956) The blood supply of developing long bones with special references to the metaphyse. J Bone Joint Surg Br 38:928–933

Mankin HJ (1992) Nontraumatic necrosis of bone (osteonecrosis). N Engl J Med 326:1473–1479

Mitchell MD, Kundel HL, Steinberg ME et al (1986) Avascular necrosis of the hip: comparison of MR, CT, and scintigraphy. Am J Radiol 147:67–71

Morris L, McGibbon KC (1962) Osteochondritis dissecans following Legg-Calvé-Perthes disease. J Bone Joint Surg Br 44:562–564

Nelson GG, Kelly PJ, Peterson LEA, Janes JM (1961) Blood supply of the human tibia. J Bone Joint Surg Am 42:625–636

Patterson RJ, Bickel WH, Dahlin DC (1964) Idiopathic avascular necrosis of the head of the femur. A study of fifty-two cases. J Bone Joint Surg Am 46:267–282

Persson M (1945) Pathogenese und Behandlung der Kienböckschen Lunatummalazie. Acta Chir Scand 92 [Suppl 98]:1–158

Pich G (1936) Histopathologic study in a case of Perthes' disease of traumatic origin. Arch Surg 33:609–629

Platt H (1921/22) Pseudo-Coxalgia (Osteochondritis deformans juvenilis coxae: quiet hip disease). Br J Surg 9:366–407

Ponseti IV (1956) Legg-Perthes disease. J Bone Joint Surg Am 38:739–750

Poppel MH, Robinson WT (1956) The roentgen manifestation of caisson disease. Am J Roentgenol 76:74–80

Ratliff AHC (1967) Osteochondritis dissecans following Legg-Calvé-Perthes' disease. J Bone Joint Surg Br 49:108–11

Rhinelander FW (1982) Circulation of bone. In: Bourne GH (ed) The physiology and biochemistry of bone, 2nd edn, vol 2. Academic Press, New York, pp 1–76

Riniker P, Huggler A (1971) Idiopathic necrosis of the femoral head. In: Zinn WM (ed) Idiopathic ischemic necrosis of the femoral head in adults. Thieme, Stuttgart, p 67

Rutishauser E, Rhoner A, Held D (1960) Experimentelle Untersuchungen über die Wirkung der Ischämie auf den Knochen und das Mark. Virchows Arch 333:101–118

Rüttner JR (1946) Beiträge zur Klinik und pathologischen Anatomie der Kienböckschen Krankheit (Lunatummalazie). Helv Chir Acta 13 [Suppl 1]:1–44

Ryu KN, Kim EJ, Yoo MC et al (1997) Ischemic necrosis of the entire femoral head and rapidly destructive hip disease: potential causative relationship. Skeletal Radiol 26:143–149

Salter RB (1966) Experimental and clinical aspects of Perthes' disease. J Bone Joint Surg Br 48:393–394

Salter RB, Harris WR (1963) Injuries involving the epiphyseal plate. J Bone Joint Surg Am 45:587–622

Sanchis M, Zahir A, Freeman MAR (1973) The experimental stimulation of Perthes disease by consecutive interruptions of the blood supply to the capital femoral epiphysis in the puppy. J Bone Joint Surg Am 55:335–342

Schinz HR, Baensch WE, Friedl E, Uehlinger E (1952) Lehrbuch der Röntgendiagnostik. Thieme, Stuttgart

Schumacher S (1935) Zur Anordnung der Gefäßkanäle in der Diaphyse langer Knochen des Menschen. Z Mikr Anat Forsch 38:145–160

Sevitt S, Thompson RG (1965) The distribution and anastomoses of arteries supplying the head and neck of the femur. J Bone Joint Surg Br 47:560–573

Shim SS (1968) Physiology of blood circulation of bone. J Bone Joint Surg Am 50:812–824

Springfield DS, Enneking WF (1976) Idiopathic aseptic necrosis. In: Ackerman LV, Spjut HJ, Abell MR (eds) Bones and joints (Int Acad Path Monogr). Williams & Wilkins, Baltimore, pp 61–87

Stähl F (1947) On lunatomalacia (Kienböck's disease). Acta Chir Scand 95[Suppl 126]:1–133

Torres FX, Kyriakos M (1992) Bone infarct-associated osteosarcoma. Cancer 70:2418–2430

Totty WG, Murphy WA, Ganz WI et al (1984) Magnetic resonance imaging of the normal and ischemic femoral head. Am J Radiol 143:1273–1280

Trueta J (1957) The normal vascular anatomy of the human femoral head during growth. J Bone Joint Surg Br 39:358–394

Trueta J (1963) The role of vessels in osteogenesis. J Bone Joint Surg Br 45:402–418

Trueta J, Cavadias AX (1964) A study of blood supply of the long bones. Surg Gynec Obstet 118:485–498

Trueta J, Harrison MHM (1953) The normal vascular anatomy of the femoral head in adult man. J Bone Joint Surg Br 35:442–461

Trueta J, Little K (1960) Vascular contribution to osteogenesis. J Bone Joint Surg Br 42:367–376

Tucker FR (1949) Arterial supply to the femoral head and its clinical importance. J Bone Joint Surg Br 31:82–93

Vaughan JM (1975) The physiology of bone, 2nd edn. Clarendon Press, Oxford

Zinn WM (1979) Die ischämischen Knochennekrosen des Erwachsenen, dargestellt am Beispiel der spontanen Femurkopfnekrose. Verb Dtsch Ges Inn Med 85:348–361

Chapter 9
Metabolic and Storage Diseases

Adler CP (1980) Granulomatöse Erkrankungen im Knochen. Verh Dtsch Ges Pathol 64:359–365

Agarwal AK (1993) Gout and pseudogout (Rev). Primary Care: Clinics in Office Practice 20:839–855

Alaren-Segovia D, Centina JA, Diaz-Jouanen E (1973) Sacroiliac joints in primary gout. Am J Roentgenol 118:438–443

Amstutz HC, Carey EJ (1966) Skeletal manifestations and treatment of Gaucher's disease. J Bone Joint Surg Am 48:670–701

Ashkenazy A, Zairov R, Matoth Y (1986) Effect of splenomegaly on destructive bone changes in children with chronic (type I) Gaucher disease. Eur J Radiol 145:138

Barthelemy CR, Nakayama DA, Carrera GF et al (1984) Gouty arthritis: a prospective radiographic evaluation of sixty patients. Skeletal Radiol 11:1–8

Bauer R (1968) Osteomyelitis urica. Fortschr Röntgenstr 108:266

Beutler E (1993) Modern diagnostic and treatment of Gaucher's disease (Rev). Am J Dis Child 147:1175–1183

Boccalatte M, Pratesi G, Calabrese G et al (1994) Amyloid bone disease and highly permeable synthetic membranes. Internat. J Artificial Organs 17:203–208

Bondurant RE, Henry JB (1965) Pathogenesis of ochronosis in experimental alkaptonuria of the white rat. Lab Invest 14:62–69

Casey TT, Stone WJ, DiRaimondo CR et al (1986) Tumoral amyloidosis of bone of beta$_2$ microglobulin origin in association with long-term hemadialysis: a new type of amyloid disease. Hum Pathol 17:731–738

Cohen PR, Schmidt WA, Rapini RP (1991) Chronic tophaceous gout with severely deforming arthritis: a case report with emphasis on histopathologic considerations. Cutis 48:445–451

Cooper JA, Moran TJ (1957) Studies on ochronosis. Arch Pathol 64:46–53

Dihlmann W, Fernholz HJ (1969) Gibt es charakteristische Röntgenbefunde bei der Gicht? Dtsch Med Wochenschr 94:1909–1911

Epstein E (1924) Beitrag zur Pathologie der Gaucherschen Krankheit. Virchows Arch 253:157–207

Fassbender HG (1972) Zur Pathologie der Gicht. Therapiewoche 22:105–108

Fisher ER, Reidbord H (1962) Gaucher's disease: Pathogenic considerations based on electron microscopic and histochemical observations. Am J Pathol 41:679–692

Foldes K, Petersilge CA, Weisman MH, Resnick D (1996) Nodal osteoarthritis and gout: a report of four new cases. Skeletal Radiol 25:421–424

Greenfield GB (1970) Bone changes in chronic adult Gaucher's disease. Am J Roentgenol 110:800–807

Hemmati A, Vogel W (1969) Schwere Knochendestruktionen bei Gicht-Arthritis. Chirurg 40:285–287

Hermann G, Shapiro RS, Abdelwahab IF, Grabowski G (1993) MR imaging in adults with Gaucher disease type I: evaluation of marrow involvement and disease activity. Skeletal Radiol 22:247–251

Hermann G, Shapiro RS, Abdelwahab IF et al (1994) Extraosseous extension of Gaucher cell deposits mimicking malignancy. Skeletal Radiol 23:253–256

Ishida T, Dorfman HD, Bullough PG (1995) Tophaceous pseudogout (tumoral calcium pyrophosphate dihydrate crystal deposition disease). Hum Pathol 26:587–593

Jaffe HL (1972) Metabolic, degenerative, and inflammatory diseases of bones and joints. Urban & Schwarzenberg, Munich, pp 479–505

Kurer MH, Baillod RA, Madgwick JC (1991) Musculoskeletal manifestations of amyloidosis. A review of 83 patients on haemodialysis for at least 10 years. J Bone Joint Surg Br 73:271–276

Lally EV, Zimmermann B, Ho G Jr, Kaplan SR (1989) Urate-mediated inflammation in nodal osteoarthritis: clinical and roentgenographic correlations. Arthritis Rheum 32:86–90

Levin B (1961) Gaucher's disease. Clinical and roentgenologic manifestations. Am J Roentgenol 85:685–696

Lichtenstein L, Scott HW, Levin MH (1956) Pathologic changes in gout: survey of eleven necropsied cases. Am J Pathol 32:871–887

Linduskova M, Hrba J, Vykydal M, Pavelka K (1992) Needle biopsy of joints: its contribution to the diagnosis of ochronotic arthropathy (alcaptonuria). Clin Rheumatol 11:569–570

MacCollum DE, Odom GL (1965) Alkaptonuria, ochronosis, and low-back pain. J Bone Joint Surg Am 47:1389

Martel W (1968) The overhanging margin of bone: a roentgenologic manifestation of gout. Radiology 91:755–756

Matoth Y, Fried K (1965) Chronic Gaucher's disease. Clinical observations on 34 patients. Israel J Med Sci 1:521

Mauvoisin F, Bernard J, Gémain J (1955) Aspects tomographiques des hanches chez un gotteux. Rev Rhum 22:336–337

Melis M, Onori P, Aliberti G, Vecci E, Gaudio E (1994) Ochronotic arthropathy: structural and ultrastructural features. Ultrastruct Pathol 18:467–471

Murray RO, Jacobson HG (1977) The radiology of skeletal disorders, 2nd edn, vol. 11. Churchill Livingstone, Edinburgh, pp 850–853

Nägele E (1957) Röntgenbefunde bei Alkaptonurie. Fortschr Röntgenstr 87:523–529

Pastores GM, Hermann G, Norton KI, Lorberboym M, Desnick RJ (1996) Regression of skeletal changes in Type I Gaucher disease with enzyme replacement therapy. Skeletal Radiol 25:485–488

Peloquin LA, Graham JH (1955) Gout of the patella: report of a case. N Engl J Med 253:979–980

Pommer G (1929) Mikroskopische Untersuchungen über Gelenkgicht. Fischer, Jena

Rosenberg EF, Arens RA (1947) Gout: clinical, pathologic and roentgenographic oberservations. Radiology 49:169–177

Rosenthal DI, Barton NW, McKusick KA et al (1992) Quantitative imaging of Gaucher disease. Radiology 185:841

Ross LV, Ross GJ, Mesgarzadeh M, Edmonds PR, Bonakdarpour A (1991) Hemodialysis-related amyloidomas of bone. Radiology 178:263–265

Rourke JA, Heslin DJ (1965) Gaucher's disease. Roentgenologic bone changes over 20 year interval. Am J Roentgenol 94:621–630

Ryan SJ, Smith CD, Slevin JT (1994) Magnetic resonance imaging in ochronosis: a rare cause of back pain. J Neuroiniaging 4:41–42

Schindelmeiser J, Radzun HJ, Munstermann D (1991) Tartrate-resistant, purple acid phosphatase in Gaucher cells of the spleen. Immuno- and cytochemical analysis. Pathol Res Pract 187:209–213

Silverstein MN, Kelly PJ (1967) Osteoarticular manifestation of Gaucher's disease. Am J Med Sci 253:569–577

Simon I (1962) Ein Fall einer durch Gicht verursachten schweren Knochenzerstörung. Fortschr Röntgenstr 96:835–836

Starer F, Sargent JD, Hobbs JR (1987) Regression of the radiological changes of Gaucher's disease following bone marrow transplantation. Br J Radiol 60:1189–1195

Talbott JH (1957) Gout. Grime & Stratton, New York

Thomas C (1973) Nierenveränderungen bei Gicht. Intern Welt 2:59

Uehlinger E (1970) Strukturwandlungen des Skeletts bei metabolischen Erkrankungen. Nova Acta Leopoldina (NF) 194/35:217–237

Uehlinger E (1976) Die pathologische Anatomie der Gicht. In: Schwiegk H (ed) Handbuch der inneren Medizin, 5th edn, vol VII/3. Springer, Berlin Heidelberg New York, pp 213–234

Zimran A, Kay A, Gelbart T et al (1992) Gaucher disease. Clinical, laboratory, radiologic, and genetic features of 53 patients. Medicine 71:337–353

Chapter 10
Bone Granulomas

Ackerman LV, Spjut HJ (1962) Tumors of bone and cartilage, Fascicle 4. Armed Forces Institute of Pathology, Washington D.C.

Adkins KF, Martinez MG, Hartley MW (1969) Ultrastructure of giant-cell lesions. A peripheral giant-cell reparative granuloma. Oral Surg 28:713–723

Adler CP (1973) Knochenzysten. Beitr Pathol 150:103–131

Adler CP (1980) Granulomatöse Erkrankungen im Knochen. Verh Dtsch Ges Pathol 64:359–365

Adler CP, Härle F (1974) Zur Differentialdiagnose osteofibröser Kiefererkrankungen. Verh Dtsch Ges Pathol 58:308–314

Adler CP, Uehlinger E (1979) Grenzfälle bei Knochentumoren. Präneoplastische Veränderungen und Geschwülste fraglicher Dignität. Verh Dtsch Ges Pathol 63:352–358

Adler CP, Schaefer HE (1988) Histiocytosis X of the left proximal femur. Skeletal Radiol 17:531–535

Augerau B, Thuilleux G, Moinet Ph (1977) Eosinophil granuloma of bones. Report of 15 cases including 10 survivals with an average follow up of 4 years. J Chir (Paris) 113:159–170

Austin IT Jr, Dahlin DC, Royer EQ (1959) Giant-cell reparative granuloma and related conditions affecting the jawbones. Oral Surg 12:1285–1295

Bergholz M, Schauer A, Poppe H (1979) Diagnostic and differential diagnostic aspects in histiocytosis X diseases. Pathol Res Pract 166:59–71

Bonk U (1976) Zur Problematik der Riesenzelltumoren und Riesenzellgranulome im Kieferknochen. In: Schuchardt K, Pfeifer G (eds) Grundlagen, Entwicklung und Fortschritte der Mund-, Kiefer- und Gesichtschirurgie, vol XXI. Thieme, Stuttgart, pp 161–164

Bopp H, Günther D (1970) Die Strahlenbehandlung des eosinphilen Granuloms. Strahlentherapie 140:143–147

Cheyne C (1971) Histiocytosis. J Bone Joint Surg Br 53:366–382

Dameshbod K, Kissane JM (1978) Idiopathic differentiated histiocytosis. Am J Clin Path 70:381–389

Dominok GW, Knoch HG (1977) Knochengeschwülste und geschwulstähnliche Knochenerkrankungen, 2nd edn. VEB Fischer, Jena, pp 223–231

Eble JN, Rosenberg AE, Young RH (1994) Retroperitoneal xanthogranuloma in a patient with Erdheim-Chester disease (Rev). Am J Surg Pathol 18:843–848

Engelbreth-Holm J, Partum G, Christensen E (1944) Eosinophil granuloma of bone – Schüller-Christian's disease. Acta Med Scand 118:292–312

Enriquez P, Dahlin DC, Hayles AB, Henderson ED (1967) Histiocytosis X: a clinical study. Mayo Clin Proc 42:88–89

Fink MG, Levinson DJ, Brown NL et al (1991) Erdheim-Chester disease. Case report with autopsy findings. Arch Pathol Lab Med 115:619–623

Fraser J (1934/35) Skeletal lipoid gramilomatosis (Hand-Schüller-Christians's disease). Br J Surg 22:800–824

Huhn D, Meister P (1978) Malignant histiocytosis. Cancer (Phila) 42:1341–1349

Jaffe HL (1953) Giant-cell reparative granuloma, traumatic bone cyst, and fibrous (fibro-osseous) dysplasia of the jawbones. Oral Surg 6:159–175

Jaffe HL (1968) Tumors and tumorous conditions of the bones and joints. Lea & Febiger, Philadelphia, pp 36–37

Jaffe HL (1972) Metabolic, degenerative, and inflammatory diseases of bones and joints. Urban & Schwarzenberg, Munich, pp 875–906

Küchemann K (1974) Congenital Letterer-Siwe disease. Beitr Pathol Anat 151:405–411

Lichtenstein L (1953) Histiocytosis X integration of eosinophilic granuloma of bone, Letterer-Siwe disease and Schüller-Christian disease as related manifestations of a single nosologic entity. Arch Pathol 56:84–102

Makley JT, Carter JR (1986) Eosinophilic granuloma of bone. Clin Orthop 204:37–44

Matus-Ridley M, Raney RB, Thawerani H, Meadows AT (1983) Histiocytosis X in children: patterns of disease and results of treatment. Med Pediatr Oncol 11:99–105

Mickelson MR, Bonfiglio M (1977) Eosinophilic granuloma and its variations. Orthop Clin N Am 8:933–945

Panico L, Passeretti U, De Rosa N et al (1994) Giant cell reparative granuloma of the distal skeletal bones. A report of five cases with inummohistochemical findings. Virchows Arch 425:315–320

Ratner V, Dorfman HD (1990) Giant-cell reparative granuloma of the hand and foot bones. Clin Orthop 260:251

Schajowicz F, Slullitel J (1973) Eosinophilic granuloma of bone and its relationship to Hand-Schüller-Christian and Letterer-Siwe syndromes. J Bone Joint Surg Br 55: 545–565

Schulz A, Märker R, Delling G (1976) Central giant cell granuloma. Histochemical and ultrastructural study on giant cell function. Virchows Arch 371:161–170

Seemann W-R, Genz T, Gospos Ch, Adler CP (1985) Die riesenzellige Reaktion der kurzen Röhrenknochen von Hand und Fuß. Fortschr Röntgenstr 142:355–360

Stull MA, Kransdorf MJ, Devaney KO (1992) Langerhans cell histiocytosis of bone. Radiographics 12:801–823

Uehlinger E (1963) Das eosinophile Knochengranulom. In: Heilmeyer L, Hittmair A (eds) Handbuch der Gesellschaft für Hämatologie, vol IV/2. Urban & Schwarzenberg, Munich, pp 56–87

Van der Wilde RS, Wold LE, McLeod RA, Sim FH (1990) Eosinophilic granuloma. Orthopedics 13:1301–1303

Wold LE, Dobyns JH, Swee RG, Dahlin DC (1986) Giant cell reaction (giant cell reparative granuloma of the small bones of the hands and feet). Am J Surg Pathol 10:491–496

Chapter 11
Bone Tumors

Chapter 11.1: General

Adler CP (1972) Probleme und Erfahrungen bei der Diagnostik von Knochentumoren. Beitr Pathol Anat 146:389–395

Adler CP (1974) Klinische und morphologische Aspekte maligner Knochentumoren. Dtsch Med Wochenschr 99:665–671

Adler CP (1980) Klassifikation der Knochentumoren und Pathologie der gutartigen und semimalignen Knochentumoren. In: Frommhold W, Gerhardt P (eds) Knochentumoren. Klinisch-radiologisches Seminar, vol X. Thieme, Stuttgart

Adler CP (1988) Diagnostic problems with semimalignant bone tumors. In: Heuck FHW, Keck E (eds) Fortschritte der Osteologie in Diagnostik und Therapie. Springer, Berlin Heidelberg New York, pp 103–118

Adler CP (1989) Klinische und morphologische Aspekte von gutartigen Knochentumoren und tumorähnlichen Knochenläsionen – Verlauf, Therapie und Prognose. Versicherungsmedizin 4:132–138

Adler CP, Klümper A (1977) Röntgenologische und pathologisch-anatomische Aspekte von Knochentumoren. Radiologe 17:355–392

Adler CP, Krause W, Gebert G (1992) Knochen und Gelenke. In: Thomas C (ed) 8. Grundlagen der klinischen Medizin. Schattauer, Stuttgart

Adler CP, Kozlowski K (1993) Primary bone tumors and tumorous conditions in children. Pathologic and radiologic diagnosis. Springer, London

Baumann RP, Lennert K, Piotrowski W et al (1978) Tumor-Histologie-Schlüssel. ICD-O-DA. Springer, Berlin Heidelberg New York

Becker W (1975) Knochentumorschlüssel. Arbeitsgemeinschaft Knochentumoren, 1975 edn. Printed at the Deutsches Krebsforschungszentrum, Heidelberg

Bullogh P, Vigorita VI (1984) Atlas of orthopaedic pathology with clinical and radiologic correlations. University Park Press, Gower Medical Publishing, New York London

Campanacci M (1990) Bone and soft tissue tumors. Springer, Berlin Heidelberg New York

Dominok GW, Knoch HG (1982) Knochengeschwülste und geschwulstähnliche Knochenerkrankungen, 3d edn. Fischer, Stuttgart

Dorfman HD, Czerniak B (1998) Bone tumors. Mosby & Mosby-Wolfe, London

Enneking WF, Spanier SS, Goodman MA (1980) A system for the surgical staging of musculoskeletal sarcomata. Clin Orthop 153:106–120

Enneking WF (1985) Staging of musculoskeletal neoplasms. Skeletal Radiol 13:183–184

Fechner RE, Mills SE (1993) Tumors of the bones and joints. AFIP, Washington DC

Freyschmidt J (1997) Skeletterkrankungen. Klinisch-radiologische Diagnose und Differentialdiagnose, 2nd edn. Springer, Berlin Heidelberg New York

Freyschmidt J, Ostertag H (1988) Knochentumoren. Klinik, Radiologie, Pathologie. Springer, Berlin Heidelberg New York

Hudson TM (1987) Radiologic-pathologic correlation of musculoskeletal lesions. Williams & Wilkins, Baltimore

Huvos AG (1991) Bone tumors. Diagnosis, treatment, and prognosis, 2nd edn. Saunders, Philadelphia

Jaffe HL (1958) Tumors and tumorous conditions of bones and joints. Lea & Febiger, Philadelphia

Johnson LC (1953) A general theory of bone tumors. Bull NY Acad Med 29:164–171

Lichtenstein L (1977) Bone tumors, 5th edn. Mosby, St. Louis

Lodwick GS, Wilson AJ, Farrell C et al (1980) Determining growth rates of focal lesions of bone from radiographs. Radiology 134:577–583

Mirra JM, Picci P, Gold RH (1989) Bone tumors: clinical, radiologic, and pathologic correlations. Lea & Febiger, Philadelphia

Nierhard FU, Pfeil J (1989) Orthopädie. Hippokrates, Stuttgart (Duale Reihe)

Resnick D (1995) Diagnosis of bone and joint disorders, 3rd edn. Saunders, Philadelphia

Richter GM, Ernst H-U, Dinkel E, Adler CP (1986) Morphologie und Diagnostik von Knochentumoren des Fußes. Radiologe 26:341–352

Schajowicz F (1994) Tumors and tumorlike lesions of bone: pathology, radiology, and treatment, 2nd edn. Springer, New York Berlin Heidelberg

Schajowicz F (1993) Histological typing of bone tumours. WHO Geneva, 2nd edn. Springer, Berlin Heidelberg New York

Schedel H, Wicht L, Tempka A et al (1995) Stellenwert der MRT bei Knochentumoren. Osteologie 4:36–43

Sissons HA (1979) Bones. In: Symmers SC (ed) Systemic pathology, 2nd edn, vol 5. Churchill Livingstone, Edinburgh, pp 2383–2489

Unni KK (1996) Dahlins bone tumors. General aspects and data on 11,087 cases, 5th edn. Lippincott-Raven, Philadelphia

Wold LE, McLeod RA, Sim FH, Unni KK (1990) Atlas of orthopedic pathology. Saunders, Philadelphia

Chapter 11.2: Cartilaginous Tumors

Adler CP (1979) Differential diagnosis of cartilage tumors. Pathol Res Pract 166:45–58

Adler CP (1985) Chondromyxoid fibroma (CMF) of the radius associated with an aneurysmal bone cyst (ABC). Skeletal Radiol 14:305–308

Adler CP (1993) Mesenchymal chondrosarcoma of soft tissue of the left foot. Skeletal Radiol 22:300–305

Adler CP, Fringes B (1978) Chondrosarkom der distalen Femurmetaphyse. Med Welt (Stuttgart) 29:1511–1516

Adler CP, Klümper A (1977) Röntgenologische und pathologisch-anatomische Aspekte von Knochentumoren. Radiologe 17:355–392

Adler CP, Klümper A, Wenz W (1979) Enchondrome aus radiologischer und pathologisch-anatomischer Sicht. Radiologe 19:341–349

Alexander C (1976) Chondroblastoma of tibia: case report 5. Skeletal Radiol 1:63–64

Anderson RL, Popowitz L, Li JKH (1969) An unusual sarcoma arising in a solitary osteochondroma. J Bone Joint Surg Am 51:1199–1204

Anract P, Tomeno B, Forest M (1994) Chondrosarcomes dedifferenciés. Étude de treize cas cliniques et revue de la litterature. Rev Chir Orthop Reparatrice Appar Mot 80:669–680

Bertoni F, Present D, Bacchini P et al (1989) Dedifferentiated peripheral chondrosarcoma: a report of seven cases. Cancer 63:2054–2059

Bessler W (1966) Die malignen Potenzen der Skelettchondrome. Schweiz Med Wochenschr 96:461–469

Bjornsson J, Unni KK, Dahlin DC et al (1984) Clear cell chondrosarcoma of bone: observations in 47 cases. Am J Surg Pathol 8:223–230

Brien EW, Mirra JM, Kerr R (1997) Benign and malignant cartilage tumors of bone and joint: their anatomic and theoretical basis with an emphasis on radiology, pathology and clinical biology. 1. The intramedullary cartilage tumors. Skeletal Radiol 26:325–353

Capanna R, Bertoni F, Bettelli G (1988) Dedifferentiated chondrosarcoma. J Bone Joint Surg Am 70:60–69

Cash SL, Habermarm ET (1988) Chondrosarcoma of the small bones of the hand: case report and review of the literature. Orthop Rev 17:365–369

Chow LTC, Lin J, Yip KMH et al (1996) Chondromyxoid fibroma-like osteosarcoma: a distinct variant of low-grade osteosacoma. Histopathology 29:429–436

Cohen J, Cahen 1 (1963) Benign chondroblastoma of the patella. J Bone Joint Surg Am 45:824–826

Crim JR, Seeger LL (1993) Diagnosis of low-grade chondrosarcoma: devil's advocate. Radiology 189:503–504

Dahlin DC (1956) Chondromyxoid fibroma of bone, with emphasis on its morphological relationship to benign chondroblastoma. Cancer 9:195–203

Dahlin DC (1976) Chondrosarcoma and its variants. In: Ackerman LV, Spjut HJ, Abell MR (eds) Bones and joints (Int Acad Path Monogr). Williams & Wilkins, Baltimore

Dahlin DC (1978) Clear cell chondrosarcoma of humerus. Case report 54. Skeletal Radiol 2:247–249

Dahlin DC, Beabout JW (1971) Dedifferentiation of low-grade chondrosarcoma. Cancer (Phila) 28:461

Dahlin DC, Ivins JC (1972) Benign chondroblastoma. A study of 125 cases. Cancer (Phila) 30:401–413

Dahlin DC, Wells AH, Henderson ED (1953) Chondromyxoid fibroma of bone. J Bone Joint Surg Am 35:831–834

De Beuckeleer LHL, Schepper AMA, Ramon F (1996) Magnetic resonance imaging of cartilaginous tumors: is it useful or necessary? Skeletal Radiol 25:137–141

Dominok GW, Knoch HG (1982) Knochengeschwülste und geschwulstähnliche Knochenerkrankungen, 3d edn. Fischer, Stuttgart

Dorfman HD (1973) Malignant transformation of benign bone lesions. Proc Nat Cancer Conf 7:901–913

Fechner RE, Mills SE (1993) Tumors of the bones and joints. AFIP, Washington, DC

Feldmann F, Hecht HL, Johnston AD (1970) Chondroxyoidfibroma of bone. Radiology 94:249–260

Frassica FJ, Unni KK, Beabout JW, Sim FH (1986) Differentiated chondrosarcoma: a report of the clinicopathological features and treatment of seventy-eight cases. J Bone Joint Surg Am 68:1197–1205

Ganzoni N, Wirth W (1965) Zur Klinik der genuinen Knochengeschwülste im Bereich der langen Röhrenknochen. Praxis 54:342–350

Goethals PL, Dahlin DC, Devine KD (1963) Cartilaginous tumors of the larynx. Surg Gynec Obstet 117:77–82

Henderson ED, Dahlin DC (1963) Chondrosarcoma of bone: a study of two hundred and eighty-eight cases. J Bone Joint Surg Am 45:1450–1458

Hohbach C, Mall W (1977) Chondrosarcoma of the pulmonary artery. Beitr Pathol Anat 160:298–307

Huvos AG (1979) Bone tumors. Saunders, Philadelphia

Huvos AG, Marcove RC, Erlandson RA, Mike V (1972) Chondroblastoma of bone. Cancer 29:760–771

Jacobs P (1976) Highly malignant chondrosarcoma of unknown origin, with tumor emboli of the inferior vena cava and main pulmonary artery: case report 7. Skeletal Radiol 1:109–111

Jaffe HL, Lichtenstein L (1948) Chondromyxoidfibroma of bone. A distinctive benign tumor likely to be mistaken especially for chondrosarcoma. Arch Pathol 45:541–551

Johnson S, Ttu B, Ayala AG, Chawla SP (1986) Chondrosarcoma with additional mesenchymal component (dedifferentiated chondrosarcoma) 1. A clinicopathologic study of 26 cases. Cancer 58:278–286

Karbowski A, Eckardt A, Rompe JD (1995) Multiple kartilaginäre Exostosen. Orthopäde 24:37–43

Kunkel MG, Dahlin DC, Young HH (1956) Benign chondroblastoma. J Bone Joint Surg Am 38:817–826

Kyriakos M, Land VJ, Penning HL, Parker SG (1985) Metastatic chondroblastoma: report of a fatal case with a review of the literature on atypical, aggressive, and malignant chondroblastoma. Cancer 55:1770–1789

Lichtenstein L, Bernstein D (1959) Unusual benign and malignant chondroid tumors of bone. Cancer (Phila) 12:1142–1157

Mainzer F, Minagi H, Steinbach HL (1971) The variable manifestations of multiple enchondromatosis. Radiology 99:377–388

Marmor L (1964) Periosteal chondroma (juxtacortical chondroma). Clin Orthop 37:150–153

Mazabraud A (1974) Le chondrosarcome mésenchymateux: A propos de six observations. Rev Chir Orthop Raparatrice Appar Mot 60:197–203

McBryde A, Goldner JL (1970) Chondroblastoma of bone. Am Surg 36:94–108

Meneses MF, Unni KK, Swee RG (1993) Bizarre parosteal osteochondromatous proliferation of bone (Nora's lesion). Am J Surg Pathol 17:691–697

Mirra JM, Gold R, Downs J, Eckardt JI (1985) A new histologic approach to the differentiation of enchondroma and chondrosarcoma of the bones: a clinicopathologic analysis of 51 cases. Clin Orthop 201:214–237

Nakashima Y, Unni KK, Shiveset TC al. (1986) Mesenchymal chondrosarcoma of bone and soft tissue: a review of 111 cases. Cancer 57:2444–2453

Nelson DL, Abdul-Karim FW, Carter JR, Makley JT (1990) Chondrosarcoma of small bones of the hand arising from enchondroma. J Hand Surg Am 15:655–659

Nojima T, Unni KK, McLeod RA, Pritchard DJ (1985) Periosteal chondroma and periosteal chondrosarcoma. Am J Surg Pathol 9:666–677

Nora FE, Dahlin DC, Beabout JW (1983) Bizarre parosteal osteochondromatous proliferations of the hands and feet. Am J Surg Pathol 7:245–250

Norman A, Steiner GC (1977) Recurrent chondromyxoid fibroma of the tibia: case report 38. Skeletal Radiol 2:105–107

O'Connor Pj, Gibbon WW, Hardy G, ButtWP (1996) Chondromyxoid fibroma of the foot. Skeletal Radiol 25:143–148

Ogose A, Unni KK, Swee RG et al (1997) Chondrosarcoma of small bones of the hands and feet. Cancer 80:50–59

Peterson HA (1989) Multiple hereditary osteochondromatosis. Clin Orthop 239:222–230

Poppe H (1965) Die röntgenologische Symptomatik der gutartige und semimalignen Knochengeschwülste. Thieme, Stuttgart (Dtsch. Röntgenkongr. 1964, Wiesbaden), pp 218–241

Ryall RDH (1970) Chondromyxoidfibroma of bone. Br J Radiol 43:71–72

Salvador AH, Beabout JW, Dahlin DC (1971) Mesenchymal chondrosarcoma: observations on 30 new cases. Cancer (Phila) 28:605–615

Salzer M, Salzer-Kuntschik M (1965) Das Chondromyxoidfibrom. Langenbecks Arch Chir 312:216–231

Schajowicz F, Gallardo H (1970) Epiphysial chondroblastoma of bone: A clinico-pathological study of sixty-nine cases. J Bone Joint Sing Am 52:205–226

Schauwecker F, Weller S, Klümper A, Anlauf B (1969) Therapeutische Möglichkeiten beim benignen Chondroblastom. Bruns' Beitr Klin Chir 217:155–159

Sirsatz MV, Doctor VM (1970) Benign chondroblastoma of bone: report of a case of malignant transformation. J Bone Joint Surg Br 52:741–745

Sissons HA (1979) Dedifferentiated chondrosarcoma of the tibia: case report 83. Skeletal Radiol 3:257–259

Springfield DS, Capanna R, Gherlinzoni F et al (1985) Chondroblastoma: a review of seventy cases. J Bone Joint Surg Am 67:748–755

Springfield DS, Gebhardt MC, McGuire MH (1996) Chondrosarcoma: a review. Instr Course Lect 45:417–124

Toshifumi O, Hillmann A, Lindner N et al (1996) Metastasis of chondrosarcoma. J Cancer Res Clin Oncol 122:625–628

Turcotte RE, Kurt AM, Sim FM et al (1993) Chondroblastoma. Hum Pathol 24:944–949

Uehlinger E (1974) Pathologische Anatomie der Knochengeschwülste (unter besonderer Berücksichtigung der semimalignen Formen). Chirurg 45:62–70

Unni KK, Dahlin DC (1979) Premalignant tumors and conditions of bone. Am J Surg Pathol 3:47–60

Unni KK, Dahlin DC, Beabout JW, Sim JH (1976) Chondrosarcoma: clear-cell variant: a report of sixteen cases. J Bone Joint Surg Am 58:676–683

Unni KK (1996) Dahlin's bone tumors: general aspects and data on 11,087 cases, 5th edn. Lippincott-Raven, Philadelphia

White PG, Saunders L, Orr W, Friedman L (1996) Chondromyxoid fibroma. Skeletal Radiol 25:79–81

Wilkinson RH, Kirkpatrick JA (1976) Low-grade chondrosarcoma of femur: case report 14. Skeletal Radiol 1:127–128

Wilson AJ, Kyriakos M, Ackerman IV (1991) Chondromyxoid fibroma: radiographic appearance in 38 cases and in a review of the literature. Radiology 179:513–518

Young CL, Sim FH, Unni KK, McLeod RA (1990) Chondrosarcoma of bone of children. Cancer 66:1641–1648

Chapter 11.3: Osseous Bone Tumors

Abudu A, Sferopoulos NK, Tillman RM et al (1996) The surgical treatment and outcome of pathological fractures in localised osteosarcoma. J Bone Joint Surg Br 78:694–698

Adler CP (1974) Osteosarkom der distalen Radius-Epi-Metaphyse mit pseudoepithelialen Ausdifferenzierungen. (Epitheloides Osteosarkom). Verh Dtsch Ges Path 58:272–274

Adler CP (1976) Knochentumoren. In: C Thomas, Sandritter W (eds) Spezielle Pathologie. Textbuch zu einem audiovisuellen Kurs. Schattauer, Stuttgart

Adler CP (1977) Histogenese und praktische Konsequenzen bei Knochengeschwülsten (Freiburger Chirurgengespräch). Gödecke, Freiburg, pp 10–62

Adler CP (1980 a) Klassifikation der Knochentumoren und Pathologie der gutartigen und semimalignen Knochentumoren. In: Frommhold W, Gerhardt P (eds) Knochentumoren. Klinisch-radiologisches Seminar, vol X. Thieme, Stuttgart, pp 1–24

Adler CP (1980 b) Parosteal (juxtacortica) osteosarcoma of the distal femur. Pathol Res Pract 169:388–395

Adler CP (1984) Osteoblastoma of the lesser trochanter of the left femur. Skeletal Radiol 11:65–68

Adler CP (1985) Aggressive osteoblastoma. Pathol Res Pract 179:437–438

Adler CP, Schmidt A (1978) Aneurysmale Knochenzyste des Femurs mit malignem Verlauf. Verh Dtsch Ges Pathol 62:487

Adler CP, Uehlinger E (1979) Grenzfälle bei Knochentumoren. Präneoplastische Veränderungen und Geschwülste fraglicher Dignität. Verh Dtsch Ges Pathol 63:352–358

Amstutz HC (1969) Multiple osteogenic sarcoma – metastasis or multicentric? Report of two cases and review of literature. Cancer 24:923–931

Bertoni F, Present DA, Enneking WF (1985) Giant-cell tumor of bone with pulmonary metastases. J Bone Joint Surg 67:890–900

Bertoni F, Present DA, Sudanese A et al (1988) Giant-cell tumor of bone with pulmonary metastases: six case reports and a review of the literature. Clin Orthop 237:275–285

Bertoni F, Donati D, Bacchini P et al (1992) The morphologic spectrum of osteoblastoma (OBL). Is its aggressive nature predictable? Lab Invest 66:3

Bieling P, Rehan N, Winkle P et al (1996) Tumor size and prognosis in aggressively treated osteosarcoma. J Clin Oncol 14:848–858

Bosse A, Vollmer E, Böcker W et al (1990) The impact of osteonectin for differential diagnosis of bone tumors. An immunohistochemical approach. Pathol Res Pract 186:651–657

Burkhardt L, Fischer H (1970) Pathologische Anatomie des Schädels in seiner Beziehung zum Inhalt. Spezielle Pathologie des Schädelskeletts. In: Uehlinger E (ed) Handbuch Spezielle Pathologie, Anatomie, Histologie, vol IX/7. Springer, Berlin Heidelberg New York, pp 259–273

Busso MG, Schajowicz F (1945) Sarcoma osteogenico a localization multiple. Rev Ortop Traumatol 15:85–96

Campanacci M, Pizzoferrato A (1971) Osteosarcoma emorragico. Chir Organi Mov 60:409–421

Chan YF, Llewellyn H (1995) Sclerosing osteosarcoma of the great toe phalanx in an 11-year-old girl. Histopathology 26:281–284

Carter SR, Grimer RJ, Sneath RS (1991) A review of 13-years experience of osteosarcoma. Clin Orthop 270:45–51

Choong PFM, Pritchard DJ, Rock MG et al (1996) Low grade central osteogenic sarcoma – a long term follow-up of 20 patients. Clin Orthop 322:198–206

Dahlin DC, Johnson EW Jr (1954) Giant osteoid osteoma. J Bone Joint Surg Am 36:559–572

Davis AM, Bell RS, Goodwin PJ (1994) Prognostic factors in osteosarcoma: a critical review. J Clin Oncol 12:423–431

Delling G, Dreyer T, Heise U et al (1990) Therapieinduzierte Veränderungen in Osteosarkomen – qualitative und quantitative morphologische Ergebnisse der Therapiestudie COSS 80 und ihre Beziehung zur Prognose. Tumordiagn Ther 11:167–174

Denictolis M, Goteri G, Brancorsini D et al (1995) Extraskeletal osteosarcoma of the mediastinum associated with long-term patient survival – a case report. Anticancer Res 15:2785–2789

Dorfman HD (1973) Malignant transformation of benign bone lesions in bone and soft tissue sarcoma. American Cancer Society, Lippincott, Philadelphia (Proc Natl Cancer Conf 7), pp 901–913

Dorfman HD, Weiss SW (1984) Borderline osteoblastic tumors: problems in the differential diagnosis of aggressive osteoblastoma and low-grade osteosarcoma. Semin Diagn Pathol 1:215–234

Dorfman HD, Czerniak B (1998) Bone Tumors. Mosby, St. Louis

Enneking WF, Kagan A (1975) Skip metastases in osteosarcoma. Cancer 36:2192–2205

Fechner RE, Mills SE (1993) Tumors of the bones and joints. AFIP Washington, DC

Frassica FJ, Sim FH, Frassica DA, Wold LE (1991) Survival and management considerations in postirradiation osteosarcoma and Paget's osteosarcoma. Clin Orthop 270:120–127

Fuchs N, Winkler K (1993) Osteosarcoma. Curr Op Oncol 5:667–671

Geschickter CF, Copeland MM (1951) Parosteal osteoma of the bone: a new entity. Arch Surg 133:790–806

Gördes W, Adler CP, Huyer C (1991) Hochmalignes teleangiektatisches Osteosarkom. Langjährige Verlaufsbeobachtung. Z Orthop 129:460–464

Gbssner W, Hug O, Luz A, Müller WA (1976) Experimental induction of bone tumors by short-lived bone-seeking radionuclides. In: Grundmann E (ed) Malignant bone tumors. Springer, Berlin Heidelberg New York

Greenspan A (1993) Benign bone-forming lesions: osteoma, osteoid osteoma, and osteoblastoma. Clinical, imaging, pathologic, and differential considerations. Skeletal Radiol 22:485–500

Grundmarm E. Hobik HP, Immenkamp M, Roessner A (1979) Histo-diagnostic remarks of bone tumors, a review of 3026 cases registered in Knochengeschwülstregister Westfalens. Pathol Res Pract 166:5–24

Grundmarm E, Ueda Y, Schneider-Stock R, Roessner A (1995) New aspects of cell biology in osteosarcoma. Pathol Res Pract 191:563–570

Grundmann E, Roessner A, Ueda Y et al (1995) Current aspects of the pathology of osteosarcoma. Anticancer Res 15:1023–1032

Heymer B, Kreidler H, Adler CP (1988) Strahleninduziertes Osteosarkom des Unterkiefers. Z Mund Kiefer Gesichtschir 12:113–119

Hochstetter AR von, Cserhati K, Cserhati MD (1996) Central low grade osteosarcoma. of >30 years' duration. Osteologie 5:25–29

Hudson TM, Springfield DS, Benjamin M et al (1985) Computed tomography of parosteal osteosarcoma. Am J Radiol 144:961–965

Huvos AG (1979) Bone tumors: diagnosis, treatment and prognosis. Saunders, Philadelphia

Huvos AG, Butler A, Bretsky SS (1983) Osteogenic sarcoma associated with Paget's disease of bone: a clinicopathologic study of 65 patients. Cancer 52:1489–1495

Huvos AG, Woodard HQ, Cahan WG et al (1985) Postradiation osteogenic sarcoma of bone and soft tissue: a clinicopathologic study of 66 patients. Cancer 55:1244

Jackson JR, Bell MEA (1977) Spurious benign osteoblastoma. J Bone Joint Surg Am 59:397–401

Jaffe N, Watts H, Fellows KE (1978) Local en bloc resection for limb preservation. Cancer Treat Rep 62:217–223

Jaffe N, Farber S, Traggis D (1973) Favorable response of osteogenic sarcoma to high dose methotrexate with citrovorum rescue and radiation therapy. Cancer 31:1367–1373

Jaffe N, Patel SR, Benjamin RS (1995) Chemotherapy in osteosarcoma. Basis for application and antagonism to implementation; early controversies surrounding its implementation. Hem Oncol Clin NY 9:825–840

Korholz D, Wirtz I, Vosberg H et al (1996) The role of bone scintigraphy in the follow-up of osteogenic sarcoma. Europ J Cancer 32 Am: 461–464

Kurt A-M, Unni KK, McLeod RA, Pritchard DJ (1990) Low-grade intraosseous osteosarcoma. Cancer 65:1418

Lee ES, Mackenzie DH (1964) Osteosarcoma. A study of the value of preoperative megavoltage radiotherapy. Br J Surg 51:252-274

Levine E, De Smet AA, Huntrakoon M (1985) Juxtacortical osteosarcoma: a radiologic and histologic spectrum. Skeletal Radiol 14:38-46

Logan PM, Munk PL, O'Connell JX et al (1996) Post-radiation osteosarcoma of the scapula. Skeletal Radiol 25:596-601

Loizaga JM, Calvo M, Lopez Barea F et al (1993) Osteoblastoma and osteoid osteoma. Clinical and morphological features of 162 cases. Pathol Res Pract 189:33-41

Lorigan JG, Libshitz HI, Peuchot M (1989) Radiation-induced sarcoma of bone: CT findings in 19 cases. AJR 153:791-794

Lowbeer L (1968) Multifocal osteosarcomatosis – rare entity. Bull Pathol 9:52-53

Lucas DR, Unni KK, McLeod RA et al (1994) Osteoblastoma: clinicopathologic study of 306 cases. Hum Pathol 25:117-134

Marcove RC, Heelan RT, Huvos AG et al (1991) Osteoid osteoma: diagnosis, localization, and treatment. Clin Orthop 267:197-201

Marsh BW, Bonfigho M, Brady LP, Enneking WF (1975) Benign osteoblastoma: Range of manifestations. J Bone Joint Surg Am 57:1-9

Matsuno T, Unni KK, McLeod RA, Dahlin DC (1976) Teleangiectatic osteogenic sarcoma. Cancer 38:2538-2547

McLeod RA, Dahlin DC, Beabout JW (1976) The spectrum of osteoblastoma. Am J Roentgenol 126:321-335

Mervak TR, Unni KK, Pritchard DJ, McLeod RA (1991) Teleangiectatic osteosaroma. Clin Orthop 270:135-139

Meyer WH (1991) Recent developments in genetic mechanisms, assessment, and treatment of osteosarcomas (Rev). Cur Op Oncol 3:689-693

Mirra JM, Kendrick RA, Kendrick RE (1976) Pseudomalignant osteoblastoma versus arrested osteosarcoma: a case report. Cancer 37:2005-2014

Murray RO, Jacobson HG (1977) The radiology of skeletal disorders, 2nd edn, vol 1. Churchill Livingstone, Edinburgh, p. 568

Ogihara Y, Sudo A, Fujinami S, Sato K, Miura T (1991) Current management, local management, and survival statistics of high-grade osteosaroma. Experience in Japan. Clin Orthop 270:72-78

{Okada K, Frassica FJ, Sim FH et al (1994) Parosteal osteosarcoma: a clinicopathologic study. J Bone Joint Surg 76 Am: 366-378

Okada K, Wold LE, Beaubout JW, Shives TC (1993) Osteosarcoma of the hand. A clinicopathologic study of 12 cases. Cancer 72:719-725

Partovi S, Logan PM, Janzen DL et al (1996) Low-grade parosteal osteosarcoma of the ulna with dedifferentiation into high-grade osteosarcoma. Skeletal Radiol 25:497

Phillips TL, Sheline GE (1963) Bone sarcomas following radiation therapy. Radiology 81:992-996

Poppe H (1977) Radiologische Differentialdiagnose bei primär malignen und potentiell malignen Knochentumoren Freiburg (Freiburger Chirurgengespräch). Gödecke, pp 75-105

Rock MG, Pritchard DJ, Unni KK (1984) Metastases from histologically benign giant-cell tumor of bone. J Bone Joint Surg 66:269-274

Rosen G, Murphy ML, Huvos AG (1976) Chemotherapy, en bloc resection, and prosthetic bone replacement in the treatment of osteogenic sarcoma. Cancer 37:1-11

Ruiter DJ, Cornelisse CJ, Rijssel TG van, Velde EA van der (1977) Aneurysmal bone cyst and teleangiectatic osteosarcoma. A histo-pathological and morphometric study. Virchows Arch Abt A 373:311-325

Sabanas AO, Dahlin DC, Childs DS Jr, Ivins JC (1956) Post-radiation sarcoma of bone. Cancer 9:528-542

Schajowicz F, Lemos D (1976) Malignant osteoblastoma. J Bone Joint Surg Br 58:202-211

Seki T, Fukuda H, Ishii Y et al (1975) Malignant transformation of benign osteoblastoma. J Bone Joint Surg 57 Am:424-426

Sheth DS, Yasko AW, Raymond AK et al (1996) Conventional and dedifferentiated. parosteal osteosarcoma. Diagnosis, treatment, and outcome. Cancer 78:136-145

Spiess H, Poppe H, Schoen H (1962) Strahleninduzierte Knochentumoren nach Thorium-X-Bestrahlung. Mschr Kinderheilk 110:198-201

Steiner GC (1965) Postradiation sarcoma of bone. Cancer 18:603-612

Stutch R (1975) Osteoblastoma – a benign entity? Orthop Rev 4:27-33

Ueda Y, Roessner A, Grundmarm E (1993) Pathological diagnosis of osteosarcoma: the validity of the subclassification and some new diagnostic approaches using immunohistochemistry. Cancer Treatm Res 62:109-124

Uehlinger E (1974) Pathologische Anatomie der Knochengeschwülste (unter besonderer Berücksichtigung der semimalignen Formen). Chirurg 45:62-70

Uehlinger E (1976) Primary malignancy, secondary malignancy and semimalignancy of bone tumors. In: Grundmann E (ed) Malignant bone tumors. Springer, Berlin Heidelberg New York

Uehlinger E (1977) Über Erfolge und Mißerfolge in der operativen Behandlung der Knochengeschwülste (Freiburger Chirurgengespräche). Gödecke, Freiburg, pp 53-74

Unni KK, Dahlin D, Beabout JW, Ivins JC (1976) Parosteal osteogenic sarcoma. Cancer 37:2466-2475

Unni KK, Dahlin DC, Beabout JW (1976) Periosteal osteogenic sarcoma. Cancer 37:2476-2485

Unni KK, Dahlin DC, McLeod RA, Pritchard DJ (1977) Intraosseous well-differentiated osteosarcoma. Cancer 40:1337-1347

Van der Heul RO, Ronnen JR von (1967) Juxtacortical osteosarcoma. Diagnosis, differential diagnosis, treatment, and an analysis of eighty cases. J Bone Joint Surg 49:415-439

Van der Griend RA (1996) Osteosarcoma. and its variants. Orthop Clin North Am 27:575-581

Vaughan J (1968) The effects of skeletal irradiation. Clin Orthop 56:283-303

Winkler K, Bieling P, Bielack SS et al (1991) Local control and survival from the cooperative osteosarcoma. Study group studies of the German Society of Pediatric Oncology and the Vienna Bone Tumor Registry. Clin Orthop 270:79-86

Winkler K, Bielack SS, Delling G et al (1993) Treatment of osteosarcoma: experience of the Cooperative Osteosarcoma Study Group (COSS). Cancer Treat Res 62:269-277

Wold LE, Unni KK, Beabout JW (1984) Dedifferentiated parosteal osteosarcoma. J Bone Joint Surg 66:53-59

Wold LE, Unni KK, Beabout JW, Dahlin DC (1984) High-grade surface osteosarcomas. Am J Surg Pathol 8:181

Wuisman P, Roessner A, Blasius S et al (1993) Highly malignant surface osteosarcoma arising at the site of a previously treated aneurysmal bone cyst. J Cancer Res Clin Oncol 119:375–378

Yunis EJ, Barnes L (1986) The histologic diversity of osteosarcoma. Pathol Ann 21:121–141

Chapter 11.4: Fibrous Tissue Bone Tumors

Adler CP (1973) Knochenzysten. Beitr Pathol Anat 150:103–131

Adler CP (1980) Granulomatöse Erkrankungen im Knochen. Verh Dtsch Ges Pathol 64:359–365

Adler CP (1980) Klassifikation der Knochentumoren und Pathologie der gutartigen und semimalignen Knochentumoren. In: Frommhold W, Gerhardt P (eds) Knochentumoren. Klinisch-radiologisches Seminar, vol X. Thieme, Stuttgart

Adler CP (1981) Fibromyxoma of bone within the femoral neck und the tibial head. J Cancer Res Clin Oncol 101:183–189

Adler CP, Härle F (1974) Zur Differentialdiagnose osteofibröses Kiefererkrankungen. Verh Dtsch Ges Pathol 58:308–314

Adler CP, Klümper A (1977) Röntgenologische und pathologisch-anatomische Aspekte von Knochentumoren. Radiologe 17:355–392

Adler CP, Stock D (1985) Zur Problematik aggressiver Fibromatosen in der Orthopädie. Orthop Grenzgeb 124:355–360

Adler CP, Reinartz H (1988) Fleckige Osteosklerose des Tibiaschaftes: Osteofibröse Knochendysplasie Campanacci der linken Tibia. Radiologe 28:591–592

Alguacil-Garcia A, Alonso A, Pettigrew NM (1984) Osteofibrous dysplasia (ossifying fibroma) of the tibia and fibula and adamantinoma: a case report. Am J Clin Pathol 82:470–474

Bauer WH, Harell A (1954) Myxoma of bone. J Bone Joint Surg Am 36:263–266

Berkin CR (1966) Non-ossifying fibroma of bone. Br J Radiol 39:469–471

Bertoni F, Calderoni P, Bacchini P et al (1986) Benign fibrous histiocytoma of bone. J Bone Joint Surg Am 68:1225–1230

Blackwell JB, McCarthy SW, Xipell JM et al (1988) Osteofibrous dysplasia of the tibia and fibula. Pathology 20:227–233

Bullough PG, Walley J (1965) Fibrous cortical defect and non-ossifying fibroma. Postgrad Med J 41:672–676

Caffey J (1955) On fibrous defects in cortical walls of growing tubular bones. Adv Pediatr 7:13–51

Campanacci M, Leonessa C (1970) Displasia fibrosa dello scheletro. Chir Organi Mov 59:195–225

Campanacci M, Laus M (1981) Osteofibrous dysplasia of the tibia and fibula. J Bone Joint Surg Am 63:367–375

Clarke BE, Xipell JM, Thomas DP (1985) Benign fibrous histiocytoma of bone. Am J Surg Pathol 9:806–815

Cohen DM, Dahlin DC, Pugh DG (1962) Fibrous dysplasia associated with adamantinoma of the long bones. Cancer 15:515–521

Cunningham JB, Ackerman IV (1956) Metaphyseal fibrous defects. J Bone Joint Surg Am 38:797–808

Dahlin DC (1967) Xanthoma of bone. In: Dahlin DC (ed) Bone tumors, 2nd edn. Thomas, Springfield, Ill., pp 97–98

Dahlin DC, Ivins JC (1969) Fibrosarcoma of bone. A study of 114 cases. Cancer 23:35–41

Dahlin DC, Unni KK, Matsumo T (1977) Malignant (fibrous) histiocytoma of bone – fact or fancy? Cancer 39:1508–1516

Delmer LP (1976) Fibro-osseous lesions of bone. In: Ackerman LV, Spjut HJ, Abell MR (eds) Bones and joints (Int Acad Pathol Monogr). Williams & Wilkins, Philadelphia, pp 209–235

Dominok GW, Knoch HG (1982) Knochengeschwülste und geschwulstähnliche Knochenerkrankungen, 3d edn. Fischer, Stuttgart

Dutz W, Stout AP (1961) The myxoma in childhood. Cancer 14:629–635

Fechner RE, Mills SE (1993) Tumors of the bones and joints. AFIP, Washington, DC

Feldman F, Lattes R (1977) Primary malignant fibrous histiocytoma (fibrous xanthoma) of bone. Skeletal Radiol 1:145–160

Feldman F, Norman D (1972) Intra- and extraosseous malignant histiocytoma (malignant fibrous xanthoma). Radiology 104:497–508

Fink B, Schneider T, Ramp U et al (1995) Riesenzell-Tumor der Patella. Osteologie 4:111–114

Fletcher CDM (1992) Pleomorphic malignant fibrous histiocytoma: fact or fiction? A critical reappraisal based on 159 tumors diagnosed as pleomorphic sarcoma. Am J Sing Pathol 16:213–228

Galli SJ, Weintraub HP, Proppe KH (1978) Malignant fibrous histiocytoma and pleomorphic sarcoma in association with medullary bone infarcts. Cancer 41:607–619

Garlipp M (1976) Non-osteogenic fibroma of bone. Zentralbl Chir 101:1525–1529

Haag M, Adler CP (1989) Malignant fibrous histiocytoma in association with hip replacement. J Bone Joint Surg Br 71:701

Hamada T, Ito H, Araki Y et al (1996) Benign fibrous histiocytoma of the femur: review of three cases. Skeletal Radiol 25:25–29

Hatcher CH (1945) The pathogenesis of localized fibrous lesions in the metaphyses of long bones. Arch Surg 122:1016–1030

Henry A (1969) Monostotic fibrous dysplasia. J Bone Joint Surg Br 51:300–306

Hiranandani LH, Chandra O, Melgiri RD, Hiranandani NL (1966) Ossifying fibromas (report of four unusual cases). J Laryngol 80:964–969

Huvos AG (1976) Primary malignant fibrous histiocytoma of bone. Clinicopathologic study of 18 patients. NY Stud J Med 76:552–559

Huvos AG (1979) Bone tumors: diagnosis, treatment and prognosis. Saunders, Philadelphia

Huvos AG, Heilweil M, Bretsky SS (1985) The pathology of malignant fibrous histiocytoma of bone: a study of 130 patients. Am J Surg Pathol 9:853–871

Inwards CY, Unni KK, Beabout JW, Sim FH (1991) Desmoplastic fibroma of bone. Cancer 68:1978–1983

Ishida T, Dorfman HD (1993) Massive chondroid differentiation in fibrous dysplasia of bone (fibrocartilaginous dysplasia). Am J Surg Pathol 17:924–930

Jaffe HL (1946) Fibrous dysplasia of bone. Bull NY Acad Med 22:588–604

Kempson RL (1966) Ossifying fibroma of the long bones. A light and electron microscopic study. Arch Pathol 82:218–233

Lautenbach E, Dockborn R (1968) Fibröse Kiefererkrankungen. Thieme, Stuttgart

Llombart-Bosch A, Pedro-Olaya A, Lopez-Fernandez A (1974) Non-ossifying fibroma of bone. A histochemical and ultrastructural characterization. Virchows Arch Pathol. Anat 362:13–21

Marks KE, Bauer TW (1989) Fibrous tumors of bone. Orthop Clin North Am 20:377–393

Mau H, Ewerbeck V, Reichardt P et al (1995) Malignant fibrous histiocytoma of bone and soft tissue – two different tumor entities? A retrospective study of 45 cases. Onkologie 18:573–579

McCarthy EF, Matsuno T, Dorfman HD (1979) Malignant fibrous histiocytoma of bone: a study of 35 cases. Hum Pathol 10:57–70

McClure DK, Dahlin DC (1977) Myxoma of bone: report of three cases. Mayo Clin Proc 52:249–253

Marcove RC, Kambolis C, Bullough PG, Jaffe HL (1964) Fibromyxoma of bone: a report of 3 cases. Cancer 17:1209–1213

Meister P, Konrad E, Engert J (1977) Polyostotische fibröse kortikale Defekte (bzw. nicht ossifizierende Knochenfibrome). Arch Orthop Unfall Chir 89:315–318

Michael RH, Dorfman HD (1976) Malignant fibrous histiocytoma associated with bone infarcts. Report of a case. Clin Orthop 118:180–183

Nguyen BD, Lugo-Olivieri CH, McCarthy EF et al (1996) Fibrous dysplasia with secondary aneurysmal bone cyst. Skeletal Radiol 25:88–91

Nilsonne U, Mazabraud A (1974) Les Fibrosarcomes de l'os. Rev Chir Orthop Reparatrice Appar Mot 60:109–122

Park YK, Unni KK, McLeod RA, Pritchard DJ (1993) Osteofibrous dysplasia of the tibia and fibula. Pathology 20:227–233

Phelan JT (1964) Fibrous cortical defects and nonosseous fibroma of bone. Surg Gynec Obstet 119:807–810

Povysil C, Matejovsky Z (1993) Fibro-osseous lesion with calcified spherules (cementifying fibromalike lesion) of the tibia. Ultrastruct Pathol 17:25–34

Reed RJ (1963) Fibrous dysplasia of bone. A review of 25 cases. Arch Pathol 75:480–495

Rodenberg J, Jensen OM, Keller J et al (1996) Fibrous dysplasia of the spine, costae and hemipelvis with sarcomatous transformation. Skeletal Radiol 25:682–684

Ruffoni R (1961) Solitary bone xanthoma. Panminerva Med 3:416–419

Ruggieri P, Sim FH, Bond JR, Unni KK (1994) Malignancies in fibrous dysplasia. Cancer 73:1411–1424

Scaglietti O, Stringa G (1961) Myxoma of bone in childhood. J Bone Joint Surg Am 43:67–80

Selby S (1961) Metaphyseal cortical defects in the tubular bones of growing children. J Bone Joint Surg Am 43:395–400

Soren A (1964) Myxoma in bone. Clin Orthop 37:145–149

Spanier SS (1977) Malignant fibrous histiocytoma of bone. Orthop Clin North Am 8:947–961

Spanier SS, Enneking WF, Enriquez P (1975) Primary malignant fibrous histiocytoma of bone. Cancer 36:2084–2098

Steiner GC (1974) Fibrous cortical defect and nonossifying fibroma of bone. Arch Pathol 97:205–210

Stout AP (1948) Myxoma, the tumor of primitive mesenchyme. Arch Surg 127:706–719

Sweet DE, Vinh TN, Devaney K (1992) Cortical osteofibrous dysplasia of long bone and its relationship to adamantinoma. A clinicopathologic study of 30 cases. Am J Surg Pathol 16:282–290

Taconis WK, Rijssel TG van (1985) Fibrosarcoma of long bones: a study of the significance of areas of malignant fibrous histiocytoma. J Bone Joint Surg Br 67:111–116

Uehlinger E (1940) Osteofibrosis deformans juvenilis (Polyostotische fibröse Dysplasie Jaffe-Lichtenstein). Virchows Arch 306:255–299

Van Horn PE Jr, Dahlin DC, Buckel WH (1963) Fibrous dysplasia. Mayo Clin Proc 38:175–189

Voytek TM, Ro JY, Edeiken J, Ayala AG (1995) Fibrous dysplasia and cemento-ossifying fibroma. A histologic spectrum. Am J Surg Pathol 19:775–781

Zimmer JF, Dahlin DC, Pugh DG, Clagett OT (1956) Fibrous dysplasia of bone: analysis of 15 cases of surgically verified costal fibrous dysplasia. J Thorac Cardiovasc Surg 31:488–496

Yabut SM, Kenan S, Sissons HA, Lewis MM (1988) Malignant transformation of fibrous dysplasia. Clin Orthop 228:281–289

Chapter 11.5: Giant Cell Tumor of Bone (Osteoclastoma)

Adler CP (1973) Knochenzysten. Beitr Pathol Anat 150:103–131

Adler CP (1977) Histogenese und praktische Konsequenzen bei Knochengeschwülsten. Spezielle Pathologie der Knochengeschwülste (Freiburger Chirurgengespräch). Gödecke, Freiburg, pp 10–62

Adler CP (1980) Klassifikation der Knochentumoren und Pathologie der gutartigen und semimalignen Knochentumoren. In: Frommhold W, Gerhardt P (eds) Knochentumoren. Klinisch-radiologisches Seminar, vol X. Thieme, Stuttgart, pp 1–24

Adler CP, Klümper A (1977) Röntgenologische und pathologisch-anatomische Aspekte von Knochentumoren. Radiologe 17:355–392

Adler CP, Uehlinger E (1979) Grenzfälle bei Knochentumoren. Präneoplastische Veränderungen und Geschwülste fraglicher Dignität. Verh Dtsch Ges Pathol 63:352–358

Campanacci M, Giunti A, Olmi R (1975) Giant-cell tumors of bone: a study of 209 cases with long-term follow-up in 130. Ital J Orthop Traumat 1:249–277

Campbell CJ, Bonfiglio M (1973) Aggressiveness and malignancy in giant-cell tumors of bone. In: Price CHG, Ross FGM (eds) Bone – certain aspects of neoplasia. Butterworth, London, pp 15–38

Dahlin DC (1977) Giant-cell tumor of vertebrae above the sacrum. A review of 31 cases. Cancer 39:1350–1356

Dahlin DC, Cupps RE, Johnson EW Jr (1970) Giant-cell tumor: a study of 195 cases. Cancer 25:1061–1070

Dahlin DC, Ghormley RK, Pugh DG (1956) Giant cell tumor of bone: differential diagnosis. Proc Mayo Clin 31:31–42

Edeiken J, Hodes PJ (1963) Giant cell tumors vs. tumors with giant cells. Radiol Clin North Aml:75–100

Fechner RE, Mills SE (1993) Tumors of the bones and joints. AFIP Washington, DC

Goldenberg RR, Campbell CJ, Bonfiglio M (1970) Giant-cell tumor of bone: an analysis of two hundred and eighteen cases. J Bone Joint Surg Am 52:619–663

Gresen AA, Dahlin DC, Peterson LFA, Pane WS (1973) Benign giant cell tumor of bone metastasizing to lung: report of a case. Ann Thorac Surg 16:531–535

Gunterberg B, Kindblom LG, Laurin S (1977) Giant-cell tumor of bone and aneurysmal bone cyst. A correlated histologic and angiographic study. Skeletal Radiol 2:65–74

Jacobs P (1972) The diagnosis of osteoclastoma (giant cell tumor): a radiological and pathological correlation. Br J Radiol 45:121–136

Jaffe HL, Lichtenstein L, Portis RB (1940) Giant cell tumor of bone: its pathologic appearance, grading, supposed variants and treatment. Arch Pathol 30:993–1031

Kossey P, Cervenansky J (1973) Malignant giant-cell tumours of bone. In: Price CHG, Ross FGM (eds) Bone – certain aspects of neoplasia. Butterworth, London

Larsson SE, Lorentzon R, Boquist L (1975) Giant-cell tumor of bone: a demographic, clinical, and histopathological study of all cases recorded in the Swedish Cancer-Registry for the years 1958 through 1968. J Bone Joint Surg Am 57:167–173

Lichtenstein L (1951) Giant-cell tumor of bone. Current status of problems in diagnosis and treatment. J Bone Joint Surg Am 33:143–150

Meister P, Finsterer H (1972) Der Riesenzelltumor des Knochens und seine Problematik. MMW 114:55–60

Mnaymneh WA, Dudley HR, Mnaymneh LG (1964) Excision of giant-cell bone tumor. J Bone Joint Surg Am 46:63–75

Serber W (1987) Radiation treatment of benign diseases. In: Perez CA, Brady LW (eds) Principles and practice of radiation oncology. Lippincott, London, pp 1248–1257

Rosai J (1968) Carcinoma of pancreas simulating giant cell tumor of bone. Electron-microscopic evidence of its acinar cell origin. Cancer 22:333–344

Schajowicz F (1961) Giant-cell tumors of bone (osteoclastoma). A pathological and histochemical study. J Bone Joint Surg Am 43:1–29

Schajowicz F (1993) Histological typing of bone tumours. WHO Geneva, 2nd edn. Springer, Berlin Heidelberg New York

Steiner GC, Ghosh L, Dorfman HD (1972) Utrastructure of giant cell tumor of bone. Hum Path 3:569–586

Sun D, Biesterfeld S, Adler CR Böcking A (1992) Prediction of recurrence in giant cell bone tumors by DNA cytometry. Analyt Quant Cytol 14:341–346

Tornberg; DN, Dick HM, Johnston AD (1975) Multicentric giant-cell tumors in the long bones: a case report. J Bone Joint Surg Am 57:420–422

Uehlinger E (1976) Primary malignancy, secondary malignancy and semimalignancy of bone tumors. In: Grundmann E (ed) Malignant bone tumors. Springer, Berlin Heidelberg New York, pp 109–119

Uehlinger E (1977) Über Erfolge und Mißerfolge in der operativen Behandlung der Knochengeschwülste (Freiburger Chirurgengespräch). Gödecke, Freiburg, pp 63–74

Chapter 11.6: Osteomyelogenous Bone Tumors

Adler CP (1974) Klinische und morphologische Aspekte maligner Knochentumoren. Dtsch Med Wochenschr 99:665–671

Adler CP, Klümper A (1977) Röntgenologische und pathologisch-anatomische Aspekte von Knochentumoren. Radiologe 17:355–392

Adler CP, Böcking A, Kropff M, Leo ETG (1992) DNS-zytophotometrische Untersuchungen zur Prognose von reaktiver Plasmozytose und Plasmozytom. Verh Dtsch Ges Path 76:303

Alexanian R (1976) Plasma cell neoplasm. CA (NY) 26:38

Ambros IM, Ambros PF, Strehl S et al (1991) MIC2 is a specific marker for Ewing's sarcoma and peripheral primitive neuroectodermal tumors. Evidence for a common histogenesis of Ewing's sarcoma and peripheral primitive neuroectodermal tumors from MIC2 expression and specific chromosome aberration. Cancer 67:1886–1893

Angervall L, Enzinger FM (1975) Extraskeletal neoplasm resembling Ewing's sarcoma. Cancer 36:240–251

Arkun R, Memis A, Akalin T et al (1997) Liposarcoma of soft tissue: MRI findings with pathologic correlation. Skeletal Radiol 26:167–172

Bataille R, Sany J (1981) Solitary myeloma: clinical and prognostic features of a review of 114 cases. Cancer 48:845–851

Braunstein EM, White SJ (1980) Non-Hodgkin's lymphoma of bone. Radiology 135:59–63

Carson CP, Ackerman LV, Maltby JD (1955) Plasma cell myeloma. A clinical, pathologic and roentgenologic review of 90 cases. Am J Clin Path 25:849–888

Catto M, Stevens J (1963) Liposarcoma of bone. J Path Bact 86:248–253

Cha S, Schultz E, McHeffey-Atkinson B, Sherr D (1996) Malignant lymphoma involving the patella. Skeletal Radiol 25:783–785

Chan JKC, Ng C, Hui P (1991) Anaplastic large cell Ki-1 lymphoma of bone. Cancer 68:2186–2191

Child PL (1955) Lipoma of the os calcis. Report of a case. Am J Clin Path 25:1050–1052

Chow LTC, Lee KC (1992) Intraosseous lipoma. A clinicopathologic study of nine cases. Am J Surg Pathol 16:401–410

Clayton F, Butler JJ, Ayala AG et al (1990) Non-Hodgkin's lymphoma of bone: pathologic and radiologic features with clinical correlates. Cancer 60:2494–2501

Dahlin DC (1973) Primary malignant lymphoma (reticulum cell sarcoma) of bone. In: Price CHG, Ross FGM (eds) Bone – certain aspects of neoplasia. Davis, Philadelphia, pp 207–215

Dahlin DC, Coventry MB, Scanlon PW (1961) Ewing's sarcoma. A critical analysis of 165 cases. J Bone Joint Surg Am 43:185–192

Dawson EK (1955) Liposarcoma of bone. J Path Bact 70:513–520

Dörken H, Vollmer J (1968) Die Epidemiologie des multiplen Myeloms. Untersuchungen von 149 Fällen. Arch Geschwulstforsch 31:18–38

Edeiken Monroe B, Edeiken J, Kim EE (1990) Radiologic concepts of lymphoma of bone. Radiol Clin North Am 28:841–864

Evans JE (1977) Ewing's tumour: uncommon presentation of an uncommon tumour. Med J Aust 1:590–591

Falk S, Alpert M (1965) The clinical and roentgen aspects of Ewing's sarcoma. Am J Med Sci 250:492–508

Fechner RE, Mills SE (1993) Tumors of the bones and joints. AFIP Washington, DC

Fuchs R, Reisner R, Hellerich U (1995) Multilobulated multiple myeloma – a rare morphological type. Onkologie 18:580–584

Goldman RL (1964) Primary liposarcoma of bone. Report of a case. Am J Clin Path 42:503–508

Güthert H, Wbckel W, Janisch W (1961) Zur Häufigkeit des Plasmozytoms und seiner Ausbreitung im Skelettsystem. MMW 103:1561–1564

Hartman KR, Triche TJ, Kinsella TJ, Miser JS (1991) Prognostic value of histopathology in Ewing's sarcoma: long-term follow-up of distal extremity primary tumors. Cancer 67:163–171

Hillemanns M, McLeod RA, Unni KK (1996) Malignant lymphoma. Skeletal Radiol 25:73–75

Howat AJ, Thomas H, Waters KD, Campbell PE (1987) Malignant lymphoma of bone in children. Cancer 59:335

Hustu HO, Pinkel D (1967) Lymphosarcoma, Hodkin's disease and leukemia in bone. Clin Orthop 52:83–93

Ivins JC, Dahlin DC (1963) Malignant lymphoma (reticulum cell sarcoma) of bone. Proc Mayo Clin 38:375–385

Kauffmann SL, Stout AP (1959) Lipoblastic tumors of children. Cancer 12:912–925

Krepp S (1965) Über ein Knochenhämangio-Lipom. Zentralbl Chir 90:1674–1677

Kropff M, Leo E, Steinfarth G et al (1991) DNA-zytophotometrischer Nachweis von Aneuploidie, erhöhter Proliferation und Kernfläche als frühe Marker prospektiver Malignität bei monoklonaler Gammopathie unklarer Signifikanz (MGUS). Verb Dtsch Ges Pathol 75:480

Kropff M, Leo ETG, Steinfurth G et al (1994) DNS-image cytometry and clinical staging systems in multiple myeloma. Anticancer Res 14:2183–2188

Kyle RA (1975) Multiple myeloma: review of 869 cases. Mayo Clin Proc 50:29–40

Levin MF, Vellet AD, Munk PL, McLean CA (1996) Intraosseous lipoma of the distal femur: MRI appearance. Skeletal Radiol 25:82–84

Lizard-Nacol S, Lizard G, Justrabo E, Turc-Carel C (1989) Immunologic characterization of Ewing's sarcoma using mesenchymal and neural markers. Am J Pathol 135:847–855

Llombart-Bosch A, Blache R (1974) Über die Morphologie und Ultrastruktur des Ewing-Tumors. Verh Dtsch Ges Pathol 58:459–466

Llombart-Bosch A, Contesso G, Henry-Amar M et al (1986) Histopathological predictive factors in Ewing's sarcoma of bone and clinicopathological correlations: a retrospective study of 261 cases. Virchows Arch A 409:627–640

Macintosh DJ, Price CHG, Jeffree GM (1977) Malignant lymphoma (reticulosarcoma) in bone. Clin Oncol 3:287–300

Melamed JW, Martinez S, Hoffman Q (1997) Imaging of primary multifocal osseous lymphoma. Skeletal Radiol 26:35–41

Mendenhall NP, Jones JJ, Kramer BS (1987) The management of primary lymphoma of bone. Radiother Oncol 9:137–145

Meyer JE, Schulz MD (1974) Solitary myeloma of bone: a review of 12 cases. Cancer 34:438–440

Milgram JW (1988) Intraosseous lipomas: a clinicopathologic study of 66 cases. Clin Orthop 231:277–302

Milgram JW (1990) Malignant transformation in bone lipomas. Skeletal Radiol 19:347–352

Moorefield WG Jr, Urbaniak JR, Gonzalvo AAA (1976) Intramedullary lipoma of the distal femur. South Med J (Birmingham, Ala.) 69:1210–1211

Ostrowski ML, Unni KK, Banks PM et al (1986) Malignant lymphoma of bone. Cancer 58:2646–2655

Peloux Y, Thevenot P, Bouffard A (1965) Le lipome intramédullaire osseux. Etude d'un nouveau cas observé au Dahomay. Presse Med 73:2057–2058

Remagen W (1974) Knochentumoren: Diagnostische Probleme – methodische Möglichkeiten. Verh Dtsch Ges Pathol 58:219–235

Retz LD (1961) Primary liposarcoma of bone. Report of a case and review of the literature. J Bone Joint Surg Am 43:123–129

Roessner A, Jürgens H (1993) Neue Aspekte zur Pathologie des Ewing-Sarkoms. Osteologie 2:57–73

Rosen BJ (1975) Multiple myeloma. A clinical review. Med Clin North Am 59:375–386

Salmon SE, Durie BGM (1975) Cellular kinetics in multiple myeloma. A new approach to staging and treatment. Arch Intern Med 135:131–138

Salter M, Sollaccio Rj, Bernreuter WK, Weppelman B (1989) Primary lymphoma of bone: the use of MRI in pretreatment evaluation. Am J Clin Oncol 12:101–105

Salzer M, Gotzmann H (1963) Parostale Lipoma. Bruns' Beitr Klin Chir 206:501–505

Salzer M, Salzer-Kuntschik M (1965) Zur Frage der sogenannten zentralen Knochenlipome. Beitr Pathol Anat 132:365–375

Salzer-Kuntschik M (1973) Zytologisches Verhalten primärer maligner Knochentumoren. Verh Dtsch Ges Pathol 57:280–283

Salzer-Kuntschik M (1974) Zur Beurteilung von Probeentnahmen bei Knochentumoren. Verh Dtsch Ges Pathol 58:235–248

Salzer-Kuntschik M, Wunderlich M (1971) Das Ewing-Sarkom in der Literatur: Kritische Studien zur histomorphologischen Definition und zur Prognose. Arch Orthop Unfall Chir 71:297–306

Schajowicz F (1959) Ewing's sarcoma and reticulum cell sarcoma of bone with special reference to histochemical demonstration of glycogen as an aid to differential diagnosis. J Bone Joint Surg Am 41:349–356

Schmidt D, Hermann C, Jürgens H, Harms D (1991) Malignant peripheral neuroectodermal tumor and its necessary distinction from Ewing's sarcoma: a report from the Kiel Pediatric Tumor Registry. Cancer 68:2251–2259

Schwartz A, Shuster M, Becker SM (1970) Liposarcoma of bone: report of a case and review of the literature. J Bone Joint Surg Am 52:171–177

Sharma SC, Radotra BD (1991) Primary lymphoma of the bones of the foot: management of two cases. Foot Ankle 11:314–316

Sherman RS, Soong KY (1956) Ewing's sarcoma: its roentgen classification and diagnosis. Radiology 66:529–539

Short JH (1977) Malignant lymphoma (reticulum cell sarcoma) of bone. Radiography 43:139–143

Silverman LM, Shklar G (1962) Multiple myeloma: report of a case. Oral Surg 15:301–309

Smith WE, Fienberg R (1957) Intraosseous lipoma of bone. Cancer 10:1151–1152

Stephenson CF, Bridge JA, Sandberg AA (1992) Cytogenetic and pathologic aspects of Ewing's sarcoma and neurodermal tumors. Hum Pathol 23:1270–1277

Stevens AR Jr (1965) Evaluation of multiple myeloma. Arch Intern Med 115:90–93

Sundaram M, Baran G, Merenda. G, McDonald DJ (1990) Myxoid liposarcoma: magnetic resonance imaging appearance with clinical and histologic correlation. Skeletal Radiol 19:359–362

Telles NC, Rabson AS, Pomeroy TC (1978) Ewing's sarcoma: an autopsy study. Cancer 41:2321–2329

Tsuneyoshi M, Yokoyama R, Hashimoto H, Enjoji M (1989) Comparative study of neuroectodermal tumor and Ewing's sarcoma of the bone: histopathologic, immunohistochemical and ultrastructural features. Acta Pathol Jpn 39:573–581

Uehlinger E, Botsztejn C, Schinz HR (1948) Ewingsarkom und Knochenretikulosarkom. Klinik, Diagnose und Differentialdiagnose. Oncologia (Basel) 1:193–245

Unni KK (1996) Dahlin's bone tumors: general aspects and data on 11,087 cases, 5th edn. Lippincott-Raven, Philadelphia

van Valen F, Prior R, Wechsler W et al (1988) Immunzytochemische und biochemische Untersuchungen an einer Ewing-Sarkom-Zellinie: Hinweise für eine neurale in-vitro Differenzierung. Klin Pädiatr 200:267–270

Vincent JM, Ng YY, Norton AJ, Armstrong PA (1992) Primary lymphoma of bone: MRI appearance with pathological correlation. Clin Radiol 45:407–409

White LM, Siegel S, Shin SS et al (1996) Primary lymphoma of the calcaneus. Skeletal Radiol 25:775–778

Whitehouse GH, Griffiths GJ (1976) Roentgenologic aspects of spinal involvement by primary and metastatic Ewing's tumor. J Canad Ass Radiol 27:290–297

Wittig KH, Motsch H (1977) Solitary plasmocytoma. Zentralbl Chir 102:410–415

Chapter 11.7: Vascular Bone Tumors
(and other Bone Tumors)

Abdelwahab IF, Hermann G, Stollman A et al (1989) Giant intraosseous schwannoma. Skeletal Radiol 18:466–469

Adler CP (1990) Adamantinoma of the tibia mimicking osteofibrous dysplasia (Campanacci). Skeletal Radiol 19:55–58

Adler CP, Klümper A (1977) Röntgenologische und pathologisch-anatomische Aspekte von Knochentumoren. Radiologe 17:355–392

Adler CP, Reichelt A (1985) Hemangiosarcoma of bone. Int Orthop 8:273–279

Adler CP, Träger D (1989) Malignes Hämangioperizytom – ein Weichteil- und Knochentumor. Z Orthop 127:611–615

Adler CP, Reinbold WD (1989) Osteodensitometry of vertebral metastases after radiotherapy using quantitative computed tomography. Skeletal Radiol 18:517–521

Agnoli AL, Kirchhoff D, Eggert H (1978) Röntgenologische Befunde beim Hämangiom des Schädels. Radiologe 18:37–41

Alguacil-Garcia A, Alonso A, Pettigrew NM (1984) Osteofibrous dysplasia (ossifying fibroma) of the tibia and fibula and adamantinoma: a case report. Am J Clin Pathol 82:470–474

Anderson WB, Meyers HI (1968) Multicentric chordoma. Report of a case. Cancer 21:126–128

Angervall L, Berlin O, Kindblom LG, Stener B (1980) Primary leiomyosarcoma of bone: a study of five cases. Cancer 46:1270–1279

Aoki J, Tanikawa H, Fujioka F et al (1997) Intaosseous neurilemmoma of the fibula. Skeletal Radiol 26:60–63

Ariel IM, Verdu C (1975) Chordoma: an analysis of 20 cases treated over a 20 year span. J Surg Oncol 7:27–44

Arnemann W, Fiegler C (1962) Über Frakturen in Metastasen. Med Monatschr 16:257–262

Assoun J, Richardi G, Railhac JJ et al (1994) CT and MRI of massive osteolysis of Gorham. J Comp Ass Tomograph 18:981–984

Bach ST (1970) Cervical chordoma. Report of a case and a brief review of the literature. Acta Otolaryngol (Stockh) 69:450–456

Bachman AL, Sproul EE (1955) Correlation of radiographic and autopsy findings in suspected metastases in the spine. Bull N Y Acad Med 31:146–164

Baker LH, Vaitkevicius VK, Figiel SJ (1974) Bone metastasis from adenocarcinoma of the colon. Am J Gatsroent 62:139–144

Barnett LS, Morris JM (1969) Metastases of renal–cell carcinoma simultaneously in a finger and a toe. J Bone Joint Surg Am 51:773–774

Batson OV (1942) The function of the vertebral vein system as a mechanism for the spread of metastases. Am J Roentgenol 48:715–718

Berrettoni BA, Carter JR (1986) Mechanisms of cancer metastasis to bone. J Bone Joint Surg Am 68:308–312

Bjornsson J, Wold LE, Ebersold MJ, Laws ER (1993) Chordoma of the mobile spine. A clinicopathologic analysis of 40 patients. Cancer 71:735–740

Bottles K, Beckstead JH (1984) Enzyme histochemical characterization of chordomas. Am J Surg Pathol 8:443–447

Brewer HB (1975) Osteoblastic bone resorption and the hypercalcemia of cancer. N Engl J Med 291:1081–1082

Brocher JEW (1973) Die Prognose der Wirbelsäulenleiden. Thieme, Stuttgart

Brooks JJ, Trojanowski JQ, Livolsi VA (1989) Chondroid chordoma: a low-grade chondrosarcoma and its differential diagnosis. Curr Top Pathol 80:165–181

Bullock MJ, Bedard YC, Bell RS, Kandel R (1995) Intraosseous malignant peripheral nerve sheath tumor. Report of a case and review of the literature. Arch Pathol Lab Med 119:367–370

Bullough PG, Goodfellow JW (1976) Solitary lymphangioma of bone. A case report. J Bone Joint Surg Am 58:418–419

Bulychova IV, Unni KK, Bertoni F, Beabout JW (1993) Fibrocartilaginous mesenchymoma of bone. Am J Surg Pathol 17:830–836

Bundens WD Jr, Brighton CT (1965) Malignant hemangioendothelioma of bone. Report of two cases and review of the literature. J Bone Joint Surg Am 47:762–772

Burger PC, Makek M, Kleihues P (1986) Tissue polypeptide antigen staining of the chordoma and notochordal remnants. Acta Neuropathol 70:269–272

Burkhardt H, Wepler R, Rommel K (1975) Diagnostik von Knochenmetastasen unter besonderer Berücksichtigung klinisch-chemischer Untersuchungsmethoden. Med Welt 26:1411–1415

Campanacci M, Cenni F, Giunti A (1969) Angectasie, amartomi, e neoplasmi vascolari dello scheletro (angiomi, emangioendotelioma, emangiosarcoma). Chir Organi Mov 58:472–496

Carroll RE, Berman AT (1972) Glomus tumors of the hand. Review of the literature and report of twenty-eight cases. J Bone Joint Surg Am 54:691–703

Charhon SA, Chapuy MC, Delvin EE et al (1983) Histomorphometric analysis of sclerotic bone metastases from prostatic carcinoma with special reference of osteomalacia. Cancer 51:918–924

Choma ND, Biscotti CV, Mehta AC, Lieata AA (1987) Gorham's syndrome: a case report and review of the literature. Am J Med 83:115

Coffin CM, Swanson PE, Wick MR, Dehner LP (1993) Chordoma in childhood and adolescence. A clinicopathologic analysis of 12 cases. Arch Pathol Lab Med 117:927–933

Cohen DM, Dahlin DC, Pugh DG (1962) Fibrous dysplasia associated with adamantinoma of long bones. Cancer 15:515–521

Czerniak B, Rojas-Corona RR, Dorfman HD (1989) Morphologic diversity of long bone adamantinoma and its relationship to osteofibrous dysplasia. Cancer 64:2319–2334

Czitober H (1968) Zur klinischen Pathologie der diffusen Karzinome im Knochenmark und Skelett. Wien Z Inn Med 49:7–17

Dahlin DC, MacCarty CS (1952) Chordoma: a study of fifty-nine cases. Cancer 5:1170–1178

Dahlin DC, Bertoni F, Beabout JW, Campanacci M (1984) Fibrocartilaginous mesenchymoma with low-grade malignancy. Skeletal Radiol 12:263–269

Daroca PJ Jr, Reed RJ, Martin PC (1990) Metastatic amelanotic melanoma simulating giant-cell tumor of bone. Hum Pathol 21:978–980

Davis E, Morgan LR (1974) Hemangioma of bone. Arch Otolaryngol 99:443–445

De La Monte SM, Dorfman HD, Chandra R, Malawer M (1984) Intraosseous schwannoma. Histologic features, ultrastructure, and review of the literature. Hum Pathol 15:551–558

Dick HJ, Senn HJ, Mayr AC, Hünig R (1974) Die Bedeutung von Knochenmarkpunktion und radiologischem Skelettstatus zum Nachweis ossärer Tumormetastasen. Untersuchungen bei 116 Patienten mit soliden Tumoren. Schweiz Med Wochenschr 104:1275–1280

Dominguez R, Washowich TL (1994) Gorham's disease or vanishing bone disease: plain film, CT, and MRI findings of two cases. Pediatr Radiol 24:316–318

Dominok GW, Knoch HG (1982) Knochengeschwülste und geschwulstähnliche Knochenerkrankungen, 3d edn. Fischer, Stuttgart

Dorfman HD, Steiner GC, Jaffe HL (1971) Vascular tumors of bone. Hum Path 2:349–376

Ducatman BS, Scheithauer BW, Dahlin DC (1983) Malignant bone tumors associated with neurofibromatosis. Mayo Clin Proc 58:578–582

Dumont J (1975) Glomus tumour of the fingers. Canad J Surg 18:542–544

Dunbar SF, Rosenberg A, Mankin H et al (1993) Gorham's massive osteolysis: the role of radiation therapy and a review of the literature. Int J Radiat Oncol Biol Phys 26:491–497

Dunlop J (1973) Primary hemangiopericytoma of bone. Report of two cases. J Bone Joint Sing Br 55:854–857

Evans DMD, Samerkin NG (1965) Primary leiomyosarcoma of bone. J Path Bact 90:348–350

Fairbank T (1956) Haemangioma of bone. Practioner 177:707–711

Fechner RE, Mills SE (1993) Tumors of the bones and joints. AFIP Washington, DC

Fornasier VL, Paley D (1983) Leiomyosarcoma in bone. Primary or secondary? Skeletal Radiol 10:147–153

Garcia-Moral CA (1972) Malignant hemangioendothelioma of bone: review of world literature and report of two cases. Clin Orthop 82:70–79

Glauber A, Juhsz J (1962) Das Adamantinom der Tibia. Z Orthop 96:523–527

Gloor F (1963) Das sogenannte Adamantinom der langen Röhrenknochen. Virchows Arch Pathol Anat 336:489

Gold GL, Reefe WE (1963) Carcinoma and metastases to the bones of the hand. J Am Med Assoc 184:237–239

Gordon EJ (1976) Solitary intraosseous neurilemmoma of the tibia: review of intraosseous neurilemmoma and neurofibroma. Clin Orthop 117:271–282

Hardegger F, Simpson LA, Segmilller G (1985) The syndrome of idiopathic osteolysis. Classification, review, and case report. J Bone Joint Surg Br 67:89–93

Hartmann WH, Stewart FW (1962) Hemangioendothelioma of bones. Unusual tumor characterized by indolent course. Cancer 15:846–854

Healey JH, Turnbull ADM, Miedema B, Lane JM (1986) Acrometastases. A study of twenty-nine patients with osseous involvement of the hands and feet. J Bone Joint Surg Am 68:743–746

Heffelfinger MJ, Dahlin DC, MacCarty CS, Beabout JW (1973) Chordomas and cartiliginous tumors at the skull base. Cancer 32:410–420

Heuck F (1978) Röntgen-Morphologie der sekundaren Knochentumoren. Radiologe 18:287–301

Higinbotham NL, Phillips RF, Farr HW, Hustu HO (1967) Chordoma: thirty-five-year study at Memorial Hospital. Cancer 20:1841–1850

Hochstetter AR von, Eberle H, Ruettner JR (1984) Primary leiomyosarcoma of extragnathic bones. Cancer 53:2194

Hübener KH, Klott KJ (1978) Chordoma lumbalis. Fortschr Röntgenstr 128:373–374

Hunt JC, Pugh DG (1961) Skeletal lesions in neurofibromatosis. Radiology 76:1–20

Huvos AG, Marcove RC (1975) Adamantinoma of long bone – a clinicopathological study of fourteen cases with vascular origin suggested. J Bone Joint Surg Am 57:148–154

Ishida T, Dorfman HD, Steiner GC, Norman A (1994) Cystic angiomatosis of bone with sclerotic changes mimicking osteoblastic metastases. Skeletal Radiol 23:247–252

Jaffe HL (1958) Tumors metastatic to the skeleton. In: Jaffe HL (ed) Tumors and tumorous conditions of the bones and joints. Lea & Febiger, Philadelphia, pp 589–618

Jaffe HL (1958) Tumors and tumorous conditions of the bones and joints. Lea & Febiger, Philadelphia, pp 240–255

Jeffrey PB, Biava CG, Davis RL (1995) Chondroid chordoma. A hyalinized chordoma without cartilaginous differentiation. Am J Clin Pathol 103:271–279

Jöbis AC, De Vries GP, Anholdt RR, Sanders GTB (1978) Demonstration of the prostatic origin of metastasis. An immun-histochemical method for formalin-fixed embedded tissue. Cancer 41:1788–1793

Johnston AD (1970) Pathology of metastatic tumors in bone. Clin Orthop 73:8–32

Jundt G, Moll C, Nidecker A, Schilt R, Remagen W (1994) Primary leiomyosarcoma. of bone: report of eight cases. Hum Pathol 25:1205–1212

Jundt G, Remberger K, Roessner A et al (1995) Adamantinoma of long bones. A histopathological and immunohistological study of 23 cases. Pathol Res Pract 191:112–120

Kahn LB, Wood FW, Ackerman IV (1969) Fracture callus associated with benign and malignant bone lesions and mimicking osteosarcoma. Am J Clin Path 52:14–24

Kaiser TE, Pritchard DJ, Unni KK (1984) Clinicopathologic study of sacrococcygeal chordoma. Cancer 53:2574

Keeney GL, Unni KK, Beabout W, Pritchard DJ (1989) Adamantinoma of long bones: a clinicopathologic study of 85 cases. Cancer 64:730–737

Köhler G, Rossner JA, Waldherr R (1974) Zur Struktur und Differentialdiagnose des sog. Tibia-Adamantinomes. Eine licht- und elektronenoptische Untersuchung. Verh Dtsch Ges Pathol 58:454–458

Kühne HH (1967) Über das sogenannte Adamantinom der langen Röhrenknochen. Singuläre Beobachtung als Beitrag zur Differentialdiagnose. Langenbecks Arch Klin Chir 318:161–177

Kulenkampff H-A, Adler CP (1987) Radiologische und pathologische Befunde beim Gorham-Stout-Syndrom (massive Osteolyse). Verh Dtsch Ges Pathol 71:574

Kulenkampff H-A, Richter GM, Adler CP, Haase WE (1989) Massive Osteolyse (Gorham-Stout-Syndrom). Klinik, Diagnostik, Therapie und Prognose. In: Willert H-G, Heuck FHW (eds) Neuere Ergebnisse der Osteologie. Springer, Berlin Heidelberg New York, pp 387–397

Kulenkampff H-A, Richter HG, Haase W, Adler CP (1990) Massive pelvis osteolysis in Gorham-Stout syndrome. Case report and literature review of a rare skeletal disorder. Int Orthop (SICOT) 4:361–366

Kuruvilla G, Steiner GC (1993) Adamantinoma of the tibia in children and adolescents simulating osteofibrous dysplasia of bone. Lab Invest 68:7

Laredo JD, Reizine D, Bard M, Merland JJ (1986) Vertebral hemangiomas: radiologic evaluation. Radiology 161:183–189

Larsson SE, Lorentzon R, Boquist L (1975) Malignant hemangioendothelioma of bone. J Bone Joint Surg Am 57:84–89

Lee S (1986) Hemangioendothelial sarcoma of the sacrum: CT findings. Comput Radiol 10:51–53

Lehrer HZ, Maxfield WS, Nice C (1970) The periosteal sunburst pattern in metastatic bone tumors. Am J Roengenol 108:154–161

Levey DS, MacCormack LM, Sartoris DJ et al (1996) Cystic angiomatosis: case report and review of the literature. Skeletal Radiol 25:287–293

Lidtholm SO, Lindbom A, Spjut HJ (1961) Multiple capillary hemangiomas of the bones of the foot. Acta Pathol Microbiol Scand 51:9–16

Livesley PJ, Saifuddin A, Webb PJ et al (1996) Gorham's disease of the spine. Skeletal Radiol 25:403–405

Lomasney LM, Martinez S, Demos TC, Harrelson JM (1996) Multifocal vascular lesions of bone:imaging characteristics. Skeletal Radiol 25:255–261

MacCarty S, Waugh JM, Coventry MB, O'Sullivan DC (1961) Sacrococcygeal chordomas. Surg Gynec Obstet 113:551–554

Markel SF (1978) Ossifying fibroma of long bone: its distinction from fibrous dysplasia and its association with adamantinoma of long bone. Am J Clin Path 69:91–97

Maruyama N, Kumagai Y, Ishida Y et al (1985) Epitheloid haemangioendothelioma of the bone tissue. Virchows Arch A 407:159–165

McLeod RA, Dahlin DC (1979) Hamartoma (mesenchymoma) on the chest wall in infancy. Radiology 131:657–661

Meis JM, Raymond AK, Evans HL et al (1987) Dedifferentiated chordoma. A clinicopathologic and immunohistological study of three cases. Am J Surg Pathol 11:516–525

Meister P, Konrad E, Gokel JMC, Remberger K (1978) Leiomyosarcoma of the humerus: case report 59. Skeletal Radiol 2:265–267

Mendez AA, Keret D, Robertson W, MacEwen GD (1989) Massive osteolysis of the femur (Gorhams disease): a case report and review of the literature. J Paediatr Orthop 9:604–608

Messmer B, Sinner W (1966) Der vertebrale Metastasierungsweg. Dtsch Med Wochenschr 91:2061–2066

Miller G (1953) Die Knochenveränderungen bei der Neurofibromatose Recklinghausen. Fortschr Röntgenstr 78:669–689

Mikuz G, MydIa F (1974) Elektronenmikroskopische und zytophotometrische Untersuchungen des Chordoms. Verb Dtsch Ges Pathol 58:447–453

Monte SM de la, Dorfman HD, Chandra R, Malawer M (1984) Intraosseous schwannoma: histologic features, ultrastructure, and review of the literature. Hum Pathol 15:551–558

Moon NF (1965) Adamantinoma of the appendicular skeleton. A statistical review of reported cases. Clin Orthop 43:189–213

Mierau GW, Weeks DA (1987) Chondroid chordoma. Ultrastruct Pathol 11:731–737

Mori H, Yamamoto S, Hiramatsu K, Miura T, Moon NF (1984) Adamantinoma of the tibia: ultrastructural and immunohistochemical study with reference to histogenesis. Clin Orthop 190:299–310

Myers JL, Bernreuter W, Dunham W (1990) Melanotic schwannoma. Clinicopathologic, immunohistochemical, and ultrastructural features of a rare primary bone tumor. Am J Clin Pathol 93:424–429

Myers JL, Arocho J, Bernreuter W, Dunham W, Mazur MT (1991) Leiomyosarcoma of bone: a clinicopathologic, immunohistochemical, and ultrastructural study of five cases. Cancer 67:1051–1056

Nathan W (1931) Hypernephrommetastase unter dem Bild eines Elfenbeinwirbels. Röntgenpraxis 3:994–997

O'Connell JX, Kattapuram SV, Mankin HJ et al (1993) Epitheloid hemangioma of bone: a tumor often mistaken for low-grade angiosarcoma or malignant hemangioendothelioma. Am J Surg Pathol 17:610–617

O'Connell JX, Renard LG, Liebsch NJ et al (1994) Base of skull chordoma. A correlative study of histologic and clinical features of 62 cases. Cancer 74:2261–2267

Odell JM, Benjamin DR (1986) Mesenchymal hamartoma of chest wall in infancy: natural history of two cases. Pediatr Pathol 5:135–146

Oeser H, Kunze H (1964) Die Beckenkamm-Metastase. Fortschr Röntgenstr 100:391–394

Overgaard J, Frederikson P, Helmig O, Jensen OM (1971) Primary leiomyosarcoma of bone: a case report. Cancer 39:1664–1671

Pasquel PM, Levet SN, De Leon B (1976) Primary rhabdomyosarcoma of bone: a case report. J Bone Joint Surg 58 Am:1176–1178

Petasnick JP (1977) Metastatic bone disaese. In: Diethelm L, Heuck F, Olsson O et al (eds) Handbuch der medizinischen Radiologie, vol V/6. Springer, Berlin Heidelberg New York, pp 553–602

Rosai J (1969) Adamantinoma of the tibia – electron microscopic evidence of its epithelial origin. Am J Clin Path 51:786–792

Rosenberg AE, Brown GA, Bahn AK, Lee JM (1994) Chondroid chordoma: a variant of chordoma. A morphologic and immunohistochemical study. Am J Clin Pathol 101:36–41

Rosenquist Q, Wolfe DC (1968) Lymphangioma of bone. J Bone Joint Surg Am 50:158–162

Ross JS, Masaryk TJ, Modic MT et al (1987) Vertebral hemangioma: MR imaging. Radiology 165:165–169

Rutherfoord GS, Davies AG (1987) Chordomas – ultrastructure and immunohistochemistry. A report based on the examination of six cases. Histopathology 11:775–787

Sahin-Akyar G, Fitöz S, Akpolat I et al (1997) Primary hemangiopericytoma of bone located in the tibia. Skeletal Radiol 26:47–50

Schinz HR, Botsztejn C (1949) Der elektive Metastasierungstypus bei Malignomen. Oncologia (Basel) 11:65

Schöppe J (1973) Vergleichende histologische Untersuchungen sekundärer Knochentumoren (Skelettmetastasen) und der zugehörigen Primärgeschwülste. Inauguraldissertation, Freiburg

Schubert GE (1980) Pathologie der sekundären malignen Knochentumoren. In: Frommhold W, Gerhardt P (eds) Knochentumoren. Klinisch-radiologisches Seminar, vol X. Thieme, Stuttgart, pp 79–89

Schultz E, Sapan MR, McHeffey-Atkinson B et al (1994) Ancient schwannoma (degenerated neurilemoma). Skeletal Radiol 23:593–595

Sherman RS, Wilner W (1961) The roentgen diagnosis of hemangioma of bone. Am J Roentgenol 86:1146–1159

Shives TC, Beabout JW, Unni KK (1993) Massive osteolysis. Clin Orthop 294:267–276

Siegel MW (1967) Intraosseous glomus tumor. A case report. Am J Orthop 9:68–69

Silverberg SG, Evans RH, Koehler AL (1969) Clinical and pathologic features of initial metastatic presentation of renal cell carcinoma. Cancer 23:1126–1132

Simon MA, Bartucci EJ (1986) The search for the primary tumor in patients with skeletal metastases of unknown origin. Cancer 58:1088–1095

Suh JS, Abenoza P, Galloway H et al (1992) Peripheral (extracranial) nerve tumors: correlation of MR imaging and histologic findings. Radiology 183:341–346

Sundaresan N (1986) Chordomas. Clin Orthop 204:135–142

Sweet DE, Vinh TN, Devaney K (1992) Cortical osteofibrous dysplasia of long bone and its relationship to adamantinoma. A clinicopathologic study of 30 cases. Am J Surg Pathol 16:282–290

Tang JSH, Gold RH, Mirra JM, Eckardt J (1988) Hemangiopericytoma of bone. Cancer 62:848–859

Tatra G, Kratochwil A (1970) Skelettmetastasen des Zervixkarzinoms. Wien Klin Wochenschr 39:676–679

Troncoso A, Ro JY, Grignon Dj et al (1991) Renal cell carcinoma with acrometastasis. Report of two cases and review of the literature. Mod Pathol 4:66–69

Tsuneyoshi M, Dorfman HD, Bauer TW (1986) Epithelioid hemangioendothelioma of bone: a clinicopathologic, ultrastructural, and immunohistochemical study. Am J Surg Pathol 10:754–764

Turk PS, Peters N, Libbey NP, Wanebo HJ (1992) Diagnosis and management of giant intrasacral schwannoma. Cancer 70:2650–2657

Turner J, Jaffe HL (1940) Metastatic neoplasms: a clinical and roentgenological study of involvement of skeleton and lungs. Am J Roentgenol 43:479–492

Ueda Y, Roessner A, Edel G, Böcker W, Wuisman P (1991) Juvenile intracortical adamantinoma of the tibia with predominant osteofibrous dysplasia-like features. Pathol Res Pract 187:1039–1044

Uehlinger E (1957) Das Skelettsynoviom (Adamantinom). In: Schinz HR, Glaumer R, Uehlinger E (eds) Röntgendiagnostik. Ergebnisse 1952–1956. Thieme, Stuttgart

Uehlinger E (1981) Sekundäre Knochengeschwülste. In: Schinz HR, Baensch WE, Frommhold W et al (eds) Lehrbuch der Röntgendiagnostik, vol 11/2, 6th edn. Thieme, Stuttgart, pp 702–758

Uhlmann E, Grossmann A (1940) Von Recklinghausen's neurofibromatosis with bone manifestation. Ann Intern Med 14:225–241

Unni KK, Dahlin DC, Beabout JW, Ivins JC (1974) Adamantinoma of long bone. Cancer 34:1796–1805

Unni KK, Ivins JC, Beabout JW, Dahlin DC (1971) Hemangioma, hemangiopericytoma, and hemangioendothelioma (angiosarcoma) of bone. Cancer 27:1403–1414

Volpe R, Mazabraud A (1983) A clinicopathologic review of 25 cases of chordoma (a pleomorphic and metastasizing neoplasm). Am J Surg Pathol 7:161–170

Walker WP, Landas SK, Bromley CM, Sturm MT (1991) Imimmohistochemical distinction of classic and chondroid chordomas. Mod Pathol 4:661–666

Walther HE (1948) Krebsmetastasen. Schwabe, Basel

Waßmann D, Barthel S, Frege J et al (1996) Das Adamantinom der langen Röhrenknochen – Einzelfalldarstellung und Literaturübersicht. Osteologie 5:221–230

Weiss SW, Dorfman HD (1977) Adamantinoma of long bone: an analysis of nine new cases with emphasis on metastasizing lesions and fibrous dysplasia-like changes. Hum Path 8:141–153

Wenz W, Reichelt A, Rau WS, Adler CP (1984) Lymphographischer Nachweis eines Wirbellymphangioms. Radiologe 24:381–388

Wojno KJ, Hruban RH, Garin-Chesa P, Huvos AG (1992) Chondroid chordomas and low-grade chondrosarcomas of the craniospinal axis. An immunohistochemical analysis of 17 cases. Am J Surg Pathol 16:1144–1152

Wold LE, Sweet RG, Sim FH (1985) Vascular lesions of bone. Pathol Amin 20/2:101–137

Young JM, Funk JF (1954) Incidence of tumor metastasis to the lumbar spine. A comparative study of roentgenographic changes and gross lesions. J Bone Joint Surg Am 35:55–64

Chapter 11.8: Tumor-like Bone Lesions

Adler CP (1973) Knochenzysten. Beitr Pathol Anat 150:103–131

Adler CP (1974) Recidivierende cortikale diaphysäre aneurysmatische Knochenzyste der Tibia. Verb Dtsch Ges Pathol 58:256–258

Adler CP (1980) Granulomatöse Erkrankungen im Knochen. Verb Dtsch Ges Pathol 64:359–365

Adler CP (1980) Klassifikation der Knochentumoren und Pathologie der gutartigen und semimalignen Knochentumoren. In: Frommhold W, Gerhardt P (eds) Knochentumoren. Klinisch-radiologisches Seminar, vol X. Thieme, Stuttgart, pp 1–24

Adler CP (1980) Case report 111: Telangiectatic osteosarcoma of the femur with features of an aggressive aneurysmal bone cyst. Skeletal Radiol 5:56–60

Adler CP (1985) Tumor-like lesions in the femur with cementum-like material. Does a cementoma of long bone exist? Skeletal Radiol 14:26–37

Adler CP (1995) Solid aneurysmal bone cyst with pathologic bone fracture. Skeletal Radiol 24:214–216

Adler CP, Klümper A (1977) Röntgenologische und pathologisch-anatomische Aspekte von Knochentumoren. Radiologe 17:355–392

Adler CP, Schmidt A (1978) Aneurysmale Knochenzyste des Femurs mit malignem Verlauf. Verh Dtsch Ges Pathol 62:487

Alles JU, Schulz A (1986) Immunocytochemical markers (endothelial and histiocytic) and ultrastructure of primary aneurysmal bone cysts. Hum Pathol 17:39–45

Amling M, Werner M, Maas R, Delling G (1994) Calcifizierende solitäre Knochenzysten – morphologische Charakteristika und Differentialdiagnosen zu sklerosierten Knochentumoren. Osteologie 3:62–69

Amling M, Werner M, Posl Met al (1995) Calcifying solitary bone cyst. Morphologic aspects and differential diagnosis of sclerotic bone tumours. Virchows Arch. 426:235–242

Apaydin A, Ozkaynak C, Yilmaz S et al (1996) Aneurysmal bone cyst of metacarpal. Skeletal Radiol 25:76–78

Bauer TW, Dorfman HD (1982) Intraosseous ganglion: a clinicopathologic study of 11 cases. Am J Surg Pathol 6:207–213

Becker F (1940) Plattenepithelzysten der Fingerknochen. Chirurg 12:275–279

Bertoni F, Bacchini P, Capanna R et al (1993) Solid variant of aneurysmal bone cyst. Cancer 71:729–734

Biesecker JI, Marcove RC, Huvos AG, Mike V (1970) Aneurysmal bone cysts: a clinicopathologic study of 66 cases. Cancer 26:615–625

Bone LB, Johnston CE, Bucholz RW (1986) Unicameral bone cysts. J Pediatr Orthop 9:1155–1161

Boseker EH, Bickel WH, Dahlin DC (1968) A clinicopathologic study of simple unicameral bone cyst. Surg Gynec Obstet 127:550–560

Campanacci M, Capanna R, Picci P (1986) Unicameral and aneurysmal bone cysts. Clin Orthop 204:25–36

Capanna R, Van Harn J, Ruggieri P, Biagini R (1986) Epiphyseal involvement in unicameral bone cysts. Skeletal Radiol 15:428–432

Clough JR, Price CHG (1968) Aneurysmal bone cysts. J Bone Joint Surg Br 50:116–127

Cohen J (1960) Simple bone cysts. Studies of cyst fluid in six cases with a theory of pathogenesis. J Bone Joint Surg 42 Am:609–616

Cohen J (1970) Etiology of simple bone cysts. J Bone Joint Surg Am 52:1493–1497

Crane AR, Scarano JJ (1967) Synovial cysts (ganglia) of bone. Report of two cases. J Bone Joint Surg Am 49:355–361

Dabska M, Buraczewski J (1969) Aneurysmal bone cyst: pathology, clinical course and radiologic appearance. Cancer 23:371–389

Diercks RL, Sauter AJM, Mallens WMC (1986) Aneurysmal bone cyst in association with fibrous dysplasia: a case report. J Bone Joint Surg Br 68:144–146

Dominok GW, Crasselt C (1967) Das intraossäre Ganglion. Z Orthop 103:250–253

Donahue F, Turkel DH, Mnaymneh W, Mnaymneh LG (1996) Intraosseous ganglion cyst associated with neuropathy. Skeletal Radiol 25:675–678

Feldman F, Johnston AD (1973) Ganglia of bone: theories, manifestations, and presentations. CRC Crit Rev Clin Radiol Nucl Med 4:303–332

Garceau GJ, Gregory CF (1954) Solitary unicameral bone cyst. J Bone Joint Surg Am 36:267–280

Goldman RL, Friedman NB (1969) Ganglia (synovial cyst) arising in unusual locations. Report of 3 cases, one primary in bone. Clin Orthop 63:184–189

Haims AH, Desai P, Present D, Beltran J (1996) Epiphyseal extension of a unicameral bone cyst. Skletal Radiol 25:51–54

Hicks JD (1956) Synovial cysts in bone. Aust N Z I Surg 26:138–143

Jaffe HL, Lichtenstein L (1942) Solitary unicameral bone cyst. With emphasis on the roentgen picture, the pathologic appearance and the pathogenesis. Arch Surg 44:1004–1025

Kretschmer H (1970) Das Epidermoid der Kalotte. Chir Praxis 14:551–554

Kyriakos M, Hardy D (1991) Malignant transformation of aneurysmal bone cyst, with an analysis of the literature. Cancer 68:1770–1780

Lodwick GS (1958) Juvenile unicameral bone cyst. A roentgen reappraisal. Am J Roentgenol 80:495–504

Makley JT, Joyce MJ (1989) Unicameral bone cyst. Orthop Clin North Am 20:407–415

Martinez V, Sissons HA (1988) Aneurysmal bone cyst: a review of 123 cases including primary lesions and those secondary to other bone pathology. Cancer 61:2291

May DA, McCabe KM, Kuivila TE (1996) Intraosseous ganglion in a 6-year-old boy. Skeletal Radiol 25:67–69

Moore TE, King AR, Travis RC, Allen BC (1989) Post-traumatic cysts and cyst-like lesions of bone. Skeletal Radiol 18:93–97

Mulder JD, Poppe H, Ronnen JR van (1981) Primäre Knochengeschwülste. In: Schinz HR, Baensch WE, Frommhold W et al (eds) Lehrbuch der Röntgendiagnostik, vol II/ 2, 6th edn. Thieme, Stuttgart, pp 529–689

Neer CS, Francis KC, Marcove RC et al (1966) Treatment of unicameral bone cyst. A follow-up study of one hundred seventy-five cases. J Bone Joint Surg Am 48:731–745

Poper TL, Fechner RE, Keats TE (1989) Intra-osseous ganglion. Report of four cases and review of the literature. Skeletal Radiol 18:185–187

Roth SI (1964) Squamous cysts involving the skull and distal phalanges. J Bone Joint Surg Am 46:1442–1450

Samerkin NG, Mott MG, Roylance J (1983) An unusual intraosseous lesion with fibroblastic, osteoclastic, osteoblastic, aneurysmal and fibromyxoid elements. Solid variant of aneurysmal bone cyst. Cancer 51:2278–2286

Schoedel K, Shankman S, Desai P (1996) Intracortical and subperiosteal aneurysmal bone cysts: a report of three cases. Skeletal Radiol 25:455–459

Sigmund G, Vinee P, Dosch JC et al (1991) MRT der aneurysmalen Knochenzyste. Fortschr Röntgenstr 155:289–293

Skandalakis JE, Godeoin JT, Mabon RF (1958) Epidermoid cyst in the skull. A report of four cases and review of the literature. Surgery 43:990–1001

Struhl S, Edelson C, Pritzker H, Seimon LP, Dorfman HD (1989) Solitary (unicameral) bone cyst: the fallen fragment sign revisited. Skeletal Radiol 18:261–265

Tam W, Resnick D, Haghighi P, Vaughan L (1996) Intraosseous ganglion of the patella. Skeletal Radiol 25:588–591

Tillmann B, Dahlin DC, Lipscomb PR, Stewart JR (1968) Aneurysmal bone cyst – an analysis of ninety-five cases. Mayo Clin Proc 43:478–495

Vergel de Dios AM, Bone JR et al (1992) Aneurysmal bone cyst: a clinicopathologic study of 238 cases. Cancer 69:2921–2931

Chapter 12
Degenerative Joint Diseases

Adler CP (1979) Hüftsgelenkserkrankungen aus radiologischer und pathologisch-anatomischer Sicht. Röntgenpraxis 32:29–43

Adler CP (1989) Pathologie der Wirbelsäulenerkrankungen. Radiologe 29:153–158

Adler CP (1992) Degenerative Gelenkerkrankungen. In: Thomas C (ed) Histopathologie, 11th edn. Schattauer, Stuttgart

Aegerter E, Kirkpatrick A Jr (1968) Orthopedic diseases. Saunders, Philadelphia

Andreesen R, Schramm W (1975) Meniskusschäden als Berufskrankheit. MMW 117:973–976

Aufdermaur M (1971) Die Bedeutung der histologischen Untersuchung des Kniegelenksmeniskus. Schweiz Med Wochenschr 101:1405–1412, 1441–1445

Aufdermaur M (1975) Meniskus. In: Büchner F, Grundmann E (eds) Spezielle Pathologie, 5th edn, vol 11. Urban & Schwarzenberg, Munich, pp 391

Aufdermaur M (1975) Bewegungsapparat. In: Büchner F, Grundmann E (eds) Spezielle Pathologie, vol IL Urban & Schwarzenberg, Munich

Beneke G (1971) Pathologie der Arthrose. In: Mathies H (ed) Arthrosen. Aktuelle Rheumaprobleme. Banaschewski, Munich (Gräfelfing)

Beneke G (1975) Störungen der Gelenkfunktion. In: Sandritter W, Beneke G (eds) Allgemeine Pathologie. Schattauer, Stuttgart, pp 700–725

Bürkle de la Camp H (1957) Meniskusverletzungen und Meniskusschaden. Wien Med Wochenschr 107:896–901

Ceelen W (1941) Über histologische Meniskusbefunde nach Unfallverletzungen. Zentralbl Chir 68:1491–1498

Ceelen W (1953) Zur Meniskuspathologie. Ärztl Wochenschr 8:337–338

Chapchal G (1966) Die Bedeutung der Fehlbelastung in der Genese der Arthrosen. In: Belart W (ed) Ursachen rheumatischer Krankheiten. Rheumatismus in Forschung und Praxis, vol III. Huber, Bern

Dettmer N (1968) Einige Aspekte zum Problem der Arthrose. Z Rheumaforsch 27:356–363

Diiasi W (1965) Zur pathologisch-anatomischen Burteilung von Meniskusschäden. In: Mauerer G (ed) Chirurgie im Fortschritt. Enke, Stuttgart

Dihlmann W (1964) Über ein besonderes Coxarthrosezeichen (Psuedofrakturlinie) im Röntgenbild. Fortschr Röntgenstr 100:383–388

Dihlmann W (1979) Degenerative Gelenkerkrankungen. In: Schinz HR, Baensch WE, Frommhold W et al (eds) Lehrbuch der Röntgendiagnostik, vol II/1, 6th edn. Thieme, Stuttgart

Edeiken J (1976) Radiologic diagnosis of joint diseases. In: Ackerman LV, Spjut HJ, Abell MR (eds) Bones and joints. Williams & Wilkins, Baltimore, pp 98–109

Egner E (1978) Meniskusdegeneration – Faserarchitektur und mechanische Festigkeit. Verh Dtsch Ges Pathol 62:483

Fehr P (1946) Die histologische Untersuchung des verletzten Meniskus nach topographischen Gesichtspunkten. Z Unfallmed Berufskr 39:5–32

Francillon MR (1957) Zur Orthopädie der Coxarthrose. Z Rheumaforsch 16:305–335

Glasgow MM, Allen PW, Blakeway C (1993) Arthroscopic treatment of cysts of the lateral meniscus. J Bone Joint Surg Br 75:299–302

Husten K (1952) Die Auswertung des geweblichen Befundes beim Meniskusschaden des Knies. Verh Dtsch Ges Pathol 35:208–215

Jaffe HL (1972) Metabolic, degenerative, and inflammatory diseases of bones and joints. Urban & Schwarzenberg, Munich

Könn G (1971) Meniskusschäden – Morphologie und Beurteilung. Folia traumatologica (Geigy) 2:9–16

Könn G, Oellig W-P (1980) Zur Morphologie und Beurteilung der Veränderungen an den Kniegelenksmenisken. Pathologe 1:206–213

Könn G, Rüther M (1976) Zur pathologischen Anatomie und Beurteilung der Meniskusschäden. H Unfallheilk 128:7–13

Krompecher S (1958) Die qualitative Adaptation der Gewebe. Z Mikr Anat Forsch 64:71–98

Lang FJ, Thurner J (1962) Erkrankungen der Gelenke. In: Kaufmann E (ed) Lehrbuch der Speziellen Pathologischen Anatomie, vol II/4. De Gruyter, Berlin

Maatz R (1979) Gelenkschäden. In: Schinz HR, Baensch WE, Frommhold W et al (eds) Lehrbuch der Röntgendiagnostik, vol 11/1, 6th edn. Thieme, Stuttgart, pp 435–491

Merkel KHH (1978) Struktur und Alterungsvorgänge der Oberfläche menschlicher Menisci. Eine kombinierte elektronenoptische Untersuchung mit dem Transmissions- und Rasterelektronenmikroskop (TEM, REM). Verh Dtsch Ges Pathol 62:482

Merker HJ (1975) Das Knorpelgewebe. In: Ferner H, Staubesand HJ (eds) Lehrbuch der Anatomie des Menschen. Urban & Schwarzenberg, Munich, pp 131–140

Moor W (1984) Gelenkkrankheiten. Thieme, Stuttgart

Ott VR (1953) Über die Spondylosis hyperostotica. Schweiz Med Wochenschr 83:790–799

Ott VR, Wurm H (1957) Spondylitis ankylopoetica (Morbus Strümpell-Marie-Bechterew), 2nd edn. Steinkopff, Darmstadt

Pauwels F (1973) Atlas zur Biomechanik der gesunden und kranken Hüfte. Prinzipien, Technik und Resultate einer kausalen Therapie. Springer, Berlin Heidelberg New York

Riede UN (1976) Die Rolle der Lysosomen bei Erkrankungen des Bindegewebes. Verh Dtsch Ges Pathol 60:133

Riede UN (1981) Störungen der Gelenkfunktion. In: Sandritter W (ed) Allgemeine Pathologie, 2nd edn. Schattauer, Stuttgart, pp 740–752

Riede UN, Schweizer W, Marti J, Willenegger H (1973) Gelenkmechanische Untersuchungen zum Problem der posttraumatischen Arthrosen im oberen Sprunggelenk. 3. Funktionell-morphometrische Analyse des Gelenkknorpels. Langenbecks Arch Chir 333:91–107

Romanini L, Calvisi V, Collodel M, Masciocchi C (1988) Cystic degeneration of the lateral meniscus. Pathogenesis and diagnosis approach. Ital J Orthop Traumatol 14:493–500

Rüttner JR, Spycher MA, Lothe K (1971) Pathomorphology of human osteoarthrosis. In: Lindner J, Rüttner JR, Miescher PA et al (eds) Arthritis – Arthrose. Experimentelle und klinische Grundlagenforschung. Huber, Bern, pp 193–202

Schallock G (1939) Untersuchungen zur Morphologie der Kniegelenksmenisci anhand von Messungen und histologischen Befunden. Virchows Arch Pathol Aanat 304:559–590

Sokoloff L (1971) Some aspects of the aging of cartilage. In: Lindner J, Rüttner JR, Miescher PA et al (eds) Arthritis – Arthrose. Experimentelle und klinische Grundlagenforschung. Huber, Bern, pp 462–466

Springorum PW (1960) Anamnese und Befunde bei Meniskusläsionen. Monatsschr Unfallheilk 63:201–206

Springorum PW (1968) Berufliche Meniskusschäden außerhalb des Bergbaues. Monatsschr Unfallheilk 71:288

Teitelbaum SL, Bullough PG (1979) The pathophysiology of bone and joint disease. Am J Pathol 96:283–353

Thurner J (1971) Altersveränderungen des Knorpels und Arthrose. In: Lindner J, Rüttner IR, Miescher PA et al (eds) Arthritis – Arthrose. Experimentelle und klinische Grundlagenforschung. Huber, Bern, pp 470–475

Wirth W (1979) Arthrographie. In: Schinz HR, Baensch WE, Frommhold W et al (eds) Lehrbuch der Röntgendiagnostik, vol II/l:, 6th edn. Thieme, Stuttgart, p 492

Zippel H (1964) Meniskusschäden und Meniskusverletzungen. Arch Orthop Unfall Chir 56:236–247

Chapter 13
Inflammatory Joint Diseases

Adler CP (1979) Hüftgelenkserkrankungen aus radiologischer und pathologisch-anatomischer Sicht. Röntgenpraxis 32:29–43

Adler CP (1985) Spondylitis – Spondylodiscitis. Pathologisch-anatomische Morphologie und diagnostische Probleme. Radiologe 25:291–298

Adler CP (1989) Pathologie der Wirbelsäulenerkrankungen. Radiologe 29:153–158

Adler CP (1992) Knochen – Gelenke. In: Thomas C (ed) Histopathologie, 11th edn. Schattauer, Stuttgart, pp 190–314

Dendrade JR, Brennan JC (1964) The morphology of the rheumatoid bone erosion. Arthritis Rheum 7:287

Aufdermaur M (1970) Die Pathogenese der Synchondrose bei der Spondylitis ankylopoetica. Dtsch Med Wochenschr 95:110–112

Aufdermaur M (1972) Die Synovialis bei der progredienten chronischen Polyarthritis. Dtsch Med Wochenschr 97:448–453

Aufdermaur M (1975) Bewegungsapparat. In: Büchner F, Grundmann E (eds) Spezielle Pathologie, vol 11, 5th edn. Urban & Schwarzenberg, Munich

Avila R, Pugh DG, Slocumb CH, Winkelmann RK (1960) Psoriatic arthritis: a roentgenologic study. Radiology 75:691–702

Bartley O, Chidekel N (1966) Roentgenologic changes in postoperative septic osteoarthritis of the hip. Acta Radiol Diagn 4:113–122

Bäumer A (1966) LE-Zellen und Sjögren-Zellen bei Arthropathien mit und ohne begleitendes Sjögren-Syndrom. Z Rheumaforsch 25:330–335

Behrend T, Hartmann F, Deicher H (1962) Über die Notwendigkeit einer Unterscheidung von primär und sekundär chronischer Polyarthritis. Dtsch Med Wochenschr 87:944–953

Berens DL, Lockie LM, Lin RK, Norcross BM (1964) Roentgen changes in early rheumatoid arthritis. Radiology 82:645–654

Bland JH, Phillips CA (1972) Etiology and pathogenesis of rheumatoid arthritis and related multisystem diseases. Semin Arthritis Rheum 1:339–359

Böni A (1970) Die progredient chronische Polyarthritis. In: Schoen R, Böni A, Miehlke K (eds) Klinik der rheumatischen Erkrankungen. Springer, Berlin Heidelberg New York, p 139

Brocher JEW (1973) Die Prognose der Wirbelsäulenleiden. Thieme, Stuttgart

Burkhardt R (1970) Farbatlas der klinischen Histopathologie von Knochenmark und Knochen. Springer, Berlin Heidelberg New York

Butenandt O, Knorr D, Stoeber E (1962) Die Ursache der Wachstumshemmung bei der rheumatoiden Arthritis (primär-chronischen Polyarthritis) im Kindesalter. Z Rheumaforsch 21:280–297

Bywaters EGL, Ansell B (1970) The rarer arthritic syndromes. In: Copeman WSC (ed) Textbook of the rheumatic diseases, 4th edn. Livingstone, Edinburgh, pp 524–554

Cawley MID (1972) Destructive lesions of vertebral bodies in ankylosing spondylitis. Ann Rheum Dis 31:345–358

Cole BC, Ward JR, Smith CB (1973) Studies on the infectious etiology of rheumatoid arthritis. Arthritis Rheum 16:191–198

Cramblett HG (1956) Juvenile rheumatoid arthritis. A review of the literature. Clin Proc Child Hosp (Wash) 12:98–114

Cruickshank B (1959) Lesions of joints and tendon sheaths in systemic lupus erythematosus. Ann Rheum Dis 18:111–119

Cruickshank B (1971) Pathology of ankylosing spondylitis. Clin Orthop 74:43–58

Dihlmann W (1962) Die Diagnostik des sehr frühen Morbus Bechterew. Fortschr Röntgenstr 97:716–733

Dihlmann W (1965) Die Veränderungen an den Extremitengelenken beim Morbus Bechterew (Diagnose, Prognose, Problematik). Fortschr Röntgenstr 102:680–689

Dihlmann W (1968) Spondylitis ankylopoetica – die Bechterewsche Krankheit. Thieme, Stuttgart

Dihlmann W (1968) Ein röntgenologisches Frühzeichen der Arthritis. Der Schwund der subchondralen Grenzlamelle. Z Rheumaforsch 27:129–132

Dihlmann W, Cen M (1969) Die ankylosierende dysostotische Arthritis. Fortschr Röntgenstr 110:246–248

Dihlmann W (1970) Zwei Aspekte der röntgenologischen Differentialdiagnose bei der Spondylarthritis ankylopoetica. Therapiewoche 20:789–794

Dihlmann W (1979) Entzündliche Gelenkerkrankungen. In: Schinz HR, Baensch WE, Frommhold W et al (eds) Lehrbuch der Röntgendiagnostik, vol II/1, 6th edn. Thieme, Stuttgart, p 655

Dorfman HD (1976) Rheumatoid and related arthritides. In: Ackerman LV, Spjut HJ, Abell MR (eds) Bones and joints. Williams & Wilkins, Baltimore, pp 130–145

Edeiken J (1976) Radiologic diagnosis of joint diseases. In: Ackerman LV, Spjut HJ, Abell MR (eds) Bones and joints. Williams & Wilkins, Baltimore, pp 98–109

Ehrlich GE (1972) Inflammatory osteoarthritis. 1. The clinical syndrome. J Chron Dis 25:317–328

Fassbender HG (1966) Pathologie des entzündlichen Rheumatismus. In: Bleat W (ed) Ursachen rheumatischer Krankheiten. Rheumatismus in Forschung und Praxis, vol 3. Huber, Bern, pp 9–15

Fehr K (1972) Pathogenese der progredienten chronischen Polyarthritis. Huber, Bern

Forestier J, Jacqueline F, Rotes-Querol J (1956) Ankylosing Spondylitis. Thomas, Springfield, Ill.

Freislederer W (1973) Rheumatische Erkrankungen beim Kind und Jugendlichen. Mkurse Arztl Fortbild 23:279–284

Gerber N, Ambrosini GC, Böni A et al (1977) Spondylitis ankylosans (Bechterew) und Gewebsantigene HLA-B 27. 1. Diagnostische Aussagekraft der HLA-Typisierung. Z Rheumatol 36:29–223

Golding FC (1936) Spondylitis ankylopoetica. Br J Surg 23:484–500

Green N, Osmer JC (1968) Small bone changes secondary to systemic lupus erythematosus. Radiology 90:118–120

Guest CM, Jacobson HG (1951) Pelvic and extra-pelvic osteopathy in rheumatoid spondylitis. Am J Roentgenol 65:760–768

Gumpel JM, Johns CJ, Schulman LE (1967) The joint disease in sarcoidosis. Ann Rheum Dis 26:194–205

Harris ED Jr (1990) Rheumatoid arthritis: pathophysiology and implications for therapy. N Engl J Med 322:1277

Hard W (1967) Moderne Vorstellungen zur Pathogenese der primär chronischen Polyarthritis. Med Welt 18:15–18

Hartmann F (1965) Differenzierung der chronischen Polyarthritis. Z Rheumaforsch 24:161–179

Hartmann F, Rohde J, Schmidt A (1969) Aktivitätsdiagnostik bei der primär-chronischen Polyarthritis. Z Rheumaforsch 28:263–270

Hegglin R (1959) Lupus erythematosus visceralis. Verb Dtsch Ges Inn Med 65:91–101

Hegglin R (1961) Die visceralen Erscheinungen der Kollagenosen. Z Rheumaforsch 20:99–114

Henssge R, Boehme A, Miller A (1970) Herzbeteiligung bei der Spondylitis ankylopoetica. Dtsch Gesundh Wes 25:391–393

Imai Y, Sato T, Yamakawa M et al. (1989) A morphological and immunohistochemical study of lymphoid germinal centers in synovial and lymph node tissues from rheumatoid arthritis patients with special reference to complement components and their receptors. Acta Pathol Jpn 39:127–134

Jaffe HL (1972) Inflammatory arthritis of undetermined origin. In: Jaffe HL (ed) Metabolic, degenerative, and inflammatory diseases of bones and joints. Lea & Febiger, Philadelphia, pp 779–846

Jesserer H (1971) Knochenkrankheiten. Urban & Schwarzenberg, Munich

Kaplan H (1963) Sarcoid arthritis: a review. Arch Intern Med 112:924–935

Kölle G (1969) Verlaufsformen des kindlichen Rheumatismus. Therapiewoche 19:240–243

Kölle G (1971) Rheumadiagnostik im Kindesalter. Diagnostik 4:7–11

Lang FJ (1962) Zur Morphologie der chronisch-rheumatoiden Polyarthritis. MMW 104:1670–1674

Leventhal GH, Dorfman HD (1974) Aseptic necrosis of bone in systemic lupus erythemadosus. Semin Arthritis Rheum 4:73–93

Martel W, Page JW (1960) Cervical vertebral erosions and subluxations in rheumatoid arthritis and ankylosing spondylitis. Arthritis Rheum 3:546–556

Martel W, Holt JF, Cassidy JT (1962) Roentgenologic manifestations of juvenile rheumatoid arthritis. Am J Roentgenol 88:400–423

Mason RM (1970) Ankylosing spondylitis. In: Copeman WSC (ed) Textbook of the rheumatic diseases, 4th edn. S Livingstone, Edinburgh, pp 344–365

Mason RM, Murray RS, Oates JK, Young AC (1959) Spondylitis ankylopoetica und Reitersche Krankheit. Z Rheumaforsch 18:233–241

Mathies H (1969) Die sog. symptomatischen Arthritiden. Therapiewoche 19:237

Matzen PF (1957) Entzündungen der Gelenke. In: Hohmann SG, Hackenbroch M, Lindemann K (eds) Handbuch der Orthopädie, vol 1. Thieme, Stuttgart

Middlemiss JH (1956) Ankylosing spondylitis. J Fac Radiol 7:155–166

Miehlke K (1961) Die Rheumafibel. Springer, Berlin Göttingen Heidelberg

Murray RO, Jacobson FIG (1977) The radiology of skeletal disorders, 2nd edn. Churchill Livingstone, Edinburgh

Norgaard F (1965) Earliest roentgenological changes in polyarthritis of the rheumatoid type: rheumatoid arthritis. Radiology 84:325–329

Norgaard F (1969) Earliest Roentgen changes in poylarthritis of the rheumatoid type: continued investigations. Radiology 92:299–303

O'Connell DJ, Bennett RM (1977) Mixed connective tissue disease – clinical and radiological aspects of 20 cases. Br J Radiol 50:620–625

Pauwels F (1973) Atlas zur Biomechanik der gesunden und kranken Hüfte. Prinzipien, Technik und Resultate einer kausalen Therapie. Springer, Berlin Heidelberg New York

Peter E, Schuler B, Dihlmann W (1964) Veränderungen der Wirbeldornfortsätze bei Arthritis mutilans. Dtsch Med Wochenschr 89:1990–1993

Reichmann S (1967) Roentgenologic soft tissue appearances in hip joint disease. Acta Radiol Diagn 6:167–176

Revell PA (1987) The synovial biopsy. In: Anthony PP, MacSween RNM (eds) Recent advances in histopathology, vol 13. Churchill Livingstone, Edinburgh

Riede UN, Schweizer G, Marti J, Willenegger H (1973) Gelenkmechanische Untersuchungen zum Problem der posttraumatischen Arthrosen im oberen Sprunggelenk. 3. Funktionell-morphometrische Analyse des Gelenkknorpels. Langenbecks Arch Chir 333:91–107

Riede UN, Adler CP (1975) Funktionelle morphometrische Analyse des alternden Gelenkknorpels. Verh Dtsch Ges Pathol 59:313–317

Romanus R, Yden S (1955) Pelvo-Spondylitis ossifians. Munksgaard, Kopenhagen, p 104

Rutishauser E, Jacqueline F (1959) Die rheumatischen Koxitiden. Eine pathologisch-anatomische und röntgenologische Studie. Geigy, Basel

Schacherl M (1969) Röntgenologische Differentialdiagnose rheumatischer Erkrankungen. Therapiewoche 19:307-314

Schaller J, Wedgwood RJ (1972) Juvenile rheumatoid arthritis: A review. Pediatrics 50:940-953

Schattenkirchner M (1969) Der chronische Streptokokkenrheumatismus. Therapiewoche 19:238-239

Schilling F (1968) Das klinische Bild der Spondylitis ankylopoetica. Med Welt 19:2334-2344

Schilling F (1969) Differentialdiagnose der Spondylitis ankylopoetica: Spondylitis psoriatica, chronisches Reiter-Syndrom und Spondylosis hyperostotica. Therapiewoche 19:249-260

Schilling F, Schacherl M, Rosenberg R (1969) Die juvenile Spondylitis ankylopoetica. Dtsch Med Wochenschr 94:473-481

Schilling F, Schacherl M, Bopp A, Gamp A, Haas JP (1963) Veränderungen der Halswirbelsäule (Spondylitis cervicalis) bei der chronischen Polyarthritis und bei der Spondylitis ankylopetica. Radiologe 3:483-501

Schmorl G, Junghanns H (1968) Die gesunde und die kranke Wirbelsäule in Röntgenbild und Klinik, 5th edn. Thieme, Stuttgart

Schoen R (1959) Die primär chronische Polyarthritis. Verh Dtsch Ges Inn Med 65:54-108

Sokoloff L (1976) Osteoarthritis. In: Ackerman LV, Spjut H1, Abell MR (eds) Bones and joints (Int Acad Pathol 17). Williams & Wilkins, pp 110-129

Sorenson KH, Christensen HE (1973) Local amyloid formation in the hip joint capsule in osteoarthritis. Acta Orthop Scand 44:460-466

Streda A, Pazderka V (1966) Vergleichende röntgenologische und anatomische Untersuchungen der Knochen und Gelenkssymptome bei der primär chronischen Polyarthritis. Radiologe 6:40-50

Thurner J (1960) Die chronisch-rheumatoide Polyarthritis und ihre Stellung im Rahmen der rheumatisch genannten Erkrankungen. Z Rheumaforsch 19:373-400

Uehlinger E (1971) Bone changes in rheumatoid arthritis and their pathogenesis. In: Müller W, Harwerth HG, Fehr K (eds) Rheumatoid arthritis. Pathogenetic mechanisms and consequences in therapeutics. Academic Press, New York

Vignon E, Arlot M, Meunier P, Vignon G (1974) Quantitative histological changes in osteoarthritic hip cartilage. Morphometric analysis of 29 osteoarthritic and 26 normal human femoral heads. Clin Orthop 103:269-278

Wagenhäuser FJ (1968) Klinik der progredient chronischen Polyarthritis des Erwachsenen. Med Welt 19:2323-2329

Wagenhäuser FJ (1973) Die klinische Differentialdiagnostik zwischen Arthrose und chronischer Polyarthritis. Schweiz Rdsch Med 62:272-281

Wagenhäuser FJ (1969) Die Rheumamorbidität. Huber, Bern

Wilkes RM, Simsarian JP, Hopps HE et al (1973) Virologic studies on rheumatoid arthritis. Arthritis Rheum 16:446-454

Zvaifer NJ (1995) Rheumatoid arthritis. The multiple pathways to chronic synovitis. Lab Invest 73:307-310

Chapter 14
Tumorous Joint Diseases

Ackerman LV, Rosai J (1974) Surgical pathology, 5th edn. Mosby, St. Louis, p 1084

Andel JG von (1972) Synovial sarcoma – a review and analysis of treated cases. Radiol Clin Biol (Basel) 419:145

Ballard R, Weiland LH (1972) Synovial chondromatosis of the temporo-mandibular joint. Cancer 30:791-795

Bertoni F, Unni KK, Beabout JW, Sim FH (1991) Chondrosarcomas of the synovium. Cancer 67:155-162

Blankestijn J, Panders AK, Vermey A, Scherpbier AJ (1985) Synovial chondromatosis of the temporo-mandibular joint: report of three cases and a review of the literature. Cancer 55:479-485

Breimer CA, Freiberger RH (1958) Bone lesions associated with villonodular synovitis. Am J Roentgenol 79:618

Cade S (1962) Synovial sarcoma. J Roy Coll Surg Edinb 8:1-51

Cadman NL, Soule EH, Kelly PJ (1965) Synovial sarcoma. An analysis of 134 tumors. Cancer 18:613-627

Chung SMK, Janes JM (1965) Diffuse pigmented villonodular synovitis of the hip joint. Review of the literature and report of four cases. J Bone Joint Surg Am 47:293

Dorwart RH, Genant HK, Johnston WH, Morris JM (1984) Pigmented villonodular synovitis of synovial joints: clinical, pathologic, and radiologic features. Am J Roentgenol 143:886-888

Dunn AW, Whisler JH (1973) Synovial chondromatosis of the knee with associated extra-capsular chondromas. J Bone Joint Surg Am 55:1747-1748

Eisenberg KS, Johnston JO (1972) Synovial chondromatosis of the hip joint presenting as an intrapelvic mass; a case report. J Bone Joint Surg Am 54:176-178

Enzinger F, Lattes R, Torloni H (1969) Histological typing of soft tissue tumors. WHO, Geneva

Fechner RE (1976) Neoplasms and neoplasm-like lesions of the synovium. In: Ackerman LV, Spjut HJ, Abell MR (eds) Bones and joints (Int Acad Pathol Monogr 17). Williams & Wilkins, Philadelphia, pp 157-186 (chap 11)

Fechner RE, Mills SE (1993) Tumors of the bones and joints. AFIP, Washington, DC

Fraire AE, Fechner RE (1972) Intraarticular localized nodular synovitis of the knee. Arch Pathol 93:473-476

Friedman M, Schwartz EE (1957) Irradiation therapy of pigmented villonodular synovitis. Bul Hosp Joint Dis (NY) 28:19-32

Gabbiani G, Kay GI, Lattes R, Majno G (1971) Synovial sarcoma: electron microscopic study of a typical case. Cancer 28:1031-1039

Granowitz SP, Mankin HJ (1967) Localized pigmented villonodular synovitis of the knee. J Bone Joint Surg Am 49:122-128

Greenfield MM, Wallace KM (1950) Pigmented villonodular synovitis. Radiology 54:350-356

Hajdu SI (1979) Pathology of soft tissue tumors. Lea & Febiger, Philadelphia, pp 183-198

Hale JE, Calder IM (1970) Synovial sarcoma of abdominal wall. Br J Cancer 24:471-474

Jaffe HL (1958) Tumors and tumorous conditions of the bones and joints. Lea & Febiger, Philadelphia, pp 532-545

Jeffreys TE (1967) Synovial chondromatosis. J Bone Joint Surg Br 49:530-534

Koivuniemi A, Nickels J (1978) Synovial sarcoma diagnosed by fine-needle aspiration biopsy. Acta Cytol 22:515–518

Lee SM, Hajdu SI, Exelby PR (1974) Synovial sarcomas in children. Surg Gynec Obstet 138:701–704

Lewis MM, Marshall JL, Mirra JM (1974) Synovial chondromatosis of the thumb: a case report and review of the literature. J Bone Joint Surg Am 56:180–183

Lewis RW (1947) Roentgen diagnosis of pigmented villonodular synovitis and synovial sarcoma of the knee joint. Radiology 49:26–38

Lichtenstein L (1955) Tumors of synovial joints, bursae, and tendon sheaths. Cancer 8:816–830

Mackenzie DH (1966) Synovial sarcoma: a review of 58 cases. Cancer 19:169–180

Mackenzie DH (1977) Monophasic synovial sarcoma – a histological entity? Histopathology 1:151–157

McMaster PE (1960) Pigmented villonodular synovitis with invasion of bone. Report of six cases. J Bone Joint Surg Am 42:1170–1183

Massarelli G, Tanda F, Salis B (1978) Synovial sarcoma of the soft palate: report of a case. Hum Path 9:341–345

Murphy AF, Wilson JN (1958) Tenosynovial osteochondroma in the hand. J Bone Joint Surg Am 40:1236–1240

Murphy AF, Dahlin DD, Sullivan CR (1962) Articular synovial chondromatosis. J Bone Joint Surg Am 44:77–86

Murray RO, Jacobson HG (1977) The radiology of skeletal disorders, 2nd edn. Churchill Livingstone, Edinburgh, pp 558–561

Mussey RD Jr, Henderson MS (1949) Osteochondromatosis. J Bone Joint Surg Am 31:619–627

O'Connell JX, Fanburg JC, Rosenberg AE (1995) Giant cell tumor of tendon sheath and pigmented villonodular synovitis. Immunophenotype suggests a synovial cell origin. Hum Pathol 26:771–775

Paul GR, Leach RE (1970) Synovial chondromatosis of the shoulder. Clin Orthop 68:130–135

Pickren JW, Valenzula L, Elias EG (1970) Synovial sarcoma. Proc Nat Cancer Conf 6:795–801

Roth JA, Enzinger FM, Tannenbaum M (1975) Synovial sarcoma of the neck: a follow-up study of 24 cases. Cancer 35:1243–1253

Schajowicz F, Blumenfeld I (1968) Pigmented villonodular synovitis of the wrist with penetration into bone. J Bone Joint Surg Br 50:312–317

Schwartz HS, Unni KK, Pritchard DJ (1989) Pigmented villonodular synovitis: a retrospective review of affected large joints. Clin Orthop 247:243–255

Scott PM (1968) Bone lesions on pigmented villonodular synovitis. J Bone Joint Surg Br 50:306–311

Shafer SJ, Larmon WA (1951) Pigmented villonodular synovitis. A report of seven cases. Surg Gynec Obstet 92:574–580

Stout AP, Lattes R (1967) Tumors of the soft tissues, 2nd series, fascicle 1. AFIT, Washington, DC, pp 164–171

Sviland L, Malcolm AJ (1995) Synovial chondromatosis presenting as painless soft tissue mass. A report of 19 cases. Histopathology 27:275–279

Swan EF, Owens WF Jr (1972) Synovial chondrometaplasia: a case report with spontaneous regression and a review of the literature. South Med J (Birmingham, Ala.) 65:1496–1500

Weidner N, Challa VR, Bonsib SM et al (1986) Giant cell tumors of synovium (pigmented villonodular synovitis) involving the vertebral column. Cancer 57:2030–2036

Wilmoth CL (1971) Osteochondromatosis. J Bone Joint Surg Br 23:367–374

Chapter 15
Parosteal and Extraskeletal Lesions

Ackerman LV (1958) Extra-osseous localized non-neoplastic bone and cartilage formation (so-called myositis ossificans). Clinical and pathological confusion with neoplasms. J Bone Joint Surg Am 40:279–298

Adler CP (1979) Extra-osseous osteoblastic osteosarcoma of the right breast. Skeletal Radiol 4:107–110

Aegerter E, Kirkpatrick JA (1968) Orthopedic diseases, 3rd edn. Saunders, Philadelphia

Allan CJ, Soule EH (1971) Osteogenic sarcoma of the soft tissues. Cancer 27:1121–1133

Angervall L, Enzinger FM (1975) Extraskeletal neoplasm resembling Ewing's sarcoma. Cancer 36:240–251

Angervall L, Enerbdck L, Knutson H (1973) Chondrosarcoma of soft tissue origin. Cancer 32:507–513

Angervall L, Stener B, Stener I, Ahrön C (1969) Pseudomalignant osseous tumor of soft tissue. J Bone Joint Surg Br 51:654–663

Aufdermaur M (1975) Bewegungsapparat. In: Büchner F, Grundmann E (eds) Spezielle Pathologie, vol 2. Urban & Schwarzenberg, Munich, pp 337–425

Barton DL, Reeves RJ (1961) Tumoral calcinosis. Report of three cases and review of the literature. Am J Roentgenol 86:351–358

Bishop AF, Destouet JM, Murphy WA, Gilula LA (1982) Tumoral calcinosis:case report and review. Skeletal Radiol 8:269–274

Blasius S, Link T, Hillmann A, Edel G (1995) Myositis assifikans mit aneurysmatischer Knochenzyste. Osteologie 4:169–172

Botham RJ, McDonal JR (1958) Sarcoma of the mammary os gland. Surg Gynec Obstet 107:55–61

Bucher O (1965) Ein Fall von extraossärem osteogenem Sarkom der Subcutis mit besonderer Berücksichtigung der Verkalkungsprobleme. Langenbecks Arch Chir 312:197–215

Burleson RJ, Bickel WH, Dahlin DC (1956) Popliteal cyst: a clinicopathological survey. J Bone Joint Surg Am 3:1265–1274

Carleton CC, Williamson JW (1961) Osteogenic sarcoma of the uterus. Arch Pathol 72:121–125

Dahlin DC, Salvador AH (1974) Cartilaginous tumor of the soft tissues of the hand and feet. Mayo Clin Proc 4:721–726

Enzinger FM, Shiraki M (1972) Extraskeletal myxoid chondrosarcoma. An analysis of 34 cases. Hum Path 3:421–43

Enzinger FM, Lattes R, Torloni H (1969) Histological typing of soft tissue tumours. WHO, Geneva

Fechner RE, Mills SE (1993) Tumors of the bones and joints. AFIP, Washinton, DC

Fine G, Stout AP (1956) Osteogenic sarcoma of the extraskeletal soft tissue. Cancer 9:1027–1043

Geiler G (1961) Die Synoviolome. Springer, Berlin Göttingen Heidelberg

Genovese GR, Jayson MIV, St J Dixon A (1972) Protective value of synovial cysts in rheumatoid knees. Ann Rheum Dis 31:179–182

Gilmer WS Jr, Anderson LD (1959) Reactions of soft somatic tissue which may progress the bone formation: circumscribed (traumatic) myositis ossificans. South Med (Birmingham, Ala.) 52:1432–1448

Goldenberg RR, Cohen P, Steinlauf P (1967) Chondrosarcoma of extraskeletal soft tissues: report of seven cases and review of literature. J Bone Joint Surg Am 49:1487–1507

Goldman RL (1967) Mesenchymal chondrosarcoma – a rare malignant chondroid tumor usually arising in bone – cases in soft tissue. Cancer 20:1494–1498

Granowitz SP, Mankin HJ (1967) Localized pigmented villonodular synovitis of the knee. J Bone Joint Surg Am 49:122–128

Guccion J, Font RL, Enzinger FM, Zimmerman LE (1973) Extraskeletal mesenchymal chondrosarcoma. Arch Pathol 95:336–340

Hajdu Sl (1979) Pathology of soft tissue tumors. Lea & Febiger, Philadelphia

Harkess JW, Peters HJ (1967) Tumoral calcinosis: a report of six cases. J Bone Joint Surg Am 49:721–731

Heffner RR, Armbrustmacher VW, Earle KM (1977) Focal myositis. Cancer 40:301–306

Henck ME, Simpson EL, Ochs RH, Eremus JL (1996) Extraskeletal soft tissue masses of Langerhans' cell histiocytosis. Skeletal Radiol 25:409–412

Hughston JC, Whatley GS, Stone MM (1962) Myositis ossificans traumatica (myo-osteosis). South Med J (Birmingham, Ala.) 55:1167–1170

Jaffe HL (1971) Metabolic, degenerative, and inflammatory diseases of bones and joints. Urban & Schwarzenberg, Munich

Kambolis C, Bullough PG, Jaffe HL (1973) Ganglionic cystic defects of bone. J Bone Joint Surg Am 55:496–505

Kauffman SL, Stout AP (1963) Extraskeletal osteogenic sarcomas and chondrosarcomas in children. Cancer 16:323–329

Kirchner R, Stremmel W, Adler CP (1979) Extraossäres osteoplastisches Osteosarkom der Mamma. Chirurg 50:456–459

Korns ME (1967) Primary chondrosarcoma of extraskeletal soft tissue. Arch Pathol 83:13–15

Kuhlenkampff HA, Meyer E, Adler CP et al. (1988) Thibièrge-Wcissenbach syndrome with tumor-like calcification of soft tissue. In: Heuck FHW, Keck E (eds) Fortschritte der Osteologie in Diagnostik und Therapie. Springer, Berlin Heidelberg New York, pp 409–417

Lafferty FW, Reynolds ES, Pearson OH (1965) Tumoral calcinosis. A metabolic disease of obscure etiology. Am J Med 38:105–118

Lagier R, Cox JN (1975) Pseudomalignant myositis ossificans. A pathological study of eight cases. Hum Path 6:653–665

Lowry WB, McKee EE (1972) Primary osteosarcoma of the heart. Cancer 30:1068–1073

Maluf HM, DeYoung BR, Swanson PE, Wick WR (1995) Fibroma and giant cell tumor of tendon sheath. A comparative histological and immunohistological study. Mod Pathol 8:155–159

Martinez S, JB Vogler, JM Harrelson, KW Lyles (1990) Imaging of tumoral calcinosis: new observations. Radiology 174:215–222

McEvedy BV (1962) Simple ganglia. Br J Surg 49:585–594

Nicolai CH, Spjut HJ (1959) Primary osteogenic sarcoma of the bladder. J Urol (Balt) 82:497–499

Norman A, Dorfman HD (1970) Juxtacortical circumscribed myositis ossificans. Evolution and radiographic features. Radiology 96:301

Ohashi K, Yamada T, Ishikawa T et al (1996) Idiopathic calcinosis involving the cervical spine. Skeletal Radiol 25:388–390

Rao U, Cheng A (1978) Extraosseous osteogenic sarcoma. Cancer 41:1488–1496

Rau WS, Adler CP (1979) Ein ungewöhnlicher Lungenherd. Extraossäres osteoplastisches Osteosarkom der Mamma. Radiologe 19:189–192

Reed RJ, RW Hunt (1965) Granulomatous (tumoral) calcinosis. Clin Orthop 43:233–240

Ruckes J (1974) Gelenke, Bursen, Sehnenscheiden und Menisken. In: Eder M, Gedigk P (eds) Lehrbuch der Allgemeinen Pathologie und der Pathologischen Anatomie, 29th edn. Springer, Berlin Heidelberg New York, pp 746–763

Schajowicz F (1994) Tumors and tumorlike lesions of bone and joints, 2nd edn. Springer, Berlin Heidelberg New York

Skajaa T (1958) Myositis ossificans. Acta Chir Scand 116:68–72

Smit GG, Schmaman A (1967) Tumoral calcinosis. J Bone Joint Surg Br 49:698–703

Stout AP, Verner EW (1953) Chondrosarcoma of the extraskeletal soft tissues. Cancer 6:581–590

Sumiyoshi K, Tsuneyoshi M, Enjoji M (1985) Myositis ossificans. A clinicopathologic study of 21 cases. Acta Pathol Jpn 35:1109–1122

Tashiro H, Iwasaki H, Kikuchi M et al (1995) Giant cell tumors of tendon sheath. A single and multiple immunostaining analysis. Pathol Int 45:147–155

Thompson JR, Entin SD (1969) Primary extraskeletal chondrosarcoma. Cancer 23:936–939

Tophoj K, Henriques U (1971) Ganglion of the wrist – a structure developed from the joint: a histological study with serial sections. Acta Orthop Scand 42:244–250

Viegas SF, Evans EB, Calhoun J et al (1985) Tumor calcinosis: a case report and review of the literature. J Hand Surg Am 10:744–748

Chapter 16
Examination Techniques

Achilles E, Padberg BC, Holl K, Klöppel G, Schröder S (1991) Immunocytochemistry of paragangliomas – value of staining for S-100 protein and glial fibrillary acid protein in diagnis and prognosis. Histopathology 18:453–458

Adler CP (1979) Differential diagnosis of cartilage tumors. Pathol Res Pract 166:45–58

Adler CP (1979) Extra-osseous osteoblastic osteosarcoma of the right breast. Skeletal Radiol 4:107–110

Adler CP, Uehlinger E (1979) Grenzfälle bei Knochentumoren. Präneoplastische Veränderungen und Geschwülste fraglicher Dignität. Verb Dtsch Ges Pathol 63:352–358

Adler CP, Wenz W (1981) Intraossäre Osteolyseherde. Radiologe 21:470–479

Adler CF, Genz T (1982) Zytophotometrische Untersuchungen von Knochentumoren. Pathologe 3:174

Adler CP, Riede UN, Wurdak W, Zugmaier G (1984) Measurements of DNA in Hodgkin lymphomas and non-Hodgkin lymphomas. Path Res Pract 178:579–589

Adler CP (1986) DNS-Zytophotometrie an Knochentumoren. In: Dietsch P, Keck E, Kruse HP, Kuhlencordt F (eds) Aktuelle Ergebnisse der Osteologie. Osteologica 1:233–239

Adler CP, Böcking A, Kropff M, Leo ETG (1992) DNS-zytophotometrische Untersuchungen zur Prognose von reaktiver Plasmozytose und Plasmozytom. Verb Dtsch Ges Pathol 76:303

Adler CP, Herget GW, Neuburger M, Pfisterer J (1995) DNS-Bestimmung von Knochentumoren mit der Flow-Zytometrie und der Einzelzell-Zytophotometrie. Vergleichende Darstellung von Methodik, diagnostischer Wertigkeit und der Interpretation von Histogrammen. Osteologie 4:1–8

Adler CP, Neuburger M, Herget GW, Pfisterer J (1995) DNS-Zytophotometrie von Weichteiltumoren – vergleichende einzellzytophotometrische und flowzytometrische Messungen an paraffin-eingebettetem Material. Tumordiagn Ther 16:102–106

Adler CP, Herget GW, Neuburger M (1995) DNS-Zytophotometrie zur Prognosebeurteilung von Osteosarkomen. Tumordiagn Ther 16:166–169

Adler CP, Herget GW, Neuburger M (1995) Cartilaginous tumors. Prognostic applications of cytophotometric DNA analysis. Cancer 76:1176–1180

Adler CP, Neuburger M, Herget GW et al (1996) Cytophotometric DNA analysis of bone tumors. New method for preparing formalin-fixed tissue and the regarding of DNA malignancy grade and its prognostic value. Pathol Res Pract 192:437–445

Adler CP, Friedburg H, Herget GW et al (1996) Variability of cardiomyocyte DNA content, ploidy level and nuclear number in mammalian hearts. Virchows Arch 429:159

Alho A, Connor JF, Mankin HJ, Schiller AL, Crawford JC (1983) Assessment of malignancy of cartilage tumors using flow-cytometry. A preliminary report. J Bone Joint Surg 65:779–785

Altmannsberger M, Alles JU, Fritz H et al (1986) Mesenchymale Tumormarker. Verh Dtsch Ges Pathol 70:51–63

Altmannsberger M, Weber K, Droste R, Osborn M (1985) Desmin is a specific marker for rhabdomyosarcomas of human and rat origin. Am J Pathol 118:85–95

Ambros IM, Ambros PF, Strehl S et al. (1991) MIC2 is a specific marker for Ewing's sarcoma and peripheral primitive neuroectodermal tumors. Evidence for a common histogenesis of Ewing's sarcoma and peripheral primitive neuroectodermal tumors from MIC2 expression and specific chromosome aberration. Cancer 67:1886–1893

Atkin NB, Kay R (1979) Prognostic significance of modal DNA value and other factors in malignant tumours, based on 1465 cases. Br J Cancer 40:210–221

Bauer HC, Kreicbergs A, Silfversward C (1989) Prognostication including DNA analysis in osteosarcoma. Acta Orthop Scand 60:353–360

Bauer HC (1993) Current status of DNA cytometry in osteosarcoma. Cancer Treatm Res 62:151–161

Bauer HC (1988) DNA Cytometry of osteosarcoma. Acta Scand 59 [Suppl 1]:1–39

Bauer TW, Tubbs RR, Edinger MG et al. (1989) A prospective comparison of DNA quantitation by image and flow cytometry. J Clin Pathol 92:322–326

Bengtsson A, Grimelius L, Johannsson H, Pontén J (1977) Nuclear DNA-content of parathyroid cells in adenomas, hyperplastic and normal glands. Acta Path Microbiol Scand [Sect A] 85:455–460

Böcking A (1981) Grading des Prostatakarzinoms. Habilitationssschrift, Freiburg

Böcking A (1982) Algorithmus für ein universelles DNS-Malignitätsgrading. Verh Dtsch Ges Path 66:540

Böcking A, Sommerkamp H (1980) Malignitäts-Grading des Prostatakarzinoms durch Analyse der Ploidieverteilung. XXXII. Kongr Dtsch Ges Urol (10–13 Sept 1980), Berlin

Böcking A (1990) DNA-Zytometrie und Automatisation in der klinischen Diagnostik. Verh Dtsch Ges Path 74:176–185

Böhm N, Sandritter W (1975) DNA in human tumors: a cytophotometric study. In: Grundmann E, Kirsten WH (eds) Current topics in pathology. Springer, Berlin Heidelberg New York, pp 151–219

Bosse A, Vollmer E, Böcker W et al. (1990) The impact of osteonectin for differential diagnosis of bone tumors. An immunohistochemical approach. Pathol Res Pract 186:651–657

Brooks JP, Pascal RR (1984) Malignant giant cell tumor of bone: ultrastructural and immunohistologic evidence of histiocytic origin. Hum Pathol 15:1098–1100

Brooks J (1982) Immunohistochemistry of soft tissue tumors. Myoglobin as a tumor marker for rhabdomyosarcoma. Cancer 50:1757–1763

Brown DC, Theaker JM, Banks PM (1987) Cytokeratin expression in smooth muscle and smooth muscle tumors. Histopathology 11:477–486

Bunn PA, Krasnow S, Makuch RW et al. (1982) Flow cytometric analysis of DNA content of bone marrow cells in patients with plasma cell myeloma: clinical implications. Blood 59:528–535

Caspersson T (1936) Über den chemischen Aufbau der Strukturen des Zellkernes. Skand Arch Physiol 73[Suppl 8]:1–151

Colvin RB, Bhan AK, McCluskey RT (1988) (eds) Diagnostic immunopathology. Raven, New York

Cuvelier CA, Roels HJ (1979) Cytophotometric studies of the nuclear DNA content incartilaginous tumors. Cancer 44:1363–1374

Dierick AM, Langlois M, van Oostveldt P, Roels H (1993) The prognostic significance of the DNA content in Ewing's sarcoma: a retrospective cytophotometric and flow cytometric study. Histopathol 23:333–339

Eneroth CM, Zetterberg A (1973) Microspectrophotometric DNA content as a criterion of malignancy in salivary gland tumors of the oral cavity. Acta Otorhinolaryngol (Stockh) 75:296–298

Engler H, Thürlimann B, Riesen WF (1996) Biochemical markers of bone remodelling. Onkologie 19:126–131

Eusebi V, Ceccarelli C, Gorza L et al. (1986) Immunocytochemistry of rhabdomyosarcoma. The use of four different markers. Am J Surg Pathol 10:293–299

Födisch HJ, Mikuz G, Walter N (1974) Cytophotometrische Untersuchungen an Knochengeschwülsten. Verh Dtsch Ges Pathol 58:425–429

Frohn A, Födisch HJ, Bode U (1986) Fluorescence cytophotometric DNA studies of Ewing and osteosarcoma. Klin Pädiatr 198:262–266

Gatter KC (1989) Diagnostic immunocytochemistry: achievements and challenges. J Pathol 159:183–190

Gatter KC, Alcock C, Heryet A, Mason DY (1985) Clinical importance of analysing malignant tumours of uncertain origin with immunohistological techniques. Lancet I:1302–1305

Genz T, Böcking A, Adler CP (1983) DNS-Malignitätsgrading an Knochentumoren. Verh Dtsch Ges Pathol 67:697

Hämmerli G, Sträuli P, Schlüter G (1968) Deoxyribonucleic acid measurements in nodular lesions of the human thyroid. Lab Invest 18:675–680

Hashimoto H, Daimaru Y, Enjoji M (1984) S-100 protein distribution in liposarcoma. An immunoperoxidase study with special reference to the distinction of liposarcoma from myxoid malignant fibrous histiocytoma. Virchows Arch A 405:1–10

Hauenstein FH, Wimmer B, Beck A, Adler CP (1988) Knochenbiopsie unklarer Knochenläsionen mit einer 1,4 mm messenden Biopsiekanüle. Radiologe 28:251–256

Helio H, Karaharju E, Nordling S (1985) Flow cytometric determination of DNA content in malignant and benign bone tumors. Cytometry 6:165–171

Hofstddter F, Jakse G, Lederer B, Mikuz G (1980) Cytophotometric investigations of the DNA-content of transitional cell tumours of the bladder. Pathol Res Pract 167:254–264

Kahn HJ, Marks A, Thom H, Baumal R (1983) Role of antibody to S-100 protein in diagnostic pathology. Am J Clin Pathol 79:341–347

Kreicbergs A, Cewrien R, Tribukait B, Zetterberg A (1981) Comparative single-cell and flow DNA analysis of bone sarcoma. Anal Quant Cytol Histol 3:121–127

Kreicbergs A, Silversward C, Tribukait B (1984) Flow DNA analysis of primary bone tumors. Relationship between cellular DNA content and histopathological classification. Cancer 53:129–136

Kropff M, Leo E, Steinfurth G et al (1991) DNA-zytophotometrischer Nachweis von Aneuploidie, erhöhter Proliferation und Kernfläche als frühe Marker prospektiver Malignität bei monoklonales Gammopathie unklarer Signifikanz (MGUS). Verh Dtsch Ges Pathol 75:480

Kropff M, Leo E, Steinfurth G et al (1994) DNA-image cytometry and clinical staging systems in multiple myeloma. Anticancer Res 14:2183–2188

Lederer B, Mikuz G, Giitter W, Nedden G zur (1972) Zytophotometrische Untersuchungen von Tumoren des Übergangsepithels der Harnblase. Vergleich zytophotometrischer Untersuchungsergebnisse mit den histologischen Grading. Beitr Pathol Anat 147:379–389

Leo E, Kropff M, Lindemann A et al (1995) DNA aneuploidy, increased proliferation and nuclear area of plasma cells in monoclonal gammopathy of undetermined significance and multiple myeloma. Anal Quant Cytol Histol 17:113–120

Leong AS-Y (1993) Applied immunohistochemistry for the surgical pathologist. Edward Arnold, London

Lizard-Nacol S, Lizard G, Justrabo E, Turc-Carel C (1989) Immunologic characterization of Ewing's sarcoma using mesenchymal and neural markers. Am J Pathol 135:847–855

Look AT, Douglass EC, Meyer WH (1988) Clinical importance of near-diploid tumor stem lines in patients with osteosarcoma of an extremity. N Engl J Med 318:1567–1572

Mason DY, Gatter KC (1987) The role of immunocytochemistry in diagnostic pathology. J Clin Pathol 40:1042–1054

Matsumou H, Shimoda T, Kakimoto S et al (1985) Histopathologic and immunohistochemical study of malignant tumors of peripheral nerve sheath (malignant schwannoma). Cancer 56:2269–2279

McElroy HH, Shih MS, Parfitt AM (1993) Producing frozen sections of calcified bone. Biotech Histochem 68:50–55

Mellin W (1990) Cytophotometry in tumor pathology. A critical review of methods and application, and some results of DNA-analysis. Pathol Res Pract 186:37–62

Michie SA, Spagnolo DV, Dunn KA et al (1987) A panel approach to the evaluation of the sensitivity and specificity of antibodies for the diagnosis of routinely processed, histologically undifferentiated human neoplasm. Am J Clin Pathol 88:457–462

Moore GW, Riede UN, Sandritter W (1977) Application of Quine's nullities to a quantitative organelle pathology. J Theor Pathol 65:633–651

Moore GW, Hutchins GM, Bulkley BH (1979) Certainity levels in the nullity method of symbolic logic: application to the pathogenesis of congenital heart malformations. J Theor Biol 76:53–81

Neuburger M, Herget GW, Adler CP (1996) Liposarcoma – Comparison of flow-cytometric and image-cytophotometric DNA measurements. Oncol Rep 3:559–562

Neumann K, Ramaswanry A, Schmitz-Moormann P (1990) Immunhistochemie der Weichteiltumoren. Tumordiagn Ther 11:120–124

Norton AJ, Thomas JA, Isaacson PG (1987) Cytokeratinspecific monoclonal antibodies are reactive with tumors of smooth muscle derivation. An immunocytochemical and biochemical study using antibodies to intermediate filament cytoskeletal proteins. Histopathology 11:487

Otto HF, Berndt R, Schwechheimer K, Möller P (1987) Mesenchymal tumor markers: special proteins and enzymes. In: Seifert G (ed) Morphological tumor markers. Curr Top Pathol 77:179–205

Overbeck J von, Staehli C, Gudat F (1985) Immunohistochemical characterization of an anti-epithelial monoclonal antibody (mAB Lu-5). Virchows Arch 407:1–12

Park YK, Yang MH, Park HR (1996) The impact of osteonectin for differential diagnosis of osteogenic bone tumors: an immunohistochemical and in situ hybridization approach. Skeletal Radiol 25:13–17

Reiser M, Semmler W (1997) Magnetresonanztomographie, 2nd edn. Springer, Berlin Heidelberg New York

Robinson M, Alcock C, Gatter KC, Mason DY (1988) The analysis of malignant tumours of uncertain origin with immunohistological techniques: clinical follow-up. Clin Radiol 39:432–434

Sandritter W (1958) Ultraviolett-Mikrospektrophotometrie. In: Graumann W, Neumann K (eds) Handbuch der Histochemie, vol 1/1. Fischer, Stuttgart, pp 220–338

Sandritter W (1961) Methoden und Ergebnisse der quantitativen Histochemie. Dtsch Med Wochenschr 45:2177

Sandritter W, Carl M, Ritter W (1966) Cytophotometric measurements of DNA content of human malignant tumors by means of the Feulgen reaction. Acta Cytol (Phila) 10:26–30

Sandritter W, Adler CP (1972) A method for determing cell number on organs with polpoid cell nuclei. Beitr Pathol Anat 146:99–103

Sandritter W, Kiefer G, Kiefer R et al (1974) DNA in heterochromatin. Cytophotometric pattern recognition image analysis among cell nuclei in duct epithelium and in carnima of the human breast. Beitr Pathol Anat 151:87

Sandritter W (1977) Zytophotometrie. Verb Anat Ges (Jena): 59–73

Sandritter W (1981) Quantitative pathology in theory and practice. Pathol Res Pract 171:2–21

Sasaki K, Murakami T (1992) Clinical application of flow cytometry for DNA analysis of solid tumors. Acta Pathol Jpn 42:1–14

Schulz A, Jundt G (1989) Immunohistological demonstration of osteonectin in normal bone tissue and in bone tumors. Curr Top Pathol 80:31–54

Schulz A, Jundt G, Berghauser KH et al (1988) Immunohistochemical study of osteonectin in various types of osteosarcoma. Am J Pathol 132:233–238

Schürch W, Skalli O, Lagacé R (1990) Intermediate filament proteins and actin isoforms as markers for soft-tissue tumor differentiation and origin. 3. Hemangiopericytomas and glomus tumors. Am J Pathol 136:771–786

Schütte B, Reynders MM, Bosman FT, Blijham GH (1985) Flow cytometric DNA ploidy level in nuclei isolated from paraffin-embedded tissue. Cytometry 6:26–30

Seidel A, Sandritter W (1963) Cytophotometrische Messungen des DNS-Gehaltes eines Lungenadenoms und einer malignen Lungenadenomatose. Z Krebsforsch 65:555

Shankey TV, Rabinovitch PS, Bagwell B (1993) Guidelines for implementation of clinical DNA cytometry. Cytometry 14:472–477

Siefert G (1987) Morphological tumor markers. Springer, Berlin Heidelberg New York

Sun D, Biesterfeld S, Adler CP, Böcking A (1992) Prediction of recurrence in giant cell bone tumors by DNA cytometry. Anal Quant Cytol 14:341–346

Tavares AS, Costa J, De Carvalho A, Reis M (1966) Tumor ploidy and prognosis in carcinomas of the bladder and prostate. Br J Cancer 20:438–441

Tienhaara A, Pelliniemi TT (1992) Flow cytometric DNA analysis and clinical correlation in multiple myeloma. Am J Clin Pathol 97:322–330

Uehlinger E (1974) Pathologische Anatomie der Knochengeschwülste (unter besonderer Berücksichtigung der semimalignen Formen). Chirurg 45:62–70

Valen F van, Prior R, Wechsler W et al (1988) Immunzytochemiche und biochemische Untersuchungen an einer Ewing-Sarkom-Zellinie: Hinweise für eine neurale Differenzierung. Klin Pddiatr 200:267–270

Weiss SW, Langloss JM, Enzinger FM (1983) Value of S-100 protein in the diagnosis of soft tissue tumors with particular reference to benign and malignant Schwarm cell tumors. Lab Invest 49:299–308

Werner M, Rieck J, Heintz A, Pösl M, Delling G (1996) Vergleichende DNA-zytometrische und zytogenetische Ploidiebestimmungen an Chondrosarkomen und Osteosarkomen. Pathologe 17:374–379

Wersto RP, Liblit RL, Koss LG (1991) Flow cytometric DNA analysis of human solid tumors: a review of the interpretation of DNA histograms. Hum Pathol 22:1085–1098

Wick MR, Siegal GP (1988) Monoclonal antibodies in diagnostic immunohistochemistry. Marcel Dekker, New York

Zollinger HU (1946) Geschwulstprobleme. Gut- und Bösartigkeit der Geschwülste. Vjschr Naturforsch Ges 91:81–94

List of Subjects

Heavily printed page numbers refer to the more detailed discussion of the subject.

Spider fingers   58
Spin density (in MRT)   492
Spinal changes, degenerative **436–440**
Spins (in MRT)   492
Spondylarthritis ankylopoetica   450
Spondylarthrosis deformans   423, 424, **436**
Spondylitis   140, 402
– Non-specific   448
– Tuberculous   448
Spondylitis ankylopoetica Bechterew (see also
  Bechterew's disease)   192, 441, 450
Spondylodiscitis   140, 448
Spondyloepiphyseal dysplasia congenita (see also
  Spranger-Wiedemann dysplasia)   **38**
Spondylometaphyseal dysplasia   31
Spondylosis   188
– Ochronotic **192**
Spondylosis deformans   192, **436**
Spongiosa   2, 16, 68, 74
Spongiosal plastic treatment   **122**
Spongiosal surface area, inactive (histomorpho-
  metry)   510
Spongiosal transplants   122, 124
Spongiosclerosis   440
Spongy degeneration of the articular cartilage (in
  arthrosis)   428
Spontaneous fracture   84, 348, 516
Spontaneous healing   408
Sporotrichosis   156
Spotted bones (see also osteopoikilosis)   108
Spranger-Wiedemann dysplasia (see also spondy-
  loepiphyseal dysplasia congenita)   **38**
Squaring (rectangular vertebral body)   450
Staining sets (kits)   506
Staining techniques   **502–505**
Starvation osteoporosis   65
Stasis, venous   162
Steeple or tower head (see also
  Turricephaly)   36
Sternberg giant cells   362
Steroid osteoporosis   76
Storage diseases of bone   **183–193**, 345
Stratum synoviale (see also synovia)   28, 168,
  441, 442, 446
Subtraction angiography, digital (DSA)   489
Sudan staining   346, 392
Sudeck's atrophy (see also sympathetic reflex dys-
  trophy, SRD)   65, **96**, 124
Summation vector of the proton spin (in
  MRT)   492
Sunburst   372
Surface density of the entire resorption area (his-
  tomorphometry)   510

Surface osteosarcoma   304
Survival period   212
Sympathetic reflex dystrophy (see also Sudeck's
  atrophy, SRD)   65, **96**, 124
Sympathicoblastoma   **388**
Synostosis   450
Synovectomy   460, 464
Synovia (see also stratum synoviale)   28, 168,
  452, 457, 464
Synovial biopsy   454
Synovial chondromatosis   254, 457, **458**
Synovial sarcoma   378, 457, 462, 464, **466–469**
– Biphasic type **466**
– Monophasic epithelioid   468
– Monophasic type **466**, 468
Synovial villi   457, 460
Synovioma, malignant   466
Synovitis   441
– Localized nodular   457, **462**, 471, 476
– Non-specific   442, 486
– Purulent granulating   454
– Tuberculoid   452
– Villonodular (see also pigmented villonodular
  synovitis)   457, **464**, 468
Syphilis (see also bone syphilis, osteochondritis
  luetica)   32, **152**
Syphilis, acquired **152**
Syphilis, congenital **152**
Syringomyelia   438

T

Tabular osteons **20**, 22
Taenia echinococcus   158
Tear of substance (meniscus)   434
Tendon sheath   418, 457, 462, 464, 472, 474
Tendosynovitis, localized nodular   462
Tendovaginitis stenosans de Quervain   457, 471,
  474
Tetracyclin double marking **511**
Tetracyclin marking, intravital   22, 82, **500**
Thanatophoric Dwarfism Type Neumoff   32, **40**
Theory of bone neoplasia   210
Thibièrge-Weissenbach syndrome **486**
Tibia recurvata   8
Tibor-PAP staining   360
Tissue differentiation, topographical and func-
  tional   210
Tissue patterns
– Angiomatous   394
– Basaloid   378
– Spindle-cell   378